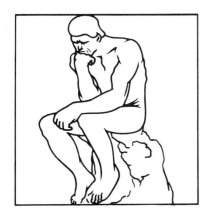

Ervin Epstein, M.D.

Associate Clinical Professor of Dermatology
    University of California Medical School
    San Francisco, California
Formerly Associate Clinical Professor of Dermatology
    Stanford Medical School
    Stanford, California
Chairman FDA Committee on Surgical and
    Rehabilitation Devices
Co-Editor Schoch Letter
Member and Former Vice-President American
    Dermatological Association

Controversies in Dermatology

W.B. SAUNDERS COMPANY   **1984**
Philadelphia London Toronto Mexico City Rio de Janeiro Sydney Tokyo

W. B. Saunders Company: West Washington Square
Philadelphia, PA 19105

1 St. Anne's Road
Eastbourne, East Sussex BN 21 3UN, England

1 Goldthorne Avenue
Toronto, Ontario M8Z 5T9, Canada

Cedro 512
Mexico 4, D.F. Mexico

Rua Coronel Cabrita, 8
Sao Cristovao Caixa Postal 21176
Rio de Janeiro, Brazil

9 Waltham Street
Artarmon, N.S.W. 2064, Australia

Ichibancho, Central Bldg., 22-1 Ichibancho
Chiyoda-Ku, Tokyo 102, Japan

Library of Congress Cataloging in Publication Data

Epstein, Ervin.
  Controversies in dermatology.

  1. Skin—Diseases—Addresses, essays, lectures.
2. Skin—Cancer—Addresses, essays, lectures. I. Title.
[DNLM: 1. Skin diseases. WR 140 C764]
RL75.E67 1984   616.5   82-25548
ISBN 0-7216-3398-6

Controversies in Dermatology   ISBN   0-7216-3398-6

Last digit is the print number: 9   8   7   6   5   4   3   2   1

Dedicated to those who made this book possible

The contributors

And to those who made the publication possible

The employees of the W.B. Saunders Company
And especially to
Mr. Carroll Cann

CONTRIBUTORS

ELIZABETH A. ABEL, M.D.
Assistant Professor, Department of Dermatology, Stanford University School of Medicine, Stanford, California. Assistant Professor, Stanford University Medical Center, Stanford, California.
Hazards of PUVA Therapy

THOMAS H. ALT, M.D.
Assistant Clinical Professor, Department of Dermatology, University of Minnesota Medical School, Minneapolis, Minnesota. Staff Member, Unity Hospital, Fridley, Minnesota; Methodist Hospital, St. Louis Park, Minnesota; Hennepin County Medical Center, Minneapolis, Minnesota.
Primary Excision of Basal Cell Epithelioma; The Value of Effective Therapeutic and Cosmetic Dermabrasion

REX A. AMONETTE, M.D.
Clinical Professor of Dermatology, University of Tennessee Center for the Health Sciences. Staff Member, University of Tennessee Medical Center, Memphis, Tennessee; Baptist Memorial Hospital, Memphis, Tennessee; City of Memphis Hospital, Memphis, Tennessee.
Microscopic Control of Skin Cancer: Chemosurgical Method

PHILIP ANDERSON, M.D.
Professor of Medicine, Chairman of Dermatology, University of Missouri–Columbia School of Medicine, Columbia, Missouri. Professor and Chairman of Dermatology, University of Missouri Medical Center, Columbia, Missouri. Professor of Medicine, Harry S. Truman Veterans Administration Hospital, Columbia, Missouri.
Peritoneal Dialysis

IRVING M. ARIEL, MD.
Clinical Professor of Surgery, New York Medical College, Valhalla, New York. Clinical Professor of Surgery, School of Medicine, State University of New York at Stony Brook, Stony Brook, New York. Attending Surgeon, Cabrini Medical Center, New York, New York; Doctors Hospital, New York, New York. Staff Surgeon, Long Island Jewish–Hillside Medical Center, New Hyde Park, New York. Consultant Surgeon, Hospital for Joint Diseases Orthopaedic Institute, New York, New York.
Chemotherapy of Malignant Melanoma

SAMUEL AYRES, JR., M.D.
Emeritus Clinical Professor of Medicine (Dermatology), University of California at Los Angeles, The Center for Health Sciences, Los Angeles, California. Attending Staff, Hospital of the Good Samaritan, Los Angeles, California. Consulting Staff, White Memorial Medical Center, Los Angeles, California. Member of Professional Staff, Los Angeles County–University of Southern California Medical Center, Los Angeles, California.
Vitamin E: An Effective Therapeutic Agent in Dermatology

RUDOLF L. BAER, M.D.
Professor of Dermatology, New York University School of Medicine, New York, New York. Attending Physician, University Hospital, New York, New York. Visiting Physician, Bellevue Hospital, New York, New York.
The Value of Academic Research in Dermatology

PHILIP L. BAILIN, M.D.
Chairman, Department of Dermatology, Head, Section of Histographic Surgery (Mohs) and Oncology, Cleveland Clinic, Cleveland, Ohio.
Use of the Carbon Dioxide Laser in Microscopically Controlled Excision (Mohs Surgery); Liquid Crystal Thermography in the Preoperative Evaluation of the Margins of Basal Cell Carcinomas

RICHARD D. BAUGHMAN, M.D.
Clinical Professor of Medicine (Dermatology), Dartmouth Medical School, Hanover, New Hampshire. Staff Member, Section of Dermatology, Mary Hitchcock Memorial Hospital and Hitchcock Clinic, Hanover, New Hampshire. Consultant, Veterans Administration Medical Center, White River Junction, Vermont.
Effect of Psychosomatic Influences on Psoriasis

BRUNO BERRETTI, M.D.
Assistant, Department of Dermatology, Polyclinique d'Aubervilliers, Aubervilliers, France.
Psoriasis: PUVA Therapy

DAVID R. BICKERS, M.D.
Professor and Chairman, Department of Dermatology, Case Western Reserve University, Cleveland, Ohio. Director of Dermatology, University Hospitals and Veterans Administration Medical Center, Cleveland, Ohio.
Squamous Cell Carcinomas of Actinic Origin Rarely Metastasize Beyond the Skin; The Etiologic Irrelevance of Diet in Acne Vulgaris

LANCE J. CAINS
Clinical Lecturer in Dermatology, University of Sydney, Sydney, Australia. Consultant Dermatologist, Sydney Hospital; Royal Alexandria Hospital for Children; Manley District Hospital. Senior Visiting Specialist, Concord Rehabilitation Hospital, Sydney, Australia.
Sun Exposure and Malignant Melanoma

JEFFREY P. CALLEN, M.D., F.A.C.P.
Associate Clinical Professor, Dermatology, University of Louisville School of Medicine, Louisville, Kentucky.
Skin Cancer: An Important Marker of Internal Neoplasia

C.V. CAVER, M.D.
Instructor, Dermatology, Queen Emma Clinic, Honolulu, Hawaii. Staff Member, Queen's Medical Center, Honolulu, Hawaii; St. Francis Hospital, Honolulu, Hawaii; Kuakini Medical Center, Honolulu, Hawaii; Kapiolani–Children's Medical Center, Honolulu, Hawaii; Wahiawa General Hospital, Wahiawa, Hawaii; Kahuku Hospital, Kahuku, Hawaii; Castle Memorial Hospital, Kailua, Hawaii; Waluhia Hospital, Honolulu, Hawaii; Hali Nani Health Center, Honolulu, Hawaii.
Primary Excision of Melanoma

EARL R. CLAIBORNE, M.D.
Diplomate, American Board of Dermatology and Syphilology. Dermatologist, Crenshaw Center Hospital, Los Angeles, California.
Adults Cannot Be Immunized Against Rhus *Sensitivity . . . And Certainly Not with Currently Available Extracts*

MARCUS A. CONANT, M.D.
Associate Professor of Dermatology and Co-Director, Kaposi's Sarcoma Clinic, University of California, San Francisco, School of Medicine, San Francisco, California.
Smallpox Vaccination Is Not a Treatment for Herpes Simplex

JOHN THORNE CRISSEY, M.D.
Division of Dermatology and Syphilology, University of Southern California School of Medicine, Los Angeles, California. Senior Attending Physician, Los Angeles County–University of Southern California Medical Center, Los Angeles, California.
Hunch, Chance, and Serendipity in Dermatologic Research

WILLIAM H. EAGLSTEIN, M.D.
Professor, University of Pittsburgh School of Medicine, Pittsburgh, Pennsylvania. Active Staff, Presbyterian–University Hospital, Pittsburgh, Pennsylvania; Children's Hospital, Pittsburgh, Pennsylvania; Veterans Administration Hospital (Oakland Branch), Pittsburgh, Pennsylvania; Eye and Ear Hospital, Pittsburgh, Pennsylvania.
Corticosteroids and the Treatment of Zoster: Systemic Administration

P. HAINES ELY, M.D.
Assistant Clinical Professor of Dermatology, University of California, Davis, School of Medicine, Davis, California. Active Staff, Roseville Community Hospital, Roseville, California. Active Staff, Sacramento Medical Center, Sacramento, California.
Clinical Research

ERVIN EPSTEIN, JR., M.D.
Associate Research Dermatologist and Associate Clinical Professor, Department of Dermatology, University of California Medical Center, San Francisco, California. Attending Staff, University of California Hospitals and Clinics, San Francisco, California; San Francisco General Hospital Medical Center, San Francisco, California.
Treatment of Acute Herpes Zoster with Intralesional Glucocorticoids; Mycosis Fungoides Is a Cancer

JOHN H. EPSTEIN, M.D.
Clinical Professor of Dermatology, University of California, San Francisco, School of Medicine, San Francisco, California. Staff Member, University of California Hospital, San Francisco, California; Mount Zion Hospital and Medical Center, San Francisco, California; Ralph K. Davies Medical Center–Franklin Hospital, San Francisco, California; San Francisco General Hospital Medical Center, San Francisco, California.
How Important Is the Role of Radiation from the Sun in the Rising Incidence of Melanomas?

KENNETH N. EPSTEIN, PH.D.
University of California, Santa Cruz, California.
Psychological Influences Are Important in Psoriasis

WILLIAM L. EPSTEIN, M.D.
Professor and Chairman, Department of Dermatology, University of California, San Francisco, School of Medicine, San Francisco, California.
Role of the Biopsy in Management of Cutaneous Malignant Melanoma; What Factors Determine Unresponsiveness to Poison Oak/Ivy?

MARK ALLEN EVERETT, M.D.
Regents' Professor and Head, Department of Dermatology, University of Oklahoma Health Sciences Center, Norman, Oklahoma. Chief of Staff, Oklahoma Memorial Hospital, Oklahoma City, Oklahoma.
The Clinical Diagnosis of Malignant Melanoma

EUGENE M. FARBER, M.D.
Professor and Chairman, Department of Dermatology, Stanford University School of Medicine, Stanford, California. Consultant, Pacific Medical Center, San Francisco, California. Consultant, United States Naval Hospital, San Diego, California.
Hazards of PUVA Therapy

LAWRENCE M. FIELD, M.D., F.I.A.C.S.
Assistant Clinical Professor, University of California, San Francisco, School of Medicine, San Francisco, California.
On the Value of Dermabrasion in the Management of Actinic Keratoses

ALEXANDER A. FISHER, M.D.
Clinical Professor, Department of Dermatology, New York University Post-Graduate Medical School, New York, New York. Associate Attending in Dermatology, University Hospital, New York University Medical Center, New York, New York.
The Safety of Patch Testing

THOMAS B. FITZPATRICK, M.D.
Professor and Chairman, Department of Dermatology, Harvard Medical School, Boston, Massachusetts. Chief of Dermatology, Massachusetts General Hospital, Boston, Massachusetts.
PUVA in Perspective

ANDREW A. GAGE, M.D.
Professor of Surgery, State University of New York at Buffalo School of Medicine, Buffalo, New York. Chief, Surgical Service and Chief of Staff, Veterans Administration Medical Center, Buffalo, New York.
Cryosurgery for Skin Disease: Variants in Technique

RICHARD G. GLOGAU, M.D.
Assistant Clinical Professor, Department of Dermatology, University of California, San Francisco, School of Medicine, San Francisco, California. Active Staff, University of California Hospital, San Francisco, California. Courtesy Staff, Peninsula Hospital and Medical Center, Burlingame, California.
Collagen for Implantation: Problems for Consideration

LEON GOLDMAN, M.D.
Professor Emeritus, Dermatology, University of Cincinnati College of Medicine, Cincinnati, Ohio. Department of Dermatology, University of Cincinnati Medical Center, Cincinnati, Ohio. Director, Laser Treatment Center, Director, Laser Research Laboratory, Jew-

ish Hospital of Cincinnati, Cincinnati, Ohio. Consultant-Dermatology, Children's Hospital Medical Center, Cincinnati, Ohio.
Is There a Controversy on the Laser Treatment of Melanoma?

HERBERT GOLDSCHMIDT, M.D.
Clinical Professor of Dermatology, Department of Dermatology, University of Pennsylvania School of Medicine, Philadelphia, Pennsylvania. Attending Physician, Hospital of the University of Pennsylvania, Philadelphia, Pennsylvania.
X-ray Therapy of Skin Cancer

JAMES H. GRAHAM, M.D.
Professor of Dermatology, Clinical Professor of Pathology, Uniformed Services University of the Health Sciences, Bethesda, Maryland. Chairman, Department of Dermatopathology, Armed Forces Institute of Pathology, Washington, District of Columbia.
Relationship Between Bowen's Disease and Internal Cancer

CHARLES GRUPPER, M.D.
Chief, Department of Dermatology, Polyclinique d'Aubervilliers, Aubervilliers, France.
Psoriasis: PUVA Therapy

JON M. HANIFIN, M.D.
Professor, Department of Dermatology, Oregon Health Sciences University, Portland, Oregon.
Herpes Zoster and Herpes Simplex Infections: The Case for Laboratory Confirmation of Recurrent Zosteriform Eruptions

NEIL HESKEL, M.D.
Private practice in dermatology, Doctors' Clinic, Vero Beach, Florida.
Herpes Zoster and Herpes Simplex Infections: The Case for Laboratory Confirmation of Recurrent Zosteriform Eruptions

STEFANIA JABLOŃSKA, M.D.
Professor of Dermatology, Chief of the Department of Dermatology, Warsaw School of Medicine, Warsaw, Poland.
Limitations of Immunofluorescence Testing

ROBERT JACKSON, M.D.
Professor of Medicine (Dermatology), University of Ottawa School of Medicine, Ottawa, Ontario, Canada. Dermatologist, Ottawa Civic Hospital, Ottawa, Ontario, Canada. Consultant, Dermatology, Ontario Cancer Treatment and Research Foundation, Ontario, Canada.
Treatment of Epitheliomas: Electrodesiccation and Curettage

ALVIN H. JACOBS, M.D.
Professor of Dermatology and Pediatrics, Emeritus (Active), Stanford University School of Medicine, Stanford, California.
The Argument for Removal of Congenital Nevocytic Nevi

DENNIS D. JURANEK, D.V.M., M.P.H., M.Sc.
Private practitioner, Atlanta, Georgia.
Treatment of Household and Sexual Contacts of Patients with Scabies

SHELDON S. KABAKER, M.D., F.A.C.S.
Assistant Clinical Professor of Otolaryngology–Head and Neck Surgery, University of California, San Francisco, School of Medicine, San Francisco, California. Active Staff, Samuel Merritt Hospital, Oakland, California; Providence Hospital, Oakland, California; Peralta Hospital, Oakland, California.
Flap Operations for Baldness

EDWIN H. LENNETTE, M.D., Ph.D.
Emeritus Chief, Viral and Rickettsial Disease Laboratory, California Department of Health Services, Berkeley, California. Senior Medical Staff, Peralta Hospital, Oakland, California.
Laboratory Differentiation of Herpes Simplex and Herpes Zoster

RONALD R. LUBRITZ, M.D., F.A.C.P.
Clinical Associate Professor of Medicine (Dermatology), Tulane University School of Medicine, New Orleans, Louisiana. Staff Physician, Charity Hospital of Louisiana, New Orleans, Louisiana; Forrest County General Hospital, Hattiesburg, Mississippi; Methodist Hospital, Hattiesburg, Mississippi.
Advantages and Disadvantages of Cryosurgery and Cryospray for Malignancies

STUART MADDIN, M.D., F.R.C.P.
Clinical Professor, Division of Dermatology, Department of Medicine, University of British Columbia Faculty of Medicine, Vancouver, British Columbia, Canada. Attending Staff, Vancouver General Hospital, Vancouver, British Columbia, Canada. Chief of Dermatology, John F. McCreary Health Sciences Centre, Vancouver, British Columbia, Canada.
Acne Surgery

HOWARD I. MAIBACH, M.D.
Professor of Dermatology, University of California, San Francisco, School of Medicine, San Francisco, California.
Patch Testing: Hazards; Treatment of Household and Sexual Contacts of Patients with Scabies

CHARLES M. McBRIDE, B.Sc., M.D., C.M.
Professor of Surgery, University of Texas System Cancer Center; Department of Surgery, University of Texas M.D. Anderson Hospital and Tumor Institute, Houston, Texas.
Treatment of Melanoma: Viewpoint of the Oncologic Surgeon

FREDERIC E. MOHS, B.Sc., M.D.
Clinical Professor of Surgery, University of Wisconsin Medical School, Madison, Wisconsin. Director of Chemosurgery Clinic, University of Wisconsin Hospital, Madison, Wisconsin.
Microcontrolled Surgery (Chemosurgery) for Skin Cancer

ROBERT J. MORGAN, M.D.
Clinical Professor, Dermatology, University of Oklahoma Health Sciences Center, Norman, Oklahoma. Chief, Department of Dermatology, St. Anthony Hospital, Oklahoma City, Oklahoma.
Metastatic Squamous Cell Cancer from the Skin

RICHARD B. ODOM, M.D.
Chief, Dermatology Service, Letterman Army Medical Center, San Francisco, California. Associate Clinical Professor of Dermatology, University of California, San Francisco, School of Medicine, San Francisco, California.
Treatment of Actinic Keratoses with Topical 5-Fluorouracil

MILTON ORKIN, M.D.
Clinical Professor, Department of Dermatology, University of Minnesota Hospitals, Minneapolis, Minnesota. Active Staff, North Memorial Medical Center, Minneapolis, Minnesota; Mount Sinai Hospital, Minneapolis, Minnesota; Metropolitan Medical Center, Minneapolis, Minnesota; Fairview Hospital, Minneapolis, Minnesota.
Treatment of Household and Sexual Contacts of Patients with Scabies

LAWRENCE CHARLES PARISH, M.D.
Department of Dermatology, Jefferson Medical College, Thomas Jefferson University, Philadelphia, Pennsylvania. Division of Dermatology, University of Pennsylvania School of Veterinary Medicine, Philadelphia, Pennsylvania. Chief of Dermatology, Frankford Hospital of the City of Philadelphia, Philadelphia, Pennsylvania; Albert Einstein Medical Center–Mt. Sinai/Daroff Division, Philadelphia, Pennsylvania. Attending Dermatologist, Thomas Jefferson University Hospital, Philadelphia, Pennsylvania; St. Agnes Medical Center, Philadelphia, Pennsylvania.
Hunch, Chance, and Serendipity in Dermatologic Research

JOHN A. PARRISH, M.D.
Associate Professor of Dermatology, Department of Dermatology, Harvard Medical School, Boston, Massachusetts. Assistant Dermatologist, Massachusetts General Hospital, Boston, Massachusetts.
PUVA in Perspective

HAROLD O. PERRY, M.D.
Professor, Mayo Graduate School of Medicine, University of Minnesota, Rochester, Minnesota. Chairman, Department of Dermatology, Mayo Clinic, Rochester, Minnesota. Consultant, Rochester Methodist Hospital, Rochester, Minnesota; St. Marys Hospital of Rochester, Rochester, Minnesota.
Psoriasis: The Goeckerman Treatment

HERMANN PINKUS, M.D.
Professor Emeritus, Wayne State University, Detroit, Michigan. Emeritus Staff Member, Detroit Receiving Hospital, Detroit, Michigan.
Bowen's Disease Is Not a Marker of Internal Cancer

PETER E. POCHI, M.D.
Professor of Dermatology, Boston University School of Medicine, Boston, Massachusetts. Visiting Dermatologist, University Hospital, Boston, Massachusetts. Visiting Physician, Dermatology, Boston City Hospital, Boston, Massachusetts.
Pathogenesis of Acne: Importance of Follicular Epithelial Changes

F. H. J. RAMPEN, M.D., D.Sc.
Senior Registrar, Department of Dermatology, University of Amsterdam, Amsterdam, The Netherlands.
Deleterious Effects of Biopsy on Survival of Patients with Melanoma

JOHN L. RATZ, M.D.
Associate Professor of Dermatology, University of Cincinnati Medical Center, Cincinnati, Ohio. Medical Staff, Department of Dermatology, Jewish Hospital, Cincinnati, Ohio.
Liquid Crystal Thermography in the Preoperative Evaluation of the Margins of Basal Cell Carcinomas

RONALD M. REISNER, M.D.
Professor and Chief, Division of Dermatology, UCLA School of Medicine, Los Angeles, California. Chief, Dermatology Service, Veterans Administration Wadsworth Medical Center, Los Angeles, California.
Some Controversial Areas in the Topical Treatment of Acne; 13-cis-Retinoic Acid in the Treatment of Acne

H. J. ROBERTS, M.D.
Director, Palm Beach Institute for Medical Research, West Palm Beach, Florida. Senior Active Staff, St. Mary's Hospital, West Palm Beach, Florida; Good Samaritan Hospital, West Palm Beach, Florida.
The Vitamin E Enigma: Perspectives for Physicians

PERRY ROBINS, M.D.
Associate Professor, Dermatology, New York University School of Medicine, New York, New York. Chief of Chemosurgery, New York University Medical Center, University Hospital, New York, New York.
Chemosurgery

JUNE K. ROBINSON, M.D.
Assistant Professor of Dermatology and Surgery, Northwestern University Medical School, Chicago, Illinois. Staff Member, Northwestern Memorial Hospital, Chicago, Illinois.
Microscopic Control of Skin Cancer Excision: Mohs Chemosurgery Versus Double-Blade Scalpel

HENRY H. ROENIGK, JR., M.D.
Walter Hamlin Professor of Dermatology, Chairman, Department of Dermatology, Northwestern University Medical School, Chicago, Illinois. Staff Member, Northwestern Memorial Hospital, Chicago, Illinois. Chairman of Dermatology, Veterans Administration Lakeside Medical Center, Chicago, Illinois.
Microscopic Control of Skin Cancer Excision: Mohs Chemosurgery Versus Double-Blade Scalpel

E. WILLIAM ROSENBERG, M.D.
Professor and Chairman, Division of Dermatology, Department of Medicine and Professor, Department of Community Medicine, University of Tennessee College of Medicine, Memphis, Tennessee.
Acne, Diet, and the Conventional Wisdom

NEVILLE R. ROWELL, M.D., F.R.C.P.
Reader in Dermatology, University of Leeds, Leeds, Yorkshire, England. Senior Consultant Physician, The General Infirmary at Leeds, Yorkshire, England.
Are Discoid and Systemic Lupus Erythematosus the Same Disease?

BIJAN SAFAI, M.D.
Associate Professor of Medicine, Cornell University Medical College, New York, New York. Adjunct Member, Rockefeller University, New York, New York. Chief, Dermatol-

ogy Service, Attending Physician, Memorial Sloan-Kettering Cancer Center, New York, New York.
Immunotherapy of Malignant Melanoma

HAROLD M. SCHNEIDMAN, M.D.
Professor of Clinical Dermatology, Stanford University School of Medicine, Stanford, California. Chairman, Department of Dermatology, Pacific Medical Center, San Francisco, California.
Treatment of Psoriasis at the Dead Sea

EUGENE P. SCHOCH, JR., M.D.
Associate Clinical Professor of Dermatology, University of Texas Southwestern Medical School at Dallas, Dallas, Texas. Senior Staff, Brackenridge Hospital, Austin, Texas; Seton Medical Center, Austin, Texas; St. David's Community Hospital, Austin, Texas.
Excisional Electrosurgery (Endothermy)

ALAN R. SHALITA, M.D.
Professor and Chairman, Department of Dermatology, State University of New York, Downstate Medical Center College of Medicine, Brooklyn, New York. Chief of Dermatology, State University Hospital, Downstate Medical Center, Brooklyn, New York; Kings County Hospital Center, Brooklyn, New York; Brookdale Hospital Medical Center, Brooklyn, New York; Woodhull Hospital Center, Brooklyn, New York. Consultant, Veterans Administration Medical Center, Brooklyn, New York; Long Island College Hospital, Brooklyn, New York; Interfaith Medical Center, Brooklyn, New York.
Systemic and Topical Antibiotics in Acne

SAM SHUSTER, M.B., B.S., Ph.D., F.R.C.P.
Professor of Dermatology, University of Newcastle Upon Tyne, Newcastle Upon Tyne, United Kingdom. Consultant Dermatologist, Newcastle Teaching Hospitals, United Kingdom.
Acne: The Ashes of a Burnt-Out Controversy

ROBERT A. SNYDER, M.D.
Clinical Instructor in Dermatology, University of California, San Francisco, School of Medicine, San Francisco, California.
Patch Testing: Hazards

SAMUEL J. STEGMAN, M.D.
Associate Clinical Professor, Dermatology, University of California, San Francisco, School of Medicine, San Francisco, California.
Zyderm

WILLIAM D. STEWART, M.D., F.R.C.P.(C.)
Professor and Chairman, Division of Dermatology, Department of Medicine, University of British Columbia Faculty of Medicine, Vancouver, British Columbia, Canada. Active Staff, Vancouver General Hospital, Vancouver, British Columbia, Canada. Courtesy Staff, John F. McCreary Health Sciences Centre, Vancouver, British Columbia, Canada; Shaughnessy Hospital, Vancouver, British Columbia, Canada.
An Appraisal of the Retinoids in the Treatment of Psoriasis

D. BLUFORD STOUGH, III, M.D.
Clinical Lecturer, Division of Dermatology, University of Arkansas College of Medicine, Little Rock, Arkansas. Staff, Division of Dermatology, St. Joseph's Mercy Medical Center, Hot Springs, Arkansas.
Hair Transplanation: Punch Autograft Method

DENNY L. TUFFANELLI, M.D.
Clinical Professor, University of California, San Francisco, School of Medicine, San Francisco, California. Active Staff, St. Francis Memorial Hospital, San Francisco, California; Presbyterian Hospital, Pacific Medical Center, San Francisco, California.
The Relationship Between Chronic Cutaneous (Discoid) and Systemic Lupus Erythematosus; Immunofluorescence Microscopy in the Diagnosis of Lupus Erythematosus

MARTIN G. UNGER, M.D., F.R.C.S.(C.)
Associate Surgeon, Institute of Traumatic Plastic and Restorative Surgery, Toronto, Ontario, Canada.
Alopecia Reduction

WALTER P. UNGER, M.D., F.R.C.P.(C.)
Assistant Professor of Medicine (Dermatology), University of Toronto Faculty of Medicine, Toronto, Ontario, Canada. Staff Clinician, Wellesley Hospital, Toronto, Ontario, Canada.
Alopecia Reduction

MORRIS WAISMAN, M.D.
Clinical Professor of Medicine (Dermatology) and of Pharmacology, University of South Florida College of Medicine, Tampa, Florida. Adjunct Professor of Dermatology, University of Miami School of Medicine, Miami, Florida. Attending Dermatologist, Tampa General Hospital, Tampa, Florida; St. Joseph's Hospital, Tampa, Florida. Consultant in Dermatology, Veterans Administration Medical Center, Bay Pines, Florida; Hillsborough County Hospital, Tampa, Florida.
Diet in Acne

ROBERT G. WALTON, M.D.
Clinical Professor of Dermatology, Stanford University School of Medicine, Stanford, California. Visiting Staff, Stanford University Hospital, Stanford, California. Staff Member, Presbyterian Hospital, Pacific Medical Center, San Francisco, California; Doctors Medical Center, Modesto, California.
Not All Congenital Nevi Should Be Removed

GERALD D. WEINSTEIN, M.D.
Professor and Chairman, Department of Dermatology, University of California, Irvine, California College of Medicine, Irvine, California.
Psoriasis and the Selection of Methotrexate for Therapy

RONALD G. WHEELAND, M.D.
Assistant Professor of Dermatology, Adjunct Assistant Professor of Pathology, University of Oklahoma Health Sciences Center, Norman, Oklahoma. Chief, Dermatology Service, Oklahoma Children's Memorial Hospital, Oklahoma City, Oklahoma.
The Clinical Diagnosis of Malignant Melanoma

R. K. WINKELMANN, M.D., Ph.D.
Professor, Dermatology and Anatomy, Mayo Medical School, Rochester, Minnesota. Consultant, Department of Dermatology, Mayo Clinic, Rochester, Minnesota.
Controversies in T Cell Skin Disease: Mycosis Fungoides and Sézary Syndrome

SETRAG A. ZACARIAN, B.Sc., M.D., F.A.C.P.
Associate Clinical Professor of Dermatology, Yale University School of Medicine, New

Haven, Connecticut. Chief of Dermatology, Baystate Medical Center, Springfield, Massachusetts.

Cryosurgery of Malignant Tumors of the Skin

HERSCHEL S. ZACKHEIM, M.D.
Clinical Professor, University of California, San Francisco, School of Medicine, San Francisco, California. Attending Physician, University of California Hospital, San Francisco, California. Consultant, Veterans Administration Medical Center, San Francisco, California. Active Staff, Sequoia Hospital District, Redwood City, California.

Treatment of Psoriasis: Use of Corticosteroids

PREFACE

Medicine is an inexact science. Therefore, there is room for differences of opinion. Each physician has his own ideas of truth and fallacies in his own field. It is true that one man's myth is another man's belief. The differences are based on the fact that each doctor has different experiences, and his intelligence allows him to interpret these experiences individually. Unfortunately, the human mind is not a computer. It does not remember everything that it learns or confronts. If a physician treats 1000 patients with a given condition, he is fortunate if he can remember 100 of them. In other words, his views are patterned by his recollection of a limited number of the experiences to which he has been exposed.

In all probability, about one half of what we believe in medicine is fallacious. The difficulty is in recognizing the truth from the errors, but this is very difficult and filled with opportunities for mistakes. If one were to review the basic literature on which the so-called truths are based and think about these accepted tenets, he would realize that some of them are false. However, when there is a difference of opinion, who can say who is right and who is wrong?

When I started in medicine, the field was ruled by giants—immortals whose word was not only law but also fact. One of the first national dermatology meetings that I attended was a clinical meeting at which patients were examined, questioned, and discussed. Dr. George Miller MacKee was head of the New York Skin and Cancer Hospital at that time and the most respected dermatologist in the country. Although many of the leaders of the specialty were present at this meeting, Dr. MacKee examined each patient and closed the discussion on each one, his words constituting the official diagnosis and recommended therapy for each patient. It is an axiom that votes do not establish scientific facts. Here, the opinions of one man, brilliant as he may have been, were accepted as the truth, the whole truth, and nothing but the truth.

The purpose of medical practice is to cure wherever possible and to alleviate suffering. Most dermatologists are clinicians caring for the sick. However, they get their training from teachers and academicians who often have limited knowledge of clinical dermatology. The difference between a clinician and an academician, basically, is the experience of 200 to 400 patient visits a week. Most academicians practice dermatology but on a limited scale. Yet the tail is definitely wagging the dog that we call dermatology. The two branches must have controversies, one based on experience, the other on accepted teachings and knowledge of the literature . . . the true and the false. This is a potent source of the controversies that exist. Only a small number of such disagreements are presented between the covers of this volume.

Inviting peers to contribute to this volume did much to make one understand his colleagues better. Some of the reasons for refusing to cooperate in this project were interesting. One retired practitioner and teacher said that he deals in facts, not controversies. Another academician asked to defend his opinion regarding a hotly debated topic said, ''I do not consider that this is a controversial subject.''

It is interesting that as knowledge increases, there are more controversies. This brings us back to the opening paragraph in this preface. As we learn more, we realize that the authoritarian approach is not all-encompassing. With increased knowledge, we realize that there is more and more that we do not know. This, however, does not stop us from making decisions and deductions—hence the well-known disagreements between experts. To paraphrase Voltaire, "I do not agree with you, but I will defend to the death your right to express your misconceptions." This is the attitude that we should adopt.

Mark Twain is credited with a quotation that perhaps sums up this problem best, to wit, "Science is a wonderful thing. For a very small input of fact you get such a large yield of theory." I am afraid that this is true.

It is hoped that this book and the discussions presented herein will increase the curiosity of the reader and will inspire him not to accept statements from authorities blindly. He should develop his own beliefs based on his analysis of his experiences. It is better to be wrong than to avoid entering into the process of decision making. Even if your interpretations are questionable, this is far better than uncritical acceptance of what a teacher, researcher, or clinician pontificates. It is said that intelligence is the difference between human beings and animals. Make use of your God-given gift of reason.

ERVIN EPSTEIN

TABLE OF CONTENTS

SECTION 1

MELANOMA

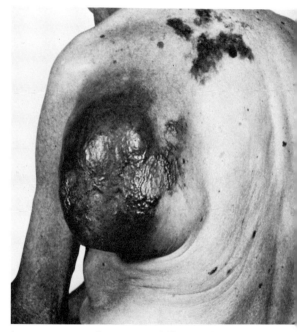

A gigantic untreated metanoma of 18 years' duration in an 88-year-old man.

CHAPTER 1

IMPORTANCE OF SUNLIGHT IN CAUSATION OF MELANOMA

SUN EXPOSURE AND MALIGNANT MELANOMA

Lance J. Cains

"White stallions get them, salamanders get them, and so do Scottish Terriers. The Pre-Columbian Incas of Peru had them. The spotted Dalamatian dog has never been recorded as having a melanoma."[2]

In human beings, melanoma seldom occurs in dark-skinned people or in mongoloid races, such as the Japanese. It is the white races that are highly susceptible to melanoma, and the risk of developing it has risen sharply since World War II. The daily hours of sunlight throughout the world do not appear to have altered, but life patterns, including those related to sun exposure, have shown remarkable changes.

This story starts with a paper by Lancaster, in which he considered that the incidence of melanoma of the skin is dependent upon some geographic or climatic feature. His data were collected from Europeans, and his conclusion was consistent with a hypothesis that excess sunlight is an important predisposing factor in melanoma.[1] This suggestion originally was made by McGovern, who noticed that there were pronounced differences among his series of malignant melanoma and others from the United Kingdom and other overseas areas with respect to site and age. It is interesting to note that neither Norman Paul[18] nor E. H. Molesworth,[19] who had written extensively and convincingly about the relationship of sunlight and basal and squamous cell carcinomas in Australia, had considered the possibility of this as a cause of malignant melanoma. Lancaster, in commenting on the mortality in Australia from 1951 to 1953, found that the true death rate in Australia was two and one half times that in England and Wales. The mortality in Queensland, the northern state, was almost three times that in Victoria and Tasmania.[1] In New Zealand, Eastcott[25] found that the death rate in the north island was higher than that in the south island. In the United States, it had been shown that the incidence of melanoma in southern areas was higher than that in the northern areas and that the coastal areas showed a higher incidence than did the inland areas. Because the population of Australia is largely on the coast, there are no comparative figures for this region. However, these findings strongly suggest that sun exposure during swimming is of significance. In South Africa, the incidence rates in Natal and the Cape of Good Hope, which are a short distance from the coast, are significantly higher than those of the Orange Free State, which is situated inland. The cause of melanoma has not been determined, but epidemiologic features strongly suggest a solar origin.

Sun exposure as a significant etiologic factor in melanoma formation is the basis for this article. In view of the rapidly changing epidemiology and the relatively sharp rise in the increase in melanoma in certain areas, an attempt has been made to present figures as current as possible.

Fitzpatrick[20] states that there has been a 340 per cent increase in malignant melanoma and that the rate has doubled in the last decade. The incidence in Australia in 1966 was 4 to 16 per 100,000, whereas the rate in 1980 was 40 per 100,000 in Queensland.[2] New Zealand, Norway, Sweden, and Israel also show a high incidence.[21] The occurrence is diminished among pigmented people in India, Japan, and Puerto Rico, and the rate in Singapore is 0.1 per 100,000. Holman, investigating the annual incidence of malignant melanoma in Western Australia, showed that in 1975 to 1976 the incidence was 4.4 per 100,000 in male subjects and 6.2 per 100,000 in female subjects in preinvasive lesions, whereas in invasive lesions the rate was 18.6 in male subjects and 18.8 in female subjects.[3] Current figures show a very significant increase in incidence of this disease in many countries, including the United States, Canada, England, Wales, and Scandinavia. The incidence of melanoma in male subjects in four northern cities in the United States was approximately half the rate in four southern cities and less than one third than that for female subjects.

Attention has been drawn to the large increase in incidence of melanoma in southern Arizona, where there is an extremely high incidence of basal and squamous cell carcinoma. The figures quoted are for the period 1969 through 1978. The 1969 incidence was 6.5, and that for 1978 was 28.5 per 100,000. The yearly rise was 34 to 37 per cent, and the total increase for the period was 340 per cent.[4] In contrast, according to the Third National Cancer Survey of the United States, the average American increase for 1965 through 1976 was 5 per cent, and that for southern Arizona was seven times as great.[5] Mortality during this period showed similar increases. Since 1931, a significant rise in the number of deaths has been recorded in Australia. Mortality has increased in individual states, with the greatest rises in those areas in proximity to the equator. Queensland, in which the center of population is closer to the equator than that of other Australian states, has the highest incidence of and mortality from melanoma of any country in the world. The mortality from 1961 to 1970 shows a change commensurate with the latitude distribution. The mortality from malignant melanomas rises despite the improved prognosis. The rate has been increasing by 3 per cent per year in white populations in the United States, Canada, England, and Wales. At present, there is probably a 7 per cent annual increase in malignant melanoma in Australia.

Geography and Climatic Factors

In his figures of 1956, Lancaster (followed by Lee and Merrill in 1970[22]) showed a strong inverse relationship between melanoma and latitude.[1] Magnus showed that there was a threefold increase in malignant melanoma in the southern part of Norway compared with the northern part.[6] It has been shown that in countries extending over many latitudes, there is an increase in incidence of malignant melanoma among whites that is greatest in individuals residing close to the equator. In the United States, Mason and associates plotted skin cancer deaths (for the period 1950 through 1969) by county and showed that the highest age-adjusted mortality in whites occurred in the southern part of the nation.[7] The distribution of deaths resulting from nonmelanoma skin cancer closely mimics that of melanoma, suggesting a common causative factor, either geography or sunlight exposure. The differences in mortality in various regions are not confined to small, limited areas. Age-adjusted death rates in Australia for the period 1961 through 1970 are shown in Table 1.[8]

The Third National Cancer Survey showed that the mortality from malignant melanoma in the United States is greatest among whites living in areas of low latitudes.[5] A survey in southern Arizona (by Schreiber and coworkers[4]) showed that meteorologic and

Table 1.   AGE-ADJUSTED DEATH RATES IN
AUSTRALIA (1961–1970)*

Latitude of Capital City (°S)		Age-Adjusted Mortality (per 100,000)
Queensland	27	44
Western Australia	32	32
New South Wales	34	34
Southern Australia	35	26
Victoria	38	25

*From Beardmore, G. L.: The epidemiology of malignant melanoma in Australia. *In* Melanoma and Skin Cancer: Proceedings of the International Cancer Conference. Syndey, Australia, 1971, p. 43. Used by permission.

geographic factors allow a greater quantity of ultraviolet radiation to reach the surface of the earth. It has been postulated that these are the important factors in the large increase in the incidence of malignant melanoma in that area.

Tucson lies on latitude 32°N and has more sunlight (a mean annual percentage of 80), more clear days (a mean annual number of 193), and fewer daytime clouds (a cumulative annual mean percentage of 38) than does any populated geographic site in North America. This leads to the wearing of lighter clothing as well as to an increase in outdoor activity. In this area, the incidence of malignant melanoma rose from 6.5 to 28.5 per 100,000 during the period 1969 to 1978. Surpassing that reported from other areas of the United States, this is an annual increase of 34 to 37 per cent and a total rise of 340 per cent for the 10 years.[4]

Pigmentary Relations

The Third National Cancer Survey in the United States showed that the incidence of malignant melanoma was 0.8 per 100,000 for blacks and 4.5 per 100,000 for whites. There was a remarkably low incidence of malignant melanoma in nonwhite groups and in whites with darkly pigmented skin. This strongly suggests that pigment protects from the effect of sunlight.

Countries with a high incidence of malignant melanoma have many light-skinned whites who are exposed to a high incidence of solar radiation (such as Australia, where there is a large Celtic population and Israel, where immigrant Jewish populations are not well pigmented). This relationship will be discussed in detail later.

Gellin and associates suggested in 1969 that there was a clear negative relationship between skin color and malignant melanoma. They found in a well-conducted survey that there was a tendency for patients with malignant melanoma to have light complexions, light eyes, and blonde or red hair and to spend a greater amount of time outdoors.[9] This was significant in relation to sun exposure, because a close correlation was found in a study of patients with basal and squamous cell carcinoma of similar phenotype. This supports the finding of a high incidence of malignant melanoma in patients who are unprotected from sunlight. These people tend to freckle readily or burn on exposure to sunlight. It is surely significant that the Queensland Melanoma Project does not have any record of a Queensland aboriginal's developing a melanoma. It further appears from this survey that people of Scottish, Irish, and Welsh descent and, to a lesser extent, those of northern European ancestry are particularly prone to develop cutaneous melanoma in Queensland.[8]

According to Wallace and Exton,[10] the development of the concept of acral lentiginous melanoma has explained to a large extent the incidence of melanoma in pigmented people. Acral melanoma is not common in high-incidence populations, but in those of low-incidence dark races, such as in the United States, Japan, and Africa, malignant melanomas are relatively common. The incidence in Japan is similar to that among American blacks. Malignant melanoma in these people was considered for years to be traumatic in nature, but this concept is no longer tenable. Urbanization and protective footwear have not diminished the incidence of malignant melanoma. Recent epidemiologic figures indicate a strong relation between nevus cell nevi in hypopigmented areas and the development of malignant melanoma. It is possible that even on these areas repeated sun exposure over a long period may play some part. The relationship of melanocytic nevi and malignant melanoma is not clearly defined and is said to vary from 20 to 66 per cent. It is significant that the aforementioned study and that of Lewis concerning Ugandan blacks[11] showed that melanomas in this area occur late in life and that the histologic pattern is largely that of Hutchinson's melanotic freckle and superficial spreading melanoma, suggesting a long cumulative sun exposure effect as a factor involving pigmented nevi in hypopigmented areas.

In a number of countries, there is evidence of high incidence of malignant melanoma in light-skinned whites compared with a low incidence in dark-skinned white Latins, Indians, and blacks. This protective pigmentary relationship is very significant.

1. Studies in New Mexico showed the incidence to be 16 per 100,000 in whites, 2.8 per 100,000 in Latins, and 1.3 per 100,000 in Indians.[12]

2. In Israel the incidence was 3.4 per 100,000 among European Jews and 2.7 per 100,000 among African Jews.[13]

3. In McDonald's study of Texans, the incidence was 3.4 per 100,000 whites and 0.27 per 100,000 nonwhites.[14]

4. In Schreiber's study of southern Arizona, the incidence was 28.5 per 100,000 in whites and nil in Latins, Indians, and blacks.[4]

This group of epidemiologic factors supports the conclusion that there is a very high correlation between malignant melanoma and sunlight exposure. In these population groups, hormonal factors would be fairly uniformly dispersed throughout these geographic areas. Other exposures, such as industrial petrochemicals and carcinogens in suntan lotions, alcohol, and arsenic, would be similarly distributed. Under these circumstances, it is difficult to associate any etiologic factor other than sunlight.

Body Area of Distribution

The body area of distribution of nonmelanoma cancer follows fairly closely a pattern of solar-dependent exposure. In both basal cell carcinoma and squamous cell carcinoma (more in the latter than in the former), the pattern leaves little room for doubt of a direct relationship. The highest incidence lies in the more exposed areas, in which both the clinical and the histologic findings are those of extensive solar damage. The age of onset seems to be increased, except in relatively unprotected persons. All of these features point quite definitely to an accumulative sun exposure effect. The relationship is not so definite in malignant melanoma, in which the exposure areas are not quite so closely related. The exposed areas, especially the face and the neck, are not the statistically common sites. The general age of onset is reduced in melanoma, and evidence of some solar damage is not so readily seen. However, on careful consideration, the effect of sunlight on body distribution of lesions is very strong evidence of a causative factor. Lentigo maligna melanoma follows the nonmelanoma pattern fairly closely: slow progress after an onset late in life with a clinical and histologically marked solar background. Inversely, malignant melanoma rarely occurs in doubly protected areas, such as the female breast and the male buttock. The common incidence sites are the trunk in male patients and the lower limbs in female patients, which are both areas of ordinary exposure. It is significant that the incidence on the commonly exposed area, the face, is equal in males and females, and this incidence has not changed greatly over the years.

The relation of malignant melanoma and sunspots has drawn attention to the possible effect of recurrent intense blistering exposures and etiologic factors, especially in untanned skin.[15] This adequately explains the favoring of sites exposed intermittently and extensively to sun during recreation, particularly the male trunk and the female legs. That is, ultraviolet radiation is not necessarily a cumulative dose-dependent carcinogen. The rise in melanoma incidence begins with persons born around 1900, a generation that first experienced substantial liberalization of recreational dress and behavior as it passed into adulthood. Anatomic areas that had not previously been exposed to sun, especially the trunk in males and the lower limbs in females, became uncovered during recreation. It was these two sites that accounted for the large general rise in the incidence of melanoma, whereas virtually no increase in melanoma of the face occurred. Studies related to the incidence of malignant melanoma in areas of historically documented blistering exposure are in progress in Australia. Investigators in this area are impressed with a history of specific sun exposure of the lower legs in females following the "healthy tan cult." This may well be more significant than the rising hemline.

Solar Exposure Patterns

Attention has been drawn to the high incidence of melanoma in countries in which there is a marked solar exposure of poorly pigmented people and a positive correlation between this and accumulated sun exposure.

In a survey of melanoma in Israel, the highest incidence was found in native-born Israelis of European extraction. The rates were intermediate in veteran foreign-born Europeans and lowest in European-born recent immigrants.[16] That is, the longer the exposure to the intense sun of Israel, the greater the age-adjusted incidence of malignant melanoma.

Anaise and coworkers reported a significantly higher incidence of melanoma in:

1. European-born Jews of the same age and ethnic background who stayed in Israel 20 to 30 years compared with those who stayed only 2 to 5 years.

2. European-born Jews compared with those born in Africa or Asia.

3. Those who worked in agricultural kibbutzim compared with those in the city (5.4 to 1.7 per 100,000).[13]

The annual incidence of malignant melanoma in Israel rose from 2 in 100,000 in 1960 to 4 in 100,000 in 1970. The age-adjusted rates in immigrants from Europe and the United States were 10 times higher than those in Jews from Africa and Asia. The incidence was higher for those living on the coast than those in the mountains. (Israelis living on the coast obviously were more exposed to sunlight, especially during recreation.)

In western Australia, Holman showed that differences in incidence between immigrants and native-born Australians (not aboriginals) is proportional to the duration of residence in an area of high exposure. In western Australia, where the annual incidence rate of melanoma is 18.6 per 100,000 in males and 18.8 per 100,000 in females, the rates in British migrants are more than double those in Britons in the British Isles.[3] Recreation involving sun exposure is common in western Australia, probably more so among well-to-do classes. Increasing incidence or mortality from malignant melanoma described in many white populations is another phenomenon that could well be attributed to increasing intermittent exposure to sunlight. The opportunity for recreation has risen with affluence and an increase in leisure hours. The differences in epidemiology of nonmelanoma and melanoma cancer also can be explained by the correlation of the former with continuous sun exposure and the latter with intermittent sun exposure.

The largest increase in malignant melanoma rates has occurred in the young. These people are among the more affluent and spend more time swimming and boating than formerly. The traditional ''healthy tan'' is an accepted philosophy among the young. As people grow older, they stand sun exposure less readily and have observed its effect. The increase is not an occupational effect, since the same gradient of risk is seen in married women classified by the status of their husbands' occupation. As industrial societies develop, the exposure of the population to sunlight becomes greater. Hours of work are fewer, vacations are longer, the opportunity for travel is greater, and clothing therefore becomes lighter.

A further observation relating solar exposure and malignant melanoma is that sunspot cycles correlate with the increase in melanoma incidence. In Connecticut, the age-adjusted incidence of melanoma has risen from 1.1 per 100,000 in 1935 to 7.4 in 1976. Superimposed on the steady rise in incidence were intervals of excessive increases occurring every 8 to 12 years. These periods of markedly increased rates peaked at 3 to 5 years, followed by a return to baseline rates. These fluctuations of melanoma incidence correlated with sunspot numbers, and the highest correlation coefficients occurred 2 years after peak sunspot activity. Melanoma incidence rates from other tumor registries (including New York state, Finland, and Denmark, but not Norway) have shown similar correlation with sunspot numbers. Wigle has confirmed the association between sunspot maxima and the rises of melanoma incidence in Alberta and Saskatchewan. It is evident that solar activity is variable and that sunspot numbers are the closest indication of this activity. This survey would seem to show that rises in melanoma incidence occur after sunspot peaks and would suggest that heavier exposures to ultraviolet radiation trigger the clinical appearance of melanoma. This further raises the question as to whether melanoma could be induced in a short period, such as 3 years. This supports the concept of early age formation of superficial spreading melanoma and nodular melanoma as tumors of nonaccumulative solar dosage dependency.

The dose-dependent carcinogen concept closely follows the high rate of malignant melanoma with the inherited autosomal recessive xeroderma pigmentosum. Those patients in whom sunlight induces numerous cutaneous tumors, such as solar keratoses, basal cell carcinoma, squamous cell carcinoma, and keratoacanthoma, have a much higher risk of developing malignant melanomas. In a study of 15 patients with xeroderma pigmentosum at the National Institutes of Health, 7 (47 per cent) were found to have malignant melanoma.[17] The relation of sun exposure to nonmelanoma cancer in this condition is widely accepted, and the finding that malignant melanoma also is involved in a high percentage is strong evidence of sun exposure as an etiologic factor in melanoma. This direct association of minimal solar radiation and multiple malignant melanomas suggests an acceleration of damage to the skin of patients with increased sensitivity to the carcinogenic potential of ultraviolet radiation.

The new measurements of ultraviolet radiation (290 to 320 mm) exposure at various locations show clearly that the amount reaching the surface of the earth peaks during the summer months and drops during the winter months in typical sinusoidal patterns. Using data from the Third National Cancer Survey for the period 1967 through 1971, Scotto and associates[26] studied seasonal patterns for whites in detail, including anatomic site, sex, age, and geographic regions. Overall, a strong seasonal pattern with a summertime peak was observed for females. It was most pronounced for females under 55 years and for those of all ages with melanomas of the upper and lower extremities. In males, a seasonal pattern with a summertime peak was observed for malignant melanomas of the upper extremity. In females, it was found that over 20 per cent of all cases were diagnosed during the summer months (June to July). Less than 14 per cent were diagnosed in the winter (between December and January). One might speculate that summer peaks and the diagnosis of malignant melanoma are related to the promotion of tumor growth by high-intensity ultraviolet radiation over short periods, but the possibility that the lesions are noticed only at the time of irritating sunlight exposure must be considered. The comparable cyclic pattern of exposure in summer is the upper extremity in females and males, but there is no cyclic exposure for the head and the neck (in which exposure is constant). The trunk is especially exposed in summer and is covered in winter. The cyclic pattern is apparent in females but not in males, that is, greater exposure of the lower extremities in the female compared with the male during the winter.

This study points to the possibility that short-term, high-intensity ultraviolet radiation promotes tumor development. Scotto and coworkers,[23] using a sunburn ultraviolet meter that measures the effectiveness of ultraviolet radiation in producing erythematous skin, took readings at half-hourly intervals for 1 year in ten geographically widespread locations in the United States. The incidence of skin cancer, including basal cell carcinoma, squamous cell carcinoma, and malignant melanoma, correlated positively with ultraviolet intensity. For the first time, actual measurements are available to support the theory that ultraviolet radiation causes skin cancer, including malignant melanoma, in human beings.

References

1. Lancaster, H. O., and Nelson, J.: Sunlight as a cause of melanoma. Med. J. Aust. 1:452, 1957.
2. Green, A.: Melanoma of the skin. Aust. Fam. Physician 11:7, 1982.
3. Holman, C. D. J., Mulroney, C. D., and Armstrong, B. K.: Epidemiology of pre-invasive and invasive malignant melanoma in Western Australia. Int. J. Cancer 25:317, 1980.
4. Schreiber, M. M., Bozzo, P. D., and Moon, T. E.: Malignant melanoma in Southern Arizona. Arch. Dermatol. 117:6, 1981.
5. Third National Cancer Survey: Incidence Data, National Cancer Institute Monograph 41. U.S. Department of Health, Education and Welfare, Public Health Service, National Institutes of Health, National Cancer Institute, Bethesda, Maryland. DHEW Publication No. (NIH) 75–787, 1975.
6. Magnus, K.: Incidence of malignant melanoma of the skin in the five Nordic countries: Significance of solar radiation. Int. J. Cancer 20:477, 1977.
7. Mason, T. J., et al.: Atlas of Cancer Mortality for U.S. counties: 1950–1969. U.S. Department of Health, Education and Welfare, Public Health Service, National Institutes of Health, Bethesda, Maryland, DHEW Publication No. (NIH) 75–780, pp. 44–47 and 91–92, 1975.
8. Beardmore, G. L.: The epidemiology of malignant melanoma in Australia. Melanoma and Skin Cancer: Proceedings of the International Cancer Conference. Sydney, Australia, 1972, p. 43.
9. Gellin, G. A., Kopf, A. W., and Garfinkel, L.: Malignant melanoma: A controlled study of possible associated factors. Arch. Dermatol. 99:43, 1969.
10. Wallace, D. C., and Exton, L. A.: Genetic predisposition to development of malignant melanoma. Melanoma and Skin Cancer: Proceedings of the International Cancer Conference. Sydney, Australia, 1972, pp. 65–79.
11. Lewis, M. G.: Malignant melanoma in Uganda. Br. J. Cancer 21:483, 1967.
12. New Mexico out to detect skin cancers: Medical news. JAMA 239:1841, 1978.
13. Anaise, D., Steinitz, R., and Ben Hur, N.: Solar radiation: A possible aetiological factor in malignant melanoma in Israel. Cancer 42:299, 1978.
14. McDonald, E. J.: Regional patterns in morbidity from melanoma in Texas. J. Invest. Dermatol. 54:91, 1970.
15. Houghton, A., Munster, E. W., and Viola, M. V.: Increased incidence of malignant melanoma after peaks of sunspot activity. Lancet 1:759, 1978.
16. Movshovitz, M., and Modan, B.: Role of sun exposure in the aetiology of malignant melanoma: Epidemiologic inference. J. Natl. Cancer Inst. 51:777, 1973.
17. Moore, C., and Iverson, P. C.: Xeroderma pigmentosum: Showing common skin cancers plus melanocarcinoma controlled by surgery. Cancer 7:377, 1954.
18. Paul, N.: The influence of sunlight in the production of cancer of the skin. London, 1918.
19. Molesworth, E. H.: An Introduction to Dermatology. Sydney, Angus & Robertson, 1944, p. 4.
20. Fitzpatrick, T. B.: Personal communication, 1982.
21. Kopf, A. W., Bart, R. S., Rodriguez-Sains, R. S., and Ackerman, A. B.: Malignant Melanoma. New York, Masson Publishing USA Inc., 1979, p. 4.
22. Lee, J. A. H., and Merill, J. M.: Sunlight and the etiology of malignant melanoma: A synthesis. Med. J. Aust. 2:846, 1970.
23. Scotto, J., Fears, T. R., and Gori, G. B.: Measurements of ultraviolet radiation in the United States and comparisons with skin cancer data. National Cancer Institute, Division of Cancer Cause and Prevention, National Institutes of Health. DHEW Publication No. (NIH) 76–1039, 1976.
24. McGovern, V. J.: Melanoblastoma. Med. J. Aust. 1:139, 1952.
25. Eastcott, D. F.: Epidemiology of Skin Cancer in New Zealand. *In* Urbach, F. (ed.): Conference on Biology of Cutaneous Cancer, National Cancer Institute Monograph No. 10. Washington, D.C., U.S. Government Printing Office, Feb. 1963, pp. 141–151.
26. Scotto, J., and Nam, J. M.: Skin melanoma and seasonal patterns. Am. J. Epidemiol. 111:309, 1980.
27. Teppo, L., et al.: Sunlight as a risk factor in malignant melanoma of the skin. Cancer 41:2018, 1978.

HOW IMPORTANT IS THE ROLE OF RADIATION FROM THE SUN IN THE RISING INCIDENCE OF MELANOMAS?

John H. Epstein, M.D.

The nonmelanoma skin cancers, basal cell epitheliomas, and squamous cell carcinomas are by far the most common human malignancies that occur in the United States. The role of sun exposure in the development of these growths initially was suggested by astute clinical observations made around the turn of the twentieth century and subsequently was confirmed by epidemiologic and experimental studies.[1,2]

The malignant melanoma represents the third most common skin cancer. There has been a significant increase in the occurrence of this type of malignancy within the past few decades. Mortality resulting from malignant melanomas essentially has doubled in the past two decades.[3] In addition, the incidence per 100,000 population has increased even more, although the figures are difficult to evaluate because of the different periods examined.[4] This suggests that improved diagnostic acumen has reduced fatality. These data are relatively consistent wherever adequate information has been available (i.e., New York state, Norway, Canada, the United States, the United Kingdom, Australia, Denmark, Sweden, and Connecticut).[4] Two other factors should be noted. First, the age of those who die of melanoma is decreasing, that is, the victims are younger. Secondly, the anatomic distribution of these tumors has changed. Although there has been a small increase in numbers of tumors on the head and the neck, there has been a striking increase in these growths on the upper back in men and on the calf in women. Also, there has been a significantly increased number on the upper limbs of both sexes.[4]

This anatomic distribution has suggested to a number of observers that sun exposure may play a dominant role in the increasing incidence of these cancers.[5] The potential importance of sun exposure in the production of malignant melanomas is supported most notably by geographic distribution. In light-skinned whites, melanomas occur most commonly in areas of high insolation, such as Australia and Israel.[6,7] Also, the incidence is generally greatest in white Europeans, North Americans, and Australians who live closest to the equator.[6,8,9] These cancers are much less common in dark-skinned people who live in the same areas. Individuals with light-colored eyes and hair and very fair complexions who sunburn easily appear to be at greatest risk.[10,11] The inference is that melanin pigment protects against the damaging effects of the sun that are responsible for the melanoma formation.

In addition, there are two types of melanoma in which sun exposure plays a dominant role.[11] The first is lentigo maligna melanoma, which occurs almost exclusively on the face in older individuals and is associated with clinical and microscopic evidence of chronic solar injury. The second is the melanoma that occurs in individuals with xeroderma pigmentosum. These patients have an inordinate susceptibility to the development of sun-induced skin cancers of all varieties, including malignant melanomas. This cancer propensity presumably results from defects in the ability of xeroderma pigmentosum patients' cells to repair DNA damaged by ultraviolet radiation. Melanomas also have been produced in pigmented hairless mice by ultraviolet irradiation of benign pigmented "blue nevi," which were induced by a single application of 7,12 dimethylbenz[a]anthracene (DMBA).[12]

Other supportive factors that have been noted include increases in melanoma incidence following greater sunspot activity. This activity is associated with greater ultraviolet radiation emission by the sun.[11] Changes in life styles and dress also have been considered potentially important, as have the possible changes in the protective influences of the ozone layer by supersonic aircraft and fluorohydrocarbons.[13]

Thus, one might conclude that the evidence supporting the dominant role of the sun as the cause for the changing melanoma rates is strong. However, if the evidence is examined closely, this relationship is unclear. Unlike the common sun-induced cancers, the increased incidence has not occurred on the head, the neck, and the hands, which are the anatomic sites that receive the greatest amount of solar exposure. Geographic distribution studies also present some confusion, as do evaluations of occupational patterns. In Australia, no relationship between proximity to the equator and melanoma incidence has been reported.[13] In England, male clerical workers and professional men have a much higher mortality rate from melanomas than do outdoor workers.[14] The relationship to sunspot activity is also unusual, in that the peak increase in melanoma occurrence appears within 2 years after the peak sunspot activity.[11,13] This would be a most rapid carcinogenic induction. Also, alteration of the ozone layer would not be responsible for the melanomas that have occurred within the past 20 to 30 years, since no consistent alterations have been recorded to date.

It has been suggested that chronic repeated exposure of the skin to the rays of the sun actually might reduce the carcinogenic effects on melanocytes, perhaps by producing a protective suntan.[15] As a corollary, intermittent intense exposures of usually unexposed parts of the body have been theoretically incriminated to explain some of the anatomic distributional occupational, and age-associated data. If these concepts were applicable, women would have as many upper back lesions as men and men as many leg lesions as women. In addition, the incidence should be higher in recent immigrants to Israel than in native-born Israelis, and this is not the case.[7]

Finally, although experimental evidence in mice indicates that melanomas can be induced by ultraviolet radiation, to date this has been possible only with chronic repeated exposures of pigmented lesions that have been initiated by the application of the potent chemical carcinogen DMBA.[12]

In summary, there is convincing evidence that certain melanomas that occur on the face (primarily lentigo maligna melanoma) and in patients with xeroderma pigmentosum are caused by sun exposure. In addition, epidemiologic and experimental data support the possible role of ultraviolet radiation in the production of melanomas. However, the evidence supporting the role of solar irradiation as the primary etiologic agent responsible for the striking increase in the incidence of this malignancy in the last few decades is, at best, difficult to support. Other factors, including hormonal influences, familial tendencies, systemic and topical carcinogens, and the like, may exert much more important influences on this most significant problem. I would suggest that we examine these other potential factors with more energy.

References

1. Urbach, F., Epstein, J. H., and Forbes, P. D.: Ultraviolet carcinogenesis: Experimental, global, and genetic aspects. *In* Fitzpatrick, T. B., Pathak, M. A., Harber, L. C., Seiji, M., and Kukita, A. (eds.): Sunlight and Man. Tokyo, University of Tokyo Press, 1974, pp. 259–283.
2. Epstein, J. H.: Photocarcinogenesis: A review. *In* Kripke, M. L., and Sass, E. R. (eds.): Ultraviolet Carcinogenesis, National Cancer Institute Monograph No. 50, 1978, pp. 13–25.
3. Jensen, O. M., and Bolander, A. M.: Trends in malignant melanoma of the skin. World Health Stat. 33:2, 1980.
4. Elwood, J. M., and Lee, J. A. H.: Recent data on epidemiology of malignant melanoma. Semin. Oncol. 2:149, 1975.

5. Houghton, A. N., Flannery, J. T., and Viola, M. V.: Malignant melanoma in Connecticut and Denmark. Int. J. Cancer 25:95, 1980.
6. Davis, N. C.: Cutaneous melanoma. The Queensland experience. Curr. Probl. Surg. 13:1, 1976.
7. Morshovitz, M., and Modan, B.: Role of sun exposure in the etiology of malignant melanoma. Epidemiologic inference. J. Natl. Cancer Inst. 51:777, 1977.
8. Elwood, J. M., Lee, J. A. H., Walter, S. D., Mo, T., and Green, A. E. S.: Relationship of melanoma and other skin cancer mortality to latitude and ultraviolet radiation in the United States and Canada. Int. J. Epidemiol. 3:325, 1974.
9. Crombie, I. K.: Variation of melanoma incidence with latitude in North America and Europe. Br. J. Cancer 40:774, 1979.
10. Gellin, G. A., Kopf, A. W., and Garfinkel, L.: Malignant melanoma. A controlled study of possible associated factors. Arch. Dermatol. 99:43, 1969.
11. Houghton, A. N., and Viola, M. V.: Solar radiation and malignant melanoma of the skin. J. Am. Acad. Dermatol. 5:477, 1981.
12. Epstein, J. H., Epstein, W. L., and Nakai, T.: Production of melanomas DMBA-induced "blue nevi" in hairless mice with ultraviolet light. J. Natl. Cancer Inst. 38:19, 1967.
13. The aetiology of melanoma. Lancet 1:253, 1981.
14. Lee, J. A. H., and Strickland, D.: Malignant melanoma: Social staus and outdoor work. Br. J. Cancer 41:757, 1980.
15. McGovern, V. J.: Epidemiological aspects of melanoma: A review. Pathology 9:233, 1977.

Editorial Comment

Enough evidence has accumulated to support the contention that sunshine can produce melanoma. However, the importance of this factor has not been established in the disease as a whole. In other words, since melanoma occurs most commonly on covered parts of the body, it is difficult to accept the claim that solar irradiation is the major etiologic contributor to the production of this malignancy. Only time and further studies will determine the truth or fallacy of the suppositions that we harbor today in the hope of explaining the increased incidence of this pigmented form of cancer.

Another important etiologic consideration concerns the possible role of ionizing radiation as a cause of melanoma. Since melanomas may be caused by sunshine and since melanomas occur at times in conjunction with epitheliomas, such as in PUVA therapy, xeroderma pigmentosum, and so forth, it seems likely that x-radiation could produce these tumors also. This has become important, since industrial exposure to these rays may be associated with the development of melanomas, such as (possibly) in the Livermore "epidemic," in which a large number of cases of melanoma were noted in individuals working in a nuclear research plant. However, it has been impossible to link these cases to actual exposure to radiation in most instances. Medical and legal entanglements have resulted in some of these instances. On the other hand, this relationship between x-radiation and melanoma has not been proved. Also, there is a paucity of reports—clinical, experimental or statistical—to relate this energy to these neoplasms.

The relationship existing between melanomas and radiation is a challenging, interesting, and unsolved problem. Today I would be inclined to sum this matter up by stating that the basic cause of melanoma has not been determined. On the other hand, it seems certain that our knowledge of the tumor is increasing, and some day the causative factors will be established.

Think It Over.

CHAPTER 2

REMOVAL OF CONGENITAL MELANOCYTIC NEVI

THE ARGUMENT FOR REMOVAL OF CONGENITAL NEVOCYTIC NEVI

Alvin H. Jacobs, M.D.

The controversy rages on! To remove or not to remove congenital melanocytic nevi, that is the question. What is the risk of malignancy in these lesions? The final answer to these questions will come only out of a long-term prospective study and therefore will not be available during the lifetime of most of us. But patients and parents want answers now—what are we to tell them? I will present my opinions based on a careful analysis of currently available data: clinical, histologic, and statistical.

The ordinary melanocytic nevi ("acquired" moles) are not present at birth but begin to appear in early childhood and continue to develop through adolescence. These moles usually measure less than 2.0 cm in greatest diameter. There are an average of approximately 25 moles per person, making them the most common tumors in humans. The congenital (present at birth) melanocytic (nevocytic) nevus, on the other hand, is much less common, occurring in approximately 1 per cent of newborn infants.[1,2] In contrast with the ordinary moles, congenital nevi vary from a few millimeters in size to gigantic lesions covering a major portion of the body. For reasons that will become apparent, the giant congenital nevocytic nevi and the small congenital nevi will be considered separately.

Giant Congenital Nevocytic Nevi

Giant congenital nevocytic nevi are relatively uncommon lesions, probably occurring less than once in 20,000 newborn infants. In spite of their rarity, there is more accurate information on their malignant potential than on that of the small congenital nevi. Giant nevi are always noted at birth, with their description and measurements recorded and often photographs taken, whereas small nevi that are present at birth often are overlooked and are not recorded. Thus, retrospective statistical studies of giant nevi are possible, whereas such studies of small nevi are not as easily performed.

How large must a pigmented nevus be to warrant the "giant" designation? Many authors have answered this question in an arbitrary fashion, e.g., 10 cm² or larger, or larger than the size of the patient's hand. I prefer the definition of the giant nevocytic nevus used by Rhodes: "A nevus so large that it could not be removed by simple excision and primary closure using adjacent tissues in a single surgical procedure."[3]

Giant pigmented nevi often have a dermatomal distribution and, since they often cover a portion of the body, are referred to as garment nevi. Their color ranges from tan to various shades of brown to black. They have an uneven verrucous or papillomatous surface and irregular margins. In almost all cases, smaller satellite nevi appear at the periphery and at some distance from the giant nevus. As the infant grows, the area becomes thicker and darker, and the surface may become rugose, warty, or nodular. The hairy component becomes more prominent in later childhood.

Four pathologic components may be found in the giant nevi: the usual nevocytic nevus with epidermal and intradermal nevus cells, the neuroid nevus with schwannian-type cells, the blue nevus with dermal melanocytes and, sometimes, cell structures similar to those seen in benign juvenile melanoma. An important feature of the giant nevus is the extension of nevus cells between collagen bundles in the lower dermis or even into the subcutaneous tissue as well as within skin appendages.

Giant nevocytic nevi are serious cosmetic problems, but more important is the potential for malignant change. Various studies have indicated a malignancy potential of from 1.8 per cent to 40 per cent, with an average of approximately 10 per cent. This is in sharp contrast with the usually accepted malignancy potential of ordinary (acquired) nevi of 1 in 1 million. However, most of these studies suffer selection bias. The most reliable data are that of Lorentzen and his associates, who retrieved 151 patients with giant pigmented nevi registered in the Danish Health System during the 60-year period 1915 through 1975.[4] They concluded that the expected incidence of malignant transformation would be 4.6 per cent during the lifetime of these patients. Rhodes and coworkers,[5] applying more accurate statistical methods to the data of Lorentzen, have arrived at a malignancy potential of 6.3 per cent. Thus, the risk of malignancy in giant congenital nevi is as high as 1 in 16 over a lifetime. This risk is not spread evenly over the lifetime, since it has been shown by Kaplan that 60 per cent of the malignancies that have occurred in giant nevi have developed in the first decade of life.[6]

Trozak,[7] in a review of metastatic malignant melanoma in prepubertal children, found 21 cases in which metastatic melanoma occurred before puberty in a giant pigmented nevus. In 5 of 21 cases, malignancy was proved before the age of 2 years. None of the 21 patients survived. Trozak found that the malignancy developed early and metastasized widely. He reasoned that since giant nevi are often nodular and rugose, a developing melanoma is difficult to distinguish. He also pointed out that these melanomas arise deep in the elements of the nevus, resulting in a delay in recognition and at the same time placing the tumors in proximity to the larger lymphatics and blood vessels, thus resulting in early metastasis.

Kaplan[8] reviewed the reported cases of giant nevocytic nevi and of malignancy occurring in giant nevi. He found that although 44 per cent of giant nevi occurred in the dorsal paravertebral area (back, buttock, posterior scalp), 84 per cent of malignancies occurred in this region. Moreover, the benign atypical neural elements occur in the back, the buttock, and the scalp close to the dorsal midline. Kaplan speculates that these embryonal neural crest nevi, which occur primarily in giant nevi of the back and the scalp, are most susceptible to malignant degeneration.

Conclusions

It is clear from the preceding discussion that the risk of malignant transformation in giant nevi is at least 1 in 16 over a lifetime, that 60 per cent of the malignancies occur in the first decade of life, and that recognition of these malignancies is difficult. In addition, metastases occur early and survival is close to zero. For these reasons, I recommend very early complete removal of giant nevocytic nevi and full-depth resection. The first stage can be accomplished as early as when the patient is 3 weeks of age. When multiple operations are necessary, it seems advisable to start with resection of that portion of the nevus involving the paravertebral, posterior scalp, or buttock area.

The suggestion that giant nevocytic nevi be treated by early dermabrasion can only be condemned. Greeley reported a patient treated by superficial excision of a congenital nevus in whom melanoma occurred in the remaining deep portion of the nevus 9 years later.[9] We have had the opportunity to study biopsy tissue from two patients approximately 1 year after early dermabrasion of giant nevi. In both cases, the deep extension of the nevus in the mid-dermis and the lower dermis as well as within appendages was still present. An advocate of dermabrasion has stated that the procedure must be done before the melanocytes start moving deeper. On the contrary, biopsies performed on newborn infants with giant nevi reveal nevus cells in the deep dermis and the subcutis as well as in appendages. The migration of melanocytes is not inward, but rather outward, from the neural crest.

Small Congenital Nevocytic Nevi

Although small congenital nevocytic nevi are much more common than the giant type, statistical information concerning malignancy potential is more difficult to obtain. It is these small nevi that generate the most controversy.

In order to determine the frequency of congenital nevi, Walton, Jacobs, and Cox examined 1058 newborn infants and performed biopsies on pigmented lesions within the first 72 hours of life.[1] None of these infants had giant nevi. Small nevocytic nevi were present in 1.01 per cent of these newborns. Alper and associates[2] examined 4611 newborn infants and, although biopsies were not performed until after the neonatal period, found that 1.1 per cent had congenital nevocytic nevi. It is important to note that in this latter study, only 40 per cent of the small nevi were recorded in the medical records, and the exact location was noted for only one nevus.

Solomon[10] estimates that at least 300 melanomas occur annually in patients under the age of 20 years, with approximately 60 of these derived from a congenital melanocytic nevus. He states that it is therefore reasonable and logical to attempt to remove congenital melanocytic nevi as a preventive measure. According to Solomon, there are three main arguments offered in opposition to this view: it is not technically feasible to remove the largest lesions, it is too expensive to do so, and it is not economical to remove all congenital nevi. "When considering what to do in a given patient, I find it most difficult to weigh the economies of expense of surgery on some poorly defined mass of patients against a risk of malignancy in the individual."[10] The larger lesions, being more dangerous, should be removed even if the risk of surgery is higher, whereas the smaller lesions are easy to remove and pose much less of a surgical risk.

In an argument against prophylactic removal of small congenital nevi, Kopf and associates,[11] using the prevalence figures of Walton, Jacobs, and Cox,[1] stated that 1.3 per cent of the 3 million infants born each year in the United States (or 39,000 infants) would have nevocytic nevi. Since we actually reported that 1.01 per cent of newborns had congenital nevi, the figure should be 30,300. Kopf and coworkers have stated that removal of this many lesions would be impractical. However, I would like to point out that there are approximately 4600 board-certified dermatologists and 2500 plastic surgeons in the United States. Thus, there would be 4.27 nevi for each of these specialists to remove each year, and since many would be removed by the 50,000 general surgeons, there would be 0.5 lesions to be removed by each in a year. This is not impractical, especially when it is considered that melanoma occurring in congenital nevi in childhood is uniformly fatal.

In order to clarify the malignancy potential of small congenital nevocytic nevi, Rhodes and colleagues have done some interesting studies and statistical analyses.[3,12] They reviewed the tumor specimens from 234 patients with primary cutaneous melanoma seeking the presence of nevocellular nevi in contiguity with the melanoma. To distinguish congenital from noncongenital nevi, they designated melanoma-associated nevocellular nevi as having congenital features if nevus cells were found within the collagen of the lower two thirds of the reticular dermis or if nevus cells were present within one or more appendages, inside perineural sheaths, within blood vessel walls, or associated with lymphatic vessels causing luminal distortion. In 27.4 per cent of the 234 melanoma specimens, a dermal nevocellular nevus was found in contiguity with the melanoma. Of the 234 specimens, 8.1 per cent had tumor-associated nevocellular nevi with congenital features. The observed frequency of histologic association was estimated to be 4000 to 13,000 times greater than expected on the basis of surface area by chance alone. They concluded that small congenital nevocytic nevi may be precursors for at least some cases of cutaneous melanoma and ought to be considered for prophylactic excision.

GENERAL CONCLUSIONS

There should no longer be controversy regarding early removal of giant congenital nevocytic nevi. Not only are these lesions serious cosmetic problems, but also the 1 in 16 risk of developing malignancy of a type carrying a high probability of fatal outcome is more than parents would wish to take.

The controversy over removal of small congenital nevi is more difficult to resolve. However, there is increasing evidence that these lesions may be precursors for an appreciable number of melanomas, and since these lesions are more easily excised, there seems to be little justification for not doing so. When faced with the individual patient, questionable economic considerations should not be allowed to influence our decision. I advise removal of all nevocytic nevi that unquestionably have been present since birth. I acknowledge that all of the answers on the small nevi are not in as yet.

Finally, I seriously condemn the practice of treating congenital nevocytic nevi by dermabrasion.

References

1. Walton, R. G., Jacobs, A. H., and Cox, A. J.: Pigmented lesions in newborn infants. Br. J. Dermatol. 95:398, 1976.
2. Alper, J., Holmes, L. B., and Mihm, M. C.: Birthmarks with serious medical significance. J. Pediatr. 95:696, 1979.
3. Rhodes, A. R., Sober, A. J., Day, C. L., Melski, J. W., Harrist, T. J., Mihm, M. C., and Fitzpatrick, T. B.: The malignant potential of small congenital nevocellular nevi. J. Am. Acad. Dermatol. 6:230, 1982.
4. Lorentzen, M., Pers, M., and Bretteville-Jensen, J.: The incidence of malignant transformation in giant pigmented nevi. Scand. J. Plast. Reconstr. Surg. 11:163, 1977.
5. Rhodes, A. R., Wood, W. C., Sober, A. J., and Mihm, M. C.: Non-epidermal origin of malignant melanoma associated with a giant congenital nevocellular nevus. Plast. Reconstr. Surg. 67:782, 1981.
6. Kaplan, E. N.: The risk of malignancy in large congenital nevi. Plast. Reconstr. Surg. 53:421, 1974.
7. Trozak, D. J., Rowland, W. D., and Hu, F.: Metastatic malignant melanoma in prepubertal children. Pediatrics 55:191, 1975.
8. Kaplan, E. N.: Incidence of malignancy in small, large and giant congenital nevi. In Williams, (ed.): Symposium on Melanotic Lesions and Vascular Malformations. St. Louis, C. V. Mosby Co., 1982.
9. Greeley, P. W., Middleton, A. G., and Curtin, J. W.: Incidence of malignancy in giant pigmented nevi. Plast. Reconstr. Surg. 36:26, 1965.
10. Solomon, L. M.: The management of congenital melanocytic nevi. Arch. Dermatol. 116:1017, 1980.
11. Kopf, A. W., Bart, R. S, and Hennessey, P.: Congenital nevocytic nevi and malignant melanomas. J. Am. Acad. Dermatol. 1:123, 1979.
12. Rhodes, A. R., and Melski, J. W.: Small congenital nevocellular nevi and the risk of cutaneous melanoma. J. Pediatr. 100:219, 1982.

NOT ALL CONGENITAL NEVI SHOULD BE REMOVED

Robert G. Walton, M.D.

By definition, the term congenital nevocytic (melanocytic) nevus refers to a cluster of cells derived from the neural crest that are present in the skin at birth and that embryonically, histologically, and biochemically are a type of melanocyte. In contrast, an acquired nevocytic nevus also consists of neural crest cells but occurs at any time after birth. Whether their differing natural histories are important is questionable, since nevus cells may be present at birth microscopically and even macroscopically but do not become clinically noticeable until some period afterward. In any case, the management of all nevocytic nevi, whether congenital or acquired, must be determined on the basis of malignant potential, cosmetic abnormality, and functional and anatomic problems, with the malignant potential being the most important criterion.

Nevocytic nevi, whether congenital or acquired, can be present with different morphologic and histopathologic patterns, and they do not necessarily have the same malignant potential. Unfortunately, the type is not always easily recognized clinically. If it could be proved that congenital nevocytic nevi were of considerable risk in forming malignant melanoma, then it would be reasonable to remove all such nevi, even though this would be a gigantic task. For example, there are 3 million babies born in the United States each year and approximately 1 per cent have congenital nevi,[1] i.e., over 30,000 nevi. In addition, approximately 4 per cent have pigmented lesions clinically compatible with congenital nevi,[1] and therefore this might necessitate an even greater surgical effort in an attempt to remove all congenital nevi.

However, the congenital giant nevus (garment nevus), which involves a major portion of an entire limb or a large paravertebral area, occurs in dermatone distribution and is easily diagnosed clinically and pathologically. Parts, and sometimes all, of this nevus have characteristic histopathologic changes. These consist of features described in detail by Mark and coworkers,[2] including nevus cells deep in the dermis and in association with appendages, vessels, and nerves. In addition, and probably more importantly, there is neurotization in the dermis, and there are many other melanocytic schwannian patterns present, such as blue nevus, lentigo, junctional nevus, and spindle cell and epithelioid cell nevi of Spitz. The cells are embryonic (which is particularly true the earlier the lesions are biopsied), and the melanoma that develops in giant nevi in children is deep and of the embryonic type.[3-5] Therefore, the histopathology is strikingly characteristic. Later in life the cells are more mature and, if melanoma develops (which is much less likely), it is usually at the epidermal/dermal junction, of the classical type, and comparatively less aggressive.

The incidence of melanoma in congenital giant nevi has been variously estimated. There is probably a lifetime risk of 6.3 per cent,[6] but approximately 70 per cent,[4] or even more, occur in giant nevi before puberty. Unfortunately, the exact incidence of giant nevi is unknown, but it is a rare disease and many exist into adulthood without malignant change; therefore, these lesions are not reported. The incidence of melanoma, however, seems significant, and when this disease occurs before puberty, it is uniformly fatal.[7] Therefore, it is necessary that all giant nevi be removed as soon after birth as practical, but for those that are seen for the first time in adulthood without change, the removal may not be required. The management of other types of congenital nevi is a different matter and should not be judged by comparison with the natural history of giant nevi.

Size has been used in an arbitrary manner in defining types of congenital nevi, and these lesions on the average are possibly larger than acquired nevi.[2] It has been postulated that size per se might be important and that the malignant potential may be increased because the melanocytes are dispersed in greater density per unit than in the surrounding skin and in smaller nevi.[8] However, many congenital nevi are under 1 cm in diameter, and some are under 0.5 cm. Also, acquired nevi over 1.5 cm in diameter have been documented. Except that there is a higher risk in cases of giant nevi, there is no adequate proof that larger congenital nevi have a higher incidence of melanoma as compared with the smaller nevi; hence, the lesions do not necessarily have to be removed on the basis of size.

Mark and associates[2] reviewed and compared clinical and histologic features of 60 congenital nevi and 60 acquired nevi. They emphasized that histologically, congenital nevi had three diagnostic features that separated them from acquired nevi. (1) Nevus cells were present in the lower two thirds of the reticular layer of the dermis; (2) nevus cells were interspersed between collagen bundles singly or in "Indian" file; and (3) nevus cells commonly concentrated around appendages, nerves, and vessels, usually in the lower two thirds of the reticular dermis and in the subcutis. Six of the 60 congenital nevi were of the giant type, but irrespective of size, the histologic features were similar. The age distribution of the 60 patients with congenital nevi was from 9 to 69 years. The age of the patient at the time of biopsy apparently did not influence the histologic findings, although it was not known how old the individuals were if they were less than 9 years of age, e.g., were any under 3 months or were any biopsies done at birth? It was found that epidermal changes in both the congenital and the acquired groups were similar and of the usual acquired type. There were 13 per cent that were 10 cm in diameter or greater, including six garment nevi, and there were 15 per cent that were less than 1.5 cm in diameter, but these data do not include how small they were, e.g., were any under 0.5 cm? The remainder were intermediate in size.

The authors concluded that because garment nevi and small congenital nevi have a similar histologic picture, then the smaller congenital nevi may be more susceptible to the same malignant change as the garment nevi and may have a greater potential for malignant degeneration than do acquired nevi. However, the investigators indicated that the giant nevi studies did show some differences from those of the small congenital nevi, including extensive neurotization and the presence of different elements of the full melanocytic schwannian system. Therefore, the question is whether one can always rely on histologic diagnosis (and to what degree the histologic features assigned to congenital nevi are important) or whether the additional histologic findings, such as neurotization and the presence of deep embryonal cells, are responsible for the increase in malignant potential. These latter findings usually are not seen in small congenital nevi.

Silvers and Helwig[9] examined the histologic features of seven congenital nevi within 3 months of birth. Six of these were biopsied within 72 hours. All seven lesions demonstrated a predilection for the nevus cells within the dermis located in proximity to the adnexal structures as described by Mark and associates.[2] The epidermal findings, however, differed in that they found a heterogeneous pattern of epidermal melanocytic hyperplasia unlike the usual junctional activity found in acquired nevi, and the melanocytic hyperplasia that they found simulated the atypical melanocytic hyperplasia seen in superficial spreading melanoma.

Walton and coworkers[10] have noted these latter findings, but the authors are not convinced that the so-called congenital features in themselves are important regarding malignant potential. Although these changes may be common in congenital nevi, they are not necessarily diagnostic. There were also contradictory findings. In a series of nevi documented at birth with biopsies taken at various ages, many did not show these signs and could not be differentiated from acquired nevi. Conversely, there was a series of acquired nevi that could be classified as congenital nevi because they had some of the histopathologic features that have been assigned to congenital nevi.

In addition, Kirschenbaum[11] stated that he had done numerous biopsies of lesions in the 1- to 3-cm range and none had the typical features described for congenital nevi. Kopf and colleagues [12,13] reported that the histologic features of congenital nevi cannot be found in the majority of melanomas in which nevus cells are present and that many congenital nevi are probably not identifiable histologically as being congenital. From a review of the literature, they concluded that there are no cogent data substantiating the existence of small congenital nevi that present a significant risk of giving rise to malignant melanoma. The authors also reported that at New York University in 25 years there were only two melanomas thought clinically to have arisen in congenital nevi 1.5 to 19.9 cm in diameter. They consider that there is insufficient evidence to justify the removal of all congenital nevi. Also, Alpers and associates [14] have stated that there is no documented evidence from either retrospective or prospective studies that small congenital nevocytic nevi are premalignant lesions.

In another report, Walton, Jacobs, and Cox [1] examined 1058 newborn infants and found that 41 (3.9 per cent) had clinically discernible pigmented lesions compatible with melanocytic nevi. Biopsies were performed on 34 of the 41, and 11 (representing 1 per cent of the infants) proved to have nevocytic nevi. No giant nevi were seen in this series. Only 2 of the 11 nevi pathologically examined showed some of the histologic changes similar to those reported by Mark and coworkers.[2] These two nevi represented a diffuse permeation of the dermal connective tissue as far as the lower reticular dermis by nevus cells. However, specific involvement of the deeper appendages, nerves, or vessels was not identified, with the exception of one of the lesions, in which there was a focus of nevus cells adjacent to the sweat glands. The remainder were histologically compatible with acquired nevi. Also, 7 of the 11 nevi were under 1.5 cm in diameter.

In excellent statistical and histopathologic studies, Rhodes and his colleagues [15,16] have estimated the relative risk of melanomas associated with small congenital nevi. They compared the frequency of histologically documented nevocellular nevi in newborn infants with a frequency of congenital nevi at the tumor site ascertained by history in 234 patients and the tumor-associated nevi with histologic features commonly connected with congenital nevi in 234 unselected melanoma specimens. A 21-fold increase in melanoma risk was estimated for persons with small congenital nevi when ascertained by history and a three- to tenfold increase in risk when ascertained by histology. Therefore, according to these studies, persons with small congenital nevi who live to the age of 60 are estimated to have a cumulative risk of melanoma of 4.9 per 100 when ascertained by history and 0.8 to 2.6 per 100 when designated by histology. These figures are therefore higher when compared with the risk of developing melanoma in the general American population, which is 0.4 per cent in individuals living to 80 years.

Whether the risk is 0.8 or 2.6 per 100 when the nevi are diagnosed histologically depends on the rigidity of the criteria for diagnosis. For example, in 27.4 per cent (64 of 234) of melanoma specimens, a dermal nevocellular nevus was found in contiguity with the melanoma. Of the 64 nevus cases, 19 (8.1 per cent of 234) had tumor-associated nevocellular nevi with one or more histologic features usually attributed to congenital nevi. Therefore, 45 (19.2 per cent of 234) appeared identical to acquired nevocellular nevi. If more strict criteria were used in assigning congenital features (such as nevus cells extending into the midreticular dermis or deeper in addition to nevus cells in one or more appendages or neurovascular structures), then this would reduce the number of congenital nevi as opposed to acquired nevi and therefore would lower the risk factor of the former. The accurate historical diagnosis of congenital nevi beyond the newborn period becomes increasingly difficult because of the increased number of acquired nevi that become noticeable during childhood, and unless there is a direct parental or medical documentation, memories lapse. Also, there is an unexplained tendency for persons with melanomas to incriminate a previous pigmented lesion. The inaccuracies of historical diagnosis of congenital nevi and the differences in histopathologic criteria certainly would account for acknowledged differences in the aforementioned figures. Even though the authors conclude that according to the findings, small congenital nevi may be precursors for at least some of the cases of cutaneous melanoma, they are careful to state that the estimated risks are highly dependent on the specificity of the methods used for detecting congenital nevi in melanoma, i.e., historical and histologic diagnoses.

In summary, arguments can be made against the removal of all small and intermediate congenital nevi. The natural history of small and intermediate nevi cannot be compared directly with that of giant nevi, because the histopathologic picture associated with melanoma that develops in giant nevi (particularly prior to puberty, when the majority of malignancies occur) consists of a variety of striking features, including neurotization and the presence of deep embryonal type of cells. These changes, which are probably significant regarding malignant potential, usually are not seen in small and intermediate congenital nevi. It is true that many congenital nevi of all sizes have histopathologic changes consisting of nevus cells deep in the reticular dermis and in the periadnexal locations, but these changes also are seen in some acquired nevi, and there is no evidence that these changes in themselves are precursors of malignant melanoma. Also, some congenital nevi do not show these changes.

It seems unreasonable to attach a great deal of significance to whether the nevus actually was present at birth or whether it became noticeable 1 week, 1 month, or even 1 year later. It is not clear how important the historical diagnosis might be. For example, a very small nevus may have been present at birth and may not have been noticed; it therefore may be assumed to be acquired. Also, nevus cells might be present microscopically at birth and might later present macroscopically. Historical evidence of the presence of nevi at birth becomes more inaccurate as the person becomes older. If the historical diagnosis is important, then there is a danger in accepting that the lesion was present at birth on the basis of anamnesis. A nevus can be classified as congenital only if it was noticed within the first 24 to 72 hours of life. There has to be direct confirmation from a parent (preferably the mother) or documentation in the hospital record. It is quite possible that those melanomas that do show nevi in contiguity and have some of the features assigned to congenital nevi in reality may not have been present at birth. Furthermore, the predisposition of malignant degeneration in nevocytic nevi, whether congenital or acquired, is possibly more likely to be related to the epidermal melanocytic dysplasia, as seen in the dysplastic nevus syndrome.[17] In those rare instances in which a small congenital nevus does become malignant, it is not the embryonal type, as seen in association with giant nevi, but a superficial spreading melanoma, such as might be seen in association with small acquired nevi.

In conclusion, in our present state of knowledge, there is sufficient evidence to support the early removal of giant nevi because of the relatively high incidence of melanoma and leptomeningeal involvement. However, there are insufficient data to advise the wholesale removal of 30,000 small and intermediate congenital nevi annually. Historical and histologic evidence of whether a nevus is congenital or acquired may be confusing. It is probable that small congenital nevi behave no differently from acquired nevi. Therefore, they should be removed, as all nevi should be if they exhibit any progressive change or show an atypical appearance. It is hoped that in the near future some simpler method, either clinical, histopathologic, or biochemical, can be used to differentiate those nevi that present a risk.

References

1. Walton, R. G., Jacobs, A. H., and Cox, A. J.: Pigmented lesions in newborn infants. Br. J. Dermatol. 95:389, 1976.

2. Mark, G. J., Mihm, M. C., Litepli, M. G., Reed, R. J., and Clark, W. H.: Congenital melanocytic nevi of the small and garment type. Hum. Pathol. 4:395, 1973.
3. Reed, W. B., Becker, S. W., Sr., Becker, S. W., Jr., and Nichel, W. R.: Giant pigmented nevi, melanoma and leptomeningeal melanocytosis. Arch. Dermatol. 91:100, 1965.
4. Kaplan, E. N.: The risk of malignancy in large congenital nevi. Plast. Reconstr. Surg. 53:421, 1974.
5. Kaplan, E. N.: Incidence of malignancy in small, large and giant congenital nevi. *In* Williams, H. B. (ed.): Symposium on Melanotic Lesions and Vascular Malformations. St. Louis, C. V. Mosby Co., 1982.
6. Rhodes, S. R., Wood, W. C., Sober, A. J., and Mihm, M. C.: Non-epidermal origin of malignant melanoma associated with a giant congenital nevocellular nevus. Plas. Reconstr. Surg. 67:782, 1981.
7. Trozak, D. J., Roland, W. D., and Funan, H.: Metastatic malignant melanoma in prepubertal children. Pediatrics 55:205, 1975.
8. Lund, H. A., and Kraus, J. M.: Melanocytic tumors of the skin. *In* Atlas of Tumor Pathology, Fascicle 3. Washington, D.C., Armed Forces Institute of Pathology, 1962, p. 1.
9. Silvers, D. S., and Helwig, E. B.: Melanocytic nevi in neonates. J. Am. Acad. Dermatol. 4:166, 1981.
10. Walton, R. G., Wood, C., and Smith, L.: Histopathological differences in congenital nevi. (To be published.)
11. Kirschenbaum, M. B.: Congenital melanocytic nevi. Arch. Dermatol. 117:379, 1981.
12. Kopf, A. W., and Bart, R. S.: Malignant melanoma: A review. J. Dermatol. Surg. Oncol. 3:1, 70, 1977.
13. Kopf, A. W., Bart, R. S., and Hennessey, P.: Congenital nevocytic nevi and malignant melanomas. J. Am. Acad. Dermatol. 1:123, 1979.
14. Alpers, J., Holmes, L. B., and Mihm, M. C.: Birth marks with serious medical significance: Nevocellular nevi, sebaceous nevi and multiple cafe au lait spots. J. Pediatr. 95:696, 1979.
15. Rhodes, A. R., Sober, A. J., Day, C. L., Melski, J. W., Harrist, T. J., Mihm, M. C., and Fitzpatrick, T. B.: The malignant potential of small congenital nevocellular nevi. J. Am. Acad. Dermatol. 6:230, 1982.
16. Rhodes, A. R., and Melski, J. W.: Small congenital nevocellular nevi and the risk of cutaneous melanoma. J. Pediatr. 100:219, 1982.
17. Reed, R. J., Clark W. H., and Mihm, M. C.: Premalignant melanocytic dysplasias. *In* Ackerman, A. B. (ed.): Pathology of Malignant Melanoma, New York, Masson Publishing USA Inc., 1981, p. 173.

Editorial Comment

Whether you agree with Dr. Jacobs or Dr. Walton depends on your philosophy: Is it preferable to remove all possibly precancerous lesions as soon as possible, or should one wait for signs of change that might herald malignant degeneration? Should every lesion of actinic keratosis, leukoplakia, chronic radiodermatitis, and so forth be eradicated on sight? This is a major controversy in medicine today. One potential contributor to this section refused an invitation to participate, saying, "I do not believe that there is any controversy about this matter!" But to examine the facts . . . if the number of physicians performing surgery is considered, it would be impossible to remove all of the melanocytic nevi encountered in newborns. Also, would it be worthwhile? There is no solid evidence that nevi developing at a later date cannot progress into melanomas. The importance of size has not been proved; that is, it may be true that larger lesions are more apt to undergo such unfortunate changes, but the evidence for this is not well established, except in the case of the "bathing suit nevus." Here, too, some authorities (Mihm, for instance) decry the gung-ho removal of these lesions because of the frequency of recurrences.

As Walton mentions, it is possible that nevi developing after delivery arise in clinically unapparent nevi that are present at birth. This might be true even for lesions that make their appearance much later, such as in adolescence or during pregnancy. The latter nevi might be just as premalignant as those already visible at gestation. Furthermore, many melanomas arise de novo, not in areas of nevus formation. Therefore, early removal of moles may minimize the problem of melanoma but will not eliminate it. One should not forget that in removing all nevi at birth, we are subjecting the infant to a certain amount of trauma. Furthermore, scarring will result if the lesions are excised. Shaving can be used only for raised lesions, and most nevi are flat at the time of birth. Whereas properly performed shaving will avoid or reduce scarring, in small children this maneuver is followed frequently by recurrences. Although there is still room for honest differences of opinion, my offspring would not have his moles excised at birth.

Think It Over.

CHAPTER **3**

CLINICAL DIAGNOSIS

THE CLINICAL DIAGNOSIS OF MELANOMA IS DIFFICULT AND UNRELIABLE

Ervin Epstein, M.D.

The field of dermatology has many gray zones. Despite theoretic discussions of diagnostic signs and symptoms, many cases defy accurate classification without laboratory tests. Melanoma is among the most difficult to diagnose clinically. Until it was recognized that lesions suspected of being melanomas could be subjected to histopathologic examination after incisional or excisional biopsy, the practitioner was forced either to remove a frozen section of a suspected lesion and then to perform radical surgery if the specimen revealed changes suggestive of malignancy or to perform the mutilating surgery in the first place. We were warned (and there are many who still preach this gospel) that conservative removal of a melanoma would result quickly in dissemination of the tumor with seeding of faraway locations and the rapid demise of the patient. Today, we can perform biopsies on melanomas without fear of damaging the individual, provided that we initiate definitive surgical treatment within 1 week if the lesion proves to be melanomatous.

Black may or may not be beautiful. However, it is certainly not a pathognomonic sign of malignancy. We have all heard many physicians, including plastic surgeons, state that every black lesion must be considered to be a melanoma until proved otherwise. Although this is an anachronism, it still lives in the cerebrum of many practitioners. In a study of 559 patients with black cutaneous lesions, only 2 per cent of the tumors proved to be melanomas. Therefore, the fact that a lesion is black hardly dictates the need for mutilating and morbidity-producing surgical procedures. The remaining 98 per cent of the black lesions studied were benign, except for approximately 12 per cent, which were superficial basal cell epitheliomas. These tumors represent a malignancy indeed, but not one to be compared with the destructiveness of a melanoma. Despite the prognostic importance that some may attach to the color, it must be remembered that the odds are 50 to 1 that a given black lesion is not a melanoma. But we must not forget that statistics do not apply to individuals.

How accurate is the clinical diagnosis of melanoma in actual practice? Reviewing my own records, I found that in all of the cases in which I entered melanoma as a diagnostic possibility or did not consider that possibility in lesions later proved to be melanomas, I was correct only 38 per cent of the time. Comparable studies by other dermatologists have resulted in similar findings. I collected a series of Kodachrome slides of black lesions and tested various groups of physicians, including dermatologists, using this collection. The percentage of correct diagnoses in these tests varied from 10 per cent to 40 per cent, hardly a figure that could be a credit to a professional.

The prognosis in melanoma is excellent if the diagnosis can be made *before metas-*

tases develop. Therefore, early diagnosis is essential—the earlier the better. Although the factors mentioned by Wheeland and Everett in the following article are presumptive, the presence of these features also can be found in benign lesions. Furthermore, malignant melanoma occurs commonly in the absence of these clues. Therefore, we must appreciate the necessity of histopathologic confirmation in the diagnosis of melanoma. Since it has been established that it is safe to perform a biopsy and that definitive surgery is not necessary before an accurate diagnosis has been obtained, there is no reason to trust clinical features in identifying this neoplasm. *It must be stressed that the diagnosis of melanoma is a microscopic one,* and one should not presume to have "made" this diagnosis without such evidence. It must be emphasized also that a biopsy of a melanoma is a safe procedure.

There are two unusual tumors that may be confused with melanomas and that should be mentioned in this discussion. First is the capillary aneurysm. This is a small, flat, intensely black lesion that grows rapidly and probably disappears spontaneously after a few months. It has no clinical resemblance to an angioma or a varix, having no purplish or bluish hue. It does not attain a great size. On biopsy, a single dilated subepidermal capillary is noted. A thrombus may be present in the vessel. There are no tortuous vessels, such as one sees in a banal varix. Serial section reveals a fusiform swelling of the involved capillary.

Another uncommon tumor is the cellular blue nevus. This neoplasm grows slowly but may reach a massive size. The tissue is dark shiny black. At surgery it nearly always is diagnosed as a melanoma because of its deep black color, which extends to the depth of the neoplasm. Histologically, it does not resemble a melanoma. As a rule, the tumors are found in the midline of the lower back and the buttocks, especially in young women, but may be found in other locations as well. Since the growth is slow, such lesions are usually of years' duration. They too are benign.

Realizing that the printed and spoken word is subject to misinterpretation, I must make it clear that this is not a treatise arguing or warning against the attempt to diagnose melanomas clinically. Of course, you should make every effort to accomplish this, and all best wishes for success go with you. However, you must realize that you are doing no more than educated guessing. The key to success is early suspicion that a given lesion is a melanoma, but this is not synonymous with establishing a diagnosis. The lesson is: Suspect a melanoma whenever this is reasonable, but prove it histologically before instituting therapy that you hope to be curative. This will minimize mutilation and morbidity while offering the patient the maximum possibility of a cure and a long life as well as minimal scarring.

THE CLINICAL DIAGNOSIS OF MALIGNANT MELANOMA

Ronald G. Wheeland, M.D.
Mark Allen Everett, M.D.

The early diagnosis of malignant melanoma remains the single most important factor in determining the prognosis for many patients. This fact has been stressed repeatedly in both lay [1,2] and professional publications. [3-6] Today, most physicians, regardless of their specialty, and many well-informed patients are aware of the common danger signals for the development of malignant melanoma. Since approximately 75 per cent of patients with melanoma recall a pre-existing nevus or other pigmented lesion at the site of later development of melanoma, much emphasis has been placed upon changes occurring in nevocellular nevi that might be suggestive of malignant degeneration.

One such warning signal is color change or variegation of color in a pre-existing pigmented lesion. Specific colors that are worrisome are shades of blue, red, or white that develop in a previously brown or black pigmented lesion. Blue colors often are a sign of poor prognosis, and white areas may represent areas of regression. [7] Leaching of pigment into normal skin at the edge of a pre-existing pigmented lesion is also a troublesome finding. Another warning signal is change in shape. This is true especially if the perimeter is irregular with notches or indentations; it even may have a serpiginous shape. A change in the size of a nevus, especially if rapid, is also a sign for concern. The development of symptoms such as itching, burning, or tenderness within a pre-existing nevus or other pigmented lesion is also disturbing. Lastly, any change in the surface texture of a nevus with areas of irregular elevation or deeper palpable nodules found within the nevus itself or the skin surrounding it is an additional warning signal.

Although none of these changes is diagnostic of malignant melanoma, each change should arouse sufficient suspicion in the patient or the examining physician to warrant careful early examination and excisional biopsy wherever possible, so that an absolute diagnosis can be made. It has been established that in over 90 per cent of clinical lesions an accurate diagnosis of primary malignant melanoma now can be made by patients, nurses, and physicians using these criteria. [7]

There are several groups of patients who are at high risk for the possible development of malignant melanoma. Because of the greater risk, these individuals should be examined more frequently and more carefully than the general population. One high-risk group is those patients who have a positive family history of malignant melanoma. This group accounts for over 12 per cent of all melanomas diagnosed annually. A second high-risk group is those patients with a past history of intense excess ultraviolet light exposure either occupationally or recreationally. A third high-risk group has been described. These individuals have a condition that is known as the dysplastic nevus syndrome. [8,9]

The dysplastic nevus syndrome, also known as the B-K mole syndrome, has been found to occur in both a familial and a sporadic form. The familial form seems to be inherited as an autosomal dominant trait having incomplete penetrance, and the lesions appear much earlier in life with this type than with the sporadic form. Both groups of patients have clinically indistinguishable nevi. These nevi are usually macular. They are larger than most acquired nevi and are often greater than 7 mm in diameter. These nevi commonly have an irregular outline and are also typically irregularly pigmented. The irregular surface may be somewhat scaly, and perilesional erythema may be present. Often, these nevi are found in doubly covered areas and may not appear until later in life, commonly when the patient is over the age of 30. Additionally, these nevi often show considerable variation in appearance, and many are pruritic. The risk of developing melanoma is 100-fold greater in these patients than in the normal population.

A fourth group also might be considered to be at greater risk for developing malignant melanoma. This group includes all patients with an unusually large number of nevi—greater than the average of 30. In order to measure this risk accurately, however, one must remember that the incidence of melanoma has been estimated to be only from 1 in 40,000 to 1 in 200,000 nevi per year. Thus, the relative incidence of malignant melanoma formation within a pre-existing nevus is quite low.

For all patients, but especially for those in the high-risk groups, some additional information may prove beneficial. First, it seems appropriate that all unnecessary sunlight exposure be avoided. When this is unavoidable, use of a sunscreen with a sun protection factor of 12 or greater should be recommended. Also, more careful examination by patients and their physicians should be advised at times of greater melanocytic activity, especially at puberty and during pregnancy or when increased activity is manifested by an increase in the size or number of nevi or a change in color. Males in one of the high-risk groups should know that primary melanoma is more common on the head and the neck, and females should be informed that the lower extremities are affected more commonly. It also has been shown that certain anatomic areas seem to have a poorer prognosis when melanoma does develop. These areas include the upper back, the posterior lateral arm, the posterior lateral neck, and the posterior scalp—the so-called BANS locations.[10-12] Perhaps this information could be used by the patient to aid in the earlier diagnosis of malignant melanoma.

Despite the positive impact of patient and physician education on the early diagnosis of malignant melanoma, a high index of suspicion must be maintained to insure continued early detection. This is especially important when one realizes that the incidence of melanoma has increased sixfold over the last four decades and that melanoma represents 2 per cent of all malignancies and accounts for over 4000 deaths annually in the United States alone.[7] However, whenever a high degree of suspicion exists for a potentially fatal malignant disease such as melanoma, mistakes inevitably will occur. We have had the opportunity to review a total of 13,231 consecutive surgical pathology data slips to determine the accuracy of the clinical diagnosis of malignant melanoma. Two basic types of errors existed: melanoma that was not diagnosed in cases in which it later was proved to have existed and benign lesions that were mistaken for melanoma. The second type of error was far more common, and although it is less important than the first type, it nonetheless is still an important problem, since needless and perhaps disfiguring surgery might be performed in the overzealous removal of a benign lesion. It almost certainly would result in excessive and unnecessary anxiety of the patient while awaiting verification of the pathology. The first type of error obviously could result in a delay in the diagnosis of a true malignancy and possibly could cause increased morbidity and mortality.

In our study, we found that the most common error made, as could be expected, involved nevocellular nevi that were incorrectly diagnosed clinically as malignant melanomas. This type of error accounted for over 40 per cent of the incorrect diagnoses. Other benign pigmented lesions that were incorrectly diagnosed included dermatofibromas, lentigo benigna, and seborrheic keratoses. These benign pigmented lesions accounted for an additional one third of the incorrect clinical diagnoses. Since dermatofibromas are usually evenly pigmented and can be palpated as firm dermal nodules, it seems that the previously discussed criteria for determining the need for biopsy were not used in these cases. Lentigo benigna is usually round without notching or indentations and typically is an evenly pigmented brown or black color with a smooth or regular surface. So, once again, it appears that the types of changes in pigmented lesions that suggest the need for biopsy were not correctly identified when these lesions were incorrectly biopsied. Seborrheic keratoses usually have a greasy or verrucous surface and, typically, a "stuck-on" appearance. Although there is great variation in color of seborrheic keratoses from one lesion to another, usually there is no variegation in color within a solitary lesion. Variegation in color within a pigmented lesion is an important clue to the possible development of malignant melanoma, and perhaps more careful clinical examination would have yielded a greater degree of accuracy in the diagnosis of these types of lesions and would have prevented the unnecessary removal of these benign lesions.

Vascular lesions accounted for 15 per cent of the incorrect clinical diagnoses of malignant melanoma. The lesions that were erroneously suspected of being melanomas included pyogenic granulomas, venous lakes, cirsoid aneurysms, capillary hemangiomas, and thrombosed blood vessels. This whole category of inaccurate diagnoses cannot really be criticized, since melanomas may indeed be nonpigmented and highly vascular and thus may resemble any of the aforementioned vascular lesions. This is especially true of nodular melanoma, in which the surface may appear smooth or may be eroded and is strikingly similar to the typical clinical presentation of pyogenic granuloma. Venous lakes usually can be distinguished as vascular lesions by compression as well as by their appearance typically on sun-exposed areas, especially the vermilion border of the lip. The variegation of color seen in thrombosed blood vessels and capillary hemangiomas probably accounts for the inaccurate diagnosis and biopsy of these benign lesions.

A variety of other lesions were included in the list of incorrectly diagnosed malignant melanoma. This group accounted for the remaining 10 per cent of the clinical errors in diagnosis. These lesions included basal cell carcinoma, squamous cell carcinoma, acanthosis nigricans, lichen simplex chronicus, and epidermoid cysts. Typically, basal cell carcinoma is translucent or opalescent in appearance and has telangiectasia on the surface or on the skin adjacent to the lesion. Basal cell carcinoma may be pigmented, however, and may contain stipples of brown pigment within the opalescent nodule. This type of color is not that usually seen in malignant melanoma, in which red, blue, black, and white coloring may exist in any combination. Squamous cell carcinoma may have an eroded surface and may be confused with an amelanotic melanoma, but usually these lesions do not have pigment and typically are found in sun-exposed areas. This may be of some help in the differentiation between squamous cell carcinoma and malignant melanoma. Acanthosis nigricans and lichen simplex chronicus usually have a velvety or a lichenified surface, and again pigmentation, when present, is usually uniform and is not irregular. Even though patients will complain of pruritus in these cases, the quality of symptoms and the clinical appearance of the lesions generally should not make it difficult to differentiate these tumors from suspicious nevi. Epidermoid cysts generally are found below the skin surface and may have an overlying punctum. Pigmentation is not a usual feature of these lesions. Again, differentiation of these cysts from a more aggressive process should not be difficult in most cases.

When these data are examined closely, one can see that dermatologists were responsible for the clinical diagnosis of 65 per cent of these lesions as malignant melanomas. However, this same group of physicians was responsible for the correct diagnoses of 80 per cent of the melanomas that were verified pathologically. The remainder of lesions that were clinically suspected of being melanomas were identified by family practitioners, surgical subspecialists, and internal medicine specialists. This group of physicians diagnosed the remaining 20 per cent of the pathologically verified malignant melanomas identified at our institution. The percentage of correct diagnoses made by dermatologists was 45 per cent, compared with only 18 per cent of the correct clinical diagnoses that were made by nondermatologists. These data support the fact that although all groups of physicians had an apparently high index of suspicion that is necessary for making an early diagnosis of malignant melanoma, dermatologists were correct in their clinical diagnosis more than twice as often as were nondermatologists. This may mean that dermatologists have a truly higher index of suspicion; however, dermatologists still were incorrect more than half of the time.

One key to the early diagnosis of malignant melanoma is frequent and careful examination of all skin and mucosal surfaces for possible changes in pre-existing pigmented lesions, especially in patients with a positive family history of melanoma, patients who are chronically exposed to the sun, or patients who have the dysplastic nevus syndrome. Early (preferably excisional) biopsy of suspicious lesions remains important. However, because of the relatively low incidence of malignant melanoma in nevi, we are of the opinion that wholesale removal of nevi is not warranted. Moreover, disfiguring surgery should not be performed as a result of the initial biopsy of a suspicious lesion. When a pre-existing pigmented lesion develops symptoms, shows color change or variegation in color, changes its shape, develops an irregularly notched border, or shows rapid growth or an irregular surface with nodularity, biopsy definitely is indicated. The accuracy of the clinical diagnosis of malignant melanoma by nondermatologic specialists suggests that further training is necessary in this important area to aid in the better recognition of benign cutaneous lesions. If physicians follow these criteria, we feel that more accurate, and even earlier, diagnoses of malignant melanoma can be obtained. It is hoped that this will lead to the prevention of established melanoma and will help control the mortality of this dreaded disease.

It should be noted that in our study only three lesions that were pathologically identified as malignant melanomas were not accurately diagnosed clinically. Fortunately, all three lesions were thin melanomas (less than 0.75 mm), and consequently they have an extremely good prognosis in spite of the inaccurate clinical diagnosis and initial treatment. It does not appear from these data that increased morbidity or mortality resulted, although this conclusion may be premature. However, the potential for harm remains unchanged, as does the need for a high level of suspicion to lessen this potential.

References

1. Clark, M., and Witherspoon, D.: Suntans and skin cancer. Newsweek 159:85, 1982.
2. How to survive a season in the sun. Consumer Reports 45:350, 1980.
3. Mihm, M. C., Fitzpatrick, T. B., Lane Brown, M. M., Raker, J. W., Malt, R. A., and Kaiser, J. S.: Early detection of primary cutaneous malignant melanoma. N. Engl. J. Med. 289:989, 1973.
4. Kopf, A. W., Bart, R. S., and Rodriguez-Sains, R. S.: Malignant melanoma: A review. J. Dermatol. Surg. Oncol. 3:41, 1977.
5. Breslow, A.: Tumor thickness, level of invasion and node dissection in stage I cutaneous melanoma. Ann. Surg. 182:572, 1975.
6. Day, C. L., Lew, R. A., Mihm, M. C., Harris, M. N., et al.: The natural breakpoints for primary tumor thickness in clinical stage I melanoma. N. Engl. J. Med. 305:1155, 1981.
7. Sober, A. J., Fitzpatrick, T. B., and Mihm, M. C.: Primary melanoma of the skin: Recognition and management. J. Am. Acad. Dermatol. 2:179, 1980.
8. Clark, W. H., Reimer, R. R., Greene, M., et al.: Origin of familial malignant melanomas from heritable melanocytic lesions (the B-K mole syndrome). Arch. Dermatol. 114:732, 1978.
9. Reimer, R. R., Clark, W. H., Jr., Greene, M. H., et al.: Precursor lesions in familial melanoma. A new genetic preneoplastic syndrome. JAMA 239:744, 1978.
10. Day, C. L.: Prognostic factors for melanoma patients with lesions 0.76 to 1.69 mm in thickness: An appraisal of thin level IV lesions. Ann. Surg. 195:30, 1982.
11. Day, C. L.: Prognostic factors for clinical stage I melanoma of intermediate thickness (1.51–3.99 mm): A conceptual model for tumor growth and metastases. Ann. Surg. 195:35, 1982.
12. Day, C. L.: A multivariate analysis of prognostic factors for melanoma patients with lesions greater than 3.65 mm in thickness: The importance of revealing alternate Cox models. Ann. Surg. 195:44, 1982.

CHAPTER 4

BIOPSY OF MELANOMAS

ROLE OF THE BIOPSY IN MANAGEMENT OF CUTANEOUS MALIGNANT MELANOMA

William L. Epstein, M.D.

A great deal has been written about the importance and value of performing biopsies of skin tumors that are suspected of being malignant melanomas. The experience at New York University,[1] where melanoma experts made correct clinical diagnoses in fewer than two thirds of cases, has occurred at other major melanoma centers as well and eloquently speaks for the need of a proper biopsy and accurate interpretation before extensive surgery is undertaken. The story of General Eisenhower's treatment before D-day, which has been widely circulated among dermatologists, is a prime example of improper surgery for a black seborrheic keratosis.

But the central questions concern what constitutes a *proper* biopsy and how one insures an accurate interpretation. Cancer surgeons have become accustomed to relying on the use of frozen sections at the time of initial resection. However, it is generally agreed[2,3] that when one deals with suspected melanomas, this technique can give misleading results and actually there is little need or justification for using it. The advice about biopsy from the Comprehensive Melanoma Clinic group at the University of California, San Francisco[2] and elsewhere[4] is to excise the tumor completely whenever possible, to fix the specimen in formalin or other suitable fixation medium immediately, and to have it processed for light microscopy by a recognized and reliable histopathology laboratory. For complete and accurate interpretation, the block or blocks should have multiple-step sections.

Furthermore, to insure the accuracy of interpretation, we dermatologists should call upon our dermatopathologist colleagues, who have had extensive experience with the vagaries of malignant melanoma. This level of expertise is neither required nor practical for the majority of melanomas encountered by the practicing clinician, but of the problem cases sent to our consulting group, many of the difficulties center on faulty interpretation of the biopsy specimen. Dermatologists by and large should rely upon competent dermatopathologists for interpretation of their biopsies. However, depending upon the region, at least half of the melanomas are removed by primary-care physicians or by surgeons, who by nature send the tissue to general pathology laboratories for processing and a report. Although pathologists are trained and competent at diagnosing tumors, many have had little experience with the histologic complexities and unusual presentations of cutaneous malignant melanoma and virtually none with odd, benign pigmented lesions. When this is combined with the limited clinical skills of most primary-care physicians, we have a dangerous situation in which physician neglect can add to the mortality figures. To remedy this, dermatologists in smaller and undeserved areas must take on the responsibility of providing clinical and histopathologic education for the community physicians, offer on-the-spot consultations, serve on tumor boards, and encourage pathologists to obtain second opinions from experts when faced with unusual or uncertain histopatologic patterns. In this respect, the strength of any medical community rests with the ability of all its members to work unselfishly together to insure a proper level of care for the entire community.

Malignant melanoma of the skin is one disease seen by dermatologists that has a real potential to be fatal. This is an area in which dermatologists can play a meaningful community leadership role. Emerging evidence[5-7] indicates that melanoma, although unquestionably malignant, may be curable in many cases if diagnosed properly and treated early. But it also should be remembered that approximately 5 per cent of the melanoma cases reported in large series fall in the category of "unknown primary with metastases,"[8] and of these half are caused by physician error either clinically or histopathologically. In other words, approximately 2.5 per cent of the 25,000 to 50,000 melanoma cases reported were associated with a failure of the medical system. From the standpoints of ethical and preventive medicine, that is too much slippage.

Another problem seen by melanoma consultants is the patient whose melanoma was first removed by shave biopsy. This procedure is done primarily by dermatologists, and because it is superficial, the cut goes through the tumor. This prevents measurement of depth of invasion or classification of level, which are guides to prognosis and therapy. The result generally is a "wait-and-see" attitude rather than more aggressive approaches, which might be advocated for high-risk primary lesions. Pathologists feel that shave biopsies are counterproductive.[2] However, we have received such specimens from highly respected clinical dermatologists who would never shave a suspected melanoma, underscoring the fact that some melanomas cannot be recognized clinically, even by experts.[1] Plastic surgeons have responded to this dilemma by routinely using a "deep shave" intended to get below all but the thickest lesions, but this compromises the cosmetic result—the reason the method was first devised was to deal with the myriad of benign nevi seen in clinical practice. One suggestion to help balance the risk/benefit ratio would be not to perform a shave biopsy on any patient in the high-risk category. These individuals include the blond, blue-eyed Celts of English, Irish, Scottish, and European descent who have fair skin that burns and that does not tan. This advice is especially relevant in sun-drenched areas in the lower latitudes. In addition, these patients often have "funny moles," which they are likely to ask to have removed. These "at-risk" individuals make up almost half the patients seen in the Comprehensive Melanoma Clinic at the University of California, San Francisco.[9]

The next issue is: How inviolate is the dictum of full surgical excision of all suspect lesions? Even the pathologists agree that "certain lesions, either because of their size or location, may require some form of partial biopsy before definitive therapy."[2] Thus, very large, neglected lesions that obviously are deeply invasive with or without clinical evidence of spread require only an incisional biopsy to assure the diagnosis before definitive surgery or other treatment is undertaken. Another example is the large, deeply or irregularly pigmented lentigo maligna (Hutchinson's freckle), which frequently occurs on exposed areas, such as the head and the neck. Usually these lesions are benign and may even regress spontaneously, so that extensive and mutilating surgery cannot be condoned. However, the tumors also have a significant potential to develop into a lentigo maligna melanoma. Conservative punch biopsies of suspicious, changing areas remain the preferred approach until malignant degeneration is unequivocally proved. Other large, pigmented tumors on exposed areas or in sites where extensive surgery is hazardous also deserve an incisional biopsy first to establish the correct diagnosis before determinative treatment is chosen. A large intradermal nevus or seborrheic keratosis in the external ear or on the lobe would be an embarrassment to the physician who totally excised it with excess tissue.

Therapeutic decisions require clinical judgment and skill. The basic rule remains that all suspicious lesions should be totally *excised* if at all possible. Dermatologic surgery techniques have greatly advanced in the past few years, so that if one does not possess the requisite surgical skills to remove a nodule fully from a difficult site, one can render the best care by referring the patient to a plastic or dermatologic surgeon for a definitive excisional biopsy.

What is the effect of an incisional biopsy? As was noted earlier, a partial biopsy frequently obscures the tumor architecture, making prognostic and therapeutic projections difficult or impossible. However, a small, clean, 3- to 4-mm punch biopsy usually does not alter the overall pathologic appearance of a large malignant melanoma, although by its nature it is proinflammatory. A more important consideration is the effect of partial biopsy on the ultimate prognosis for survival of the patient. It is now well recognized that every manipulation of a tumor, including biopsy, leads to a dislodgement of cells that enter the circulation, appear in the urine, and can be isolated in other tissues. Incisional biopsies most certainly do this, raising the possibility of enhancing metastases and reducing the outlook for life. However, three clinical and epidemiologic studies failed to support this contention. Epstein and associates[10] found no evidence that incisional biopsy, when followed by a complete surgical removal, altered the final outcome. Similarly, Jones and coworkers[11] showed that the 5-year survival was approximately the same for their patients who had incisional biopsies as for those who had excisional biopsies. Knutson's[12] extensive study, using actuarial life-table analysis, also showed no difference in the outcome of patients whose diagnosis of malignant melanoma was established by partial biopsy and that of individuals who had undergone complete removal, as long as the lesions were all adequately treated surgically.

Nevertheless, the fear of incisions lingers. In 1980, Rampen and colleagues[13] analyzed their data, which seemed to show that incisional biopsies in fact altered the prognosis for the worse. However, their study suffered from being retrospective, with very few patients in the incisional group. Also, there was no clinical input to explain why incisions were made at all. These reasons easily may have influenced the results. Rampen[14] recorded some previously unpublished studies in which B16 melanoma was injected into the footpads of 28 mice. Some animals were subjected to biopsies, and others had amputations. The findings showed that mice receiving the incision alone failed significantly to survive for as long as the group receiving amputations. However, this study does not deal with the earlier clinical proviso, namely, that all lesions had to be surgically excised adequately after histopathologic establishment of the diagnosis.[10–12] On the other hand, the experimental data generated by Paslin[15] indicated that incisional biopsies of subcutaneously implanted tumors in hamsters did not alter the incidence of subsequent pulmonary metastases.

The original clinical epidemiologic information has been criticized for lumping cases[14] and sample sizes.[2] Although the data are basically retrospective and were recorded at a time when refined classification was hardly known, they provide a suggestion that whatever the effect of manipulation of the primary tumor, it has to be rather subtle. In addition, the extensive and incisive studies of Fidler and his group,[16] who worked with B16 melanoma and other experimental tumors, focus on the distinct possibility that viable metastases occur because of the emergence of a special pre-existing population of tumor cells with a phenotype for invasion and survival in a foreign tissue site rather than as a new event occurring at the time of surgery. For instance, less than 1 per cent of malignant cells remain viable 24 hours after intravenous injection.[16] Furthermore, a substantial number of steps are required for tumor cells to produce successful metastases and this biological complexity may explain why the process is inefficient.[16] Clearly, the known genetic heterogeneity of tumor cells plays an important role. The finding that the highly metastatic B16 F_{10} melanoma cell lines produce far less prostaglandin D_2 than does the parent line[17] suggests another approach in defining those cells with metastatic potential.

Although pathologists covet every bit of tissue for analysis and classification, it may become more important in the future to send part of the excisional biopsies for analysis of prostaglandin synthesis, cell surface markers, or other proteins in order to define the functional phenotype of the primary melanoma. In the meantime, small incisional biopsies of some melanomas in certain situations will continue and cannot be condemned. One should, however, be sure to use good clinical judgment and to make certain that adequate surgery is carried out as soon as the correct diagnosis has been established.

References

1. Kopf, A. W., Mintzis, M., and Bart, R. S.: Diagnostic accuracy in malignant melanoma. Arch. Dermatol. 111:1291, 1975.
2. Sagebiel, R. W.: Biopsy of the cutaneous pigmented lesion. Cutis 21:215, 1978.
3. Levene, A.: On the histological diagnosis and prognosis of malignant melanoma. J. Clin. Pathol. 33:101, 1980.
4. Kopf, A. W., Bart, R. S., and Rodriguez-Sains, R. S.: Malignant melanoma: A review. J. Dermatol. Surg. Oncol. 3:41, 1977.
5. Wanebo, H. J., Woodruff, J., and Fortner, J. G.: Malignant melanoma of the extremities: A clinicopathologic study using levels of invasion (microstage). Cancer 35:666, 1975.
6. Breslow, A., and Macht, S. D.: Optimal size of resection margin for thin cutaneous melanoma. Surg. Gynecol. Obstet. 145:691, 1977.
7. Epstein, E., and Bragg, K.: Curability of melanoma: A 25-year retrospective study. Cancer 46:818, 1980.
8. Giulano, A. E., Moseley, H. S., and Morton, D. S.: Clinical aspects of unknown primary melanoma. Ann. Surg. 191:98, 1980.
9. Epstein, W. L.: Malignant melanoma in perspective. In Epstein, E. H., and Epstein, E. H., Jr. (eds.): Skin Surgery, 5th ed. Springfield, IL, Charles C Thomas, 1982, p. 1031.
10. Epstein, E., Bragg, K., and Linden, G.: Biopsy and prognosis of malignant melanoma. JAMA 208:1369, 1969.
11. Jones, N. M., Williams, W. J., Roberts, M. M., and Davies, K.: Malignant melanoma of the skin: Prognostic value of clinical features and the role of treatment in 111 cases. Br. J. Cancer 22:437, 1968.
12. Knutson, C. O., Hori, J. M., and Spratt, J. S., Jr.: Melanoma. Curr. Probl. Surg. 3–55, Dec. 1971.
13. Rampen, F. H. J., van Houten, W. A., and Hop, W. C. J.: Incisional procedures and prognosis in malignant melanoma. Clin. Exp. Dermatol. 5:313, 1980.
14. Rampen, F. H. J.: Changing concepts in melanoma management. Br. J. Dermatol. 104:341, 1981.
15. Paslin, D. A.: The effects of biopsy on the incidence of metastasis in hamsters bearing malignant melanoma. J. Invest. Derm. 61:33, 1973.
16. Hart, I. R., and Fidler, I. J.: The implications of tumor heterogeneity on the biology and therapy of cancer metastasis. Biochim. Biophys. Acta 651:37, 1981.
17. Fitzpatrick, F. A., and Stringfellow, D. A.: Prostaglandin D_2 formation by malignant melanoma cells correlates inversely with cellular metastatic potential. Proc. Natl. Acad. Sci. USA 76:1765, 1979.

DELETERIOUS EFFECTS OF BIOPSY ON SURVIVAL OF PATIENTS WITH MELANOMA

F. H. J. Rampen, M.D.

"Mine's a melanoblastoma, a real merciless bastard. As a rule, it's eight months and you've had it. . . . But the point is that even if I'd come earlier they still wouldn't have been able to operate. A melanoblastoma is such a swine you only have to touch it with a knife and it produces secondaries. . . ."

VADIM, IN SOLZHENITSYN, *Cancer Ward*

The question of whether biopsies should be performed in lesions suspected of being malignant melanomas is of great interest. Fear of dissemination of tumor cells as a result of the mechanical disruption of the neoplasm is the main argument of the opponents to biopsy. However, a fruitful discussion of the subject requires a proper definition of the problem. If biopsies are to cause tumor cell dislodgement, it is conceivable that only *incisional* procedures will do so. *Excisional* biopsies beyond the borders of the tumor are unlikely to enhance metastases. In this respect, the width of the tumor free resection margin, whether a few millimeters or several centimeters, is less relevant to the present debate.

From the tumor-biological scene, the question we raise is of little importance. Metastasis is commonly promoted by increasing cell release from the primary tumor. Although most circulating tumor cells perish in the bloodstream, some (probably less than 1 per cent) will stop and will grow at distant sites. Shearing forces, like body movements and external forces, may enhance tumor cell dislodgement. Therefore, any undue disturbance of the normal architecture of the tumor should be avoided. Why, then, are clinicians so at loggerheads about incision in malignant melanoma?

Evidence from the Literature

It is interesting to note that the American school is somewhat opinionated as to the safety of (incisional) biopsy. "Biopsy is essential for a positive diagnosis and is attended by no danger if properly performed."[1] "Dermal punch biopsy . . . is simple, safe, and reliable. Such a technique is ideal in suspected melanoma."[2] On the other hand, biopsies have been deplored by most European authors as jeopardizing the patient's survival.

Many studies have failed to reveal any detrimental effect of biopsy on prognosis. Most sources refer to the studies of Epstein and associates[3] and Epstein and Bragg,[4] who corroborated that pretreatment biopsy did not adversely affect survival rates. However, Epstein's data do not constitute valid evidence that incomplete removal of a melanoma is not hazardous, because the investigators' "biopsy" group was not divided according to incisional and excisional procedures. Drzewiecki and coworkers[5] studied similar patient categories: One group had pretreatment nonradical "biopsy" under local anesthetic, and the second group was treated with primary radical surgery. No differences in survival were observed between the two categories. Again, this study does not allow firm conclusions, because incisional and exisional biopsies were not analyzed separately. Casual mention of the influence of biopsy or incision upon survival has been made by several other investigators. Of

111 patients studied by Jones and colleagues,[6] 18 underwent incisional biopsy; 5-year survival was similar to the overall survival rate for the entire series. Cochran[7] claimed that the fate of 20 patients with incisional biopsy was no different from that of the whole study population. Knutson and associates[8] maintained that pretreatment biopsy (incisional and excisional) did not compromise 5-year survival. Everall and Dowd[9] found that diagnostic incision had no adverse effect. Lastly, incisional biopsy was performed in 22 of 103 patients examined by Bagley and coworkers[10] without influencing the prognosis.

It is not surprising that reviewers of the subject cast doubt on the dictum that pretreatment biopsy should be incriminated as a risk factor.[11,12] However, it should be reiterated that in some of the papers quoted no discrimination was made between incisional and excisional procedures, whereas in other series the data are too concise to permit definite pronouncements.

Other reports indicate that (incisional) biopsy may be fraught with considerable hazard. Olsen[13] emphasized that of her total series of 323 determinate cases, 19 underwent "biopsy" before definitive therapy; prognosis in this group was poorer than in the radical treatment group. Excisional and incisional biopsy yielded 48 per cent and 30 per cent survival rates, respectively, in the study of Fitzpatrick and colleagues.[14] This difference could be accounted for because more lesions in the incision category were greater than or equal to 2 cm in diameter (39 per cent), compared with the excision group (15 per cent). However, there was no real difference in crude survival for lesions less than 2 cm and greater than or equal to 2 cm across. Thus, the difference in survival between the incision and excision categories might have been genuine. Inadequate pretreatment procedures, including incisional biopsy, were performed in 13 out of 195 patients studied by Tonak and associates.[15] This category exhibited a 2-year survival of 38 per cent, against 79 per cent for the adequate treatment group. These authors noted that inadequate procedures were carried out in smaller lesions that were not very suspicious. On the other hand, Tonak's patient groups were not entirely comparable with regard to stage distribution, which makes the study inconclusive. A most interesting account of this subject was presented at the Fourth International Symposium on Malignant Melanoma in Lyon in 1977, when van Slooten and van der Esch[16] reported on a statistically significant reduction in survival for patients with incomplete excisions as the initial treatment approach. Unfortunately, detailed data on this series never have been published.

Personal Observations

We have studied the prognostic impact of incisional and punch biopsies in 14 patients with Stage I melanoma, comparing these individuals with 62 patients who received primary radical treatment.[17] Multivariate statistical analysis revealed that survival was markedly reduced following incisional procedures. Admittedly, our retrospective study was based on a relatively small number of cases. Moreover, it can be argued that if tumor cell dislodgement takes place at the time of incision, clinical manifestation of metastasis would become evident only after many years. However, the tumor volume doubling time of metastatic melanoma ranges from 10 to 200 days.[18] Minute tumor emboli with a doubling time of 10 to 20 days may kill the host within 1 or 2 years. In our series, survival curves diverged from approximately 1½ to 2 years after diagnosis, which is entirely compatible with the aforementioned oncobiological fundamentals.

Another debatable facet of our study is the delay between diagnostic incision and definitive surgery. Epstein and associates[3] stressed that biopsy does not affect survival if followed within 1 week by radical surgical treatment. In our incision category definitive treatment was delayed by more than 1 week in 10 of 13 cases (1 unknown), against only 6 out of 58 cases (4 unknown) in the excision category. Of the 10 patients in the incision category who had a delay in final treatment, only 4 survived 5 years with no evidence of disease (40 per cent), against 5 of 6 patients (83 per cent) in the excision group. It is concluded that incisional biopsy bears more severely upon survival than an additional delay in final treatment up to 4 weeks. A further point of consideration is the fact that in our excision group 4 patients died intercurrently, which renders the superiority in survival of this category even more striking. Nevertheless, our findings ought to be reproduced by other investigators before definite conclusions can be advanced. Furthermore, prospective studies are now indicated to address this problem.

We also have studied the influence of physical maltreatment on the life span of tumor-bearing animals.[19] B16 melanoma suspensions were injected into the gastrocnemius muscles of C57BL mice. The effect of repeated preoperative palpation and that of preoperative incisional biopsy were compared with the effect of amputation without any preoperative intervention. The median survival time of the control group (simple amputation) was 48 days. In the preoperative palpation group, the median survival time was 39 days, and in the biopsy category, the median life span was 35 days. The differences in survival time between the control and experimental groups were statistically significant ($P = 0.01$). These data demonstrate an increased risk of tumor cell dissociation after physical trauma to the primary tumor.

Other Arguments Against Incision

An additional drawback of incision through the primary melanoma is the difficulty that may arise in diagnosis. Differentiation of this tumor from, for instance, an "active" nevocytic nevus or from a juvenile melanoma (Spitz nevus) may be extremely difficult or impossible if only punched-out specimens are available for diagnosis. Removing part of the tumor will not allow a reliable distinction of the Clark-Breslow microstaging minutiae or of the histogenetic tumor type. Even if a "representative" sample is obtained from the most nodular part of the lesion, the tissue-damaging effect of the procedure itself may have a serious impact on, for example, the measurement of tumor thickness. Moreover, post-biopsy excisions may be difficult to interpret because of secondary infection. If misdiagnosis (and mismanagement) is to be avoided, clinicians should refrain from incisional biopsy in cutaneous melanoma.

Exceptions

There is often no alternative to biopsy on such sites as the face, the hands, the feet, or the external genitalia. If primary radical excision of a suspicious lesion entails a disfiguring surgical approach, then incisional or punch biopsy may be warranted. Some authors advocate incisional biopsy through the central part of the neoplasm. Others recommend two biopsies, one from the edge and one from the thickest part of the lesion. In our opinion, there is no reason to take a biopsy specimen from the central portion of a suspicious lesion. Usually, a 3- to 4-mm punch biopsy from the edge allows an accurate distinction between a melanomatous and a nonmelanomatous growth. If the lesion has to be removed in a second attempt, precise assessment of melanoma microstages is then still possible.

Incision may promote metastases, and this danger is greatest when the central part of the tumor is traumatized. First of all, biopsy through the thickest part of the tumor increases the tumor mass that is maltreated by the procedure. This, in its turn, increases the number of circulating tumor cells in comparison with incision through a more peripheral part of the lesion. The formation of metastatic foci can be considered as a probabilistic population balance. The risk of metastatic secondary neoplasms is directly proportional to the number of tumor cells released. So, the greater the area of maltreatment (central part of the primary tumor), the greater the risk of metastatic spread. Secondly, an increased growth rate facilitates cell detachment. It is generally accepted that the nodular part of cutaneous melanoma harbors the most aggressive cell clones with the highest mitotic count. These tumor characters entail an increased potential of cell release. Thirdly, circulating tumor cells from the central part of the lesion, with its more "malignant" cell clones, are more likely to be arrested in target organs with subsequent metastasis formation than are cells from the more "benign" peripheral part, which may perish in the blood before lodging can occur. These characteristics of increased ability of cell detachment and subsequent arrest at distant sites represent serious risk factors. So, not only the number of cells released but also the aggressiveness and metastatic potential of such cells should caution against incision through the nodular portion of cutaneous melanoma.

CONCLUSIONS

There is strong evidence that incision through a melanoma compromises survival. A serious plea has been made that total excisional biopsy be performed in all suspected melanomas excising a tumor free margin of approximately 1 cm. Preferably, the procedure should be accomplished under field block anesthesia. Usually, general anesthesia is not necessary. It is incomprehensible that infiltration anesthesia at a certain distance from the primary tumor should enhance tumor cell detachment when one considers the continuous daily "trauma" from pressure, rubbing, scratching, and body movements that may exist for years before the diagnosis is established. If the lesion proves to be a melanoma, then radical surgery may be performed in a second session.

If the lesion is very large or is so anatomically situated that total excisional biopsy with a margin of 1 cm would be mutilating or disfiguring, two alternative approaches are recommended. (1) If the index of suspicion is "high," total excisional biopsy remains the treatment of choice. If this is not feasible, then the excision margin may be smaller than 1 cm. Only in exceptional cases is an incisional biopsy advocated, preferably from the edge of the lesion. (2) If the index of suspicion is "low," minor excisions are preferred. Usually, a tumor free margin of a few millimeters is sufficient. In selected cases, incisional diagnostic biopsy will be unavoidable.

What has been said about incision also applies to cytologic procedures. Although direct imprints are less dangerous than abrasion techniques or fine needle aspirations, it is stressed that cytodiagnosis of any kind has no place in the routine management of primary melanoma. In exceptional instances, however, especially when diagnostic excision would be mutilating, cytology is certainly justified.

The viewpoint that primary excision as the sole correct diagnostic procedure may result in many biopsies' not being performed, which may be counterproductive to the early detection of melanoma, is invalid as an argument in favor of incision. If there is only a slight suspicion of melanoma, the lesion has to be excised in toto anyway, since partial removal may not insure certainty of diagnosis.

Finally, I would like to voice my concern about the trend noticed by Roses and associates.[20] In the period 1949 through 1975, of 881 melanoma patients seen at the New York University School of Medicine, 166 (19 per cent) were subjected to incisional biopsy. This figure rose to 41 per cent (103 of 252 patients) over the period 1976 through 1978. Why this changing attitude? Is it because dermatologists have erroneously interpreted the recommendations of Epstein and coworkers[3] as applicable to *incisional biopsy* instead of *biopsy* in general? Or is it because they are too busy nowadays to do prompt, appropriate excisional biopsy on the spot or because they are reluctant to send every vaguely suspicious mole to their overworked fellow surgeons, afraid of a queue "from here to the dark side of the moon" ?[21] Where do we end up? And to whose benefit?

References

1. Sachs, W., MacKee, G. M., Schwartz, O. D., and Pierson, H. S.: Junction nevus—nevocarcinoma; the so-called melanoma group. JAMA 135:216, 1947.
2. Cady, B.: Changing concepts in melanoma management. Med. Clin. North Am. 59:301, 1975.
3. Epstein, E., Bragg, K., and Linden, G.: Biopsy and prognosis of malignant melanoma. JAMA 208:1369, 1969.
4. Epstein, E., and Bragg, K.: Curability of melanoma: A 25-year retrospective study. Cancer 46:818, 1980.
5. Drzewiecki, K. T., Ladefoged, C., and Christensen, H. E.: Biopsy and prognosis for cutaneous malignant melanomas in Clinical Stage I. Scand. J. Plast. Reconstr. Surg. 14:141, 1980.
6. Jones, W. M., Williams, W. J., Roberts, M. M., and Davies, K.: Malignant melanoma of the skin: Prognostic value of clinical features and the role of treatment in 111 cases. Br. J. Cancer 22:437, 1968.
7. Cochran, A. J.: Malignant melanoma; a review of 10 years' experience in Glasgow, Scotland. Cancer 23:1190, 1969.
8. Knutson, C. O., Hori, J. M., and Spratt, J. S.: Melanoma. Curr. Probl. Surg. 3–55, Dec. 1971.
9. Everall, J. D., and Dowd, P. M.: Diagnosis, prognosis and treatment of melanoma. Lancet 2:286, 1977.
10. Bagley, F. H., Cady, B., Lee, A., and Legg, M. A.: Changes in clinical presentation and management of malignant melanoma. Cancer 47:2126, 1981.
11. Lee, Y-T. N.: Malignant melanoma: To biopsy or not to biopsy. CA 24:104, 1974.
12. Kopf, A. W., Bart, R. S., and Rodriguez-Sains, R. S.: Malignant melanoma: A review. J. Dermatol. Surg. Oncol. 3:90, 1977.
13. Olsen, G.: The malignant melanoma of the skin. New theories based on a study of 500 cases. Acta Chir. Scand. Suppl. 365:1, 1966.
14. Fitzpatrick, P. J., Brown, T. C., and Reid, J.: Malignant melanoma of the head and neck: A clinicopathological study. Can. J. Surg. 15:90, 1972.
15. Tonak, J., Hermanek, P., Hornstein, O. P., and Weidner, F.: Therapie des malignen Melanoms der klinischen Stadien I und II; Ergebnisse bei 195 Patienten. Dtsch. Med. Wschr. 101:435, 1976.
16. van Slooten, E. A., and van der Esch, E. P.: Surgical treatment of primary cutaneous melanoma; a retrospective study on 130 patients. 4th International Symposium on Malignant Melanoma, Lyon, 1977.
17. Rampen, F. H. J., van Houten, W. A., and Hop, W. C. J.: Incisional procedures and prognosis in malignant melanoma. Clin. Exp. Dermatol. 5:313, 1980.
18. Rampen, F. H. J., and Mulder, J. H.: Malignant melanoma: An androgen-dependent tumour? Lancet 1:562, 1980.
19. Mulder, J. H., Rampen, F. H. J., and van der Lugt, L.: The influence of physical maltreatment on the life span of tumour bearing mice. REP-TNO Annual Report, 1978, p. 175.
20. Roses, D. F., Ackerman, A. B., Harris, M. N., Weinhouse, G. R., and Gumport, S. L.: Assessment of biopsy techniques and histopathologic interpretations of primary cutaneous malignant melanoma. Ann. Surg. 189:294, 1979.
21. Pereira, F. A.: Biopsy of melanoma. JAMA 240:2434, 1978.

Editorial Comment

In medical school I was taught that one should never cut into a melanoma or this highly malignant tumor would enter the blood stream or the lymphatic circulation and be seeded all over the body. This would certainly lead to an untimely demise for the sufferer. After observing the mutilation caused by the radical excision of benign lesions because of the possibility that they might have been melanomas, I developed a growing black lesion on my face. I insisted on a conservative removal rather than a sacrifice of half of my face because some clinicians insisted that the lesion could be a melanoma. Simple excision established the benign nature of the lesion.

However, I wondered if I would have compromised my chances for survival had the growth been a true melanoma. Therefore, I gathered 193 patients with primary melanoma treated by excision and now have followed the members of this group for 25 years. The survival figures for the members of this group compared with those who had conservative removals or incisional biopsies and with those treated by radical surgery in the first place are shown in Table 1.

Table 1. COMPARISON OF SURVIVAL RATES IN PATIENTS WITH AND WITHOUT BIOPSIES*

Number of Patients		Years After Diagnosis				
		5	10	15	20	25
Biopsy	115	79.0	65.3	51.0	46.4	39.7
No biopsy	55	75.4	55.8	51.7	47.3	44.5

*Figures represent percentages of survival at each date.

The figures in the table indicate that a biopsy followed by definitive removal, even 1 week after the original surgical experience, had no effect on the survival rate of these individuals.

Some time ago, I presented my studies of these patients at a European dermatologic center. I was assured that my audience was well-versed in the English language and would have no trouble understanding me.

At the conclusion of my presentation, the professor inquired, "Does anyone agree with you?"

I assured him that this philosophy regarding the safety of taking a biopsy from a lesion that is suspected of being a melanoma was well accepted in the United States. With that he turned and faced the members of the audience and talked for 10 minutes in his native tongue. At the conclusion of his harangue he turned toward me and stated that he was explaining what I had said, since "the members of the audience did not understand English so well." Some of the younger members of the staff came up after the meeting was adjourned and told me that he had warned them that if they were caught performing a biopsy of a melanoma, they would be dismissed immediately. Ideas backed by the authority of academicians perish slowly.

Think It Over.

CHAPTER 5

TREATMENT OF MELANOMAS

PRIMARY EXCISION OF MELANOMA

C. V. Caver, M.D.

Surgical excision remains the principal form of treatment for melanoma; all other treatment modalities are merely helpers and adjuncts. There is still a great deal of contention among those who treat melanoma about the precise principles and rationales; for example, concerning "how many centimeters of margin" for each level, thickness, or type and whether or not to remove fasciae. The more stringent the rules, the more difficult they are to follow, and it behooves us to realize that there are some differences between ideals and practice. There has even arisen lately some dissension over who should do the surgery. Some dermatologists will not even perform a biopsy of suspected melanoma and characteristically will refer all lesions to general surgeons and general plastic surgeons. The organized general plastic surgeons have taken the published position that dermatologists are not qualified to perform or capable of executing this simple surgery. The truth is that anyone who can do a simple excision should be prepared to excise recognizable melanoma.

It formerly was thought that incisional biopsy would increase the rate of metastasis, but this now has been disproved.[1] Yet, the diagnostic process of incisional biopsy takes time and may not give all necessary information on the total character of the tumor, missing some of the more malignant features. Therefore, the punch, or incisional, biopsy should give way to total excision of the lesion in order to (1) enable the physician to study the total histologic features and get confirming opinions, and (2) decrease mortality by removing the main threat—the visible tumor load.

Margins

Bagley and associates[2] found that the survival rate after simple excision is much higher than formerly was thought. The concepts of wide excision and radical dissections stem from the "doom-and-gloom" days of the early twentieth century, when all malignant melanomas seen were nodular level fives with satellites and when no classification or staging was done.[3] The incidence of low-risk melanoma has risen 53 per cent and that of high-risk melanoma has decreased 10 per cent since 1955 at the Lahey Clinic.[2] Margins of less than 3 to 5 cm may increase local recurrence slightly but do not adversely affect survival rates; however, such conservation of tissue does allow more primary closures and flaps and lessens the need for skin grafting and disfiguring donor areas. Day and coworkers found that magnitude of margins has no effect on survival, even for high-risk melanoma.[4] Thus, the previously enforced dicta of arbitrarily wide margins cannot be clinically or statistically justified.

Breslow and Macht[5] showed, and Kopf confirmed,[6] that for malignant melanomas of less than 0.76 mm thickness any margin, no matter how small, seemed sufficient to protect from local recurrences. A European study of 588 cases of primary Stage I cutaneous malignant melanomas reported by the German Melanoma Study Group at the European Society for Dermatological Research by Schmoeckel and colleagues[7] showed that patients with excision margins of 5 cm developed metastasis at a higher rate (50 per cent) than did those with excision margins of less than 5 mm (24 per cent). Thus, the rate of metastasis was independent of the width of excision.

One may perform more definitive and proven procedures, such as wider excision, removal of fasciae, dissection of regional lymph nodes, and amputation of a digit and its nearest metatarsal or metacarpal, after examination of a complete tumor and consultation with the appropriate experts in the regional disciplines of otorhinolaryngology, ophthalmology, dentistry, gynecology, proctology, urology, general surgery, general plastic surgery, and so forth.[8] Early and total cold steel excision of necessity will decrease the need for radical procedures, such as chemotherapy, radiation, Mohs chemosurgery, laser surgery, hyperthermia, cryotherapy, regional node dissection, and immunotherapy. Fortner and associates[9] showed that with wide excision alone the 5-year survival rate was 82 per cent and the 10-year rate was 81 per cent.

Technique

If patients are known to be taking anticoagulant medications, the appropriate tests for prothrombin activity should be performed. Patients should be informed in this case and in all other surgery that there is a possibility that re-excision and even more extensive procedures may have to be done later in order for an acceptable result to be achieved and that this will depend on the exact findings during the surgery and the interpretation by the pathologists. Only with this information can the patient have a full concept of the nature and the extent of the problem.

The surgical site is prepared with the antiseptic agent of the surgeon's choice and is draped as necessary. The presence of any sensitivity to drugs or anesthetics should be determined by careful questioning, and any of these substances should be removed from the room. The excision that has been planned is marked with a suitable dye oriented in the direction of the probable pathway of the lymphatic drainage. The site is shown to the patient in a mirror for approval and is photographed prior to the infiltration of the local anesthetic agent in order to avoid distortion of the tissues. Should re-excision become necessary after the diagnosis has been established, the entire scar or the biopsy site and its underlying bed to the fascia should be removed, since the patient already should have been apprised of the possibility that the biopsy may be only the first in a series of operations designed for the total treatment of the tumor. A total excision biopsy probably will be done by a fusiform resection or a double m-plasty, if possible in the relaxed or favorable skin lines with a border of 3 to 5 mm. Dissection should be down to the fat or under the tumor limits by direct visual control, but no fasciae need be removed at this point. To assist in the planning of later surgical extirpations, one should point the incision and the scar toward the regional or draining lymph node group. Reasonable exceptions to these rules are cases in which the lesion is too large for direct closure or incorporates or is too near a vital structure, such as the eye. At these times, an incisional biopsy through the deepest part is indicated.[10,11]

The technique of the biopsy has been dealt with by Castrow and Chernosky[12] but may be varied somewhat, according to the situation and the type of tumor. The authors emphasize that even incomplete removal of a malignant melanoma does not reduce the rate of survival, provided that the definitive treatments chosen are not delayed by more than 1 month.[13] Total excision is preferred over the partial scalpel technique, which in turn is preferred over the punch, and shave biopsy is condemned as inadequate and misleading.

An excision biopsy, properly and adequately carried out, can be the diagnostic and the curative procedure at the same time in many cases. Castrow and Chernosky point out that the newer data (previously cited) do not support their criteria that biopsy should be performed only on "thin primary cutaneous malignant melanomas without local spread or metastasis" and with margins of 3 to 5 cm. Relapses and death rates do not appear to be affected by the excision method as much as by the site, the thickness, the presence of microscopic satellites, the gross type,[14,15] and the degree of mitotic activity.[16]

James T. Helsper, of the University of Southern California School of Medicine and Comprehensive Cancer Center, believes in a "no-touch" technique of excision biopsy.[17] He appears to advocate this method more to preserve the histologic architecture of the lesion than to prevent the dislodging of small clusters of malignant cells, as Frederic E. Mohs so often has described. The anesthetic agent is injected outside the borders of the specimen, so that the needle does not penetrate it. No sponge or hemostatic instrument is allowed to touch the specimen as it is being removed for diagnostic study. Helsper also advocates a margin equal to the diameter of the lesion and the use of clean instruments for closure—an admirable surgical technique in any event. He confirms Pack's[13] theory of the safe period for delay of definitive removal from the time of diagnosis without a decrease in the survival rate but sets it at 3 weeks instead of 1 month.

The specimen should be clearly oriented for the laboratory by placement of marking sutures of different colors in one or more margins of the specimen. These should be identified on a drawing, and the material should be submitted with a complete gross description, a short clinical history and, if possible, a photograph of the marked surgical site. Only with this information can a pathologist give a truly meaningful interpretation of the tumor.

Harris and Gumport[11] state that 81 per cent of malignant melanomas are lentigo melanomas or superficial spreading melanomas of 5 to 20 mm and thus are subject to total excision biopsy, but equal to the biopsy in importance is photography of the lesions by ordinary or infrared methods. Total excision biopsy offers the patient the best chance of a favorable result with the least amount of surgery.

Accuracy

Three factors contribute to the accuracy of the biopsy as a main diagnostic effort: the surgeon, the technique, and the pathologist. Winkelmann[18] has pointed out that malignant melanoma is among the most accessible tumors for diagnosis, yet it is misdiagnosed more frequently than any other skin tumor.

The practice of dermatology encourages a high index of suspicion of malignant melanoma that is not necessarily seen in other disciplines. Kopf and coworkers[6] found that the preoperative impression of malignant melanoma for dermatologists and residents was 96 per cent in those cases correctly diagnosed, even though the histologic accuracy was only 64 per cent. Epstein found that in the same type of personnel, malignant melanoma was suspected in 31 cases but was proved histologically in only 12 cases. Thus, the most successful and beneficial factor in the overall treatment of malignant melanoma is the adequate clinical examination and proper biopsy of suspected lesions. The factor of technique has been discussed earlier and should be total excision when possible. The pathologist (the third factor) is critical in that he must be well-versed in the features of melanomas and their many variations. He must have access to other pathologists for consultations and must not be too proud to submit slides to specialty centers, such as the Armed Forces Institute of Pathology. He also must realize that time is of the essence and must submit his interpretation as soon as possible in order to relieve the anxiety of the patient and the surgeon.

Melanocytic Nevi

The important question of which melanocytic nevi to remove and which to watch or ignore frequently arises. There is general agreement that all congenital and large nevi should be removed and that the earlier in life, the better—in undeniable cases, even in infancy, at which time removal of these lesions (under light sedation and local anesthesia) is comparable with or less annoying than circumcision. The older the child at presentation, the less excuse there is for waiting to excise congenital or large nevi, since even infants and young children have been known to develop melanoma in congenital nevi. Kopf[19] advocates removal of all large lesions, which he defines as those in which the largest diameter is 20 cm or more. For smaller nevi, patients or parents, or both, should be informed of the data associating these lesions with melanoma and should be allowed to decide whether to have them removed.

Rhodes and his associates[20] found that the rate of nonselected proven melanomas associated with dermal nevi was 7.3 per cent. This frequency was estimated to be more than 8000 times greater than expected on the basis of surface area considerations and the 1 per cent prevalence of small congenital nevi in the general population. Rhodes does not, however, recommend the removal of all congenital nevi; rather, he states that only those with recent change or those that are very dark or darkening should be removed. Harris and Gumport[11] estimate that for the whole population there is only one nevus in 1 million that becomes malignant, since most melanomas arise de novo.

Certainly no one advocates the removal of all nevi at all ages; our economy could not bear it. A high index of suspicion among dermatologists probably will result in ten excisions for every four histologically confirmed melanomas. This is consistent with my recorded experience in practice, but I have never yet regretted excising a suspicious lesion. No matter how many times I have been wrong, if all my excisions have prevented a single death from that one-in-a-million malignant melanoma, it was worth it.

SUMMARY

A survey of all current published studies indicates a definite trend away from the mutilating radical excisions and explorations of the past toward a more conservative extirpation, in a single stage if possible. The view of most dermatologists and combined groups of specialists tends to be that the width of margins is not as important in affecting a recurrence and survival rates as are the thickness and level of the tumors. Since surgical treatment has changed very little in the last half-century and since no generally acknowledged effective adjuvant therapy has been developed, today's high survival rates almost certainly evolve from earlier detection and diagnosis, better staging, and total primary excision.

When presented with a questionable lesion, the beloved old family physician might have said, "Let's watch that thing for a while, and if it starts to look bad I will spark it off with my electrodesiccator." Our attitude today should be that a small, suspicious lesion is like a small, suspicious fire in the house; we should not wait until it is a big fire but should put it out entirely while it is still small. Leave the electrodesiccator hanging on the wall and do a total excision as early as possible.

References

1. Epstein, E., Bragg, K., and Linden, G.: Biopsy and prognosis of malignant melanomas. JAMA 208:1369, 1969.

2. Bagley, F. H., Cody, B., Lee, A., and Legg, M. A.: Changes in clinical presentation and management of melanoma. Cancer 47:2126, 1981.
3. Handley, W. S.: The pathology of melanotic growths in relation to their operative treatment. Lancet 1:927–933 and 996–1003, 1907.
4. Day, C., Mihm, M., Sober, A., Fitzpatrick, T., and Walt, R.: Narrower margins for clinical stage I malignant melanoma. N. Engl. J. Med. 306:479, 1982.
5. Breslow, A., and Macht, S. D.: Optimal size of resection margin for thin cutaneous melanoma. Surg. Gynecol. Obstet. 145:691, 1977.
6. Kopf, A. W., Mintzis, M., and Bart R. S.: Diagnostic accuracy in malignant melanoma. Arch. Dermatol. 111:1292, 1975.
7. Schmoeckel, C., Bockelbrink, A., Bockelbrink, H., Kistler, H., and Braun-Falco, I.: Is wide excision necessary in malignant melanoma? J. Invest. Dermatol. 76:424, 1982.
8. Kopf, A. W., Bart, R., Rodriguez-Sains, R., and Ackerman, A. B.: Malignant Melanoma. Paris, Masson, 1979, p. 180.
9. Fortner, J. G., Woodruff, J., Shottenfeld, D., and Maclean, B.: Biostatistical basis of elective node dissection for malignant melanoma. Ann. Surg. 186:101, 1977.
10. Harris, M. N., and Gumport, S. L.: Total excisional biopsy for primary malignant melanoma. JAMA 226:354, 1973.
11. Harris, M. N., and Gumport, S. L.: Biopsy technique for malignant melanoma. J. Dermatol. Surg. 1:24, 1975.
12. Castrow, F. F., 2nd, Chernosky, M. E.: Scalpel excision of primary cutaneous malignant melanomas without metastasis. J. Dermatol. Surg. Oncol. 5:109, 1979.
13. Pack, G. T., Gerber, D. M., and Scharnagel, T. M.: End results in the treatment of malignant melanoma. Ann. Surg. 136:905, 1952.
14. Jones, W. M., Williams, W. J., Roberts, M. M., and Davies, K.: Malignant melanoma of the skin: Prognostic value of clinical features and the role of treatment in 111 cases. Br. J. Cancer 22:452, 1968.
15. Knutson, C. O., Hori, J. M., and Spratt, J. S.: Melanoma. Curr. Probl. Surg. 3–55, Dec. 1971.
16. Day, C.: Derm. Capsule and Comment, vol. 4, no. 3, March 1982.
17. Helsper, J. T.: Skin and Allergy News, vol. 12, no. 12, Dec. 1981, p. 9.
18. Winkelmann, R. L.: The differential diagnosis of malignant melanoma. In Melanoma and Skin Cancer: Proceedings of the International Cancer Conference, Sydney, Australia, 1972.
19. Kopf, A. W.: Congenital nevocytic nevi and malignant melanomas. J. Am. Acad. Dermatol. 1:123, 1979.
20. Rhodes, A. R., Sober, A. J., Day, C. L., Melski, J. W., Harrist, T. J., Mihm, M. C., Jr., and Fitzpatrick, T. B.: The malignant potential of small congenital nevocellular nevi. J. Am. Acad. Dermatol. 6:230, Feb. 1982.

TREATMENT OF MELANOMA: VIEWPOINT OF THE ONCOLOGIC SURGEON

Charles M. McBride, M.D.

The oncologic surgeon who treats patients with malignant melanoma usually is at a disadvantage in that he seldom sees the patient with the primary lesion intact. For this reason, he must rely entirely on the description given by the patient, the referring physician, and the pathologist in an attempt to determine the stage of the disease and which ancillary therapies may be required. Surgeons still see patients whose pigmented lesions were excised and were not sent for pathologic examination or patients with pigmented lesions that were shaved and their bases electrocoagulated, although this has been occurring less frequently. The disadvantage of the latter procedure is that the pathologist can determine only a minimum depth of invasion or a minimum level of disease; he cannot assign a definitive microstage. Re-excision of the area usually does not help definitive staging, because electrocoagulation changes the tissues at the base in such a way that further information cannot be obtained; however, when all the data that are available concerning a given patient have been collected, the surgeon tries to determine a stage of disease and to formulate his plan of treatment.

For malignant melanomas perhaps more than for any other cancer, the staging system relies on the opinion of the pathologist more than on the clinical examination of the patient, although both are important. Since the studies by Clark and his group[1] describing the levels of penetration of the skin by malignant melanomas and the work by Breslow,[2] who pointed out the importance of measuring the depth of invasion of the lesion, it has been possible to determine the stage of primary malignant melanomas with more accuracy. At the University of Texas System Cancer Center, M.D. Anderson Hospital and Tumor Institute, primary melanomas of Level I or II involvement or those of Level III involvement invading less than 1 mm are considered superficial lesions. Level III melanomas that invade more deeply than 1 mm and those of Level IV and V involvement are considered invasive melanomas.[3] Superficial lesions should not be able to spread beyond the local area, and therefore therapy is aimed at control of the primary lesion. Invasive lesions may be expected to involve the lymphatic system and, in fact, 15 per cent of them already will have spread by way of the hemopoietic system. Hence, they require more extensive therapy or, at the least, a closer follow-up regimen.

Superficial lesions, which can be expected to recur locally only, require excisions that encompass any areas of microscopic disease that would not be obvious on inspection. There are many theories about the exact required size of the excision,[4] but these lesions certainly do not necessitate the 5-cm excision that has been the classical therapy for melanoma.

For patients with invasive malignant melanoma, spread toward the regional lymph nodes may be expected, and hence it has been our practice to excise a portion of the skin in the direction of the suspected nodal drainage basin; two thirds of the excision is made in that direction.[5] In-transit metastases, regional lymph node metastases, and dissemination are managed by other therapies. To some extent, the form of the final excision is dictated by the physician who saw the patient first. If a large transversal incision or small skin graft has been performed, it is more difficult to locate the subsequent incision properly. If the patient has been referred with an intact primary tumor or after a small incisional biopsy, however, the lesion is usually relatively easy to treat.

Even after a careful staging workup, published series show that 25 per cent to 80 per cent of patients with primary malignant melanoma already have either regional or disseminated disease that goes undetected at the time of the primary treatment. The main controversies center on what further therapy should be employed to prevent the subsequent appearance of this microscopic disease. Most of the attempted immunologic alterations of the patient and prophylactic systemic chemotherapy regimens have not stood the test of time. For primary malignant melanoma of the limbs, regional chemotherapy may be used in an attempt to ablate any disease in transit between the primary site and the first nodal basin and to treat any metastatic disease in the proximal nodal basin.

Although no concurrent investigations to date have carefully compared patients treated by surgery alone with those managed with regional chemotherapy, reported studies of regional chemotherapy show survival to be increased with this form of treatment.[3,6] Our policy has been to treat patients with invasive malignant melanoma (as defined earlier) in which the primary site is on an arm or a leg with prophylactic regional chemotherapy using phenylalanine mustard. When compared with historical controls, patients treated by isolation-perfusion have had a significant survival advantage;[3] however, all the problems associated with studies that lack concurrent controls must be taken into account. It would appear that treatment of the limb by regional chemotherapy not only reduces recurrences but also makes secondary therapies more likely to succeed. This suggests that for patients whose disease is not completely ablated, the volume of melanoma can be reduced by regional chemotherapy so that secondary surgical therapy may be more effective.

There is considerable controversy concerning the role of prophylactic lymph node dissections for patients with primary malignant melanomas. The large study by Veronesi and associates[7] suggests that for patients with malignant melanomas of the limbs, prophylactic lymph node dissection does not produce a survival advantage. Work by others, such as Balch,[8] however, suggests that there may be a group of patients in whom this procedure does provide a better chance for cure. This group would appear to comprise those patients with malignant melanomas invading to a depth of more than 1.5 mm and less than 4 mm of tissue. These patients may have an excessively high risk of lymph node metastases that are not clinically detectable at the time the primary tumor is treated; however, the melanoma may not have been invasive to the depth at which generalized dissemination occurs. The question arises whether one can produce a survival advantage by dissecting lymph nodes prophylactically rather than waiting to dissect them until the disease declares itself clinically.[5] In addition, up to 15 per cent of lymph nodes containing microscopic metastases never will become clinically positive.

In essence, the question is: Should one expose 100 per cent of patients to regional lymph node dissection and its subsequent morbidity in the hope of salvaging 5 per cent of the patients, or could one salvage an equivalent number by careful follow-up, performing the dissection only in cases of clinical recurrence? This is a particular problem for trunk melanomas, since up to five different lymph node basins may be at risk for drainage from some primary melanomas; it is difficult to know how many to dissect. The work by Morton and his group,[9] who injected an isotope at the primary site and subsequently scanned the patient to determine which lymph node basins were at risk for drainage from the area, has been useful in this regard. Their follow-up showed that in no case did metastatic disease occur in a nodal basin that was not detected by the isotope; however, some patients had three or four nodal groups that contained an isotope. Consequently, three or four regional lymph node dissections would be required in these patients to encompass the possible areas of drainage. At present, several research efforts are under way to identify patients with a high risk of regional metastases and to select the most likely areas of drainage. The aim is to reduce unwarranted morbidity and to increase the overall salvage, albeit in a selected group.

There is clear agreement that when nodal disease is clinically palpable, a regional lymph node dissection is in order; however, if there is simultaneous spread to two or more lymph nodal basins, the chances of cure are extremely small. For therapeutic lymph node dissection patients who have less than five nodes positive, the salvage rate may be expected to be 38 per cent. Again, attempts are being made to combine surgery with both immunotherapy and chemotherapy, but at this time these combined therapies produce no clear survival advantage.

For patients with cutaneous metastases on an arm or a leg (in transit between the site of the primary origin and the regional nodal basin), isolation-perfusion[10] or infusion chemotherapy may be considered.[11] A response rate of better than 50 per cent may be expected for both forms of therapy; however, isolation-perfusion totally ablates disease in a percentage of patients, whereas eventual recurrence is the usual outcome for patients treated by infusion chemotherapy. For patients with tumor growths metastatic in the lymphatics of a limb, intralesional immunotherapy with bacille Calmette Guérin or other destructive agents may be expected to control the disease for prolonged periods in up to 25 per cent of patients. Major amputations of the limbs may be expected to produce only 10 per cent long-term survival.

When patients present with disseminated malignant melanoma, surgery has only a palliative role; however, in many cases palliation may be important. The common sites of dissemination are the liver, the lungs, the brain, and the gastrointestinal tract. Many patients with metastatic gastrointestinal melanoma will obtain alleviation of their symptoms for a period of 18 months to 2 years following bowel resection. If pulmonary and brain metastases appear to be solitary, both should be treated by resection; again, some long-term survival may be expected. Patients with hepatic metastases from malignant melanoma have not fared as well. The rate of response to systemic chemotherapy, primarily dimethyltriazenoimidazole carboxamide, is low, and the treatment does not prolong life. Even the use of intra-arterial hepatic chemotherapy has not prolonged life significantly. Melanoma metastatic to skin often produces bulky tumors that tend to break down and become infected, decreasing the quality of life. Marked improvement may be obtained by converting these open, infected wounds to closed wounds, a frequent task for the oncologic surgeon.

In summary, the extent of the primary excision for malignant melanoma is controversial, but certainly most cases do not need the classical 5-cm excision in all directions. When available, regional chemotherapy by isolation-perfusion seems to have an advantage over surgery alone, but this view is not accepted by all investigators. Prophylactic lymph node dissections may be indicated for a selected group of patients, but this group has not been adequately defined yet. Nodal dissections for more than five positive nodes carry a dismal prognosis that has not been improved by ancillary therapies. At this time, the only reasonably successful therapy for in-transit metastases has been regional chemotherapy. The oncologic surgeon plays an important role in increasing the quality of life for the melanoma patient with disseminated disease.

References

1. Clark, W. H., Jr., From, I., et al.: The histogenesis and biologic behavior of primary human malignant melanomas of the skin. Cancer Res. 29:705, 1969.
2. Breslow, A.: Thickness, cross sectional areas and depth of invasion in the prognosis of cutaneous melanoma. Ann. Surg. 172:902, 1970.
3. McBride, C. M., Smith, J. L., Jr., et al.: Primary malignant melanoma of the limbs: A re-evaluation using microstaging techniques. Cancer 48:1463, 1981.
4. Bagley, F. H., Cady, B., et al.: Changes in clinical presentation and management of malignant melanoma. Cancer 47:2126, 1981.
5. McBride, C. M., Sugarbaker, E. V., et al.: Malignant melanoma of the trunk. In McBride, C. M., and

Smith, J. L. (eds.): Neoplasms of the Skin and Malignant Melanoma. Chicago: Year Book Medical Publishers, 1976, p. 363.

6. Krementz, E. T., Carter, R. D., et al.: The use of regional chemotherapy in the management of malignant melanoma. World J. Surg. 3:289, 1979.

7. Veronesi, U., Adamus, J., et al.: Inefficacy of immediate node dissection in stage I melanoma of the limbs. N. Engl. J. Med. 297:627, 1977.

8. Balch, C. M., Soong, S.-J., et al.: Prognostic factor analysis of melanoma patients with regional lymph node metastases (stage II). Proc. Am. Assoc. Cancer Res. 21:676, May, 1980.

9. Robinson, D. S., Sample, W. F., et al.: Recurrent lymphatic drainage in primary malignant melanoma of the trunk determined by colloidal gold scanning. Surg. Forum 28:147, 1977.

10. McBride, C. M.: Advanced melanoma of the extremities: Treatment by isolation-perfusion with a triple drug combination. Arch. Surg. 101:122, 1970.

11. Pritchard, J. D., Mavligit, G. M., et al.: Regression of regionally advanced melanoma after arterial infusion with cis-platinum and actinomycin-D. Clin. Oncol. 5:179, 1979.

CHEMOTHERAPY OF MALIGNANT MELANOMA

Irving M. Ariel, M.D.

In 1958, the late Dr. George Pack and I edited nine volumes of books entitled *The Treatment of Cancer and Allied Diseases*. In the foreword to the entire series, we wrote the following:

> The editors paradoxically hope that these volumes may soon become obsolete with the discovery of more efficient means of curing cancer such as a chemotherapeutic remedy or better yet by the creation of an immunity against the disease. In the meantime, these manuals of present day therapy are offered with the wish that the best treatment plan now available can be instituted for any patient bearing any form of cancer.[1]

Today, chemotherapy of malignant melanoma remains provocative, and some encouraging results are being reported. The fact that malignant melanomas will respond to chemotherapy with objective shrinkage of the tumor and marked but often transient palliation to the patients evokes hope that these beneficial results may be consolidated and improved by more efficient drugs and immunotherapy.

The accomplishments of cancer chemotherapy must be judged in the light of the natural history of malignant melanoma, which is one of the most unpredictable diseases afflicting the human being. On one hand, there is a constant ebb and flow of tumor growth and spread, and on the other, there are immunologic attempts by the host to counter the growth. The cancer may lie dormant after local excision of the primary lesion, only to manifest itself in another organ, blood-borne to that organ, after a prolonged period (as long as 27 years in one of our patients) and then to grow wildly throughout the body and to kill the host (in a period as short as 6 weeks).

Age and sex of the patient, location of the primary tumor, genetic factors, and other as yet unknown features play a role in determining the natural history of a given melanoma. In fact, the same host may bear several primary melanomas, e.g., one that may be slow-growing and remain localized and another that may grow vertically, infiltrate deeply, and metastasize early.

Judging the effectiveness of cancer chemotherapy at present is further complicated by the fact that this treatment is mainly used for patients with far-advanced disease. Aust[2] calls attention to the fact that if a tumor weighs approximately 10 gm, it will have approximately 10 billion cells. If an agent is 99.9 per cent effective in killing the tumor, it still leaves 1 million cells for regrowth. This clearly demonstrates the burden placed upon cancer chemotherapy for patients with far-advanced disease that is located in different organs.

This article will describe the following types of melanoma chemotherapy: (1) systemic prophylactic (adjuvant) chemotherapy following hoped-for surgical cure of the primary neoplasm; (2) systemic chemotherapy for advanced cancer; (3) isolated perfusion for prophylaxis (adjuvant) therapy and for treatment of regional metastases in the offending limb; and (4) intra-arterial infusion cancer chemotherapy.

History

Many agents (immunologic and chemotherapeutic toxins and hormones) have been used in an attempt to treat malignant melanoma.[3] One of the first was the mixed toxins used by Coley in 1894,[4] which consisted of killed cultures of streptococci from patients with erysipelas. This method produced some mild, temporary results. Another was the Shear's polysaccharide, which consisted of bacterial filtrates of *Bacillus prodigiosus* and produced regression but was abandoned because of its severe toxicity.[5] Pack[6] noted a patient who had been bitten by a dog and who received rabies vaccine in treatment of the bite. The patient's disseminated melanoma spontaneously disappeared. Accordingly, Pack advocated rabies vaccine for treatment of melanoma. This method was used rather extensively by us for a while but since has been largely abandoned.[6] Various antibiotics were used in earlier years, including an endotoxin from killed *Trypanosoma cruzi* (K-R). Tamoxifen is now being intensely investigated as an anticancer agent, in view of the fact that estrogen receptors are often found on melanoma cells.

Chemotherapeutic Agents

Bellet and associates in 1977 used statistical methods to evaluate the observed rates of response to treatment.[7] Their search of the literature from 1950 to 1975 yielded 232 references. Their criterion for a minimum acceptable response was a 50 per cent decrease in the sum of the products of the perpendicular diameters of all measured lesions for at least 1 month. On this basis, only 128 articles and abstracts were acceptable for evaluation. They assessed 28 single agents that met the aforementioned criteria, of which six were alkylating agents, four were antimetabolites, four were antibiotics, and three were spindle inhibitors. Eleven agents had unknown or miscellaneous actions.

The pooled response data for each single agent were subjected to analysis in order for those agents that were therapeutically effective (i.e., at least a 95 per cent probability of the true response rate equal to or greater than 29 per cent) to be identified. Results of the analyses yielded only one drug, dacarbazine (DTIC), that met this requirement. In 1188 evaluable patients, 278 objective responses were reported, yielding an observed response rate of 23.4 per cent. Since none of the other drugs met the criterion, the authors concluded that DTIC is the most effective single agent in the treatment of malignant melanoma and stated that it can serve as a benchmark for other single- and multiple-drug therapy regimens. They further found that carmustine (BCNU), semustine (MeCCNU), and thiotepa revealed a probability of a true response rate equal to or greater than 10 per cent and therefore classified these drugs as potentially useful. Drugs that were classified as possibly useful were trimethylcolchicnic acid (TMCA), triethylenephosphoramide (TEPA), melphalan (L-PAM), dibromodulcitol (DBD), mitomycin-C (Mito-C), and methotrexate (MTX). Eight drugs were listed as probably not useful alone: streptozocin (STREPTZ), cyclophosphamide (TIC-Must), cyclophosphamide (CTS), cytosine arabinoside (ARA-C), chlorambucil (Leukeran), vinblastine (VLB), vincristine (VCR), and lomustine (CCNU). Drugs that were considered to have had adequate clinical trials and that were found not to be useful were 5-fluorouracil (5-FU), 6-mercaptopurine (6-MP), hexamethylmelamine (HXM), nitrogen mustard (HN_2), hydroxyurea (HU), bleomycin (BLEO), doxorubicin hydrochloride (ADRIA), actinomycin-D (ACT-D), and pregnanetrione (Pregnane).

Bellet and associates selected a 5 per cent improvement by a combined regimen as the minimum improvement and response rate that would justify subjecting patients to the additional toxicity and other nonacceptable factors involved in drug therapy. Of the 22 combination drug regimens that they tested for objectivity, 15 contained DTIC. They felt that of the 22 combination drugs tested, only the combination consisting of DTIC plus BCNU plus VCR plus HU could be classified as having a superior activity. Three combinations were classified as active: (1) DTIC plus BCNU plus VCR plus HU, (2) VLB plus procarbazine (Procarb) plus ACT-D, and (3) CCNU plus VCR.

Their final recommendation for current treatment is as follows: At present, DTIC is the drug of first choice in the treatment of patients with metastatic malignant melanoma. A nitrosourea (BCNU or MeCCNU) constitutes a second-line treatment. The authors currently recommend the addition of VCR to BCNU or MeCCNU because of the data suggesting some improvement in response rate without additive toxicity. The third-line treatment is problematic. The clinician can choose from among the following: (1) thiotepa or one of the potentially useful single agents; (2) a combination regimen that does not contain either DTIC or a nitrosurea; or (3) administration of untried drugs.

I have found 323 studies of melanoma chemotherapy reported between 1966 and 1982. With the exception of a few new drugs, such as *cis*-platinum dismine dichloride (CIS PT), ADRIA, piperzinedione, estramustine, cyclocytidine, azelaic acid, and others, as well as different combinations, no significant new advances have been reported since Bellet's study. Interferon has for the most part been disappointing. Certain drugs that had been frequently reported, such as L-PAM, MTX, and thiotepa, are now being used less commonly.

Systemic Chemotherapy

Systemic chemotherapy by the intravenous route is the form most frequently used. Since approximately 9000 individuals develop cutaneous melanoma in the United States each year, in a 5-year period there would be approximately 45,000 cases of melanoma. Because approximately 50 per cent of these people are not cured, there exists a period, from the time that curative surgical therapy has been found to be unsuccessful until the patient eventually succumbs to the cancer, during which there would be approximately 25,000 people in the United States bearing melanomas, practically all incurable, who would be candidates for systemic chemotherapy. The great demand for systemic chemotherapy makes this method an extremely important socioeconomic factor as well as a crucial medical modality.

Adjuvant Therapy

Systemic chemotherapy has been used for adjuvant therapy with various drugs (e.g., treating a patient with high-risk melanoma by the administration of various cancer chemotherapeutic agents systemically administered over a prolonged period).[8]

Kaufman and associates[9] randomized patients to receive DTIC, bacille Calmette Guérin (BCG), or both. In their report, there were 5 recurrences and 4 deaths in 19 patients treated with DTIC alone, 4 recurrences and 2 deaths in 24 patients receiving BCG, and no recurrences or deaths in patients receiving the combination. El Domeiri and coworkers[10] reported 5 of 15 patients alive and free of disease after 2 years of being treated with DTIC, in contrast with 8 of 15 who received BCG alone. McPherson[11] compared combination therapy of DTIC and oral BCG with a combination of BCNU, HU and DTIC plus BCG in 30 patients. The survival rate of those receiving the combination chemotherapy was superior to that of a historical control group, but neither group showed a prolongation of the disease-free interval.

Hill and colleagues,[12] in a composite evaluation, studied the effects of adjuvant DTIC. The disease-free survival period for treated patients was 40 weeks, versus 73 weeks for the control group—i.e., a better survival for the control group. Benjamin[13] believes that the poor results of this study might be caused by the fact that the DTIC was given only every 3 months and only for four courses. He also calls attention to the fact that nine protocols involving immunotherapy and chemotherapy showed an overall response rate of 28 per cent, somewhat higher than the 22 per cent for DTIC alone or the 24 per cent for nitrosoureas. There is no definite evidence that systemic chemotherapy destroys melanoma micrometastases, effects cures, or prolongs life.

Table 1. DRUG ABBREVIATIONS AND FULL
NAMES*

DTIC	Dacarbazine
DBD	Dibromodulcitol
MTX	Methotrexate
L-PAM	Melphalan
STREPTZ	Streptozocin
TMCA	Trimethylcolchicnic acid
VCR	Vincristine
TIC-Must	Cyclophosphamide
ARA-C	Cytosine arabinoside
Mito-C	Mitomycin-C
VLB	Vinblastine
6-MP	6-mercaptopurine
HXM	Hexamethylmelamine
HN_2	Nitrogen mustard
HU	Hydroxyurea
BLEO	Bleomycin
ADRIA	Doxorubicin hydrochloride (Adriamycin)
ACT-D	Actinomycin-D
Procarb	Procarbazine
6-TG	6-Thioguanine
DDP	*Cis*-diaminedichloroplatinum
Pregnane	Pregnanetrione
CIS PT	*Cis*-platinum dismine dichloride

*Modified from Bellet, R. D., et al.: Chemotherapy of metastatic melanoma. *In* Clark, W. H. (ed.): Human Malignant Melanoma. New York, Grune & Stratton, 1979, p. 325.

Palliation Therapy

Every conceivable drug has been used for the treatment of disseminated melanoma. Table 1 lists many of these drugs with their abbreviations, which are the terms most commonly used in clinical cancer chemotherapy.

All chemotherapeutic agents attempt to destroy the cell during its life cycle, and efforts are made to adapt certain agents to affect the cell during different periods of its cycle. The cycles are shown in Table 2, and the times that have been estimated for the various functions of the different cycles to be completed are also shown in this table (determined by two separate investigators). Thus, the alkylating agents affect rapidly multiplying cells, causing abnormalities in DNA. This therapy has not been successful, for the most part, for melanomas. The antimetabolites act during the S phase (DNA synthesis) and have also not proved to be very active. The Vinca alkaloids act on G-2 protein and on RNA synthesis and mitosis and have shown some activity against melanoma.

The drug that has shown the most effectiveness against melanoma is DTIC, which is also probably an alkylating agent; its response rates range from 17 per cent to 35 per cent.

Table 2. HUMAN MELANOMA CELL CYCLE
TIME

G.O. (resting)	
G.I. (DNA synthesis; ingredients)	16.3 hours*
S (replication of genome)	
G-2 (RNA and protein synthesis)	5.3 hours†
Mitosis	21.0 hours†

*Entire cycle + 36 hours. Data from Shirakawa, S., et al.: Cell proliferation in human melanoma. J. Clin. Invest. 49:1188, 1970.

†Data from Hagemann, R. F., and Schiffer, L. M.: Cell kinetic analyses of a human melanoma in vitro and in vivo-vitro. J. Natl. Cancer Inst. 47:519, 1971.

Various unknowns exist pertaining to the use of DTIC. For example, smaller doses produced better results than did larger doses in one series; females respond better than males to the drug; and patients with visceral metastases respond more poorly than do those with nonvisceral metastases. But the results, for the most part, seem to be transient. An interesting observation is that some lesions shrink or disappear, whereas others continue to progress. This suggests a variable population of cells.

Systemic Chemotherapy with Autogenous Marrow Transfusion

Between 1972 and 1982, a number of studies were performed using DTIC in combination with other drugs for patients with Stage IV melanoma, with relatively poor response rates.[7,14] Cohen and coauthors reported a response rate of 20 to 30 per cent lasting for over 30 weeks, with some patients living over a year. They believe their combination of drugs is not significantly better than DTIC alone.[15]

Several studies using combinations of chemotherapy, not including DTIC, have shown results similar to those with DTIC.[16] Didolker and colleagues, using a combination of CCNU and Procarb, had a response rate of approximately 25 per cent.[17] A combination of 5-FU and Procarb used by Nordman and associates[18] and a combination of DTIC, TIC-Must, VCR, and Procarb used by Byrne,[19] as well as a regimen of CCNU, VCR, and BLEO by DeWasch,[20] have shown response rates of between 35 and 48 per cent.

Accordingly, a number of drugs and drug combinations are available for systemic administration to offer meaningful palliation and, possibly, some prolongation of life, but these results are not too dramatic.

Gutterman and associates[21] have reported on 89 patients with disseminated melanoma who were treated with DTIC intravenously and BCG administered by scarification. These individuals were compared with 111 patients treated with DTIC alone. The chemoimmunotherapy-treated patients with metastases to the lymph nodes had a remission rate of 55 per cent, compared with 18 per cent for those treated with chemotherapy alone (P = 0.025). The duration of the remissions was longer, and chemoimmunotherapy was well tolerated without serious morbidity. The authors advocate this combination instead of chemotherapy as the sole modality. The addition of immunotherapy appears to enhance the effects of chemotherapy.

Neidhart and Dixon,[22] reporting on the Southwest Oncology Study, noted important variables in patients receiving combined chemotherapy and BCG. They observed a significant improvement in survival in patients whose purified protein derivative converted from negative to positive during therapy.

Presant and Bartolucci[23] reported from the Southeastern Cancer Study Group favorable prognostic variables to aid in stratification for further investigation.

Ariel and Pack[24,25] treated 31 patients with phenylalanine mustard. In order to administer a high dosage of the drug without hematologic complications, they withdrew 300 to 500 ml of bone marrow containing blood prior to administration and retransfused it intravenously 6 hours after giving the chemotherapeutic agent. Most of the phenylalanine mustard had been absorbed in the 6-hour period, and studies with tagged cells revealed that most of the intravenously administered marrow found residence in the bone marrow. Approximately two thirds of the patients benefited, both subjectively and objectively, from the treatment, but the improvement was all temporary, lasting from 1 to 10 months without significantly affecting longevity. Histologic studies of melanoma after this treatment revealed acute necrosis in metastatic melanoma within lymph nodes. Adding methotrexate to this regimen did not improve the results.[25]

McElwain and coworkers[26] performed a similar procedure and readministered the bone marrow 8 hours later without incident, except for one complete remission, in the eight patients treated. Cryopreserved marrow redelivered to the patient after a complete course of chemotherapy is now being investigated.

Regional Arterial Perfusion

The principle of this technique is to administer, for a short period, a large dose of a cancer chemotherapeutic agent introduced into the artery, which is attached to a pump oxygenator. The limb is perfused with the drug for approximately 2 hours. It was hoped that isolation could be accomplished, but there was always some escape, and therefore the term "regional perfusion" is preferred. This technique has been used for the arm (forequarter), the leg (hindquarter), the head and the neck (carotid artery infusion), and the pelvic area and the lower extremities (aortic infusion). The drug most frequently used has been phenylalanine mustard (Alkeran). Most of the reports describe the surgical removal of the primary lesion, with the perfusion used as adjuvant therapy to prevent metastases from occurring. In some instances, the patient suffered from Stage III melanoma, and the limb contained numerous deposits of melanoma. Hyperthermia has been used to enhance the effectiveness of the drug perfusion (Table 3).[27,28]

Rochlin, Wagner, and Rochlin reported before the 1972 International Melanoma Project in Sydney, Australia, on a study involving a total of 452 patients, of whom 238 were without evidence of metastases (Stage I). In 44 individuals, local recurrence was present within a distance of 5 cm (Stage II); 142 cases were classified as Stage III with multiple recurrent lesions scattered throughout the area included in the regional perfusion; and 28 patients had melanoma that had spread. The authors were quite optimistic about their results: There was a 92 per cent response of the Stage I group, who were free of melanoma; a 71 per cent response in the Stage II group; and a 43 per cent response of the Stage III group at the 3-year period.[29]

Krementz and associates reported on 714 patients with malignant melanoma who were treated, from 1957 through 1977, by chemotherapy administered by isolated regional perfusion of the limbs. The study also involved 56 patients who were treated by intra-arterial infusion.[30] The authors stated:

Excisional surgery and adjunctive perfusion in 286 patients with stage I disease resulted in cumulative survival rates of 87 per cent at five years and 75 per cent at ten and fifteen years. With recurrent or metastatic regional disease treated by perfusion alone or in combination with surgical excision, the survival rates were 36 per cent, 34 per cent, and 31 per cent at five, ten, and fifteen years, respectively. Even in the least favorable group, those with nodal and soft

Table 3. COLLECTED RESULTS OF TREATMENT OF PRIMARY MELANOMA OF LIMBS BY EXCISION AND CHEMOTHERAPY BY REGIONAL PERFUSION *

Author(s)	Number of Patients	Regional Lymph Node Dissection	Per Cent Survival
Stehlin (1975)	70	No	83.5 (5 yrs.)
Koops (1975)	30	NS†	77.0 (4 yrs.)
Sugarbaker and McBride (1976)	199	14/199	88.0 (5 yrs.)
Golomb (1976)	61	No	72.0 (5 yrs.)
Wagner (1976)	133	NS	94.0 (5 yrs.)
Davis (1976)	72	NS	90.0 (4 yrs.)
Jochimsen (1977)	21	Yes	100.0 (2 yrs.)

*From Krementz, E. T., et al.: The use of regional chemotherapy in the management of malignant melanoma. World J. Surg. 3:289, 1979. Used by permission.
†NS = Not stated.

tissue involvement, the survival rates were 27 per cent at five years and 22.5 per cent at ten and fifteen years. Analysis of 121 patients with stage I melanoma according to level of dermal invasion showed recurrence in 2 of 42 (4 per cent) patients with level III lesions, 11 of 75 (15 per cent) with level IV tumors, and 2 of 4 (50 per cent) with level V lesions. Recurrence rates by pathologic type were 2 of 49 (4 per cent) patients with superficial spreading melanoma, 6 of 30 (20 per cent) with nodular melanoma, and 5 of 14 (36 per cent) with acral lentiginous melanoma, the latter including subungual, plantar, or palmar lesions.[30]

Recurrences developed after perfusion in 35 patients. The mean length of time before recurrences was 2 years, with a range up to 9 years, from the date of perfusion. The investigations state that the rate of complications was relatively high and consisted of lymph sloughing and edema, which may have been related to the surgery. Five amputations were the direct result of complications of perfusion, and five additional patients had significant loss of limb function as a result of muscle contractures and sympathetic dystrophy. No patient had bone marrow depression severe enough to produce secondary infection or breathing difficulties. In 18 patients, further surgical procedures were necessary for management of the complications. Of the 111 patients who were available for analysis, 78 survived 4 to 13 years after their initial perfusion. Complications developed in 94 patients and were permanent in 34. Survival was correlated with both the depth of invasion of the primary lesion and the stage of the disease at the time of perfusion.

At the Ninth International Pigment Cell Conference, at which the aforementioned data were presented, the authors stated that this procedure is no longer being used at the Mayo Clinic. It should be noted that, in the Mayo experience, hyperthermia has been induced to increase the efficacy of the chemotherapeutic agents. In 1967, Cavaliere and associates[31] suggested that hyperthermia be used without chemotherapy. Stehlin[27] believes that hyperthermic perfusion is superior, and Golomb[32] uses it exclusively, increasing the circulating blood temperature to 43°C. He also increases the duration of perfusion up to 2 hours, and his complication rate is an acceptable one.

Stehlin and coworkers,[28] who instituted the method of hyperthermia, have reported the benefits as follows:

> Since 1967, we have used a system of hyperthermic perfusion with melphalan to treat patients with melanoma of the extremities. This report presents additional follow-up data on 165 patients, first reported on in 1975, who underwent 185 perfusions. The 70 patients classified as stage I (Stehlin classification system) had a 5-year survival rate of 86.3 per cent. The 5-year survival rate for the 73 patients with stage II and stage III disease was 52.5 per cent. There was a dramatic increase in the 5-year survival rate for patients with stage IIIA disease, from 22.2 per cent prior to the use of heat to 74 per cent for 30 patients undergoing hyperthermic perfusion.[28]

Sugarbaker and McBride[33] conducted an analysis of the results of treatment at the M.D. Anderson Hospital in Houston, Texas, where isolation perfusion with L-phenylalanine mustard was performed on 199 patients with invasive Stage I melanoma of the extremities. The survival rate of patients followed for 5 to 15 years was determined to be 83 per cent. The authors state that the survival rates were 98 per cent in 2 years, 88 per cent in 5 years, and 84 per cent in 10 years. Failures involved local recurrence in 2 per cent of the cases. Three per cent of the patients developed in-transit recurrence, 13 per cent developed positive regional lymph nodes, 8 per cent developed systemic metastases, and one patient developed a local recurrence plus positive regional nodes. Of the 49 patients failing treatment, 14 (31 per cent) are surviving after treatment of their recurrence. Sugarbaker and McBride believe that survival has probably been improved by their therapy. Their method of therapy was further evaluated in a study involving 14 patients treated by perfusion alone, without local excision. The authors state that in the regional control the survival was poor, and they conclude that the primary tumor should be locally excised, widely, but that the regional perfusion may be effective in controlling regional subclinical disease.

Table 4. COLLECTED RESULTS OF CHEMOTHERAPY OF METASTATIC MELANOMA CONFINED TO THE LIMB BY REGIONAL PERFUSION*

Author(s)	Stage†	Number of Patients	Surgical Therapy	5-Year Survival Percentage
McBride (1971)	II		Excision	57
Koops (1975)	II and III	35	RLND‡ in some; number not stated	23
Shingleton (1975)	III	43	RLND if not done previously	28
Stehlin et al. (1975)	II and III	73	Excision if appropriate	48.2
Golomb (1976)	III	85	Excision if appropriate	22
Wagner (1976)	II	41	Most with RLND	68
Davis (1976)	III	39	Excision and RLND	33.3
McBride (1978)	IIIA	40	Excision if appropriate	51
	IIIB	16	Excision if appropriate	33
	IIIAB	14	Excision if appropriate	14

*From Krementz, E. T., et al.: The use of regional chemotherapy in the management of malignant melanoma. World J. Surg. 3:289, 1979. Used by permission.
†M. D. Anderson staging.
‡RLND = Regional lymph node dissection.

In Golomb's series,[40] 66 patients with recurrent melanoma limited to one extremity were perfused. Forty-four (60 per cent) had complete disappearance of detectable tumor. The disease eventually recurred in two thirds of these patients, but 13 (30 per cent) are still free of tumor 6 to 176 months later. Seventeen per cent were alive 5 to 14 years after recurrent disease was perfused. Eleven of those whose disease recurred were perfused a second or third time (Table 4).

I have found 20 references in the English literature written between 1966 and 1982 dealing with isolation perfusion.

It does seem that regional perfusion of cancer chemotherapeutic agents plays a role in delaying the onset of metastases and, possibly, in curing small metastases. The method is of limited use, however, because it is cumbersome and has a high rate of complications. It has been used for over 20 years, but in relatively few institutions. Certain institutions that used this technique in the past, such as the Mayo Clinic, have abandoned it. Apparently, the morbidity and complexity of the treatment were considered as outweighing its accomplishments.

Ariel developed a simple pump by which he perfused phenylalanine mustard without the bubble-oxygenation of the perfusate. He treated 40 patients with this technique, perfusing for ± 30 minutes. Eighteen of the patients treated had Stage I or II melanomas, and 22 had regional satellitoses (Stage III). The results were more or less similar to those advocated by physicians who used oxygenation.[34]

Intra-arterial Infusion

Intra-arterial infusion differs from intra-arterial perfusion in that a catheter is placed in an artery proximal to the area to be infused. Using a pressure pump, one gives a continuous infusion to the extremity over a prolonged period, which varies from several days to several months. Techniques have been described by Creech and associates,[35] Bierman and coworkers,[36] and Golomb and colleagues.[40] The sites most suitable for infusion are the extremities and the pelvic region. The technique originated and advocated by Sullivan[37] is to infuse a dose of 500 mg of methotrexate over 24 hours and to give 6 mg of citrovorum factor (Leucovorin) intramuscularly every 4 to 6 hours. Many drugs have been used for infusion, but the one we have used most frequently is phenylalanine mustard. More recently, we have been using *cis*-platinum.

Complications that may occur are dislodging of the catheter and sepsis. The use of a heparinized infusate will prevent clogging of the catheter. Systemic toxicity is greater with infusion than with perfusion.[38]

Clark[39] reported on 17 patients with advanced regional malignant melanoma who were treated with intra-arterial infusion therapy with DTIC for isolated inoperable lesions. There were six partial objective responses and one complete remission in his study, for an overall response rate of 41 percent. Toxicity was less than that usually seen with systemic chemotherapy using DTIC, and the local response was higher.

We have treated 55 patients with intra-arterial infusion for extensive melanoma of the extremities. There was an objective response in 35 individuals and an apparent complete response in 5. There was no increased longevity. We have not used infusion as an adjuvant following surgery for the primary lesion with or without lymphadenectomy. The results of treatment by intra-arterial infusion are shown in Table 5.

Intra-arterial infusion can be used for those patients in whom isolation perfusion therapy is not suitable, such as those with an unacceptable operative risk or those who have failed to respond to perfusion or direct intralesional immunotherapy or chemotherapy. Intra-arterial infusion is the treatment of choice for disease confined to a region that cannot be isolated by tourniquet, such as the head and neck area, the proximal limb, or the liver. It is preferable for drugs requiring prolonged or continuous administration, such as the antimetabolites, and it can be used for palliation of regional diseases and, at times, for making advanced diseases operable.

Golomb[40] has treated 62 patients with primary melanoma by surgery plus infusion. Seven melanomas were of the upper extremity, and 54 involved the lower extremity. Today, 54 patients (72 per cent) are free of disease, 8 (13 per cent) are living with disease, and 9 (15 per cent) have died of recurrent melanoma with distant metastases. Of the 35 patients treated more than 5 years ago, 23 (66 per cent) are living. Of these patients, 19 were in Stage III (that is, with regional lymph node metastases) at the time of operation 5 or more years ago. Of these Stage III patients, eight (42 per cent) are living. Ten of the patients received actinomycin-D as a chemotherapeutic agent; of these, cancer recurred in two. Five were given thiotepa alone, and four were given thiotepa and melphalan combined. The rest received melphalan alone.

Table 5. COLLECTED RESULTS OF CHEMOTHERAPY OF MELANOMA BY INTRA-ARTERIAL INFUSION*

Author(s)	Drug	Patients Treated	Complete Response	Percentage of Objective Responses
Westburg (1967)	Epodyl, mitopodozide (podophyllin derivative), procarbazine	75	4	69 (32/46)
Oberfield and Sullivan (1969)	MTX, 5-FU	33	1	59 (17/29)
Savlov, Hall, and Oberfield (1971)	DTIC	6	2	33 (2/6)
Einhorn et al. (1973)	DTIC	17	1	41 (6/17)
Jortnay (1977)	DTIC	4	—	50 (2/4)

*From Krementz, E. T., et al.: The use of regional chemotherapy in the management of malignant melanoma. World J. Surg. 3:289, 1979. Used by permission.

Jonsson and coworkers[41] treated 17 patients with intra-arterial infusion using DTIC both as an adjunct and for palliation and observed minimal effects.

Banzet and colleagues[13] gave intra-arterially combined chemotherapy to a group of patients who had lesions categorized as Clark's levels III and IV. They noted an 81 per cent survival at 21 months among those patients receiving intra-arterial therapy in contrast with 68 per cent survival among those receiving surgery alone. Preoperative chemotherapy had no beneficial effect.

With this mode of treatment, there is accordingly moderate palliation and a suggestion that the onset of metastases is delayed, or even prevented, but there is no spectacular curing of metastases. It has been suggested that some micrometastases can be destroyed by this technique.

We are now applying a tourniquet distally to the lesion for adjuvant treatment of local metastases and injecting a bolus of 100 mg DTIC, 50 mg ADRIA, and 50 mg CIS PT with pressure maintained on the artery and vein proximal to the site of injection. It is too early to remark on the efficacy of this regiment.

SUMMARY

1. Chemotherapy does produce objective responses by shrinking and partially destroying melanoma, but no cures of existing melanomas can be attributed to chemotherapy.

2. A wide variety of drugs have been used. DTIC appears to be the best available agent to date. Other drugs, either in combination with or instead of DTIC, have been useful.

3. Systemic adjuvant chemotherapy has not been successful in controlling dissemination of melanoma but does offer moderate palliation.

4. Regional perfusion may be useful in delaying or preventing regional metastases from developing. It has also proved useful in controlling some cases of regional spread. Because of the complexity of the method, it is used in relatively few institutions.

5. Intra-arterial infusion has resulted in debatable accomplishments both as an adjuvant and as a therapeutic method of chemotherapy.

6. A combination of chemotherapy and immunotherapy appears promising. The accomplishments of chemotherapy in controlling or combating malignant melanoma are meager to date.

7. The use of regional chemotherapy for in-transit metastases or for satellitoses has been a welcome substitute for amputation, which previously was often used for treating these lesions.

References

1. Pack, G. T., and Ariel, I. M.: Principles of treatment. *In* Pack, G. T., and Ariel, I. M. (eds.): The Treatment of Cancer and Allied Diseases, vol 1. New York, Paul Hoeber & Co., 1958, p. 18.
2. Aust, J. B.: Melanoma and chemotherapy. *In* Ariel, I. M. (ed.): Progress in Clinical Cancer, vol 6. New York, Grune & Stratton, 1975, pp. 199–204.
3. Gutterman, J. U., Mavligit, G., McBridge, C., et al.: Active immunotherapy with BCG for recurrent malignant melanoma. Lancet 1:1208, 1973.
4. Coley, W. B.: The treatment of inoperable malignant tumors with the toxins of erysipelas and the *Bacillus prodigiosus*. Trans. Am. Surg. Assoc. 12:183, 1894.
5. Shear, M. J., and Turner, F. C.: Chemical treatment of tumors: Nature of hemorrhage-producing fraction from *Serratia marcescens* (*Bacillus prodigiosus*) culture filtrate. J. Natl. Cancer Inst. 5:81, 1943.
6. Pack, G. T.: A note on the experimental use of rabies vaccine for melanomatosis. Arch. Dermatol. Syphilol. 62:694, 1950.
7. Bellet, R. D., Mastrangelo, N. J., Berd, D., and Lustbader, E.: Randomized prospective phase III trial of

methyl-CCNU (NSC-95441) alone versus methyl-CCNU plus vincristine (NSC-67574) in the treatment of patients with metastatic malignant melanoma. Proc. Am. Soc. Clin. Oncol. 18:284, 1977.

8. Wood, W. C., Cosimi, A. B., Carey, R. W., and Kaufman, S. D.: Randomized trial of adjuvant therapy for "high-risk" primary malignant melanoma. Surgery 83:677, 1978.

9. Kaufman, S. D., Carey, R. W., Cosimin, A. B., and Wood, W. C.: Randomized trial of adjuvant therapy for high-risk primary malignant melanoma. Proc. Am. Assoc. Cancer Res. 19:374, 1978.

10. El Domeiri, A. A., Das Gupta, T. K., Trippon, M., et al.: Adjuvant therapy of melanoma. Proc. Am. Assoc. Cancer Res. 18:178, 1977.

11. McPherson, T. A., Paterson, A. H., Willans, D., and Watson, M.: Malignant melanoma (stage IIIB): A pilot study of adjuvant chemo-immunotherapy. In Salmon, W. E., and Jones, S. E. (eds.): Adjuvant Therapy of Cancer, Amsterdam, Elsevier/North Holland Biomedical Press, 1977, pp. 439–446.

12. Hill, G. J., Moss, S., Fletcher, W., et al.: DTIC melanoma adjuvant study: Final report. Proc. Am. Assoc. Cancer Res. 18:309, 1978.

13. Benjamin, R. X.: Chemotherapy of malignant melanoma. World J. Surg. 3:321, 1979.

14. Banzet, P., Jacquillat, D., Civatte, J., et al.: Adjuvant chemotherapy in the management of primary malignant melanoma. Cancer 41:1240, 1978.

15. Cohen, S. M., Greenspan, E. M., Weiner, N. J., and Karakow, B.: Triple combination chemotherapy of disseminated melanoma. Cancer 29:1489, 1972.

16. Bellet, R. D., Mastrangelo, D. B., and Lustbader, E.: Chemotherapy of metastatic melanoma. In Clark, W. H., et al. (eds.): Human Malignant Melanoma, New York, Grune & Stratton, 1979, pp. 325–354.

17. Didolkar, M. S., Baffi, R. R., Catane, R., et al.: Use of methyl-CCNU and procarbazine in advanced malignant melanoma resistant to DTIC therapy. Cancer Treat. Rep. 61:1738, 1977.

18. Nordman, E. M., and Mantyla, M.: Treatment of metastatic melanoma with combined 5-fluorouracil and procarbazine. Cancer Treat. Rep. 61:1709, 1977.

19. Byrne, N. J.: Cyclophosphamide, vincristine and procarbazine in the treatment of malignant melanoma. Cancer 38:1922, 1976.

20. DeWasch, G., Bernheim, J., Michel, J., et al.: Combination chemotherapy with three marginally effective agents, CCNU, vincristine, and bleomycin, in the treatment of stage III melanoma. Cancer Treat. Rep. 60:1273, 1976.

21. Gutterman, J. U., Mavligit, G., Gottlieb, J. A., et al.: Chemoimmunotherapy of disseminated malignant melanoma with dimethyl triazeno imidazole carboxamide and Bacillus Calmette-Guerin. N. Engl. J. Med. 291:592, 1974.

22. Neidhart, J., and Dixon, D.: Combination chemotherapy plus BCG in the treatment of disseminated malignant melanoma: A Southwest Oncology Group study. Med. Pediatr. Oncol. 10:251, 1982.

23. Presant, C. A., and Bartolucci, A. A.: Prognostic factors in metastatic malignant melanoma: The Southeastern Cancer Study Group experience. Cancer 49:2192, 1982.

24. Ariel, I. M., and Pack, G. T.: Treatment of disseminated melanoma with phenylalanine mustard (melphalan) and autogenous bone marrow transplants. Surgery 51:583, May 1962.

25. Ariel, I. M., and Pack, G. T.: Treatment of disseminated melanoma with systemic melphalan, methotrexate and autogenous bone marrow transplants. Cancer 20:77, Jan. 1967.

26. McElwain, T. J., Hedley, D. W., Burton, E., et al.: Marrow autotransplantation accelerates haematological recovery in patients with malignant melanoma treated with high-dose melphalan. Br. J. Cancer 40:72, 1979.

27. Stehlin, J. S., Jr.: Hyperthermic perfusion with chemotherapy for cancer of the extremities. Surg. Gynecol. Obstet. 129:305, 1969.

28. Stehlin, J. S., Jr., Giovanella, B. C., Ipolyi, P. D., and Anderson, R. F.: Eleven years' experience with hyperthermic perfusion for melanoma of the extremities. World J. Surg. 3:305, 1979.

29. Rochlin, D. B., Wagner, D. E., and Rochlin, S.: The therapy of malignant melanoma as treated by regional perfusion. In Melanoma and Skin Cancer: Proceedings of the International Cancer Conference. Sydney, Australia, Government Printer, 1972, pp. 443–451.

30. Krementz, E. T., Carter, R. D., Sutherland, C. M., and Campbell, M.: The use of regional chemotherapy in the management of malignant melanoma. World J. Surg. 3:289, 1979.

31. Cavaliere, R., Ciogatto, E. C., Giovanella, B. C., et al.: Selective heat sensitivity of cancer cells: Biochemical and clinical studies. Cancer 20:1351, 1967.

32. Golomb, F. M.: Invited commentary on: Krementz, E. T., et al.: Chemotherapy for malignant melanoma. World J. Surg. 3:302, 1979.

33. Sugarbaker, E. V., and McBride, C. M.: The results of isolation-perfusion for invasive image I melanoma of the extremities. Cancer 37:188, 1976.

34. Ariel, I. M.: A simplified method of isolation perfusion of anticancer drugs. Am. J. Surg. 104:82, 1962.

35. Creech, O., Jr., Krementz, E. T., Ryan, R. F., and Winblad, J. N.: Chemotherapy of cancer: Regional perfusion utilizing an extracorporeal circuit. Ann. Surg. 148:616, 1958.

36. Bierman, H. R., Shimkin, M. B., Buron, R. L., Jr., et al.: The effects of intra-arterial administration of nitrogen mustard, abstracted. Paris, Fifth International Cancer Congress, 1950, p. 186.

37. Sullivan, R. D., Miller, E., and Sykes, M. P.: Antimetabolite-metabolite combination cancer chemotherapy. Effects of intra-arterial methotrexate–intramuscular citrovorum factor therapy in human cancer. Cancer 12:1238, 1959.

38. Savlov, E. D., Hall, T. C., and Oberfield, R. A.: Intra-arterial therapy of melanoma with dimethyl triazeno imidazole carboxamide (NSC-45388). Cancer 28:1161, 1971.

39. Clark, R. H.: The evolution of therapy for malignant melanoma at the University of Texas, M. D. Anderson

Hospital and Tumor Institute: 1950 to 1975. *In* Riley, V. (ed.): Melanoma: Basic Properties and Clinical Behavior, New York, S. Karger, 1977, pp. 365–378.

40. Golomb, F. M.: Perfusion. *In* Andrade, R., et al. (eds.): Cancer of the Skin: Biology, Diagnosis, and Management, vol 2. Philadelphia, W.B. Saunders, Co., 1976, p. 1623.
41. Jonsson, P. E., Agrup, G., Arnbjornsson, E., et al.: Treatment of malignant melanoma with dacarbazin (DTIC/DOME) with special reference to urinary excretion of 5-S-Cysteinyldopa. Cancer 45:245, 1980.
42. Bellet, R. D., Mastrangelo, M. J., Laucius, J. F., and Bodurtha, A. J.: Randomized prospective trial of DTIC (NSC-45388) alone versus BCNU (NSC-409962) plus vincristine (NSC-67574) in the treatment of metastatic malignant melanoma. Cancer Treat. Rep. 60:595, 1976.
43. Banzet, P., Jacquillat, C., Civatte, J., et al.: Adjuvant chemotherapy in the management of primary malignant melanoma. Cancer 41:1240, 1978.
44. Creagan, E. T., Ingle, J. N., Ahmann, D. L., and Green, S. H.: Phase II study of high-dose tamoxifen (NSC-180973) in patients with disseminated malignant melanoma. Cancer 49:1353, 1982.
45. Davis, C. D., Ivins, J. C., and Soule, E. H.: Mayo Clinic experience with isolated limb perfusion for invasive malignant melanoma of the extremities. *In* Melanomas: Basic Properties and Clinical Behavior, vol. 2, Proceedings of the Ninth International Pigment Cell Conference, Houston, Texas, 1975. New York, S. Karger, 1976, p. 379.
46. Davis, N. C.: Invited commentary on: Hersh, J. T., et al.: Combined modality therapy of malignant melanoma. World J. Surg. 3:329, 1979.
47. Herbst, W. P.: Malignant melanoma of choroid with extensive metastasis treated by removing secreting tissue of testicles. JAMA 122:597, 1943.
48. Hersh, E. M., Jordan, W., Gutterman, M. D., and McBride, C. M.: Combined modality therapy of malignant melanoma. World J. Surg. 3:329, 1979.
49. Howes, W. E.: Castration for advanced malignant growth—short historical review and case report. Radiology 43:272, 1944.
50. Howes, W. E.: Removal of testes in treatment of melanoma. JAMA 123:304, 1943.
51. Krieger, H., Abbott, W. E., Levey, S., and Babb, L.: Bilateral total adrenalectomy in patients with metastatic carcinoma. Surg. Gynecol. Obstet. 97:569, 1953.
52. Leichman, C. G., Samson, M. K., and Baker, L. H.: Phase II trial of tamoxifen in malignant melanoma. Cancer Treat. Rep. 66:1447, 1982.
53. McCune, W. S.: Discussion of: Ochsner, A., and Harpole, D. H.: Malignant melanoma. Ann. Surg. 155:636, 1962.
54. Schraffordt, J., Koops, H., Beekhuis, H., et al.: Local recurrence and survival in patients with (Clark Level IV/V and over 1.5 mm thickness) Stage I malignant melanoma of the extremities after regional perfusion. Cancer 48:1952, Nov. 1981.
55. Shimkin, M.: Effects of surgical hypophysectomy in many with malignant melanoma. J. Clin. Endocrinol. 12:439, 1952.
56. Shingelton, W. W., Seigler, H. F., Stocks, L. H., and Dows, R. W., Jr.: Management of recurrent melanoma of the extremity. Cancer 35:574, 1975.
57. Theirs, B. H.: Chemotherapy of malignant melanoma. J. Am. Acad. Dermatol. 6:412, 1982.

IMMUNOTHERAPY OF MALIGNANT MELANOMA*

Bijan Safai, M.D.

The natural history of malignant melanoma suggests that the tumor growth is under host control and that patients with melanoma respond immunologically to their tumor. Because of this, melanoma has been the subject of many immunologic investigations. Clinical observations suggesting that immunologic factors affect the course of melanoma include: (1) waxing and waning of melanoma lesions and considerable individual differences in the rate of progression;[1] (2) spontaneous disappearance of the primary tumor with or without malignant cells' remaining in the regional lymph nodes;[2-10] (3) regression of the tumor following a blood transfusion;[11] (4) spontaneous regression of metastatic melanoma lesions;[12,13] and (5) an increased incidence of melanoma in patients who are immunosuppressed. In addition, lymphocytic or histiocytic infiltrates in primary melanoma, which often are associated with regression of the tumor and are correlated with a good prognosis,[14] further indicate the role of host defense in this disease.

These observations clearly suggest (but do not prove) that immunologic factors affect the course of melanoma. Conclusive evidence will be provided only by the demonstration that melanoma cells carry melanoma-specific antigens and that these antigens elicit an immune response in the host. Because of this anticipated demonstration and the observations enumerated previously, melanoma has been an important disease for the investigation of tumor immunology in humans, and extensive work, including research into the immunotherapy of melanoma, already has been done with interesting results. Since these investigations are too extensive for inclusion here, readers are referred to the available literature on tumor immunology of melanoma. This review will provide only a brief description of current knowledge of the immunotherapy of melanoma.

Although the majority of primary melanomas can be cured surgically (depending on the type of melanoma, the thickness and level of the tumor, the location, and the size), recurrent or metastatic tumors in regional or distant sites present a poor prognosis, and available conventional therapies can provide only palliative measures. Thus, interest in the immunotherapy of melanoma has developed because of both the absence of an effective therapy and the existence of clinical and laboratory data suggesting that melanoma cells express tumor-associated antigens and that these antigens elicit a host immune response.

Local Immunotherapy

Local immunotherapy actually started with observations by Coley that direct inoculation of extracts of streptococci and *Serratia* into various human sarcomas resulted in local regression of metastatic solid tumors.[15] Klein and his coworkers have applied these principles in the last two decades and have demonstrated a high cure rate for basal cell epithelioma and squamous cell cancer.[16,17] In melanoma, partial or complete resolution of metastatic tumors has been reported following delayed-hypersensitivity reactions to dinitrochlorobenzene,[17] with regression observed in challenged as well as unchallenged lesions.[17,18]

*The author wishes to acknowledge Dr. S. Blum's valuable advice and editorial assistance, Ms. N. Peralta's help in compiling the literature cited, and Ms. L. Asadorian's expert technical assistance.

In 1970, Hunter-Craig reported that local injection of live vaccinia virus resulted in complete regression in six, and partial regression in three, of the ten treated lesions of malignant melanoma,[19] thus suggesting that the delayed hypersensitivity reaction to vaccinia virus can lead to regression of melanoma lesions. In the same year, Morton demonstrated that direct injection of bacille Calmette Guérin into cutaneous melanoma lesions could induce tumor regression in immunocompetent patients.[20] Following these initial observations, intralesional bacille Calmette Guérin therapy for metastatic melanoma was adopted by a large number of investigators, who have reported generally similar findings.[21–40]

Histologic studies of treated lesions have identified melanin-laden macrophages and a chronic granulomatous reaction. Mastrangelo and coworkers have reported that even in uninoculated subcutaneous metastases, which show no clinical regression, lymphocytic infiltration in the fibrous tissue surrounding the nodules may be seen.[25] Lieberman and coworkers reported an increased lymphocyte proliferative response to phytohemagglutinin in all and to melanoma antigens in most patients who have responded to intratumoral inoculation with bacille Calmette Guérin.[26] In contrast, the nonresponders did not show increased lymphocyte stimulation. Leukocyte migration inhibition to melanoma antigens converted from negative to positive in 50 per cent of the cases after therapy, whereas a marked increase was seen in active rosette-forming cells in all responders. The histopathologic response to bacille Calmette Guérin resembled the histologic changes seen in a halo nevus.[26,41,42]

The work of Seigler and coworkers[28] on the immunotherapy of melanoma, which confirms that of other investigators, showed that regression of established tumors occurred in 65 to 70 per cent of patients with melanoma. Thirty-one per cent of these patients experienced a 2-year tumor-free survival. Although there appears to be specific cytotoxicity to melanoma-associated tumor antigens in patients receiving bacille Calmette Guérin, in vitro incubation of melanoma patients' leukocytes with melanoma cells did not augment cytotoxicity.[27] The data from 14 investigators who have been pooled by Mastrangelo[43] reveal that approximately 66 per cent of patients treated with intralesional bacille Calmette Guérin showed regression of injected nodules, whereas 21 per cent showed regression of uninjected nodules as well. Approximately 27 per cent of treated individuals demonstrated complete remission of all clinically measurable tumors. These patients were all immunocompetent, with small tumor burdens limited to the cutaneous tissues. It is concluded that the regression of injected and uninjected metastasis is seen only in patients with dermal disease and that the regressed uninjected lesions are located in proximity to the injected ones and in the same body region.

Other immunostimulants also have been used topically and intralesionally in the treatment of dermal lesions of recurrent melanoma. A variety of antigens, such as purified protein derivative,[44] methanol-extracted residue,[45,46] cell wall skeleton,[47] Corynebacterium parvum,[39] dinitrochlorobenzene,[48] vaccinia virus,[19,49] and smallpox vaccine,[50] have been used. The results of the trial with these agents appear to be similar to those obtained with bacille Calmette Guérin, and it is believed that they have mechanisms of action similar to that of bacille Calmette Guérin. The advantage of using these agents over bacille Calmette Guérin is the absence of serious systemic complications, which include the development of fever, chills, reversible hepatic dysfunction, jaundice and noncaseating granulomas, and systemic bacille Calmette Guérin disease.[29,51–53] Thus, the use of nonviable fractions of bacterial adjuvants has a strong appeal for local immunotherapy.

Local immunotherapy also has been used preoperatively in the treatment of the primary melanoma. Vaccinia virus,[54] dinitrochlorobenzene,[55] and bacille Calmette Guérin[56] all have been used prior to definitive surgical therapy, and the results of these studies suggest that preoperative treatment with these agents has been advantageous to patients. However, the number of subjects is too small to allow for generalization of the therapeutic benefit, and further investigation of presurgical intralesional therapy in the treatment of high-risk melanoma patients is warranted.

Adoptive Immunotherapy

Adoptive immunotherapy is based on the use of subcellular fractions or immune lymphocytes. Among subcellular fractions, transfer factor and immune RNA should be mentioned. Promising results have been reported by Oettgen and coworkers,[57] who have used transfer factor in the treatment of patients with breast cancer and by Spitler and his colleagues,[58] who have used this factor for the treatment of melanoma. Results of trials with immune RNA also appear to be promising.[59] Following immunization of sheep or guinea pigs with human malignant melanoma, immune RNA was extracted from the lymphoid organ of these animals. Such immune RNA has been shown to convert nonimmune human lymphocytes into cytotoxic cells effectively against human melanoma cells. Immune RNA extracted from lymphocytes of cured melanoma patients also has been reported to help normal human lymphocytes kill malignant melanoma cells.[60] Interferon also can be considered among the subcellular fractions and has been used in the treatment of malignant melanoma.[61,62] Although further studies are under way, preliminary data do not appear to be promising.

In vitro phytohemagglutinin-activated lymphocytes have been used intravenously by Frenster in the treatment of patients with lung metastasis,[63] among whom tumor regression was noted. A decrease in the size of melanoma nodules and a rise of tumor-specific antibodies were described by Lewis and his coworkers, who used intravenous injections of phytohemagglutinin.[64] In vitro sensitization of lymphocytes against melanoma-associated antigens also has been reported.[65] In general, adoptive immunotherapy using immune lymphocytes or subcellular fractions may provide an effective approach to the treatment of malignant melanoma and other types of cancer.

Passive Immunotherapy

Heterologous, allogeneic, and autologous sera have been used in the treatment of a large number of cancer patients, but careful documentation of clinical responses has not been carried out.[66-70] Some reports are of historical interest, however. Summer and Foraker reported a complete response of a patient with disseminated melanoma who received 250 ml of whole blood from another melanoma patient whose tumor had undergone spontaneous regression,[71] and Teimourian and McCune also have reported on a similar melanoma case.[72] Transient but definite responses have been reported in patients with chronic lymphocytic leukemia to infusions of allogeneic plasma or sera.[73-75] A favorable response to heterologous antithymocyte globulin has been reported in a patient with cutaneous T-cell lymphoma.[76] There is no evidence that these tumor responses resulted from the presence of antibody in the sera that was directed against tumor cell surface antigens.

Although passive administration of antibodies to cancer patients has a long history, careful and controlled studies have been hindered by the absence of the specific antibody, the irreproducibility of batches, and the scarcity of supplies. In addition, toxicity produced by large doses of heterologous sera may be quite severe, requiring extensive therapy. The hybridoma technology, however, has resulted in a revival of the possible use of antibodies in cancer therapy. The availability of monoclonal antibodies will allow careful and reproducible in vitro and in vivo studies.

Monoclonal antibodies that react with human tumor cells have become available over the past few years. These include monoclonal antibodies to colon cancer,[77] renal cancer,[78] lung cancer,[79] breast cancer,[80] neuroblastoma,[81] and malignant melanoma.[82-88] To date, none of these mouse monoclonal antibodies are tumor-specific, and most have been shown to react with at least a few normal cell types. It is conceivable that mouse B cells might recognize only certain antigens or tumor cells; therefore, human monoclonal antibodies produced by human × human or human × mouse hybrids may recognize different determinants from those of mouse monoclonal antibodies. In addition, human × human monoclonal antibodies may be free of some of the potential for development of hypersensitivity reactions to heterologous protein.[89,90] The major problem with human × human hybrids is the choice of appropriate fusion partners. In addition, the ethical and practical considerations involved in immunizing humans with cancer cells must be taken into account.

Passive immunotherapy using mouse monoclonal antibodies is still in the experimental stage. Studies of laboratory animals have demonstrated that transplanted leukemias in mice can be cured if treatment with monoclonal antibodies is started 1 to 2 days after tumor inoculation,[91,92] and it also has been shown that metastatic spread can be prevented at the inoculation site.[91] The growth of human colorectal cancers transplanted into nude mice was successfully suppressed with monoclonal antibodies raised against this tumor when the antibody was administered immediately after tumor inoculation.[93]

Mouse monoclonal antibodies have been used for the treatment of human leukemia and lymphomas.[94-97] These early reports demonstrated some transient antitumor effects for the monoclonal antibodies and showed that toxicity produced by hypersensitivity to heterologous proteins will not limit therapeutic trials of mouse monoclonal antibodies. The mechanism of therapeutic effects of these monoclonal antibodies is not clear, but it may be a result of direct inhibition of cell proliferation by blocking surface receptors or of some other mechanism, such as antibody-dependent cell-mediated cytotoxicity.[98]

For many years, attempts have been made to detect tumors by means of radiolabeled heterologous antibody. The difficulties encountered include: (1) lack of specificity, low purity, and weak titer of antibody; (2) instability of radiolabeled antibody complex and modification of the antibody combining site; and (3) location of the tumor, vascularity, density of the cell surface antigen, and concentration of circulating tumor antigen. Several reports, however, have been more encouraging.[99-103] In addition to their use for tumor detection, radiolabeled and drug-labeled antibodies have been used for therapeutic purposes.[104] An interesting observation was made by Ghose and coworkers,[105] who used cell surface heterologous antibodies against a human malignant melanoma bound to chlorambucil. The antibody-chlorambucil complex resulted in complete remission in a patient with disseminated malignant melanoma.

Some other reports[106,107] have described the use of antibodies directed against tumor-associated antigens, coupled with cytotoxic agents, to improve the therapeutic index.[108,109]

Active Specific Immunization

The basis of tumor immunology is the hypothesis that transition to the malignant state results in changes in the cell surface antigens. It is believed that the cancer cell can be distinguished from the normal cell by the presence of these distinctive antigens on its surface and that these antigens are targets for recognition and rejection by the immune system (immunosurveillance). The evidence supporting this assumption comes primarily from transplantation experiments on laboratory animals with tumors induced by chemical carcinogens or viruses, although not all tumors among experimental animals are immunogenic in transplantation experiments. The lack of such immunogenicity, however, does not necessarily imply the absence of tumor-specific antigens but rather may be related to the complex interactions involved in immunologic recognition and rejection by the host. In addition, certain antigens may not elicit the production of antibody, and their detection therefore may depend on the methods used to measure cellular immunity.

Despite the vast amount of literature dealing with the question of tumor-specific surface antigens of human cancers, the existence of such antigens still must be considered to be in the realm of speculation. The critical issue is that of specificity and demonstration of tumor-specific surface antigens by serologic or cell-mediated immune reactions. To date, candidate human tumor-specific antigens, defined by heterologous sera or even monoclonal antibodies, on further analysis have turned out to belong to the category of differentiation antigens, which characterize normal cells at some phase of differentiation, rather than to the category of antigens that are restricted to neoplastic cells.

Old and his coworkers,[110] using serologic methods, have described three categories of melanoma surface antigens: Class 1—individually distinct or unique melanoma antigens, which show an absolute restriction to autologous melanoma cells; Class 2—shared melanoma cells as well as some allogeneic tumors, which cannot be detected on normal autologous, allogeneic, or xenogeneic cells; and Class 3—antigens that are not restricted to melanoma cells and that are expressed on an extensive range of normal and malignant cells of human and animal origin. On the basis of available information, Class 1 and 2 antigens can be considered to be tumor-restricted antigens capable of eliciting tumor immunity in the autologous host, and it is possible that Class 1 and 2 melanoma antigens represent restricted differentiation antigens. In patients with malignant melanoma, the occurrence of antibodies to Class 1 and 2 antigens is infrequent, whereas those against Class 3 antigens are very common. The absence of demonstrable serologic reactivity to Class 1 and 2 antigens does not necessarily imply the lack of immunogenicity but rather may indicate that immunologic recognition of melanoma tumor-specific antigens may be restricted to cellular immunity.

The idea of a human cancer vaccine is very old. A rational approach for the treatment of cancer, based on experience with vaccination for infectious diseases, is to augment the specific immune response of patients against cancer cells by immunizing them with appropriate tumor antigens. As was discussed earlier, however, the existence of tumor-specific antigens capable of eliciting immunologic reactions is not as yet well documented. Regardless of existing problems in tumor vaccination, substantial numbers of cancer patients have been injected with autologous or allogeneic tumor cell preparations over the past 50 years, with mixed results reported. Active specific immunization for malignant melanoma has been reported by several investigators. In one report, doses of more than 2×10^8 irradiated tumor cells have been shown to increase cytotoxic antibody levels against melanoma cells.[111] In aother report, autoimmunization with irradiated tumor cells in human malignant melanoma has demonstrated an increased lymphocyte cytotoxicity against autologous melanoma cells.[112] In addition, it has been reported that immunization with autologous melanoma cells plus bacille Calmette Guérin has decreased serum inhibitor activity and has increased lymphocyte cytotoxic responses.[113] In another trial, increased lymphocyte blastogenic responses to autologous tumor cells have been reported in 6 of 11 patients treated with bacille Calmette Guérin and immunized with melanoma cells.[114]

Another interesting approach is vaccination with virally infected irradiated cultured autologous or allogeneic melanoma cells. This therapy is based on the observation that the immunogeneity of tumor antigens appears to be augmented following infection of tumor cells with certain viruses. Total tumor destruction has been reported after the infection of tumor-bearing mice with West Nile virus[115] or influenza A virus.[116] The animals that survived this procedure were found to be resistant to subsequent challenge with the corresponding tumor. Later studies showed that homogenates prepared from tumors infected with virus were more effective than those prepared from noninfected tumor cells in inducing transplantation immunity.[117–119] In humans, the two viruses used include vesicular stomatitis virus[120] and vaccinia virus.[121] It has been shown that vesicular stomatitis virus–infected melanoma cells elicit delayed hypersensitivity reactions in patients with melanoma but not in patients with other types of cancer. Uninfected melanoma cells or fibroblast membrane preparations were inactive in these studies.

Augmentation of the immunogenicity of tumor cells also has been achieved by direct chemical or enzymatic modification of the cell surface.[122] In a series of experiments, Lachmann and Sikora[123] studied the effect of purified protein derivative bound to the tumor cell surface in hosts who had a pre-existing delayed hypersensitivity to bacille Calmette Guérin.

Old and his coworkers[124] have recommended the use of melanoma autologous vaccine because Class 1 antigens appear to be restricted to autologous melanoma. If such antigens are important for the immunologic control of melanoma, then the use of autologous vaccines would seem to be logical. This obviously is not practical at the beginning, because several weeks must pass before sufficient numbers of autologous melanoma cells can be cultured. It therefore is reasonable to use allogeneic melanoma cells for initial immunization, followed by autologous melanoma cells as soon as the autologous cell line is established. The development of monoclonal antibodies against various melanoma cell lines might allow serologic definition of systems of shared melanoma antigens and may provide the rationale for the use of allogeneic melanoma vaccine and the means for selection of the appropriate allogeneic melanoma cell line.

Assessment of the value of these experiments for cancer therapy is very difficult, mainly because of the complexity and design of the studies and the advanced disease stage of these patients. Other difficulties encountered in the development of melanoma vaccine include uncertainties about the type, dose, route, and frequency of vaccination as well as the selection of the patients and the evaluation of clinical responses.

Combination Immunochemotherapy

Active specific or nonspecific immunotherapy in patients with advanced disease has been shown to be considerably less efficacious than conventional chemotherapy. This is not at all surprising, because the experimental immunotherapy in animal models has demonstrated this approach to be effective only against small tumor burdens.[125–131] Based on these observations, several investigators have combined immunotherapy with tumor-reductive chemotherapy regimens.[132–145]

The use of dimethyl-triazeno-imidazole-carboxamide plus bacille Calmette Guérin by scarification has been reported by Gutterman and his coworkers,[132] who observed statistically significant response rates in patients receiving dimethyl-triazeno-imidazole-carboxamide and bacille Calmette Guérin when compared with those treated with dimethyl-triazeno-imidazole-carboxamide alone. Patients with lymph node disease but without visceral metastasis benefited more from this chemoimmunotherapy than did those with metastasis. In a prospective study by Costanzi,[133] however, improvements resulting from chemoimmunotherapy were less encouraging than those obtained from chemotherapy alone. In other series, the use of chemotherapy combined with immunotherapy with bacille Calmette Guérin, levamisole, or *Corynebacterium parvum* has not shown additional benefit.[134–136] Mastrangelo and his coworkers[137] also failed to demonstrate increased responses to bacille Calmette Guérin, allogeneic tumor cells, and chemotherapy. Aranha and associates[138] reported on the use of a vaccine made of irradiated *Vibrio cholerae* neuroaminidase–treated autochthonous tumor cells plus bacille Calmette Guérin in combination with surgery or with chemotherapy for Stage II and Stage III malignant melanoma. No substantial benefit was observed in patients treated with this protocol when compared with those receiving conventional therapy. Other reports indicate that no difference in response or survival was observed in patients treated with *Corynebacterium parvum* alone or in combination with dimethyl-triazeno-imidazole-carboxamide when compared with those receiving dimethyl-triazeno-imidazole-carboxamide or cyclophosphamide alone.[139-141] However, in a randomized prospective trial *C. parvum* immunotherapy appeared to be associated with an improved disease-free survival rate in the subgroup of patients with melanoma less than 3 mm thickness.[142] These authors further concluded that a prognostic factor analysis is critically important in adjuvant trials of melanoma in order to determine which dominant variables should be used for analyzing patient subgroups.

Prolonged survival has been reported by Gonzalez and colleagues[143] in patients with a small residual tumor burden treated with transfer factor. In another study,[144] the results of immunotherapy with transfer factor are reported to be promising and suggest that this agent may be a valuable adjunct in the treatment of patients with high-risk Stage I melanoma. Schwarz and associates[145] have reported that transfer factor therapy did not enhance the clinical effects of dimethyl-triazeno-imidazole-carboxamide and bacille Calmette Guérin, although it augmented delayed-type hypersensitivity to recall antigens.

In general, much work remains to be done before an effective adjuvant therapy for malignant melanoma can be developed. At present, the major problem with adjuvant studies is the inability to identify the high-risk group.

CONCLUDING REMARKS

Perhaps nothing is more desirable for investigators in the field than the development of an effective therapy for malignant melanoma, especially since its incidence is rising faster than all other malignant tumors except lung cancer and the mortality rate from this disease is higher than ever.

The use of conventional and experimental chemotherapy and radiotherapy so far has been quite unsatisfactory, and greater attention to the immunotherapy of melanoma has resulted. Although the outcome of various immunotherapeutic approaches has been encouraging, many obstacles to the development of an effective program of immunotherapy for melanoma remain. Advances in nonspecific as well as adoptive immunotherapies for melanoma and other human cancers appear to be quite promising, and it is hoped that these approaches eventually may provide adequate means for the prevention and treatment of these malignancies. New developments in hybridoma technology and the availability of monoclonal antibodies give promise that in the very near future drug or radiolabeled monospecific antibodies may play a major role in selective tumor reduction and destruction. In addition, the availability of improved hybridoma technology may finally allow for the determination of the presence of tumor-specific antigens, paving the way for the development of an effective and specific tumor vaccine. Although progress toward these goals appears to be slow, it is quite clear that the future holds the key to an understanding of the host's own defense mechanism and the manner in which manipulation of this mechanism can benefit the host by the prevention and cure of cancers and infections.

References

1. Fraumeni, J. F., and Hoover, R.: Immunosurveillance and cancer: Epidemiologic observations. NCI Monograph 47. Washington, D.C., U.S. Department of Health, Education, and Welfare, 1975, pp. 121–126.
2. Lewis, M. G.: Immunology of human malignant melanoma. Ser. Haematol. 5:44, 1972.
3. Coley, W. B., and Hoquet, J. P.: Melanotic cancer. Ann. Surg. 64:206, 1916.
4. Das Gupta, T., Dowden, L., and Berg, T. W.: Malignant melanoma of unknown primary origin. Surg. Gynecol. Obstet. 117:341, 1963.
5. Milton, G. W.: Malignant melanoma: Early and late. Med. J. Aust. 1:1, 1968.

6. Smith, J. L., and Stehlin, J. S.: Spontaneous regression of primary malignant melanoma with regional metastases. Cancer 18:1399, 1965.

7. Allen, E. P.: Malignant melanoma—spontaneous regression after pregnancy. Br. Med. J. 2:1067, 1955.

8. Everson, T. C.: Spontaneous regression of cancer. Ann. N.Y. Acad. Sci. 114:721, 1964.

9. Todd, D. W., Spencer, P. W., Farrow, G. M., and Winkleman, R. K.: Spontaneous regression of primary malignant melanoma with regional metastases: Report of a case with photographic documentation. Mayo Clin. Proc. 41:672, 1966.

10. Bodurtha, A. J., Berkelhamner, J., Kim, Y. H., Laucius, J. P., and Mastrangelo, M. J.: A clinical, histologic and immunologic study of a case of metastatic malignant melanoma undergoing spontaneous remission. Cancer 37:735, 1976.

11. Sumner, W. C.: Spontaneous regression of melanoma: Report of a case. Cancer 6:1040, 1953.

12. Everson, T. C., and Cole, W. H.: Spontaneous Regression in Cancer. Philadelphia, W. B. Saunders Co., 1966, pp. 1–560.

13. Smithers, D. W.: Spontaneous regression of cancer. Ann. R. Coll. Surg. Engl. 41:160, 1967.

14. Thompson, P. G.: Relationship of lymphocytic infiltration to prognosis in primary malignant melanoma of skin. Pigm. Cell 1:285, 1973.

15. Coley, W. B.: A report of recent cases of inoperable sarcoma successfully treated with mixed toxins of erysipelas and *Bacillus prodigiosus*. Surg. Gynecol. Obstet. 13:174, 1911.

16. Klein, E.: Tumors of the skin. X. Immunotherapy of cutaneous and mucosal neoplasms. N.Y. State J. Med. 68:900, 1968.

17. Klein, E., and Holterman, O. A.: Immunotherapeutic approaches to the management of neoplasms. Natl. Cancer Inst. Monogr. 35:379, 1972.

18. Stjernsward, J., and Levin, A.: Delayed hypersensitivity-induced regression of human neoplasms. Cancer 28:628, 1971.

19. Hunter-Craig, I., Newton, K. A., Westbury, G., et al.: Use of vaccinia virus in the treatment of metastatic malignant melanoma. Br. Med. J. 2:512, 1970.

20. Morton, D. I., Eilber, F. R., Malmgren, R. A., et al.: Immunological factors which influence response to immunotherapy in malignant melanoma. Surgery 68:158, 1970.

21. Cheema, A. R., and Hersh, E. M.: Local tumor immunotherapy with in vitro activated autochthonous lymphocytes. Cancer 29:982, 1972.

22. Nathanson, L.: Regression of intradermal malignant melanoma after intralesional injection of mycobacterium bovis strain BCG. Cancer Chemother. Rep. 56:659, 1972.

23. Pinsky, C. M., Hirshaut, Y., and Oettgen, H. F.: Treatment of malignant melanoma by intratumoral injection of BCG. Natl. Cancer Inst. Monogr. 39:225, 1973.

24. Bornstein, R. S., Mastrangelo, M. J., Sulit, H., et al.: Immunotherapy of melanoma with intralesional BCG. Natl. Cancer Inst. Monogr. 39:213, 1973.

25. Mastrangelo, M. J., Kim, Y. H., Bornstein, R. S., et al.: Clinical and histologic correlation of melanoma regression after intralesional BCG therapy: A case report. J. Natl. Cancer Inst. 52:19, 1974.

26. Lieberman, R., Epstein, W., and Fudenberg, H. H.: Immunopathologic changes in patients with cutaneous malignant melanoma following intratumoral inoculation of BCG: Correlation with cell-mediated immunity. Int. J. Cancer 14:401, 1974.

27. Levy, N. L., Seigler, H. F., and Shingleton, W. W.: A multiphase immunotherapy regimen for human melanoma: Clinical and laboratory results. Cancer 34:1548, 1974.

28. Seigler, H. F., Shingleton, W. W., Metzgar, R. S., et al.: Immunotherapy in patients with melanoma. Ann. Surg. 178:352, 1973.

29. Sparks, F. C., Silverstein, M. J., Hunt, J. S., et al.: Complications of BCG immunotherapy in patients with cancer. N. Engl. J. Med. 289:827, 1973.

30. Krementz, E. T., Samuels, M. S., Wallace, J. H., et al.: Clinical experiences in immunotherapy of cancer. Surg. Gynecol. Obstet. 133:209, 1971.

31. Levy, N. L., Mahaley, M. S., Jr., and Dav, E. D.: Serum-mediated blocking of cell-mediated antitumor immunity in a melanoma patient: Association with BCG immunotherapy and clinical deterioration. Int. J. Cancer 10:244, 1972.

32. Mastrangelo, M. J., Sulit, H. L., Prehn, L. M., et al.: Intralesional BCG in the treatment of metastatic malignant melanoma. Cancer 37:684, 1976.

33. Smith, G. V., Morse, P. A., Jr., Deraps, G. D., et al.: Immunotherapy of patients with cancer. Surgery 74:59, 1973.

34. Minton, J. R.: Mumps virus and BCG vaccine in metastatic melanoma. Arch. Surg. 106:503, 1973.

35. Baker, M. A., and Taub, R. N.: BCG in malignant melanoma. Lancet 1:1117, 1973.

36. Klein, E., Holterman, O. A., Papermaster, B., et al.: Immunologic approaches to various types of cancer with the use of BCG and purified protein derivatives. Natl. Cancer Inst. Monogr. 39:229, 1973.

37. Lieberman, R., Wybran, J., and Epstein, W.: The immunologic and histopathologic changes in BCG mediated tumor regression in patients with malignant melanoma. Cancer 35:756, 1975.

38. Grant, R. M., Mackie, R., Cochran, A. J., et al.: Results of administering BCG to patients with melanoma. Lancet 2:1096, 1974.

39. Cohen, M. H., Felix, E., Jessup, J., et al.: Treatment of metastatic melanoma by intralesional injection of BCG, organic chemicals and *C. parvum*. In Crispen, R. G. (ed.): Neoplasm Immunity Mechanism. Philadelphia, Franklin Institute Press, 1975, pp. 121–134.

40. Nathanson, L., Schoenfeld, D., Regelson, W., Colsky, J., and Mittelman, A.: Prospective comparison of intralesional and multipuncture BCG in recurrent intradermal melanoma. Cancer 43:1630, 1979.

41. Epstein, W. L., Sagebeil, R., Spitler, L., et al.: Halo nevi and melanoma. JAMA 225:373, 1973.
42. Lewis, M. G., and Copeman, P. W. M.: Halo nevus—a frustrated malignant melanoma? Br. Med. J. 2:47, 1972.
43. Mastrangelo, M. J., Rosenberg, S. A., Baker, A. R., and Katz, H. R.: Cutaneous melanoma. In Devita, V., Jr., Hellman, S., and Rosenberg, S. (eds.): Cancer Principles and Practice of Oncology. Philadelphia, J. B. Lippincott Co., 1982, pp. 1124–1170.
44. Tisman, G., Wu, S. J. G., and Safire, G. E.: Intralesional PPD in malignant melanoma. Lancet 1:161, 1975.
45. Krown, S. E., Hilal, E. Y., Pinsky, C. M., et al.: Intralesional injection of the methanol extraction residue of Bacillus Calmette Guérin (MER) into cutaneous metastases of malignant melanoma. Cancer 42:2648, 1978.
46. Lokich, J. J., Garnick, M. B., and Legg, M.: Intralesional immune therapy, methanol extraction residue of BCG or purified protein derivative. Oncology 36:236, 1979.
47. Vosika, G. J., Schmidtke, J. R., Goldman, A., et al.: Intralesional immunotherapy of malignant melanoma with mycobacterium smegmatis cell wall skeleton combined with trehalose demycolate (P3). Cancer 44:495, 1979.
48. Klein, E., Holterman, O. A., Helm, F., et al.: Immunologic approaches to the management of primary and secondary tumors involving the skin and soft tissues. Review of a ten year program. Transplant Proc. 7:297, 1975.
49. Burdick, K., Hawk, W. A.: Vitiligo in a case of vaccinia virus-11 melanoma. Cancer 17:708, 1964.
50. Milton, G. W., and Brown, M. M. L.: The limited role of attenuated smallpox virus in the management of advanced malignant melanoma. Aust. N.Z. J. Surg. 35:286, 1966.
51. Hunt, J. S., Silverstein, J. M., Sparks, F. C., et al.: Granulomatous hepatitis: A complication of BCG immunotherapy. Lancet 2:820, 1973.
52. Rosenberg, E. B., Kanner, S. P., Schwartzman, R. J., et al.: Systemic infection following BCG therapy. Intern. Med. 134:769, 1974.
53. Richman, S. P., Mavligit, G. M., Wolk, R., et al.: Epilesional scarification. Preliminary report of a new approach to local immunotherapy with BCG. JAMA 234:1233, 1975.
54. Everall, J. D., O'Doherty, C. J., Ward, J., et al.: Treatment of primary melanoma by intralesional vaccinia before excision. Lancet 2:583, 1975.
55. Castermans-Elias, S., Simar, L., Vanijek, R., et al.: Immunosurgical treatment of Stage I malignant melanoma. Cancer Immunol. Immunother. 2:179, 1977.
56. Rosenberg, S. A., Rapp, H., Terry, W., et al.: Intralesional BCG therapy of patients with primary Stage I melanoma. Proceedings, Second International Conference on Immunotherapy of Cancer. Bethesda, Maryland, April 28–30, 1980, p. 8.
57. Oettgen, H. F., Old, L.. J., Farrow, J. H., et al.: Effect of dialyzable transfer factor in patients with breast cancer. Proc. Natl. Acad. Sci. U.S.A. 71:2319, 1974.
58. Spitler, L. E., Wybran, J., Fudenberg, H. H., et al.: Transfer factor therapy of malignant melanoma. Clin. Res. 21:221, 1973.
59. Pilch, Y. H., Ramming, K. P., and Deckers, P. J.: Studies in mediation of tumor immunity with "immune" RNA. In Busch, H. (ed.): Methods in Cancer Research, New York, Academic Press, 1973, pp. 195–254.
60. Pilch, Y. H., Veltman, L. I., and Kern, D. H.: Immune cytolysis of human tumor cells mediated by xenogeneic "immune" RNA. Arch, Sug. 109:30, 1974.
61. Langvad, E., Hyden, H., Kjaer Petersen, J., et al.: Extracorporeal interferon therapy in malignant melanoma. Arzneim.-Forsch./Drug Res. 30:1245, 1980.
62. Golub, H., Dorey, F., Hara, D., et al.: Systemic administration of human leukocyte interferon to melanoma patients. I. Effects on natural killer function and cell populations. J.N.C.I. 68:703, 1982.
63. Frenster, J. H., and Rogoway, W. M.: Clinical use of activated autologous lymphocytes for human cancer immunotherapy. In Cumley, R. W., and McKay, J. E. (eds.): Oncology 1970. Chicago, Year Book Medical Publishers, 1970, p. 327.
64. Lewis, M. G., Humble, J. G., Lee, E. S., et al.: The effects of intravenous phytohemagglutinin in a patient with disseminated malignant melanoma: A clinical and immunological study. Eur. J. Clin. Biol. Res. 9:924, 1971.
65. Golub, S. H., and Morton, D. L.: Sensitization of lymphocytes in vitro against human melanoma associated antigens. Nature 251:161, 1974.
66. Rosenberg, S. A., and Terry, W. D.: Passive immunotherapy of cancer in animals and man. Adv. Cancer Res. 25:323, 1977.
67. Wrigert, P. W., Hellstrom, K. E., et al.: Serotherapy of malignant disease. Med. Clin. North Am. 60:607, 1976.
68. Wright, P. W., and Bernstein, I. D.: Prog. Exp. Tumor Res. 25:140, 1980.
69. Fefer, A.: Experimental approaches to immunotherapy of cancer. Recent Results Cancer Res. 36:182, 1971.
70. Currie, G. A.: Eighty years of immunotherapy: A review of immunological methods used for the treatment of human cancer. Br. J. Cancer 26:141, 1972.
71. Sumner, W. C., and Foraker, A. G.: Spontaneous regression of human melanoma. Cancer 13:79, 1960.
72. Teimourian, B., and McCune, W. S.: Surgical management of malignant melanoma. Am. Surg. 29:515, 1963.
73. Lazlo, J., Buckley, C. E., et al.: Infusion of isologous immune plasma in chronic lymphocytic leukemia. Blood 3:104, 1968.
74. Herberman, R. B., Rogentine, G. N., et al.: Bioassay of anti-tumor effects of human alloanti-sera. Clin. Res. 17:328, 1969.

75. Fisher, R. I., Kubota, T. T., et al.: Regression of a T-cell lymphoma after administration of antithymocyte globulin. Ann. Intern. Med. 88:799, 1978.

76. Edelson, R. L., Raafat, J., et al.: Antithymocyte globulin in the management of cutaneous T-cell lymphoma. Cancer Treat. Rep. 63:675, 1979.

77. Herlyn, M., Steplewski, Z., et al.: Colorectal carcinoma-specific antigen: Detection by means of monoclonal antibodies. Proc. Natl. Acad. Sci. U.S.A. 76:1438, 1979.

78. Ueda, R., Ogata, S.-I., et al.: Cell surface antigen of human renal cancer defined by mouse monoclonal antibodies. Identification of tissue-specific kidney glycoproteins. Proc. Natl. Acad. Sci. U.S.A. 78:5122, 1981.

79. Cuttitta, F., Rosen, S., et al.: Monoclonal antibodies that demonstrate specificity for several types of human lung cancer. Proc. Natl. Acad. Sci. U.S.A. 78:4591, 1981.

80. Colcher, D., Hand, P. H., et al.: A spectrum of monoclonal antibodies reactive with human mammary tumor cells. Proc. Natl. Acad. Sci. U.S.A. 78:3199, 1981.

81. Bechtol, K. B., Jonak, Z. L., and Kennett, R. H: Germ cell–related and nervous system–related differentiation and tumor antigens. In Kennett, R. H., et al. (eds.): Monoclonal Antibodies. New York, Plenum Press, 1980, pp. 171–184.

82. Koprowski, H., Steplewski, Z., et al.: Study of antibodies against human melanoma produced by somatic cell hybrids. Proc. Natl. Acad. Sci. U.S.A. 75:3404, 1978.

83. Yeh, M. Y., Hellstrom, I., et al.: Cell surface antigens of human melanoma identified by monoclonal antibody. Proc. Natl. Acad. Sci. U.S.A. 76:2927, 1979.

84. Woodbury, R. G., Brown, J. P., et al.: Identification of a cell surface protein, p 97, in human melanoma and certain other neoplasms. Proc. Natl. Acad. Sci. U.S.A. 77:2183, 1980.

85. Dippold, W. G., Lloyd, K. O., et al.: Cell surface antigens of human malignant melanoma: Definition of six antigenic systems with mouse monoclonal antibodies. Proc. Natl. Acad. Sci. U.S.A. 77:6114, 1980.

86. Morgan, A. C., Galloway, D. R., et al.: Human melanoma associated antigens: Role of carbohydrate in shedding and cell surface expression. J. Immunol. 126:365, 1981.

87. Carrell, S., Accolla, R. S., et al.: Common melanoma associated antigen(s) detected by monoclonal antibodies. Cancer Res. 40:2523, 1980.

88. Natali, P. G., Imai, K., et al.: Structural properties and tissue distribution of the antigen recognized by the monoclonal antibody 653.40 S to human melanoma cells. J.N.C.I. 67:591, 1981.

89. Olsson, L., and Kaplan, H.: Human-human hybridomas producing monoclonal antibodies of predefined antigenic specificity. Proc. Natl. Acad. Sci. U.S.A. 77:5429, 1980.

90. Schlom, J., Wunderlich, D., et al.: Generation of human monoclonal antibodies reactive with human mammary carcinoma cells. Proc. Natl. Acad. Sci. U.S.A. 77:6841, 1980.

91. Bernstein, I. D., Tam, M. R., et al.: Mouse leukemia: Therapy with monoclonal antibodies against a thymus differentiation antigen. Science 207:68, 1979.

92. Krich, M. E., and Hammerling, U.: Immunotherapy of murine leukemias by monoclonal antibody. J. Immunol. 127:805, 1981.

93. Herlyn, D., Steplewski, Z., et al.: Inhibition of growth of colorectal carcinoma in nude mice by monoclonal antibody. Cancer Res. 40:717, 1980.

94. Nadler, L. M., Stashenko, P., et al.: Serotherapy of a patient with a monoclonal antibody directed against a human lymphoma-associated antigen. Cancer Res. 40:3147, 1980.

95. Ritz, J., Pesando, J. M., et al.: Serotherapy of acute lymphoblastic leukemia with monoclonal antibody. Blood 58:141, 1981.

96. Miller, R. A., Maloney, D. G., et al.: In vivo effects of murine hybridoma monoclonal antibody in a patient with T-cell leukemia. Blood 58:78, 1981.

97. Miller, R. A., and Levy, R.: Response of cutaneous T-cell lymphoma to therapy with hybridoma monoclonal antibody. Lancet 2:226, 1981.

98. McGrath, M. S., Pillemer, E., et al.: Murine leukemogenesis: Monoclonal antibodies to T-cell determinants arrest T-lymphoma cell proliferation. Nature 285:259, 1980.

99. Goldenberg, M. D., Deland, F., et al.: Use of radiolabeled antibodies to carcinoembryonic antigen for the detection and localization of diverse cancer by external photoscanning. N. Engl. J. Med. 298:1384, 1978.

100. Hine, K. R., Bradwell, A. R., et al.: Radioimmunodetection of gastrointestinal neoplasms with antibodies to carcinoembryonic antigen. Cancer Res. 40:2993, 1980.

101. Kim, E. E., Deland, F. H., et al.: Radioimmunodetection of cancer with radiolabeled antibodies to α-fetoprotein. Cancer Res. 40:3008, 1980.

102. Mach, J. P., Carrel, S., et al.: Tumor localization of radiolabeled antibodies against carcinoembryonic antigen in patients with carcinoma. N. Engl. J. Med. 303:5, 1980.

103. Goldenberg, D. M., Kim, E. E., et al.: Clinical radioimmunodetection of cancer with radioactive antibodies to human chorionic gonadotropin. Science 208:1284, 1980.

104. Order, S. E., Klein, J. L., et al.: Phase I-II study of radiolabeled antibody integrated in the treatment of primary hepatic malignancies. Int. J. Radiat. Oncol. Biol. Phys. 6:703, 1980.

105. Ghose, T., Norvell, S. T., Guclu, A., et al.: Immunochemotherapy of cancer with chlorambucil-carrying antibody. Br. Med. J. 3:495, 1972.

106. Rubens, R. D.: Antibodies as carriers of anticancer agents. Lancet 1:498, 1974.

107. Rubens, R. D., and Dulbecco, R.: Augmentation of cytotoxic drug action by antibodies directed at cell surface. Nature 248:81, 1974.

108. Amon, R., Hurwitz, E., et al.: Antibodies as carriers for oncostatic materials. Recent results Cancer Res. 75:236, 1980.

109. Latif, Z. A., Lozzio, B., et al.: Evaluation of drug antibody conjugates in the treatment of human myelo-sarcoma transplanted in nude mice. Cancer 45:1326, 1980.
110. Watanabe, T., Shiku, H., Li, L.T.C., Oettgen, H. F., and Old, L. J.: Detection of a tumor-restricted melanoma cell surface antigen by allogeneic typing. Proc. Am. Assoc. Cancer Res. 21:241, 1980.
111. Ikonopisov, R. L., Lewis, M. G., Hunter-Craig, I. D., et al.: Autoimmunization with irradiated tumor cells in human malignant melanoma. Br. Med. J. 2:752, 1969.
112. Currie, G. A., LeJeune, F., and Fairley, G. H.: Immunization with irradiated tumor cells and specific lymphocyte cytotoxicity in malignant melanoma. Br. Med. J. 2:305, 1971.
113. Currie, G. A.: Effect of active immunization with irradiated tumor cells on specific serum inhibitors of cell mediated immunity in patients with disseminated cancer. Br. J. Cancer 28:25, 1973.
114. Gercovich, F. G., Gutterman, J. U., Mavligit, G. M., et al.: Active specific immunization in malignant melanoma. Med. J. Pediatr. Oncol. 1:277, 1975.
115. Koprowski, H., Love, R., and Koprowski, I.: Enhancement of susceptibility to viruses in neoplastic tissues. Tex. Rep. Biol. Med. 15:559, 1957.
116. Lindenmann, J., and Klein, P.A.: Viral oncolysis: Increased immunogenicity of host cell antigen associated with influenza virus. J. Exp. Med. 126:93, 1967.
117. Axler, D.A., and Girardi, A. J.: SV 40 tumor specific transplantation antigen (TSTA) in NDV lysates of SV40 transformed cells. Proc. Am. Assoc. Cancer Res. 11:4, 1970.
118. Boone, C. W., Paranjpe, M., Orme, T., and Gillette, R.: Virus-augmented tumor transplantation antigens: Evidence for a helper antigen mechanism. Int. J. Cancer 13:543, 1974.
119. Lindenmann, J.: Viruses as immunologic adjuvants in cancer. Biochim. Biophys. Acta 355:49, 1974.
120. Boone, C. W., Austin, F. C., Gail, M., Case, R., and Klein, E.: Melanoma skin test antigens of improved sensitivity prepared from vesicular stomatitis virus–infected tumor cells. Cancer 41:1781, 1978.
121. Wallack, M. K., Steplewski, Z., Koprowski, H.: A new approach in specific active immunotherapy. Cancer 39:560, 1977.
122. Prager, M.D., and Baechtel, F. S.: Methods for modification of cancer cells to enhance their antigenicity. Methods Cancer Res. 9:339, 1973.
123. Lachmann, P.J., and Sikora, K.: Coupling PPD to tumor cells enhances their antigenicity in BCG-primed mice. Nature (London) 27:463, 1978.
124. Houghton, A. N., Oettgen, H. F., and Old, L. J.: Malignant melanoma; current status of the search for melanoma-specific antigens. In Safai, B., and Good, R. A. (eds.): Immunodermatology. New York, Plenum Press, 1981, pp. 557–576.
125. Laucius, J. F., Bodurtha, A. J., Mastrangelo, M. J., et al.: A Phase II study of autologous irradiated tumor cells plus BCG in patients with metastatic melanoma. Cancer 40:2091, 1977.
126. Arlen, M., Hollinshead, A., and Scherrer, J.: Tumor-specific immunity in patients with malignant mela-noma. Surg. Forum 28:168, 1977.
127. Orefice, S., Cascinelli, N., Vaglini, M., et al.: Intravenous administration of BCG in advanced melanoma patients. Tumori 64:437, 1978.
128. Israel, L., Edelstein, R., Depierre, A., et al.: Daily intravenous infusions of Corynebacterium parvum in twenty patients with disseminated cancer. J.N.C.I. 55:29, 1975.
129. Falk, R.E., Mann, P., and Largen, B.: Cell-mediated immunity to human tumors. Arch. Surg. 107:261, 1973.
130. Murray, D. R., Cassel, W. A., Torbin, A. H., et al.: Viral oncolysate in the management of malignant melanoma. Cancer 40:680, 1977.
131. Israel, L., Edelstein, R., Mannori, P., et al.: Plasmapheresis in patients with disseminated cancer. Clinical results and correlations with changes in serum protein. Cancer 40:3146, 1977.
132. Gutterman, J. U., Mavligit, G., Gottlieb, J. A., et al.: Chemoimmunotherapy of disseminated malignant melanoma with dimethyltriazeno-imidazole-carboxamide and Bacillus Calmette-Guerin. N. Engl. J. Med. 529:291, 1974.
133. Costanzi, J. J., Al-Saraf, M., and Dixon, D. O.: Chemoimmunotherapy of disseminated melanoma. Proc. Am. Assoc. Clin. Oncol. 19:362, 1979.
134. Jacquillat, C., Banzet, P., et al.: Clinical trials of chemotherapy and chemoimmunotherapy in primary malignant melanoma. Recent Results Cancer Res. 80:254, 1982.
135. Czarnetzki, B. M., Macher, E., et al.: Current status of melanoma chemotherapy and immunotherapy. Recent Results Cancer Res. 80:264, 1982.
136. Thatcher, N., Blackledge, G., et al.: Chemoimmunotherapy for metastatic malignant melanoma using vin-cristine (NSC-67574), DTIC (NSC-45388) and Bacillus Calmette-Guerin. Eur. J. Cancer 17:465, 1981.
137. Mastrangelo, M. J., Bellet, and R. E., and Berd, D.: A Phase II comparison Methyl-CCNU + vincristine with or without BCG + allogen tumor cells in malignant melanoma. Cancer Immunol. Immunother. 6:231, 1979.
138. Aranha, G. V., Mokhavu, C. F., et al.: Adjuvant immunotherapy of malignant melanoma. Cancer 43:1297, 1979.
139. Presant, C. A., Bartolucci, A. A., Smalley, R. V., et al.: Cyclophospham plus 5-(3.3-dimethyl-1-triazeno) imidazole-4-carboxam (DTIC) with or without Corynebacterium parvum in metastatic malignant melanoma. Cancer 44:899, 1979.
140. Clumie, G. J. A., Gough, I. R., et al.: A trial of imidazole carboxamide and Corynebacterium parvum in disseminated melanoma. Cancer 46:475, 1980.
141. Hilal, E. Y., Pirsky, C. M., et al.: Surgical adjuvant therapy of malignant melanoma with Corynebacterium parvum. Cancer 48:245, 1981.

142. Balch, C. M., Smalley, R. V., et al.: A randomized prospective clinical trial of adjuvant *C. parvum* immunotherapy in 260 patients with clinically localized melanoma (Stage 1). Cancer 49:1079, 1982.
143. Gonzalez, R. L., Wong, P., et al.: Adjuvant immunotherapy with transfer factor in patients with melanoma metastatic to lung. Cancer 45:57, 1980.
144. Blume, M. R., Rosenbaum, E. H., et al.: Adjuvant immunotherapy of high risk Stage 1 melanoma with transfer factor. Cancer 47:882, 1981.
145. Schwarz, M. A., Gutterman, J. U., et al.: Chemoimmunotherapy of disseminated malignant melanoma with DTIC-BCG transfer factor + melphalan. Cancer 45:2506, 1980.

IS THERE A CONTROVERSY ON THE LASER TREATMENT OF MELANOMA?

Leon Goldman, M.D.

It is quite appropriate to ask: Is laser treatment necessary? In the case of certain cancers, yes. For example, melanoma has been an indication for laser treatment since 1962.[1]

Because of its characteristic color, this capricious tumor has continued to offer a challenge not only to lasers in the visible light range but also to all lasers now used in the laser surgery program. Lasers can do two things for the treatment of cancer: They can volatilize an inoperable tumor and excise a tumor such as a melanoma. A melanoma has an added advantage because it is black and therefore is more affected by lasers in the visible light range than by the ordinary knife, high-frequency electrosurgery, cryosurgery, or even chemotherapy. It has been shown repeatedly that, especially with the ruby laser, melanoma can be selectively removed amidst other tumors, such as metastatic masses in the neck, with protection of the other structures because of the specific activity of the laser in the pigmented areas. In microsurgery with the ruby lasers, it has been shown that tissue cultures of melanoma cells are specifically affected by the microbeam. The amelanotic melanoma does not show this. Other cells in tissue culture are unaffected. Other clear cells and unpigmented cells are unresponsive to the power densities that can destroy the pigmented melanoma cells. Attempts to use the irradiated melanoma cells as tumor antigen so far have been unsuccessful.

Lasers in the visible light range therefore can be used where the particular color qualities of the melanoma allow it to be treated specifically with regard to the adjacent tissues. They also have value in melanoma of the eye and, to some extent, melanoma involving neural tissue. Such lasers also have been used in melanoma on the genitalia.

The arguments for the treatment of melanoma by a photoexcision scalpel are supposedly related to the effect of the laser beam, which seals off lymphatics during the excision procedure. The carbon dioxide, far infrared, near infrared, and neodymium yttrium aluminum garnet (YAG) laser have been used in photoexcision.

More studies will have to be done with labeled cells in order to prove the theory that the thermocoagulation of photoexcision seals off adjacent blood vessels so tumor cells cannot be transported by way of the vascular system from the excision area. In addition, controlled histologic and electron microscopy tissue studies are needed. Another problem in photoexcision therapy is the adequacy of graft replacement of the photoexcision area.[2,3]

In the laser treatment of burns, it has been shown by Fidler that there is less blood loss in excision of eschars with the carbon dioxide laser than in excision with the scalpel. It also has been shown that there is no graft rejection on the laser irradiant area, even with the thin skin of infants. There have been some conflicting reports of the healing of the graft replacement area in extensive laser photoexcision, especially in cases of large melanoma tumor areas. In the volatilization treatment of melanoma, at least with the ruby laser (the laser in the visible light range), the cosmetic results have been excellent because of the relative resistance of the sebaceous area to the thermocoagulation of the volatilization technique. Use of the ruby laser in the normal mode (milliseconds' duration) or in the Q-switched mode (nanoseconds' duration) raises some questions concerning the dispersion of plumed fragments containing viable cells. Such dispersion has not been established for humans but has been shown in animal experimentation. It may be that the elastic recoil and pressure waves attendant upon these techniques are responsible for dispersion of plumed fragments, which may contain viable cells. Tissue culture collectors are arranged around the site of laser treatment to detect the viability of any tissue fragments. With the continuous wave lasers, such as the carbon dioxide and neodymium YAG lasers, there is local thermocoagulation necrosis which, in spite of the site-specificity of the heat radiation transmission, can cause tissue damage in adjacent areas.

As yet, there is no evidence of any immune response to melanoma tissue treated by lasers. In our experiments,[3] which were limited to uncontrolled studies, there was increased stimulation of tissue culture cells when they were exposed to lasers of low output power. This is in accord with vague suggestions of overstimulation by lasers.

At present, photoexcision techniques have been used more frequently for early treatment of melanoma. The volatilization procedures have been limited to metastatic masses in areas on which it is difficult to operate and to melanoma metastases (in mostly academic investigative procedures). Most experiments have been done chiefly with multiple cutaneous metastases which, as in any form of metastasis, carry a very poor prognosis. Different power densities of various laser systems are used in localized areas. One untreated nodule is used as the control, and the effects of the different treatment procedures are evaluated locally. At times, the local treatment has been very effective in near eradication of the local accessible lesions but has no effect on the prognosis of metastases. For nodules that are deep in the tissue, the response to laser impacts has been much less certain. It is not possible to get adequate energy densities from the surface to the metastatic nodule with conventional laser therapy without causing severe tissue destruction of the superficial layers of the skin. Occasionally, it has been possible to make the metastatic nodules accessible by exposure to the direct beam high-output laser systems. Sometimes the results are partial; a particular nodule may even disappear completely. Such localized treatment does not have any immunologic significance for the patient. At present, metastatic nodules may be diagnosed and treated by laser (630 nm) induced by fluorescence of hematoporphyrin derivative (Hpd). This fluorochrome, absorbed especially by cancer cells and traumatized tissue, may be injected parenterally or, less effectively, implanted directly into accessible metastases.

Laser surgery also may be used as an adjuvant to all the conventional forms of treatment. If a mass is bound down where multiple adhesions are covered with major vessels and nerves and this mass is exposed by scalpel surgery, the laser volatilization technique can be used with carbon dioxide, neodymium YAG, or even high-output argon laser systems and ruby lasers in the Q-switched mode, if they are available. The thermocoagulation necrosis that results from such procedures is not significantly different from other types of induced thermocoagulation necrosis; there is less tendency to secondary infection with laser surgery. There is no evidence that laser treatment has any significant effect on melanuria.

Improved techniques of photoexcision may give rise to better cosmetic results and may allow for more careful observation of the patient. Laser treatment of melanoma may be obligatory, preferred, or contraindicated. For example, laser therapy can be used in treatment of a large superficial melanoma in an elderly individual who cannot take excisional surgery with graft transfer. A large nodule on the lower leg in a patient with severe congestive heart failure, in whom surgery and, to some extent, chemotherapy are ruled out, also can be treated with the laser.

In the future, a new field of internal laser surgery may cover metastases, especially of the nervous system. For melanomas of the eye, laser therapy also is indicated.

Laser treatment is preferred when the cosmetic results of effective laser therapy may be superior to those of other forms of treatment. The physical condition of the patient may not allow vigorous therapy.

Laser treatment need not be used on superficial melanoma that can be adequately excised. The results of excision can be checked for proper classification of the extent of the melanoma.

It should be remembered that laser therapy can be used in addition to any other modality that is used in cancer treatment. The ever-repeated dogma remains: If you don't need the laser, don't use it. If you use the laser, use it adequately.

References

1. Goldman, L.: Laser Cancer Research. New York, Springer-Verlag, 1966, p. 33.
2. Goldman, L.: The Biomedical Laser—Technology and Clinical Applications. New York, Springer-Verlag, 1981.
3. Goldman, L.: Surgery by laser for malignant melanoma. J. Dermatol. Surg. Oncol. 5:2, 1979.

SECTION 2

EPITHELIOMAS

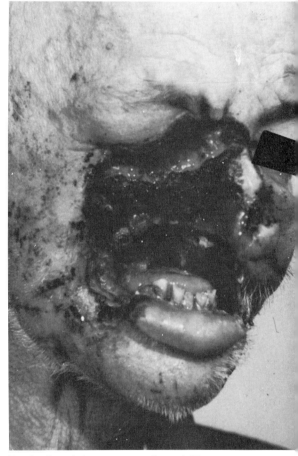

Basal cell epitheliomas are not benign! (Courtesy of Dr. Robert Jackson.)

EPITHELIOMA OF SKIN AND ITS ASSOCIATION WITH INTERNAL CANCER

SKIN CANCER: AN IMPORTANT MARKER OF INTERNAL NEOPLASIA

Jeffrey P. Callen, M.D.

The nature of the relationship of cutaneous and visceral malignancies is at least a two-part issue. First, is cancer of the skin a marker of internal malignancy? And, second, what is the exact nature of this association; i.e., how should the patient with cutaneous malignancy be evaluated for internal disease? In this paper I will attempt to address both of these controversial issues for the multitide of types of skin cancer that exist. I believe that it is not uncommon to have a visceral malignancy in the presence of cutaneous cancer.

There are many types of malignancies that occur on the skin. The most common forms seen in a dermatologist's office are the basal cell epithelioma and the squamous cell carcinoma. In addition, Kaposi's sarcoma, melanoma, and keratoacanthomas may be seen on occasion. This paper will deal mainly with basal cell epitheliomas and squamous cell epitheliomas of the skin; however, the other types of skin cancer must be mentioned.

Basal Cell Epithelioma

Basal cell epithelioma is the most common cancer occurring in humans. Its frequent presence on exposed surfaces allows for early diagnosis and, usually, definitive and curative therapy. Only rarely in the basal cell–nevus syndrome has internal malignancy been found, and the only reports are of ovarian carcinomas and medulloblastomas.[1] The relationship of the noninherited basal cell epithelioma to internal neoplasia has been examined systematically and reported in the literature by Carpenter and associates.[2] They found a 9.8 per cent incidence of internal malignancies in patients with basal cell epitheliomas. The possibility that the relationship of basal cell epithelioma to malignancy was dependent upon the age of the patient was ruled out by comparison of the subjects with age-matched patients. In a study of lung cancer as a second primary malignancy, Reynolds and coworkers found that basal cell epithelioma was the first malignancy in 8 of their 403 cases.[3] Although this is not a high percentage, it may be representative of a general phenomenon whereby patients with basal cell epitheliomas are more prone to internal malignancies. On the other hand, Møller and colleagues found an increased incidence of visceral neoplasia only when arsenic was an etiologic factor.[4] Thus, to summarize, the existing data point toward an increased frequency of internal malignancy in the patient with basal cell epithelioma.

Despite this positive relationship, there has not been an analysis of the temporal occurrence of basal cell epithelioma with other cancers. Further study is necessary in order to clarify the procedure for evaluation of the patient with a basal cell epithelioma. Most dermatologists seem to ignore these data and do not evaluate patients or refer them for evaluation.

Squamous Cell Carcinoma

Squamous cell carcinomas, including the histologic variant of Bowen's disease, do seem to be associated with visceral malignancy in a frequency greater than expected for the general population. This relationship has been studied in patients with Bowen's disease more thoroughly than in those with any other type of squamous cell epithelioma. Bowen's disease therefore will be discussed separately.

Bowen's disease is a squamous intraepidermal neoplasia with characteristic histologic features.[5] It differs from other forms of in situ squamous cell carcinoma in that it demonstrates marked cellular atypia, numerous multinucleated and vacuolated cells, and a multitude of mitotic figures. In 1959 Graham and Helwig first noted the association between Bowen's disease and internal malignancy.[6] Other authors since have reported varying incidences, but in general it seems that roughly 25 per cent of the cases of Bowen's disease occur in conjunction with an internal malignancy at some time during the patient's lifetime.[7-9] In a study of 130 patients with squamous intraepidermal neoplasia (in situ squamous cell carcinoma of the skin), Callen and Headington found a 29.1 per cent incidence of internal malignancy.[5] The rate was slightly higher in those cases classified as Bowen's disease compared with non-Bowen's squamous cell carcinomas, but this was not statistically significant. An important phenomenon, however, was that in approximately 15 per cent of the cases the malignancy was concurrent with or subsequent to the diagnosis of Bowen's disease. Data regarding the location of the skin lesion are mixed; Peterka reported that covered surfaces were more frequently associated with visceral malignancy,[7] whereas Callen could not demonstrate a difference between exposed and nonexposed surfaces.[5]

Carpenter and associates[2] also reviewed patients with squamous cell carcinoma but did not evaluate Bowen's disease separately. In their group there was an 8 to 10 per cent incidence of internal malignancy. The data collected from these patients were compared with results from a control group, and it was found that the incidence was nine times greater in patients with skin cancer. In 64 per cent of the patients with skin cancer and internal malignancy, the former occurred simultaneously with or prior to the latter. The investigators concluded that one should take a thorough history and should perform physical examinations and perhaps laboratory evaluations and radiologic studies for patients with skin cancers.

Two studies from Copenhagen have addressed the relationship between Bowen's disease and internal cancer and that of squamous cell carcinoma and internal cancer.[10,11] In both studies the authors concluded that the incidence of internal cancer was not increased among patients with squamous cell carcinoma and Bowen's disease. The methods of both investigations were similar, involving questionnaires, data from the Danish Cancer Registry, and death certificates. Although these methods appear thorough, it is possible that the questionnaires were not filled out properly or that some malignancies were not reported on the death certificates. The investigators explain the differences between their studies and those of American populations by postulating that in our more diffuse society exposure to carcinogens may lead to the concurrence of external and visceral malignancies.

The relation of internal and cutaneous malignancies is not uniform. In our study there was no evidence that any particular internal neoplasm was present more frequently than others.[5] The temporal relationship also was not uniform. In addition, the treatment of one malignancy had no demonstrable effect on the second malignancy. We felt that because of the lack of a pattern, evaluation should be minimal and thus recommended that only a thorough history and a physical examination be performed for these patients. Subsequently, I have seen over 100 individuals with squamous cell carcinoma of the skin and have yet to realize any benefit from such evaluation.

In summary, I believe that squamous cell carcinoma and, in particular, Bowen's disease are markers of malignant internal neoplasia. However, there is no uniformity to the relationship, and extensive evaluation cannot be recommended.

Cutaneous Melanoma

The data concerning malignant melanoma and internal neoplasia are less controversial. Three well-designed studies all have concluded that the incidence of second malignancies in a patient with one cutaneous melanoma is not different from the frequency of neoplasia in the general population.[12-14] However, the frequency of breast cancer approaches a significant level, and therefore careful breast examination is indicated for melanoma patients. The picture is less clear for patients with multiple cutaneous melanomas. Bellet and co-workers have concluded that the occurrence of internal malignancies in these patients is a random event.[12]

Kaposi's Sarcoma

Kaposi's sarcoma is a malignant proliferation of endothelial cells and pericapillary fibroblasts.[15] It has become more common in the last several years as a result of an increasing number of cases among immunosuppressed transplant patients and homosexuals. Kaposi's sarcoma may be localized to the skin or may involve visceral lesions. The visceral lesions may be represented by the typical histology of Koposi's sarcoma or may be a secondary malignancy. In particular, neoplasms of the lymphoreticular system have been reported on many occasions. Hanno and Owen found 53 lymphoreticular malignancies and 11 solid tumors reported in the world's literature.[16] The only incidence figures are presented by Safai and colleagues in their analysis of 92 cases of Kaposi's sarcoma.[15] They found that 37 per cent (34 of the cases) of patients with this disease had another primary malignancy. The second primary malignancy occurred prior to the Kaposi's sarcoma (12 cases), simultaneously with it (8 cases), or following the diagnosis (14 cases). Eighteen of the secondary malignancies involved the lymphoreticular system. In conclusion, it appears that Kaposi's sarcoma is indeed an important marker of visceral neoplasia and that most often the malignancy is a lymphoma or leukemia.

Keratoacanthoma

A keratoacanthoma is an epithelial neoplasm that may exhibit aggressive behavior.[17] Its etiology is unknown, but the main theories are that either viral or actinic induction is involved. Individual cases of either multiple or aggressive keratoacanthomas have been reported in association with internal malignancies.[17-19] In addition, the keratoacanthoma is a part of Torre's syndrome, a genetic disorder characterized by sebaceous carcinomas, adenomas, and multiple keratoacanthomas in association with visceral malignancy (often colonic).[20] In cases of Torre's syndrome, it is not known whether the keratoacanthoma is of any major diagnostic importance. To date, there has not been a study of keratoacanthomas that examines the incidence of internal malignancy systematically. Thus, no conclusion can be drawn at this time.

References

1. Lynch, H. T., Guirgis, H. A., Lynch, P. A., Lynch, J. F., and Harris, R. E.: Familial cancer syndromes: A survey. Cancer 39:1867, 1977.
2. Carpenter, C. L., Derbes, V. J., and Jolly, H. W.: Carcinoma of the skin—a guidepost to internal malignancy? JAMA 186:621, 1963.
3. Reynolds, R. D., Pajak, T. F., Greenberg, B. R., Shirley, J. H., Lucas, R. N., Hill, R. P., and Schacht, L. R.: Lung cancer as a second primary. Cancer 42:2887, 1978.
4. Møller, R., Nielsen, A., and Reymann, F.: Multiple basal cell carcinoma and internal malignant tumors. Arch. Dermatol. 111:584, 1975.
5. Callen, J. P., and Headington, J. T.: The relationship of Bowen's and non-Bowen's squamous intraepidermal neoplasia of the skin to internal malignancy. Arch. Dermatol. 116:422, 1980.
6. Graham, J. H., and Helwig, E. B.: Bowen's disease and its relationship to systemic cancer. Arch. Dermatol. 80:133, 1959.
7. Peterka, E. S., Lynch, F. W., and Goltz, R. W.: An association between Bowen's disease and internal cancer. Arch. Dermatol. 84:139, 1961.
8. Epstein, E.: Association of Bowen's disease with visceral cancer. Arch. Dermatol. 82:349, 1960.
9. Hugo, N. E., and Conway, H.: Bowen's disease: Its malignant potential and relationship to systemic cancer. Plast. Reconstr. Surg. 39:190, 1967.
10. Andersen, S. L. C., Nielsen, A., and Reymann, F.: Relationship between Bowen's disease and internal malignant tumors. Arch. Dermatol. 108:367, 1973.
11. Møller, R., Nielsen, A., Reymann, F., and Hon-Jensen, K.: Squamous cell carcinoma of the skin and internal malignant neoplasms. Arch. Dermatol. 115:304, 1979.
12. Bellet, R. E., Vaisman, I., Mastrangelo, M. J., and Lustbader, E.: Multiple primary malignancies in patients with cutaneous melanoma. Cancer 40:1974, 1972.
13. Fletcher, W. S.: The incidence of other primary tumors in patients with malignant melanoma. Pigment Cell 1:255, 1973.
14. Fraser, D. G., Bull J. G., and Dumphy, J. E.: Malignant melanoma and co-existing malignant neoplasma. Am. J. Surg. 122:169, 1971.
15. Safai, B., Mike, V., Giraldo, G., Beth, E., and Good, R. A.: Association of Kaposi's sarcoma with second primary malignancies. Cancer 45:1472, 1980.
16. Hanno, R., and Owen, L. G.: Kaposi's sarcoma. In Callen, J. P. (ed.): Cutaneous Aspects of Internal Disease. Chicago, Year Book Medical Publishers, 1981, pp. 291–298.
17. Fathizaden, A., Medenica, N. M., Soltani, K., Lorincz, A. C., and Griem, M. L.: Aggressive keratoacanthoma and internal malignant neoplasm. Arch. Dermatol. 118:112, 1982.
18. Chapman, R. S., and Finn, O. A.: Carcinoma of the larynx in two patients with keratoacanthoma. Br. J. Dermatol. 90:685, 1974.
19. Poleksic, S.: Keratoacanthoma and multiple carcinomas. Br. J. Dermatol. 91:461, 1974.
20. Housholder, M. S., and Zeligman, I.: Sebaceous neoplasms associated with visceral carcinomas. Arch. Dermatol. 116:61, 1980.

SKIN CANCER HAS NO EFFECT ON THE INCIDENCE OF INTERNAL CANCER

Ervin Epstein, M.D.

For many years there has been disagreement among dermatologists, oncologists, pathologists, and other specialists as to whether the appearance of a skin cancer predisposes to the development of an internal malignancy or whether it offers protection against this unfortunate occurrence. Most investigators have felt that the individual who manifested such a superficial malignancy would be *more* likely to suffer from a visceral cancer than one whose skin was free of such degenerative changes.[1] On the other hand, Peller was so convinced that skin cancer protects against internal cancer that he advised the purposeful production of a cutaneous malignancy as a "vaccination" to protect against the more serious internal type of neoplasm.[2] He even claimed that the immunity would persist long after the primary tumor had been eradicted and stated that cancer morbidity and mortality could be decreased by 90 per cent by the adoption of such a policy.

Hoping to establish the truth of this matter, this author studied 3006 individuals with skin cancer through the cooperation of the California Tumor Registry.[3] Of these patients, 180 (5.9 per cent) were known to have developed one or more primary malignant neoplasms *not* affecting the skin. Twelve hundred and forty-six (41.4 per cent) of these patients had died by the time of the study, but only 22.6 per cent of the latter group were known to have had postmortem examinations.

Establishing that approximately 6 per cent of this group had developed internal cancer at the time of the study did not resolve the question of the effect of skin cancers on more serious malignancies. After all, numbers by themselves have no meaning. To explain this statement, two illustrations should suffice. Is 1 million a lot? Well, it would represent an extreme excess of white blood cells, but, conversely, it would represent an extreme deficiency of red blood cells. If we found that 6 per cent of blue-eyed people died in automobile accidents, would this mean that those with eyes of this color were more or less apt to perish in such incidents? If 25 per cent of all persons succumbed after an automobile accident, then blue-eyed people would be able to ride more safely in cars than could the general population. However, if only 1 per cent of all passengers died in such accidents, then blue-eyed individuals should avoid automobile transportation. Furthermore, if it is established that a high-risk group has more of a certain peculiarity than do other, low-risk groups, it does not prove that changing that group's distinctive feature will lower its risk. After all, if red-heads have more freckles than do brunettes, you cannot prevent the appearance of freckles by dyeing the hair of a red-head brown.

Therefore, to establish the significance of the 6 per cent incidence of internal cancer in association with skin cancer in the studied group, we must have controls. Furthermore, these controls must be significant, and the significance of the controls may be more important than the findings in the studied group. By the judicious (or injudicious) selection of the control subjects, it can be shown that the 6 per cent incidence is high, low, or average. In other words, one can prove anything with figures if he choses the appropriate control to establish his thesis.

If normal population rates are selected, then the incidence of visceral cancer in individuals between the ages of 45 and 64 is 2.665 per 100,000, or 0.25 per cent. In persons over the age of 65, this figure rises to 900.1 per 100,000, or 0.9 per cent. Therefore, if one selects these figures as his control, he will reach the conclusion that skin cancer predisposes to internal cancer.

On the other hand, should life expectancy figures be selected, the incidence of internal cancer is 14.79 per cent in men and 20.48 per cent in women. This had risen to 20.6 per cent by 1978, the last year for which these figures are available.[4] Death statistics for the United States in 1949 were 13.2 per cent and 16 per cent in those over 45 years of age. In Alameda County in 1952 (the time and place of this study), the incidence was 15.5 per cent. If the investigator used one of these figures, he could justifiably claim that cutaneous cancer protects against visceral malignancies.

Another control used in this study was people discharged from the local county hospital. The figures revealed that 2.9 per cent of these individuals had an internal cancer when they left the hospital (dead or alive). This percentage rose to 9.0 in those over 45 years of age. This series eliminated many of the modifying factors, such as geography, time, and some socioeconomic features. The results compare reasonably well with the finding of 6 per cent reported in this series and suggest the possibility that skin cancers have no effect on the incidence of internal malignancies.

Another series involved the findings of the tumor board at the same county hospital. Eight hundred seventy-nine patients with histologically proven mucocutaneous cancers were studied. Fifty-one of these individuals with skin malignancies developed visceral cancer simultaneously with or subsequently to their epitheliomas. These patients constituted 5.8 per cent of the entire group.

To carry this one step further, approximately 60 per cent of those in the skin cancer group were still alive at the time this study was conducted. If we assume that visceral cancer will develop in an orderly manner, then when all of the 3006 individuals in this group have died, thereby exhausting all opportunities to manifest such internal malignancies, we could expect internal cancers to have appeared in 15 per cent of the patients with cutaneous malignancies. This figure, of course, compares favorably with the life expectancy and death statistics quoted earlier in this discussion. This would lead to the conclusion that the incidence rates for the two types of neoplasms were not related from a statistical viewpoint.

The findings did not vary significantly when the two common types of skin cancer were examined separately. Each type of epithelioma was associated with a deeper malignancy in a nearly equal proportion of cases. Of course, the association was noted more often with basal cell epitheliomas than with squamous cell epitheliomas, since the former tumors occur more commonly than the latter. The association was rare with melanoma. Two explanations for this finding are that melanomas occur more often in younger people and that these pigmented malignancies have a poorer prognosis.

The best method of diagnosing cancer would be at autopsy. In this series, only 22 per cent of those who died were subjected to postmortem examination. Therefore, clinical and laboratory examinations of living individuals must furnish most of the statistics.

No evidence was found to support the contention that multiple primary tumors improve the prognosis. In 37 fatal cases of associated mucocutaneous and internal cancer in the "closed file," death occurred within 3.3 years of medical observation for the first malignant tumor.

On the basis of this study, two statements can be made with reasonable certainty:

1. Skin cancer may be associated with internal cancer, so it is doubtful if "vaccination" as recommended by Peller would prevent the later development of internal cancer.

2. It is probable that skin cancer has no effect on the incidence of visceral cancer.

References

1. Warren, S., and Gates, O.: Cancer of the skin in relation to multiple malignant growth, JAMA 115:1705, 1940.
2. Peller, S.: Carcinogenesis as a means of reducing cancer mortality. Lancet 2:552, 1936.
3. Epstein, E.: Association of mucocutaneous and visceral cancers. A.M.A. Arch. Dermatol. Syph. 69:58, 1954.
4. Silverberg, E. : Cancer Statistics 1982. Cancer 32:15, 1982.

CHAPTER 7

IS BOWEN'S DISEASE A MARKER OF INTERNAL CANCER?

RELATIONSHIP BETWEEN BOWEN'S DISEASE AND INTERNAL CANCER*

James H. Graham, M.D.

Some cutaneous disorders lead to the development of carcinoma often enough to be referred to as premalignant diseases, and it is generally accepted that Bowen's disease represents such an entity. The significant criteria for referring to Bowen's disease as precancerous are based on the microscopic cytologic features of carcinoma in situ involving the epidermis and the pilary complex structures. Invasive adnexal carcinoma occurs in a significant number of patients. The presence of an extracutaneous malignant neoplasm in a patient with Bowen's disease was recorded by Bowen in 1920.[1] The patient died of cancer of the pylorus after having had skin lesions for 34 years. Twenty-six years of personal observations as well as information published since 1959 support the conclusion that Bowen's disease is indeed associated with carcinoma of the skin and extracutaneous cancer. Publications by Callen and Headington,[2] Callen,[3] Braverman,[4] and Miki and associates[5] document additional observations that individuals with Bowen's disease tend to develop cancer of the skin and internal organs.

During the past decade, only the study by Anderson and coworkers[6] gives data that seem to dispute the findings of an association between Bowen's disease and internal malignant tumors. Opinions are sometimes published; Pinkus has written that "I have never been impressed with this relationship and have not advised any thorough investigation of a patient with Bowen's disease for internal cancer. The higher incidence of cancer in the older age group must be kept in mind. Bowenoid lesions in sun exposed areas are solar keratoses, rather than Bowen's disease, and the nature of genital lesions with bowenoid histology remains to be determined."[7]

Bowen's disease affects both sexes but predominantly occurs in fair-complexioned white men who live in the southern regions of the United States. Twenty per cent of patients with Bowen's disease are women. Bowen's disease also affects other ethnic groups, including blacks, Orientals, Latin Americans, and American Indians, although there is a definite predilection for the disorder among sun-sensitive Celtic-speaking individuals of the British Isles or people of Anglo-Saxon ancestry. The disease afflicts older individuals predominantly. The lesions occur equally on covered and exposed skin. Typical lesions appear as plaques that are round to irregular, lenticular, polycyclic, erythematous, pigmented, scaly, keratotic, fissured, crusty, nodular, and eroded. The plaques are free of hair and

---

*The opinions or assertions herein are the private views of the author and are not to be construed as official or as reflecting the views of the Department of the Army or the Department of Defense.

usually appear sharply demarcated from the surrounding skin. Areas of normal-appearing skin may be present within the boundaries of larger lesions of Bowen's disease. Lesions of short duration appear as small, scaly, nonelevated keratoses. Lesions in the anogenital area, particularly in women, may appear verrucous and polypoid and frequently are pigmented.

Excision of Bowen's lesions is the treatment of choice, since at least 75 per cent of them recur after ionizing irradiation, curettage, and desiccation. In general, more than 50 per cent of patients with Bowen's disease treated for short periods with topical 1 to 5 per cent fluorouracil show evidence of regrowth after the applications are stopped. Bowen's lesions of the palms of the hands and the soles of the feet are particularly resistant to topical fluorouracil. When this cytotoxic agent is used for treating patients with multiple lesions of Bowen's disease, the therapy is most effective if used for a period of 8 to 12 weeks.

Treatment of Bowen's disease is necessary, because at least 5 per cent of patients with this disorder show clinical and microscopic evidence of an invasive adnexal carcinoma, which is more prone to occur in larger lesions. In 2 per cent of all patients with Bowen's disease, there is evidence of metastasis to extracutaneous organs, but this occurs only after in situ atypical keratinocytes disrupt the dermoepidermal basement membrane and the confines of the pilary complex to invade the dermis as adnexal carcinoma. Once adnexal carcinoma develops in a Bowen's disease lesion, up to 30 per cent of affected patients for whom long-term follow-up is performed will show metastasis. In a group of 77 patients diagnosed as having Bowen's disease with adnexal carcinoma who have been under short-term follow-up at the Armed Forces Institute of Pathology, 10 (or 13 per cent) showed evidence of metastasis from their primary skin lesions. The lower figure of 13 per cent (rather than 30 per cent) is interpreted as being a result of the short-term follow-up and early diagnosis and treatment of the affected patients. On an average of 6 to 7 years after onset of Bowen's disease, at least 42 per cent of the patients develop other skin and mucocutaneous premalignant and malignant lesions. At least 14 per cent of patients with Bowen's disease show multiple combinations of other premalignant and malignant skin and mucocutaneous lesions. Metastasis from cutaneous lesions of de novo squamous cell carcinoma and malignant melanoma occurs in 2 per cent of patients with the disorder. At least 25 per cent of 155 patients in a study of Bowen's disease reported by Helwig and Graham in 1961 had primary extracutaneous cancers.[8] In a study of 75 patients who have been followed at the Armed Forces Institute of Pathology, 19 (or 25 per cent) showed evidence of extracutaneous malignant neoplasms.

Early adequate treatment of Bowen's disease has no preventive effect on the subsequent development of systemic premalignant and malignant lesions. The systemic malignant tumors are detected usually on an average of 5 to 6 years after the onset of Bowen's disease. There is no correlation between the anatomic location of the Bowen's lesion and the absence or presence of systemic cancer. Observations indicate that at least 38 per cent of women with anogenital Bowen's disease show evidence of regional skin and extracutaneous cancer, including extramammary Paget's disease and carcinoma of the cervix, the vagina, the uterus, the ovary, the anus, the rectum, the urethra, and the urinary bladder.[13]

Anogenital Bowen's disease with an associated regional premalignant and malignant epithelial neoplasm shows a predilection for involving women. There is a general tendency for women with Bowen's disease to manifest their systemic cancers in the pelvic organs. In men with this disease, the locations of primary systemic cancer in order of frequency of involvement are the respiratory system, the gastrointestinal tract, the genitourinary organs, the reticuloendothelial system, the oral cavity, the breast, the endocrine system, the soft tissues, and the mucous membranes of the lip, the eye, and the anus.

At least 5 per cent of patients have multiple systemic cancers involving one or more anatomic sites. Occult cancer may occur in 5 per cent of the patients. This latter finding stresses the importance of long-term follow-up of patients and the necessity of an autopsy to complete the search for associated malignant disease. If thorough studies are carried out from the time of diagnosis to the death of the patient, at least 70 per cent of affected individuals show evidence of primary systemic cancer. The aggressive biology of systemic cancer in Bowen's disease is verified by distant metastasis from the primary neoplasm in 80 per cent of the patients. The median survival for patients with Bowen's disease is 12 years after the diagnosis has been established. Since the average patient with Bowen's disease dies at age 67, life expectancy for these individuals is comparable with that of the general population. The significant difference is that patients with Bowen's disease are more cancer-prone and die of neoplastic disease. Hereditary predisposition for the development of cancer is supported by the occurrence of skin tumors and internal malignant neoplasms in one or more family members in half of the patients with Bowen's disease.

The typical microscopic features of Bowen's disease are hyperkeratosis, parakeratosis, hypogranulosis, (rarely) hypergranulosis, plaque-like acanthosis, and an inflammatory infiltrate in the upper corium. The epidermis exhibits total or focal loss of normal polarity and progression of keratinocyte maturation. The loss of normal epidermal architecture is characterized by atypical keratinocyte proliferation, windblown appearance, hyperchromatic nuclei, multinucleated cells, vacuolated epithelium, malignant dyskeratosis, and abnormal mitotic figures. These changes occur at all epidermal levels but may be focal and are confined by an intact dermoepidermal basement membrane. The nuclei of atypical epithelial cells show variation in their size, shape, and staining characteristics. The malignant keratinocytes show prominent nucleoli, hyperchromasia, and some pyknosis and often are surrounded by a clear halo. Examination of multiple and serial sections of Bowen's disease lesions from hair-bearing areas invariably show involvement of the pilary acrotrichium, infundibulum, and sebaceous gland. The atypical cellular proliferation involves all levels of the outer root sheath and eventually replaces the sebaceous gland cells. Rudimentary and fragmented hairs sometimes are seen in the pilosebaceous canal. In some lesions, the majority of the atypical epithelial cells appear vacuolated and sometimes are contrasted with hyperchromatic undifferentiated keratinocytes that replace the epidermal basal layer and the pilary outer root sheath, and this gives the appearance of cellular nesting.

Bowen's disease of the palms of the hands and the soles of the feet shows essentially the same histologic features as lesions involving other anatomic sites, except for the absence of pilosebaceous follicle involvement. The acrosyringium generally is not involved but follows a straight course rather than the normal, spiral one. The lateral epidermal margins are sharply demarcated from areas that show the atypical keratinocyte proliferation. Sometimes, extensive skip areas of uninvolved epidermis are present in sections, although focal areas may show a few clones of atypical epithelial cells. Small clones of anaplastic keratinocytes occur at various epidermal levels, and these are surrounded by normal-appearing squamous cells. Serial sections usually demonstrate that these small foci of atypical keratinocytes are extensions from abnormal-appearing pilary outer root sheath epithelium. The microscopic features of small clones of atypical keratinocytes and uninvolved epidermal skip areas account for normal-appearing skin in gross lesions of Bowen's disease. An inflammatory infiltrate of lymphocytes, histiocytes and, sometimes, plasma cells is seen in the upper corium subjacent to the Bowen's disease lesion. The density and composition of the cellular infiltrate are variable, both within the same plaque and from lesion to lesion, depending on the anatomic site. A common feature in the upper corium is capillary-endothelial proliferation, and some of the small vessels are dilated. Lesions located on sun-exposed areas of the body show prominent solar elastosis.

When excised lesions are examined histologically 1 month or less after diagnostic biopsy specimens have been taken, they show re-establishment of epidermal continuity by normal keratinocytes or atypical epithelial cells, but there is no histologic evidence of adnexal carcinoma. Studies of wounds healing from biopsy sites, recurrent lesions, and large and small keratoses of Bowen's disease show that in hair-bearing areas, the atypical epithelial changes appear first in undifferentiated germinative cells of the pilary outer root sheath. Vacuolated cells normally present in the pilary outer root sheath and the sebaceous glands are involved. With continuous proliferation of these abnormal cells, the upper normal pilary outer root sheath epithelium and epidermal keratinocytes eventually are replaced. The origin of Bowen's disease from pilary outer root sheath cells at the sebaceous gland level helps explain in part the high recurrence rate of lesions after treatment with x-ray, superficial curettement and desiccation, and topical 5-fluorouracil. In lesions showing invasive adnexal carcinoma, the basement membrane is disrupted at the dermoepidermal interface or the junction of the dermis with the pilary outer root sheath. Irregular prolongations and isolated nests of pleomorphic cells extend into the corium. In general, when multiple sections of Bowen's disease with invasive carcinoma are studied, there is evidence of pilary complex differentiation of tumor cells toward follicular epithelium, sebaceous cells, and apocrine structures. Bowen's disease with adnexal carcinoma and distant spread shows abnormal histologic features in the metastatic lesions, which are similar to those seen in the dermis. Electron microscopy of Bowen's disease lesions shows abnormal cell division of malignant dyskeratotic cells, abnormal mitotic figures, decrease in tonofilament-desmosome attachments, absence of keratohyalin, aggregate tonofilaments and nuclear substances, and multiple disruptions of the dermoepidermal basement membrane.

The atypical vacuolated keratinocytes are routinely negative for cytoplasmic mucin. Some of the vacuolated atypical cells contain glycogen. There are variable amounts of epithelial hyaluronic acid in the interstices of the abnormal epidermis and the pilary outer root sheath. An argyrophilic basement membrane is present at the junction of the dermis with the epidermis and the hair follicle outer root sheath. There is a prominent proliferation of reticular fibers in areas of inflammation. The collagen and elastic fibers show general thinning in the same location. Most Bowen's disease lesions exhibit melanin granules in the atypical epithelial cells. In lesions showing solar elastosis, the elastic tissue is increased, and many fine reticular fibers are present. There are few or no collagen fibers in the areas of solar elastosis. Variable abnormal amounts of hyaluronic acid are present in the upper corium of lesions from exposed and unexposed sites. Alkaline phosphatase demonstrates striking capillary abnormalities in the papillary corium immediately beneath areas of plaque-like acanthosis. Sections show that the abnormal keratinizing cells in the pluripotential epidermis, the acrotrichium, the pilary infundibulum, and the sebaceous glands are intensely reactive with glucose-6-phosphate dehydrogenase. This enzyme method is excellent for demonstrating small clones of abnormal keratinocytes and clearly localizes atypical cells arising from the pluripotential epidermis and the pilary structures. The sections show that Bowen's disease of hair-bearing skin affects pilary adnexal keratinocytes, which proliferate from the follicle epithelium to involve the epidermis. The abnormal hair follicle keratinocytes show evidence of proliferation upward, outward, and laterally to cover over and replace the epidermis gradually.

The pathogenesis of Bowen's disease, as determined from small keratoses, recurrent lesions, and healing biopsy sites, shows development of an umbrella effect similar to that seen in lesions of solar keratosis. The principal difference in Bowen's disease is that the cells covering and replacing the epidermis represent abnormal pilary adnexal keratinocytes or pluripotential ectodermal epithelium originating from the primary epithelial germ. Frozen sections stained with oil-red-0 demonstrate lipids within atypical vacuolated cells and, particularly, those involving the pilosebaceous follicles. Papanicolaou-stained tissue imprints exhibit a few atypical keratinocytes or clumps of these cells when Bowen's disease shows microscopic features of carcinoma in situ. Multiple anaplastic tumor cells are seen when there is evidence of invasive adnexal carcinoma.

The clinical features of patients with arsenical keratoses and cancer are indistinguishable from those of patients with Bowen's disease, and there is also an identical natural history in individuals with these disorders. The association of arsenical keratosis with skin and internal cancer is generally accepted. The microscopic and histochemical features of Bowen's disease and arsenical keratosis are the same. All evidence indicates that Bowen's disease and arsenical keratosis represent the same entity. Microscopically, erythroplasia of Queyrat shows atypical epithelial changes similar to those seen in Bowen's disease, but some distinguishing features are hypokeratosis and fewer multinucleated cells. In addition, malignant dyskeratosis is not as prominent, and inflammation in the penile submucosa contains large numbers of plasma cells.

Histologically, anogenital bowenoid papulosis shows varying degrees of hyperkeratosis, frequent parakeratosis, foci of hypergranulosis, vacuolated keratinocytes, irregular acanthosis, and occasional papillomatosis. The stratum corneum and the granular cell layer often contain inclusion-like bodies that are basophilic, rounded, and sometimes surrounded by a halo. They can be easily distinguished from the flattened pyknotic parakeratotic nuclei in the altered stratum corneum. There is a relatively orderly background of keratinocyte maturation, with superimposed scattered hyperchromatic nuclei, dysplastic cells, and mitotic figures. Numerous keratinocytes containing mitotic figures in the same stage of development, particularly in metaphase, often are observed. The acrotrichium and the follicular infundibulum may show some epithelial atypia, but full-thickness involvement of these structures is not seen. The dysplastic cells frequently involve the acrosyringium. The papillary dermis or submucosa shows lymphocytes, histiocytes, and telangiectasia. Melanin pigment is free and within melanophages. Eosinophils and neutrophils sometimes are present, but plasma cells are uncommon. The most important microscopic feature that distinguishes bowenoid papulosis from Bowen's disease and erythroplasia of Queyrat is the lack of full-thickness epidermal or mucosal involvement by the atypical keratinocytes.

In sections of bowenoid papulosis, the dermoepidermal junction or mucosal basement membrane is intact, and features of invasive squamous cell cancer, Bowen's disease with adnexal carcinoma, or erythroplasia of Queyrat with carcinoma have not been observed. Sections of Bowen's disease involving hair-bearing skin characteristically show full-thickness pilosebaceous follicle involvement and sparing of the eccrine acrosyringium by the atypical keratinocytes. These features are not seen in bowenoid papulosis. Plasma cells are present in the inflammatory infiltrate in sections of Bowen's disease, and there are large numbers in the submucosa of erythroplasia of Queyrat. The significant histochemical features of bowenoid papulosis include Feulgen-positive, inclusion-like ovoid bodies surrounded by a clear halo in the stratum corneum and the foci of follicular hyperkeratosis, an intact periodic acid–Schiff-positive basement membrane, and only minimal amounts of cytoplasmic glycogen in atypical keratinocytes in the areas of dysplastic epithelial hyperplasia.

The nuclear morphology and cytoplasmic organelles in the keratinocytes of bowenoid papulosis and Bowen's disease show some common electron microscopic features. Significantly, foci of the basal lamina show disruption and decreased desmosomal attachments in Bowen's disease, but these structures are intact in bowenoid papulosis. Ultrastructural studies of lesions from patients with bowenoid papulosis show occasional keratinocytes, particularly in the stratum corneum, with uniform, rounded, intranuclear, electron-dense structures resembling viral particles that range from 30 to 35 nm in diameter. The electron microscopic observations correlate with detectable intranuclear human papilloma virus antigens that are demonstrated in tissue from patients with bowenoid papulosis by an immunoperoxidase technique. The immunoperoxidase-positive keratinocytes are present in the stratum granulosum and the horny layer and correlate with the location of Feulgen-positive inclusion-like bodies identified by light microscopy. Solar keratosis with bowenoid features can mimic the histologic changes seen in Bowen's disease, but pilary outer root sheath involvement distinguishes the latter disease. The cellular nesting of vacuolated pagetoid cells in some lesions of Bowen's disease can cause histologic confusion with malignant melanoma of the superficial spreading type, intraepidermal epithelioma, extramammary Paget's disease, and mammary Paget's disease.

The similarities of Bowen's disease and arsenical keratosis can be demonstrated through chemical analysis of typical keratoses and plaques, which shows that arsenic is present in significantly greater amounts than are found in a variety of control diseases affecting the skin. There is an abundance of arsenic in our environment. Arsenic, a known strong chemical carcinogen, can be found in water, air, soil, food, tobacco, sprays, and medicinal agents. Many occupational groups, particularly industrial workers, still have ample opportunity to be exposed to arsenic. Large amounts of arsenic still are used annually in agriculture in areas such as Orange County, California, near the University of California, Irvine. A significantly greater number of patients with Bowen's disease are seen at this institution than at hospitals in Philadelphia.[13] The intake of arsenic in small amounts for long periods can produce a general neoplastic tendency. More than 50 per cent of the arsenic taken into the body is deposited in tissues and gradually eliminated over time. The possibility that increased tissue storage of arsenic may be an individual metabolic trait has been proposed to account for the increased tendency toward carcinogenesis in some patients. The overall evidence strongly suggests that arsenic is a cause of Bowen's disease. The cutaneous and internal cancers present in patients with Bowen's disease represent the systemic manifestation of arsenic carcinogenesis. Because of the clinical, histopathologic, histochemical, chemical, and carcinogenic similarities of Bowen's disease and arsenical keratosis, arsenic is considered to represent a common etiologic factor. Patients with Bowen's disease are prone to develop cancer of multiple organ systems. Before or at the time of death, more than 80 per cent of patients have primary premalignant and malignant neoplasms in one or more locations.

Etiologic factors other than inorganic arsenic are exposure to sunlight, petroleum byproducts, or other elements; trauma; cutaneous injury from ionizing irradiation; and an inherited tendency to develop the disease. The association of Bowen's disease with cutaneous and internal cancer undoubtedly represents a systemic carcinogenic process. Women with anogenital Bowen's disease show a definite tendency toward development of internal malignant epithelial tumors involving pelvic girdle organs, which suggests a carcinogenic field effect relationship of carcinoma of the skin and extracutaneous cancer. The pathogenesis of Bowen's disease suggests that the germinal cells of the pilary outer root sheath and the pluripotential epidermis are affected. The affinity of arsenic for keratinizing epithelium is well recognized. Involvement of the epidermis and the pilosebaceous follicles in the carcinogenesis of Bowen's disease seems logical, since these structures are rich keratin producers.

In recent years, only one report has appeared that seems to dispute the association of Bowen's disease with systemic cancer.[6] It is difficult to reconcile the lack of association of systemic cancer and Bowen's disease in this Danish study with the many other investigations that seem to verify the observations reported in this paper. No clinical pictures or photomicrographs were available for study in the Danish publication, and it is possible that some of the patients actually may not have had Bowen's disease. A good example of this is the abundance of misdiagnoses of bowenoid papulosis as Bowen's disease during the past decade. Twenty-nine years of knowledge about patients with bowenoid papulosis, which are summarized in a report by Kao and Graham,[9] give no evidence that the disease represents a precancerous entity with the potential for the development of invasive squamous cell carcinoma. Patients with bowenoid papulosis show no evidence of cancer proneness. The clinicopathologic, histochemical, immunochemical, and electron microscopic changes, along with the biological behavior, natural history, follow-up data, and young age of the affected individuals, favor the theory that bowenoid papulosis represents a benign reactive disorder involving anogenital skin and mucous membranes. The occurrence of this disorder in children 1 to 2 years of age and the benign natural course indicate that bowenoid papulosis represents a reversible reactive atypical cytologic process rather than a precancerous disorder capable of invading the dermis or the submucosa.

The cause of bowenoid papulosis is not definite, but emerging scientific evidence favors human papilloma virus or herpes simplex virus type 2 as probable etiologic agents. Until proved otherwise, it is preferable not to diagnose bowenoid papulosis as Bowen's disease. Until a specific etiologic agent is identified, the term bowenoid papulosis is acceptable but should be used to designate a biologically benign disease. Treatment should be conservative.

Results of the Danish study[6] should make the authors and all others reappraise their data in an objective, candid way now and in the future in an attempt to reach a correct answer regarding the association of Bowen's disease and systemic cancer. A review of the Danish study suggests some defects in data collection: The methods used may not identify all cancers, since disorders that were cured might not have been recorded. It is recommended that until the matter is clear, every patient initially diagnosed as having Bowen's disease should be studied for systemic cancer. Experience during the past 26 years also emphasizes the importance of follow-up studies of patients with Bowen's disease, since they may continue to develop other lesions, including any type of skin cancer. The presence of internal cancer in patients with Bowen's disease may be the terminal event or may not be detected unless an autopsy is performed. At least 5 per cent of patients with Bowen's disease have occult internal cancer. Experience has emphasized that the history supplied by the patient is often unreliable with regard to exposure to agents such as arsenic. Patients still are seen who have Bowen's disease and systemic cancer but who give a negative history regarding ingestion of or exposure to arsenic, although it is well known that considerable amounts of this carcinogen continue to be present in our environment.

SUMMARY

The association of Bowen's disease with cutaneous and systemic cancer is generally accepted. Arsenic is a common etiologic agent in Bowen's disease and arsenical keratosis, and these premalignant diseases are considered to represent the same entity. The pathogenesis of Bowen's disease suggests that the germinal cells of the pilary outer root sheath and the pluripotential epidermis are affected. The affinity of arsenic for keratinizing epithelium is well recognized. Involvement of the epidermis and the pilosebaceous follicles in the carcinogenesis of Bowen's disease seems logical, since these structures are rich keratin producers. Patients with bowenoid solar keratoses show some tendency to develop cancer, and the common occurrence of these keratoses in patients with Bowen's disease suggests a common etiology and a similarity in biological behavior with regard to cutaneous and systemic malignant neoplasms. There is a striking histologic resemblance between erythroplasia of Queyrat and Bowen's disease, but the natural history and biology indicate that the penile disease is a separate entity. Cancer proneness is not a prominent feature in patients with erythroplasia of Queyrat. Caution should be taken regarding the overdiagnosis of bowenoid papulosis as Bowen's disease.

References

1. Bowen, J. T.: Precancerous dermatoses: The further course of 2 cases previously reported. Arch. Dermatol. Syph. 1:23, (Jan.) 1920.
2. Callen, J. P., and Headington, J.: Bowen's and non-Bowen's squamous intraepidermal neoplasia of the skin. Arch. Dermatol. 116:422, (Apr.) 1980.
3. Callen, J. P.: Cutaneous Aspects of Internal Disease. Chicago, Year Book Medical Publishers, 1981, pp. 209–212.

4. Braverman, I. M.: Skin Signs of Systemic Disease, 2nd ed., Philadelphia, W. B. Saunders Company, 1981, pp. 67–77.
5. Miki, Y., Kawatsu, T., Matsuda, K., Machino, H., and Kubo, K.: Cutaneous and pulmonary cancers associated with Bowen's disease. J. Acad. Dermatol. 6:26, (Jan.) 1982.
6. Anderson, S. L. C., Nielsen, A., and Reymann, F.: Relationship between Bowen's disease and internal malignant tumors. Arch. Dermatol. 108:367, (Sept.) 1973.
7. Pinkus, H.: Opinions: What is the relationship between Bowen's disease and internal cancer? Schoch Letter 31:9, (Mar.) 1981.
8. Graham, J. H., and Helwig, E. B.: Bowen's disease and its relationship to systemic cancer. Arch. Dermatol. 83:738, (May) 1962.
9. Kao, G. F., and Graham, J. H.: Bowenoid Papulosis. Int. J. Dermatol. 21:445, (Oct.) 1982.
10. Graham, J. H., and Helwig, E. B.: Bowen's disease and its relationship to systemic cancer. Arch. Dermatol. 80:133, (Aug.) 1959.
11. Graham, J. H., Mazzanti, G. R., and Helwig, E. B.: Chemistry of Bowen's disease: Relationship to arsenic. J. Invest. Dermatol. 37:317, (Nov.) 1961.
12. Graham, J. H., and Helwig, E. B.: Premalignant cutaneous and mucocutaneous disease. In Graham, J. H., Johnson, W. C., and Helwig, E. B.: Dermal Pathology, Hagerstown, MD, Harper and Row, 1972, pp. 581–597 and 621–624.
13. Graham, J. H.: Selected precancerous skin and mucocutaneous lesions. In Neoplasms of the Skin and Malignant Melanoma. Chicago, Year Book Medical Publishers, 1976, pp. 86–99 and 118–121.

BOWEN'S DISEASE IS NOT A MARKER OF INTERNAL CANCER

Hermann Pinkus, M.D.

Bowen's disease is the development of sharply defined intraepidermal foci of malignant cells anywhere on the surface of the body. These cells multipy more quickly than do epidermal basal cells, and the foci grow in size. After a variable time, often lasting a number of years, the foci of Bowen's disease grow into the dermis, and Bowen's carcinoma, which is a slowly growing squamous cell cancer, results. Metastasis of Bowen's carcinoma occurs occasionally, again after a delay of several years.

In the last few years, a debate has arisen concerning Bowen's disease of the genitalia in young people, especially in men. Lesions of this type have been designated as bowenoid papulosis and have been said to be prone to spontaneous involution rather than malignant. This controversy is not resolved, and we are not dealing with it in this discussion. A controversy of much longer duration, however, is whether people suffering from other types of Bowen's dermatosis are more prone to develop systemic forms of cancer than are normal persons. This question was raised in a paper by Graham and Helwig in 1959,[1] and it has caused considerable fear among many pathologists and dermatologists. It is difficult to answer this question; such an investigation would require a large group of persons with and without Bowen's disease who would have to be observed for many years and watched for the development of malignancy in internal organs. In addition, there is the practical question of whether a patient who has a superficial spot of Bowen's disease should be subjected to a thorough investigation for cancer that may not become clinically apparent until many years later. For a practicing dermatopathologist, this decision is a very difficult one. A positive answer burdens the patient for the rest of his life with the fear of cancer. Also, a study of this nature may expose the individual to a number of expensive medical examinations that are almost certain to be negative at the time they are done. I have not considered myself entitled to recommend intensive physical examination for cancer to a patient or a physician who sent me a specimen of skin that I diagnosed as exhibiting Bowen's disease.

In conclusion, I must state that in my opinion there is inadequate evidence to support the exposure of a patient with Bowen's disease to an expensive and inconvenient search in an attempt to demonstrate an internal cancer at the time the cutaneous lesions are present.

Reference

1. Graham, J. H., and Helwig, E. B.: Bowen's disease and its relationship to systemic cancer. Arch. Dermatol. 80:133, 1959.

Editorial Comment

If one accepts the definition that a cutaneous marker of internal cancer is a skin lesion that presents simultaneously with an internal malignancy, then Bowen's disease is not a marker. The patient with this cutaneous condition may or may not have hidden neoplastic disease. However, he is more susceptible to cancer than is a member of the general population. Approximately 16 per cent of all patients who die succumb to cancer. The percentage of people with Bowen's disease who eventually develop cancer is much higher than this figure. However, there does not seem to be a relationship between the two conditions at any given time. In other words, the patient with Bowen's disease is at a higher risk for eventually developing such a tumor than is the individual who has never suffered from Bowen's disease. On the other hand, the presence of Bowen's disease does not indicate that the patient is harboring a malignancy at that time, as in the case of adult acanthosis nigricans.

Basically, the diagnosis of Bowen's disease is established by histopathologic criteria. There are differences of opinion among dermatopathologists as to the features that are essential for this diagnosis. Bowenoid lesions may be simulated by cellular or dyskeratotic actinic keratoses, for instance. In most series, true Bowen's disease is not considered to be a common condition. Thu number of cases of this dermatosis in a series varies inversely with the stringency with which the pathology consultant conforms to strict guidelines. Errors in diagnosis can be made by both the clinician and the pathologist.

In this chapter, we have two of the most respected dermatohistopathologists in the world disagreeing on the significance of Bowen's disease. Certainly a clinician can not officiate in such a contest.

Think It Over.

CHAPTER 8

DERMABRASION VERSUS 5-FLUOROURACIL IN PRECANCEROUS SKIN

ON THE VALUE OF DERMABRASION IN THE MANAGEMENT OF ACTINIC KERATOSES

Lawrence M. Field, M.D.

The value of dermabrasion in the therapy of actinic keratoses and superficial epitheliomas was initially suggested by Kurtin[1] in 1953. Epstein first established this in 1958 in ten cases.[2] A follow-up study 10 years later further confirmed the value of this procedure. The fears expressed by Gibson concerning "the possibility of dissemination or stimulation of unrecognized squamous cell carcinoma should this be present"[3] have not been observed. An extensive literature has evolved worldwide, time and again reaffirming the value of dermabrasion in the therapy of premalignant cutaneous changes and of the prophylactic value of this treatment.[1,2,4-11] In 1958, Epstein[2] reported and subsequently published responses obtained from 120 dermatologists to whom he had sent a questionnaire on their use of dermabrasion of precancerous skin. At that time the majority did not use dermabrasion for this purpose, but 30 of 33 respondents were "enthusiastic" or deemed their results to be "satisfactory" with over 1300 accumulated cases of facial dermabrasion. There was "relatively little disagreement among those with experience in the treatment of such cases" that precancerous skin was "one of the prime indications for dermabrasion." It was agreed that new or recurrent keratoses were "much less frequent than the adjacent unplaned skin, or than in the patient prior to the performance of this procedure."[2] Even at that time, many dermatologists were quoted as believing that planing for premalignant actinic and senile skin would eventually become even more important than the cosmetic dermabrasion done for scarring.

Another survey was carried out by Epstein in 1961.[7] Of the 1075 dermatologists who answered the questionnaire, 194 had used planing in the management of cutaneous precanceroses. Seventy-eight per cent reported their results as "excellent" or "good."

Burks and associates[12] reported on the results of half-face planings after 5 years, finding "a degree of improvement of planed over un-planed sides of the face based upon the opinions of seven inspectors was 85% cosmetically and 92% therapeutically." They found that more than two thirds of their patients subsequently developed fewer premalignant lesions on the dermabraded side and that "no patient had more suspicious lesions on the planed side" than on the unplaned side. Long-term follow-up of those patients in New Orleans revealed continued pressure on the operators to dermabrade the unplaned side for the benefits expected.[3] To 1963, Epstein[7] had "never seen an epithelioma develop in planed skin,'' although Burks had observed this phenomenon. I have seen epitheliomas develop as well, but only in patients with the most severe and advanced change.

In 1961, Spira and coworkers[13] compared chemical peeling, dermabrasion, and 5-fluorouracil (5-FU) in the treatment of senile keratoses. Small numbers of patients were followed from ''four months to three years.'' Eight patients were treated using phenol solution occluded for 48 hours on the entire face or on half the face while the other half was dermabraded. Dermabrasion was carried out ''into the reticular area of the dermis.'' After this procedure, a nonocclusive gauze dressing was used. A 1 per cent 5-fluorouracil solution in propylene glycol was applied twice daily for a period up to 6 weeks, with a well-developed ''inflammatory reaction'' as the end point of treatment. They found it ''obvious that 5-FU applications are superior to chemical peeling or to dermabrasion in the treatment of widespread senile keratoses . . . despite recurrences. . . .'' These conclusions followed the statement ''the judging of overall effectiveness of treatment, in terms of preventing future keratoses, was difficult in this small series.'' Identification and separation of patients according to prognosis was not done. Although these authors believed 5-fluorouracil to be a ''more effective screening agent than peeling or dermabrasion in uncovering cancer,'' it is the observation of many that this agent is capable of obscuring deeper malignancies. Furthermore, 5-fluorouracil is not as efficacious as dermabrasion in long-term prevention of recurrent dyskeratotic and malignant cutaneous disease.[2,5-10,14-25] This may be because 5-fluorouracil does not penetrate the orthokeratotic stratum corneum and subsequently fails to reach the deeper dysplastic cells, which are adequately reached by the brush or the fraise.[43]

There has been ongoing controversy concerning whether sufficient improvements can be rendered by removal of the sun-damaged epidermis alone or whether one must also remove the degenerated elastic and collagen material of the upper dermis physically in the act of planing, thus permitting new fibers to regenerate. These have been matters of conjecture for 20 years, and no one yet is certain. Whereas Baker and Gordon[23] believe that the dermis does not undergo specific alteration following dermabrasion and that the part of the dermis that is removed by the act of dermabrasion does not regenerate, Stegman[27] has confirmed Behin's previous observation[14] that the postdermabraded injury extends deeper than the fraise removal itself. Stegman believes that the ''replacement of collagen that is injured but not actually removed by dermabrasion may account for much of the benefit achieved by dermabrasion in diminishing scars and smoothing out the surface of scars and skin.'' In studies comparing multiple chemical escharotic agents and dermabrasion,[28] he reported that dermabrasion as well as occluded and nonoccluded Baker's phenol solution all produced similar wounds in which the epidermis was lost and replaced. Subsequently, there resulted the constant development of a clear zone of enlarged papillary dermis beneath the epidermis—''the thickness of this grenz zone directly related to the amount of wounding.'' Epidermal thickness measured 0.08 mm 120 days after dermabrasion and 0.09 mm after being occluded with Baker's phenol mixture. However, the clear grenz zone beneath the epidermis measured 0.5 mm 120 days after dermabrasion and 0.12 mm after occlusion with Bakers phenol mixture, and the permanent band of fibers beneath the grenz zone (which he termed the ''dermal scar'') measured 0.5 mm after dermabrasion and 0.45 mm after chemical peel. After the occluded peel, the number of rete pegs in the epidermis returned to pretreatment levels, whereas the dermabraded epidermis rete remained almost flat. The dermal response and the histochemical quality were very similar after both types of injury; the primary variation was in increased thickness following dermabrasion.

To all who perform this procedure it is obvious that the nonplaned areas of the posterior and lateral neck, the hair-bearing margin of the scalp, and the ear continue to develop premalignant and malignant lesions at a rate far in excess of that of the dermabraded area. Even though I use a phenol-containing solution to feather the edges for pigmentary blending, chemexfoliative methods in these areas have not been sufficient to prevent further lesions. Hill[18] calls attention to the striking increase in lesions "at the margins of the dermabrasion and hair line areas." He considers dermabrasion "the treatment of choice in almost every patient" save those who are too ill to undergo surgical procedures.

In follow-ups of dermabraded patients for a period greater than 10 years, Kirschbaum[19] reported "remarkable results" from dermabrasion. Recurrences were seen in only two patients, one after 7 years and the second after 10 years. Caver[29] believes that "practically all premalignant disease and to some extent a few carcinomas in situ may be effectively treated with dermabrasion and that the recurrence rate is extremely low." Lewis[20] observed "close to miraculous" improvement in patients with xeroderma pigmentosum using facial dermabrasion. In the case of another patient with xeroderma pigmentosum reported by Epstein, Jr., and associates,[16] facial dermabrasion was followed by the absence of tumor development for a 7-year follow-up period. The authors felt the result of their dermabrasion to be cosmetically superior to the outcome in a case of xeroderma pigmentosum reported by Gleason,[30] in which the entire face was resurfaced with full-thickness skin grafts taken from less damaged areas. Additionally, Epstein, Jr., found dermatome shaving of the lower legs to be of assistance in reducing the numbers of lesions evolving in this xeroderma pigmentosum patient. Thus, with either dermatome shaving or dermabrasion, repopulation of the epidermis by cells arising in deeper areas of the follicles and glands, with their attendant reduced exposure to ultraviolet radiation, allows a greater chance that the epithelium will be restored by more normal cells.[41] Pinkus, who holds that senile keratoses originate in the epidermis and not in hair follicles or other adnexae,[31] believes that the "removal of damaged but not definitely diseased tissue and its replacement by "new skin" can prevent further development of keratoses and cancers for a prolonged period." He felt dermabrasion to be "definitely beneficial."[45]

Although Epstein[6] used dermabrasion in multiple anatomic areas, Lewis[20] believes that "it should be limited to facial skin." After 26 years of using the procedure, he finds that "the skin is far less prone to develop keratoses and lentigines than prior to dermabrasion." Stagone[23] offers photographs showing uniform actinic keratoses over the face except in the previously abraded areas. Yarborough[25] believes dermabrasion to be the "singularly most effective modality" known to him, with many patients relatively free of lesions 5 to 10 years after full face planing. He has called attention to a woman whose adolescent acne had been treated with x-radiation of unknown dose. The patient had had 44 epitheliomas removed from her face and was being treated with 5-fluorouracil every 6 to 9 months. Dermabrasion was performed 6 years ago, and no malignancies have occurred since, although new keratoses had been developing.

Stegman[24] feels that the procedure is "definitely helpful" in the prevention of "actinically induced basal cell epitheliomata." His work[27,28] shows that phenol peeling did not provide the same benefit. The primary difference was in epidermal rather than dermal changes. Barkoff,[32] following 15 years of progressive discouragement with topical 5-fluorouracil because of the rate of dyskeratotic recurrence, feels that dermabrasion is absolutely advantageous when compared with 5-fluorouracil. He employs dermabrasion when treating lentigines on the face and the dorsum of the hands and ponders its value in prevention of lentigo maligna. Stough[33] has become "very disappointed in 5-FU, and it has become less useful over the years." He states that "dermabrasion is certainly superior to the use of 5-FU in the treatment of actinic keratoses, though it is more traumatic in the elderly due to slower healing." Tromovitch[34] also believes that "dermabrasion is the preferred treatment for patients with extensive keratoses and/or multiple basal cell carcinomas or squamous cell carcinomas developing at different facial sites," provided that the patients are informed of the alternatives and disadvantages. Luikart[21] states that dermabrasion "is superior to other treatments because the dermabraded areas rarely show recurrence of actinic keratoses." He further calls attention to the excellence of "spot planing" for focal lesions but also mentions the sequela of permanent color change, especially in the elderly.

In my opinion, and in the opinion of all my consultants,[18–21,23–25,29,32–36] the superiority of dermabrasion over 5-fluorouracil in the treatment of premalignant and malignant lesions is established. In the fifth edition of Epstein's *Skin Surgery,* the author states, "It should be remembered that planing has a much greater prophylactic effect than has the popular 5-FU." He further states, "These have the best prophylactic results obtained . . . by any approach."[37] Because of the relevance of the procedure, let us review some of the important facets of this modality.

It should be understood that generally the face responds best and heals most rapidly with the least morbidity, the scalp responds to a lesser degree, and the back heals even less, with most other areas best avoided unless the operator is extremely experienced. After dermabrasion, skin color is altered by temporary erythema, and as the newly formed layers of collagen realign themselves, the planed skin appears younger.[3,4,11,28] Similarly, 5-fluorouracil works best on the face. The next best results are obtained on the scalp, and the outcome is relatively poor elsewhere, even when topical tretinoin with or without occlusion is being used to facilitate the penetration of 5-fluorouracil.[35,38,39] Since the action of 5-fluorouracil is selective on epidermal cells, little if any change occurs in the dermis. This failure to alter the elastotic dermis does not provide the facial rejuvenation that is of such important physical and emotional benefit to patients.

Actinically induced fine wrinkling around the lips and the periorbital areas may be improved by both dermabrasion and chemical peeling.[3,11,13,23,26] Diffuse fine wrinkling alone, without keratoses and without a history of epitheliomatous degeneration, might be better served by chemical peel than by dermabrasion.[42]

Although dermabrasion can be used in the treatment of chronic radiodermatitis and radiation keratoses, some presence of adnexal activity (hair, acne, sebaceous hyperplasia, seborrhea, oil production, and so forth) should be clinically evident. In the absence of this adnexal activity, the deeper germ cells of the epithelial pegs may be decreased in such number as to compromise re-epithelialization following dermabrasion. Epstein[5] believes that the extended healing time in such cases must be weighed against the possible prophylactic benefits, especially in the patient with extensive radiodermatitis who has already developed multiple epitheliomas. I use multifocal test sites before attempting full-face dermabrasion in such cases.

The usual course following dermabrasion is well known.[44] Transient edema and erythema take weeks to resolve. Milia occur in the majority of patients but often are few in number. I use topical tretinoin for a period of 3 to 4 weeks prior to dermabrasion and continue its administration postoperatively as soon as the patient can tolerate its effects. Mandy[35] taught me that this shortens healing time and lessens the number of subsequent milia. Hypertrophic scars, keloids, and ridging at the dermabrasion margins can, but rarely do, occur. Areas of bony prominence (the mandibular, mental, and zygomatic areas and, less commonly, the forehead) require less pressure because of both scarring[40] and superficial purpura.[4] Infection is extremely rare, especially when patients are placed in their own home bacteriologic milieu rather than a hospital environment. I have never seen infection of systemic import.

Postdermabrasion pigmentary disturbances are to be expected in geographic areas of increased actinic exposure. Relative hypopigmentation in planed skin areas and the contrast of that skin with unplaned surface areas may be apparent. All prospective dermabrasion patients, especially males, must be made aware of a variation in color that may persist. I have never known one of my patients to regret the dermabrasion when comparing a slight variation in color with the improvement obtained. I use a Baker's phenol solution at the periphery of the dermabrasion to accomplish a gradual transition in color change. By the use of a drier applicator, a more superficial peel should be performed on the ears, the lateral neck, and the eyelids when indicated. I do not use occlusive taping in any of these areas because of reported scarring following occlusion.

Fortunately, diffuse actinic dyskeratotic change is infrequent in Oriental peoples,[3,29] because these individuals have the greatest difficulty with postoperative variations in pigmentation. Dermabraders having extensive experience with black patients treat them with the same method used for white patients, and the pigmentary sequelae have been acceptable.[36] In general, permanent pigmentary disturbances are seen to a lesser degree with darker patients. The early application of depigmenting agents combined with nonfluorinated steroids and tretinoin is of assistance in the treatment of postinflammatory hyperpigmentation. A history of past herpes simplex or herpes zoster has not deterred me from a dermabrasion when indicated, since no convincing evidence to the contrary has been presented.

In selected patients, dermabrasion is the treatment of choice for diffuse premalignant changes. The original success with topical chemotherapy has not stood the test of time in a large percentage of patients treated. In my experience, the more severe the actinic damage and the greater the degree of hyperkeratotic change, the less likely the success of 5-fluorouracil. In general, the lighter the complexion and the more delicate the skin, the greater the degree of discomfort to be expected with 5-fluorouracil. The necessity of self-application despite continued and progressive pain in many individuals is an insurmountable barrier. Lengthening the treatment time by using intermittent applications and by administering steroids topically to reduce the inflammatory response has not, in my experience, lessened discomfort to the point of acceptability for many patients. Unlike dermabrasion, in which discomfort may be controlled during a procedure that lasts a finite number of minutes, many or most individuals must experience progressively increasing pain for weeks with 5-fluorouracil. The recovery course after dermabrasion is one of continuous improvement, whereas 5-fluorouracil requires progressively more commitment. Treatment and recovery time in most patients receiving 5-fluorouracil therapy lasts 1 month or longer.

In previous decades, depending on depth and severity, most of my dermabraded patients required 7 to 14 days to re-epithelialize, with social acceptability occurring in 2 to 4 weeks. With the advent of the new biological dressings, such as Op-Site (T. J. Smith & Nephew Ltd., England), Biobrane (Hall-Woodruff, Inc., California), Bioclusive (Johnson & Johnson Products Inc., New Jersey), and Vigilon (Bard Home Health Division, C. R. Bard, Inc., New Jersey), which are applied for the first 2 to 3 days, we see a definite decrease in discomfort and a significant shortening of the healing time. Patients should be told that according to experience, re-treatment may be required 1 to 3 years after 5-fluorouracil therapy, regardless of how successfully they prevent further actinic exposure. The usual dermabraded patient can look forward to many years of relative freedom from new lesions. Even in fair-skinned patients with the most severe changes, the numbers of new lesions occurring after the treatment should be significantly decreased. Furthermore, I believe that the dermabraded patient pays greater attention to subsequent self-protection, perhaps because of the general feeling of well-being from the younger, more normal appearance that follows the procedure.

In my patients who have been previously treated with 5-fluorouracil under my supervision or elsewhere and who exhibit widespread recurrence, full-face dermabrasion has been uniformly accepted and preferred when compared with a repeated course of 5-fluorouracil.[17] According to those who have undergone both procedures, dermabrasion has the advantages of being less painful and having a shorter recovery period.

In dermabrasion, the mid-dermis is the therapeutic end point. With 5-fluorouracil, at what anatomic depth do we cease therapy? In practice, we must judge the adequacy of a surface reaction as our therapeutic end point without knowledge of the depth change achieved.

To deny the benefits of dermabrasion because of its cost is to employ the weakest argument of all. It is impossible to compare the relative dollar values of a single procedure performed quickly and efficiently and the weeks to months of suffering and relative incapacitation experienced by a patient undergoing one or more courses of 5-fluorouracil therapy. The inability of the patient to work because of course repetitions has a great economic impact. In addition, how does one measure the cost of the multitude of lesions that would not have to be treated or excised against the cost of a single therapeutic and prophylactic dermabrasion? And who will place a dollar value on the many nights of burning discomfort experienced with 5-fluorouracil therapy?

In summary, for the patient who has widespread severe actinic damage and dyskeratotic change and in whom there is a history of epitheliomatous degeneration, I believe that dermabrasion is the treatment of choice. The course of topical chemotherapy with 5-fluorouracil is prolonged, painful, and frequently repetitive. On the other hand, a full-face dermabrasion and combined chemabrasion of the forehead, the ears, and the neck involves only putting on a biological dressing for several days and undergoing a healing time of 7 to 14 days. The result of dermabrasion is a face devoid of keratoses that is relatively wrinkle-free and looks one or two decades younger. The expectation of considerable (but less than total) prophylaxis against the development of further keratoses and carcinomas with dermabrasion is statistically valid. Dermabrasion, therefore, is the treatment of choice for those informed patients who prefer its long-term advantages.

References

1. Kurtin, A.: Corrective surgical planing of skin. Arch. Dermatol. Syphilol. 88:389, Oct. 1953.
2. Epstein, E.: Planing for precancerous skin. Arch. Dermatol. 77:676, June 1958.
3. Gibson, E. W. : Malignant tumors of the skin. In Grabb, W. C., and Smith, J. W. (eds.): Plastic Surgery, 2nd ed. Boston, Little, Brown & Co., 1973, p. 664.
4. Burks, J. W.: Dermabrasion and Chemical Peeling. Springfield, IL, Charles C Thomas, 1979, pp. 20, 76, 159, 162, and 210.
5. Epstein, E.: A discussion of Burks' paper of half-face planing of precancerous skin after five years. Arch. Dermatol. 88:150, Nov. 1963.
6. Epstein, E.: Planing for precancerous skin—a ten year evaluation. Calif. Med. 105:26, July 1966.
7. Epstein, E.: Present status of dermabrasion. Calif. Med. 98:79, Feb. 1963.
8. Field, L. M.: Dermabrasion for prevention of premalignant and malignant lesions. Cutis 2:186, Aug. 1971.
9. Field, L. M.: Dermabrasion for treatment and prevention of solar keratoses and epitheliomas. Schoch Letter 31:35, Sept. 1981.
10. Kraemer, K. H.: Xeroderma pigmentosum. In Demis, D. J., et al. (eds.) Clinical Dermatology, 9th ed. New York, Harper & Row, 1982.
11. Rees, T. D.: Chemabrasion and dermabrasion. In Rees, T. D.: Aesthetic Plastic Surgery, vol. 2. Philadelphia, W. B. Saunders Co., 1980, pp. 749–769.
12. Burks, J. W., Marascalo, J., and Clark, W. N., Jr.: Half-face planing of precancerous skin after five years. Arch. Dermatol. 88:572, Nov. 1963.
13. Spira, M., Freeman, R., Arfai, P., Erow, F. J., and Hardy, F. B.: Clinical comparison of chemical peeling, dermabrasion, and 5-FU for senile keratoses. Plast. Reconstr. Surg. 46:61, 1970.
14. Behin, F., Feuerstein, S. S., and Marovitz, W. F.: Comparative histological study of mini pig skin after chemical peel and dermabrasion. Arch. Otolaryngol. 103:271, 1977.
15. Cataldo, M. S., and Doku, H. C.: Solar chelitis. J. Dermatol. Surg. Oncol. 7:989, Dec. 1981.
16. Epstein, E. H., Jr., Burk, P. G., Cohen, I. K., and Deckers, P.: Dermatome shaving in the treatment of xeroderma pigmentosum. Arch. Dermatol. 105:589, April 1972.
17. Field, L. M.: Dermabrasion vs. 5-FU for actinic damage. J. Am. Acad. Dermatol. 6:269, Feb. 1982.
18. Hill, T.: Personal communication, Dec. 16, 1981.
19. Kirschbaum, J. A.: Personal communication, Nov. 13, 1981.
20. Lewis, A.: Personal communication, Dec. 2, 1981.
21. Luikart, R.: Personal communication, April 18, 1982.
22. Menn, H.: Personal communication, Jan. 18, 1982.
23. Stagnone, J. J.: Personal communication, Dec. 7, 1981.
24. Stegman, S.: Personal communication, Nov. 18, 1981.
25. Yarborough, J.: Personal communication, Feb. 9, 1982.
26. Baker, T. J., and Gordon, H. L.: Chemical face peeling and dermabrasion. Surg. Clin. North Am. 51:387, 1971.
27. Stegman, S.: A study of dermabrasion and chemical peels in an animal model. J. Dermatol. Surg. Oncol. 6:490, June 1980.

28. Stegman, S.: A comparative histologic study of the effects of three peeling agents and dermabrasion on normal and sun-damaged skin. American Society for Dermatologic Surgery annual meeting, Philadelphia, Oct. 1981.
29. Caver, C. V.: Personal communication, Nov. 18, 1981.
30. Gleason, M. C.: Xeroderma pigmentosum—five-year arrest after total resurfacing of the face. Plast. Reconstr. Surg. 46:577, 1970.
31. Pinkus, H.: Personal communication, Jan. 21, 1982.
32. Barkoff, J. R.: Personal communication, Nov. 9, 1981.
33. Stough, B.: Personal communication, March 20, 1982.
34. Tromovitch, T. A.: Reply. J. Am. Acad. Dermatol. 6:270, Feb. 1982.
35. Mandy, S. H.: Retin-A in the treatment of dermabrasion and chemabrasion. American Society for Dermatologic Surgery meeting, Las Vegas, NV, March 29, 1980.
36. Pierce, H.: Personal communication, Jan. 14, 1982.
37. Epstein, E.: Dermabrasion. *In* Epstein, E., and Epstein, E., Jr. (eds.): Skin Surgery, 5th ed. Springfield, IL, Charles C Thomas, 1982, pp. 593–610.
38. Dillaha, C. J., Jansen, G. T., and Honeycutt, W. M.: Selective cytotoxic effect of topical 5-fluorouracil. Arch. Dermatol. 88:247, 1963.
39. Goette, D. K.: Topical chemotherapy with 5-fluorouracil. J. Am. Acad. Dermatol. 4:633, 1981.
40. Alt, T.: Personal communication, Jan. 18, 1982.
41. Belisario, J. C.: Cancer of the skin. London, Butterworth & Co., Ltd., 1959, p. 165.
42. Campbell, R. M.: Surgical chemical planing of the skin. Plast. Reconstr. Surg. 1:442, 1977.
43. Dillaha, C. J., Jansen, G. T., and Honeycutt, W. M.: Further studies with topical fluorouracil. Arch. Dermatol. 92:420, 1965.
44. Goulian, D., and Courtiss, F. H.: Dermabrasion procedure. Abstracted from the Symposium on Surgery of the Aging Face, vol. 19. St. Louis, C. V. Mosby Co., 1978.
45. Pinkus, H.: Actinic keratosis—actinic skin. *In* Andrade, R., et al. (eds.): Cancer of the Skin, vol. 1. Philadelphia, W. B. Saunders Co., 1976, p. 456.

TREATMENT OF ACTINIC KERATOSES WITH TOPICAL 5-FLUOROURACIL

Richard B. Odom, M.D.

The significance of actinic keratoses is twofold, involving their potential for malignant degeneration and their unsightly appearance. The problems associated with their removal when the lesions are multiple and extensive are often major. A variety of methods have been proposed for the treatment of actinic keratoses, including simple excision, desiccation and curettage, emollient applications, dry ice or liquid nitrogen application, chemoexfoliation or chemical peeling, dermabrasion, and topical applications of solutions of 5-fluorouracil.

The treatment method for actinic keratoses must be individualized and depends upon the number of lesions present, the region(s) involved, the objectives of the therapy, the safety of the modality, the side effects and complications of the treatment, the acceptance of the therapy by the patient, the efficacy of the procedure, and cost-effectiveness.

For the patient with only a few actinic keratoses, cryotherapy with liquid nitrogen is effective and feasible. Lesions on any cutaneous surface, even on the vermilion of the lips, may be treated with this modality. The individual lesion is frozen for a certain time by means of a cotton-tipped applicator stick dipped into liquid nitrogen. The length of this period depends upon many variables. Initially, the lesion becomes edematous, and occasionally a blister or a bulla will develop. After 48 to 72 hours, the swelling subsides and an adherent necrotic crust develops. After 7 to 10 days, the necrotic surface separates, with an underlying intact epithelium.

For patients with multiple actinic keratoses, 5-fluorouracil therapy is the treatment of choice. In addition to clearing visible lesions and lesions that are microscopically present but not yet evident, topical fluorouracil unmasks and outlines malignant lesions, such as basal cell and squamous cell carcinomas.

The concentration of fluorouracil, the frequency of application, and the duration of treatment depend largely on the extent, the severity, and the location of the lesions. The guidelines for the choice of fluorouracil concentration and the duration of the therapy according to the site are as follows: face and lips, 1 to 2 per cent fluorouracil for 3 weeks; scalp and neck, 5 per cent fluorouracil for 4 weeks, back and chest, 5 per cent fluorouracil for 4 to 6 weeks; arms and hands, 5 per cent fluorouracil for 6 to 8 weeks.

The patient is instructed to apply fluorouracil twice daily after the skin has been thoroughly washed. Early signs of inflammation appear on the face within 3 to 5 days and on the scalp, the neck, the back, and the chest within 4 to 7 days following application; 10 to 14 days may elapse before a reaction is visible on the dorsa of the hands and the forearms. For particularly hyperkeratotic lesions, pretreatment with a keratolytic preparation for 1 to 2 weeks is helpful. Occlusion under polyethylene wrap enhances absorption and promotes more rapid clearing of the lesions. Occasionally, a 5 per cent fluorouracil preparation may be advantageous for hypertrophic lesions of the face.[1] Following the initial erythematous reaction, scaling, tenderness, erosion, and superficial ulceration occur in areas of the keratoses.

Evaluation of therapy at 7- to 10-day intervals by the physician will allow him to determine when a maximum reaction has occurred and when the keratoses have been destroyed. After a brisk inflammatory reaction has occurred, therapy with fluorouracil is discontinued, and a corticosteroid ointment is applied two to four times daily.

Severe irritant dermatitis during the course of treatment is common and necessitates a reduction in the frequency of application or in the concentrations of fluorouracil or temporary interruption and use of emollients or topical steroid preparations.

Once the erythema has subsided, usually approximately 2 weeks after discontinuation of fluorouracil, the skin appears smooth and free of keratoses. There may be slight depressions in the areas of reaction, but these responses are not recognizable as a scar. The degree of eradication is directly proportional to the amount of inflammatory reaction produced. Therefore, the patient who experiences the most pronounced reaction will have the best overall result and will have the least number of keratoses developing or recurring in subsequent months. It should be kept in mind that some keratoses may persist and other new ones may appear as time passes. This can easily be managed by cryotherapy or electrosurgery. Two to three years after therapy, a patient may require re-treatment with topical fluorouracil because of the redevelopment of a number of keratoses, but this poses no problem, and a response comparable with the initial result can be expected.[2]

The principal undesirable effects of topical fluorouracil therapy are the unsightly appearance of the skin and the local discomfort of the patient during and shortly after the course of treatment. Other side effects include hyperpigmentation and hypopigmentation, allergic contact dermatitis, photosensitivity, onycholysis and onychodystrophy, and telangiectasia.

The overall efficacy, economy, patient acceptance, good therapeutic and cosmetic results, and low incidence of side effects with topical fluorouracil make it an almost ideal drug for treatment of patients with multiple and diffuse actinic keratoses.

The use of dermabrasion as a prophylactic or therapeutic measure in the treatment of patients with actinic keratoses has been advocated by dermatologists. The planed skin with its new layers of collagen appears younger than the unplaned adjacent skin, in which long years of exposure to sun have resulted in marked collagen degeneration. When the entire face is planed, the whole appearance is more youthful, since the skin becomes pinker and plumper. The so-called rejuvenation of the skin is said to retard the onset of premalignant change by several years.[3]

Dermabrasion undoubtedly has a degree of prophylactic effect against precancerous actinic keratoses and skin cancer. The preventive effect, even though it may be substantial, is not absolute, and the persistent relative hypopigmentation or complete depigmentation that may occur following dermabrasion in older, fair-skinned patients who have previously acquired considerable suntan, freckling, lentigines, and a weather-beaten skin texture may constitute a formidable cosmetic problem. This is especially true in men, in whom the use of makeup may not be practical, inasmuch as a marked contrast, especially in color and, to some degree, in texture between treated and untreated areas may persist indefinitely.

The basic therapeutic mechanism in dermabrasion is a wound-healing process, with replacement in sun-damaged skin down to the reticular layer of the dermis by young fresh epidermis over a layer of new collagen. Dermabrasion partially removes rhytids, tightens up redundant skin, and improves abnormal pigmentations. Thus, if the therapeutic desire is to improve the degree of wrinkling and the weather-beaten texture of the skin, particularly in women, dermabrasion could be considered.[4] In addition, patients who do not tolerate topical fluorouracil because of extreme irritation or allergic contact dermatitis are candidates for dermabrasion.

If proper selection of patients has been combined with the appropriate skill and care in the execution of dermabrasion, serious complications are relatively infrequent. There are, however, fairly frequent complications of annoying but generally temporary nature. These include edema and erythema, milia, linear scarring, hypertrophic scarring, infection, and ridging. Inadequate planing of the affected areas may result in incomplete removal of lesions. The healing process following dermabrasion may cover up a carcinoma and may lull both the physician and the patient into a sense of false security. Actinic keratoses may recur, and new lesions are common in patients several months following dermabrasion.

When the prevalence of actinic keratoses and the morbidity and cost of treatment are considered, it is obvious that topical fluorouracil treatment is superior to dermabrasion in the management of this condition. Fluorouracil is inexpensive and easy to apply and, despite recurrences, is the treatment of choice. New lesions and some recurrences and treatment failures will be encountered with its use; however, these areas are easily re-treated.

Fluorouracil is more effective than dermabrasion in screening for cancer, since established carcinoma generally will not clear up under this treatment. Thus, a tumor can be isolated from adjacent keratoses, identified, and treated by an appropriate method. If the cosmetic improvement of wrinkled, actinically damaged skin is also an important consideration, dermabrasion could be performed with supplementation on a long-term basis by fluorouracil treatment of new or recurrent lesions.

References

1. Goette, D. K.: Topical chemotherapy with 5-fluorouracil. J. Am. Acad. Dermatol. 4:633, 1981.
2. Jansen, G. T.: Topical therapy with 5-fluorouracil. J. Surg. Oncol. 3:317, 1971.
3. Converse, J. M.: Reconstructive Plastic Surgery, 2nd ed. Philadelphia, W. B. Saunders Company, 1977.
4. Spira, M., Freeman, R., Arfai, P., et al.: Clinical comparison of chemical peeling, dermabrasion, and 5-FU for senile keratoses. Plast. Reconst. Surg. 46:61, 1970.

Editorial Comment

There is less of a controversy than one might imagine regarding the comparative value of dermabrasion and 5-fluorouracil in the management of precancerous skin. Each has a different function and produces unique results. Each is supreme for performing its particular task. The choice in an individual case depends on the abilities of the physician and the wishes of the patient. It is much simpler to write a prescription for a 5-fluorouracil lotion or ointment than to learn how to perform dermabrasion expertly and then apply that treatment to the skin that is damaged, usually as a result of solar irradiation. Furthermore, the prescription will eliminate the keratoses that are developing but still subclinical. However, it will not prevent recurrences. For the patient, it is a method of avoiding the trauma of a comparatively major surgical procedure.

Dermabrasion is not an operation to be taken lightly. It results in approximately 2 weeks of incapacity. There is a certain amount of discomfort, and the bleeding and crusting that result are unsightly. Although the reaction produced by 5-fluorouracil also is disfiguring, the effect is much less drastic than that of the surgical procedure. Dermabrasion will remove the keratoses and will destroy many smaller epitheliomas by acting as an electric curet. However, its main advantage is that it has undoubted and profound prophylactic effects. If a patient is weary of being a dermatologic cripple and is tired of having to have lesions removed at varying intervals, then dermabrasion is for him. On the other hand, if he is satisfied with repeating the 5-fluorouracil treatment as new lesions and recurrences appear, then he should avoid the traumatic experience of submitting his face and hands to planing.

Incidentally, one can perform dermabrasion for treatment of individual lesions by raising them on a subcutaneous injection of lidocaine or procaine and then brushing the lesion off. This is particularly applicable to single (or even multiple) lesions on the hands and the forearms. With this technique, freezing is unnecessary and should be avoided.

Think It Over.

CHAPTER 9

TREATMENT OF EPITHELIOMAS

PRIMARY EXCISION OF BASAL CELL EPITHELIOMA

Thomas H. Alt, M.D.

Types of Treatment

Dermatologic surgeons have many excellent methods for the effective treatment of a basal cell epithelioma. The most common techniques in order of probable decreasing frequency are (1) curettage and cautery, (2) primary excision with closure or resurfacing using skin flaps or skin grafts, (3) Mohs chemosurgery or the modified fresh tissue technique, (4) cryosurgery using liquid nitrogen, and (5) radiation therapy. A new, but less common, technique is laser beam therapy. Uncommon modes of therapy include systemic chemotherapy, perfusion therapy, and immunotherapy. These three treatment modalities are not within the realm of this discussion.

Criteria for Ideal Treatment

I tentatively propose the following criteria for an ideal method of treatment of basal cell epithelioma: The ideal method should (1) eliminate the offending tumor with positive microscopic identification of tumor-free borders, preferably at the time of surgery; (2) employ surgical techniques that are logical and easily understood and that require a beginning or intermediate level of surgical expertise; (3) require a minimal amount of special surgical instrumentation; (4) minimize the time required for postoperative recovery and employ simple postoperative care requiring minimal patient involvement and compliance; (5) provide excellent cosmetic results, preferably with a nearly imperceptible scar; and (6) be economically time-saving for the patient and the physician and entail modest to moderate costs.

None of the aforementioned methods employed in dermatologic surgery meets all of these criteria. Some rate higher and therefore are generally more appropriate.

Consideration of Alternative Methods. In my own practice, which is limited to dermatologic surgery, there is great emphasis on the cosmetic aspects of surgery. Therefore, although the complete excision of any offending tumor is the criterion of paramount concern, I place great emphasis on the final cosmetic result. Although a significant segment of my patient population has selected me because of my attitude regarding physical appearance, there is another group of patients who do not express a need to obtain a superior cosmetic result. I therefore discuss with them the value of an attractive postoperative appearance. Although most patients claim that a scar will not bother them, I believe this stance is taken because of their fear of the term "skin cancer." They are intent on ridding themselves of the offending cancer at all expense because they do not understand the relative benignity of basal cell epithelioma. Most patients will comply with any method proposed by the treating physician because they are unsophisticated in their knowledge of alternative modes of treatment. Although as a group they rely on our advice, more patients are becoming assertive in their questioning concerning treatment alternatives. I support this attitude and feel that inquisitive patients who are adequately informed regarding the methods of treatment, the usual postoperative course, the prognosis, the side effects, and the complications will generally approach their surgery with a sense of security and will participate in the postoperative care with a compliant attitude.

Validity of Postoperative Statistics.   The proponents of any surgical method for basal cell epithelioma will probably claim a greater than 90 per cent cure rate and will be capable of producing more than one series supporting this stance. I believe that statistics as they are currently collected are not without some faults. To be accurate a series must encompass at least a 5-year follow-up period. The initial presence or recurrence of an epithelioma is usually confirmed by microscopic examination, but the lack of recurrence is almost invariably reported as the absence of clinical signs or symptoms suggestive of basal cell epithelioma and does not involve the use of microscopic examination. We have been repeatedly made painfully aware by Mohs chemosurgeons that the extent of an existing lesion cannot be adequately evaluated by clinical examination alone. Careful microscopic examination is essential in establishing the presence or absence of an epithelioma. As clinicians we must therefore recognize that basal cell epithelioma may recur more commonly than we perceive clinically.

One may then logically ask, Is it appropriate to include a microscopic examination using the punch biopsy technique as a routine screening device in the long-term postoperative evaluation of patients having confirmed basal cell epitheliomas? This hardly seems reasonable or cost-effective and, I suspect, would be met with considerable patient resistance. Further, it would be difficult to select a specific area adjacent to the previous surgical site that could routinely identify a recurrent epithelioma, since we all recognize that these lesions may recur in any quadrant around a previously treated tumor.

Elimination of Epithelioma with Tumor-Free Borders

Using the criteria that I have proposed, I feel that primary surgical excision followed by immediate primary closure or resurfacing with a skin flap or a skin graft is usually the most appropriate mode of treatment. I doubt that many could argue that the most important aspect of treatment is the total ablation of the offending tumor. Only three of the six commonly employed treatment methods provide a high degree of assurance that the tumor has been completely removed. Microscopic confirmation of tumor-free borders is available only with Mohs chemosurgery or the fresh tissue technique, laser beam surgery, and primary excision. It is difficult for me to believe that, in view of the inability of the clinician to predict the limit of malignancy accurately without the aid of microscopic studies, dermatologists continue to propose curettage and cautery, cryosurgery using liquid nitrogen, or radiation therapy as adequate modes for definitive treatment. Some of these methods may be applicable in special instances, such as when palliation is desired in a debilitated elderly patient. Although curettage provides the surgeon with some idea of the extent of tumor involvement when the tumor mass is soft (such as lesions seen in nodular basal cells) it offers little guidance, particularly in the case of the sclerosing basal cell types of tumors. Cryosurgery techniques and radiation therapy are based solely on clinical evaluation using the visual and tactile senses of the surgeon. It has been well documented that these methods do not provide proper evaluation.

Mohs chemosurgery and the modified fresh tissue technique provide excellent microscopic evaluation of the tumor borders. These methods are particularly helpful in recurrent tumors and in lesions in specific locations, such as the nasolabial fold, the inner canthus, the external auditory canal, the scalp, and the glans penis. These methods of specimen evaluation are not well understood by most general pathologists and require a specially trained laboratory technician to orient the specimens properly. In order to be fully qualified for admission as a fellow to the American College of Chemosurgery, a surgeon must now complete a 1-year fellowship devoted specifically to Mohs chemosurgery and the modified fresh tissue technique. This will greatly limit the availability of these fine methods in the near future. I feel that 1 year's training is disproportionate to the skill required to become competent in this technique. This artificial limitation of supply will be detrimental rather than beneficial to the vast number of patients who could be helped by these fine methods.

Laser beam therapy, although not in its infancy, has very limited availability because of the major capital investment necessary to acquire the machines that are used in this form of treatment. Large clinics and university settings are currently the only available sources of this modality. Although laser provides a bloodless field with less damage to tissue than that produced by the scalpel, it seems that at present only a very small number of patients can receive its benefits. Microscopic evaluation is not hindered by artifactual damage when laser therapy is employed.

Tumor-free borders can be identified readily with the technique of primary excision. For many years I have successfully used a combination method of curettage followed by excision and evaluation with frozen tissue techniques to identify the extent of malignant lesions. The method is simple, straightforward, and logical. These procedures were employed long before I was familiar with the techniques of Mohs chemosurgery.

The lesion is first cureted using a Number 3 sharp Buck's curet. This is particularly beneficial in nodular basal cell epitheliomas. The lesion is then excised, usually in a rectangular fashion. Careful attention is taken to identify the four sides in their anatomic position. Staining of these borders in a manner similar to that used in Mohs chemosurgery assists in the positive identification of the sides.

Since the central portion of the excised tissue should have been positively identified by previous biopsy, our concern is to establish tumor-free borders on all four sides and the base. Therefore, from the specimen a small strip of skin is excised. The strip should measure approximately 2 to 3 mm in width and should encompass the entire border of the rectangle. Since four sides form the borders of a rectangle, four pieces corresponding to these sides are prepared for frozen section. A fifth piece comprising the remaining base is also prepared. Thus, all four borders and the base can be examined using the frozen section technique. Segments that are too long to be examined in toto are divided into smaller portions and identified. Areas that continue to be involved may be further excised and evaluated microscopically. This avoids excessive loss of normal tissue and provides a high degree of positive identification of involved segments. The rectangle is generally fashioned in a diamond form roughly corresponding in shape to that of an ellipse, the most commonly used configuration for closure. A straight edge with distinct corners is used rather than a curving ellipse, allowing the ends of each segment to be readily identified. A triangle may be much more appropriate when a rotation flap is anticipated, and a five- or six-sided excision may be more appropriate when the lesion is large and requires a skin graft.

I am pleased to see that some chemosurgeons using the fresh tissue technique are now advocating more frequent use of skin flaps, skin grafts, and simple primary closure to resurface the defects. It is not logical to require that all patients heal by secondary intention, but aggressive recurrent tumors should be managed in this manner. This method produces high cure rates and therefore will allow the chemosurgeon to resurface the defect with greater confidence than is attained with most other methods. If there is concern regarding the possibility of recurrence, a thin split-thickness graft provides immediate resurfacing and will bury a recurrence no deeper than that which is seen following healing by secondary intention.

Simplicity of Technique

The second criterion that I have proposed for the ideal method of correction of a basal cell epithelioma is that the technique must be logical and easily understood and should require a beginning or intermediate level of surgical expertise. I feel that primary excision rates high in this category. Certainly it has a logical basis for its approach and can be understood easily and taught to those who have only a rudimentary understanding of simple primary excision techniques. Primary excision does not require a high level of surgical expertise and therefore does not necessitate an additional period of fellowship training. Curettage and cautery and cryosurgery using liquid nitrogen would fall into the category of being easily understood and requiring a beginning or intermediate level of expertise. However, as pointed out earlier, I do not feel that these are logical approaches to the cure of epitheliomas because they do not provide positive identification of the tumor-free borders. Radiation therapy, Mohs chemosurgery, and laser beam surgery all require more knowledge, which necessitates more training.

Amount of Special Instrumentation

The availability of some of the aforementioned methods is limited because of the necessity of special instrumentation. Curettage and cautery and primary excision require the least amount of technical equipment. Therefore, both methods rate high in this category. A modest amount of equipment (namely, the delivery apparatus and the cryoprobes) is required for cryosurgery. Ready access to a cryostat is necessary for Mohs chemosurgery. Radiation therapy and laser beam surgery obviously involve a considerable capital investment.

Miminal Postoperative Recovery Phase with Simple Patient Care

This aspect of treatment is important for patient comfort. A treatment schedule or recovery phase that is protracted is economically inefficient for both the physician and the patient. Primary excision fulfills the requirement of simplicity of patient care, because it involves primary closure of the defect or resurfacing with a skin flap or a skin graft. The postoperative care is minimized, since the skin acts as a natural cover for the defect. In contrast, in the methods of cautery and curettage, cryosurgery, radiation therapy, and Mohs chemosurgery using the fresh tissue technique in which the defect is allowed to heal by secondary intention, there is a protracted period of re-epithelialization, during which the lesion is exudative and susceptible to secondary infection. This extended period of recuperation can require a considerable amount of patient participation and compliance (e.g., in changing dressings). With the advent of modern dressings, such as Op-Site, Biobrane, and Vigilon, some of these disadvantages have been minimized. However, in primary excision, laser beam surgery, and Mohs chemosurgery using the fresh tissue technique in which primary closure or immediate resurfacing is employed, the postoperative care is less complex and is shorter in duration.

Cosmetic Results

Primary closure performed by a skilled practitioner will provide a more pleasing cosmetic result than will closure by secondary intention. Primary excision rates high in this category because it is adaptable to the primary closure technique. Primary closure also can be used with laser beam therapy and, in certain cases, with the fresh tissue technique of Mohs chemosurgery. In some instances, resurfacing with skin flaps or skin grafts may be necessary when these three methods are used. Skin flaps usually produce a satisfactory cosmetic result, as do some skin grafts. In curettage and cautery, cryosurgery, radiation therapy, and Mohs chemosurgery using zinc paste, the defects are generally allowed to close by secondary intention. In areas where the basal layer of the epidermis is penetrated or destroyed in the process of correcting a basal cell epithelioma, the scar from the resulting secondary intention may have altered pigmentation. It usually will be hypopigmented and may be atrophic, hypertrophic, or keloidal in nature.

Economically Time-Saving and Moderate in Cost

Surgical procedures that are time-saving for the patient and the physician are cost-efficient. Primary excision, curettage and cautery, and cryosurgery rate high in this category. The duration of surgery is usually quite short when these three procedures are employed. Laser surgery is generally performed in a hospital surgical suite; the method therefore is costly and time-consuming. Mohs chemosurgery requires repeated sessions when several levels of frozen sections are necessary. Radiation therapy, when the radiation is properly fractionated, also will require multiple sessions. When the protracted recuperative phase of healing from secondary intention that is involved in curettage and cautery and in cryosurgery is considered, primary excision is comparatively advantageous.

SUMMARY

In conclusion, I feel that primary excision of basal cell epitheliomas is the most appropriate method of treatment. It rates high in all the criteria that I have proposed for the evaluation of an ideal surgical method. I hope that my bias favoring primary excision has not significantly affected my selection of appropriate criteria and my evaluation of the aforementioned methods of treatment based on these criteria. For each method, there are proponents who have observed a high degree of success when the technique has been applied properly. We must all remember that no one method is an ideal treatment selection. We must all attempt to be honest and complete in our evaluation and advice concerning these methods. They are all proven modes of therapy, and each has its proper place in our armamentarium.

TREATMENT OF EPITHELIOMAS: ELECTRODESICCATION AND CURETTAGE

Robert Jackson, M.D.

To support and endorse a technique, it is essential first to define the procedure involved. The method that I use for biopsy, electrodesiccation, and curettage is as follows:

The lesion is infiltrated with local anesthetic by means of a clean surgical technique. A biopsy is obtained with scissors, a scalpel, or a biopsy punch. The visible tumor is electrodesiccated, and then the lesion is cureted. It should be noted that basal cell epitheliomas have a soft, mushy, gelatinous texture and bleed freely and diffusely. Squamous cell epitheliomas are somewhat firmer. The main portion of the tumor is removed by curettage. The electrodesiccation and the curettage then are repeated. The central portion of the tumor usually comes away without difficulty. Attention must be paid to the periphery of the lesion. With the skin extended under rather firm pressure, the curet is pulled across all of the borders, thus removing any little peripheral pockets of tumor. After all of the tumor has been removed, the type of bleeding changes from a diffuse laking to pin-point capillary bleeding. This capillary bleeding can be readily stopped by slight tautening of the skin. Frequent bleeding should be almost stopped by the time the procedure is completed. When no more tumor can be felt with the curet, the operative site is examined with a magnifying glass for residual tumor. If none can be seen, the whole lesion is electrodesiccated, including 1 to 2 mm of the normal-appearing periphery. This is important, because most lesions recur at the periphery. The number of times a tumor has to be electrodesiccated and cureted will vary, depending on its size and location. At the end of the procedure, the operative site will present a dry sterile eschar. No bandage is necessary.

Indications

The technique of electrodesiccation and curettage can be used for small (1 to 1.5 cm), localized basal or squamous cell carcinomas. It is excellent for patients with multiple lesions either in the face or in the torso. This includes those lesions arising on severely sun-damaged skin, on skin damaged by improper use of ionizing radiation, and in patients with the basal cell nevus syndrome. In the restless, agitated, or confused patient, large, well-defined exophytic skin cancers can be removed, in stages if necessary, on certain areas, such as the pinna of the ear, the torso, and the hand. There is often no other treatment for these patients. Large superficial multicentric basal cell epitheliomas on the torso can be treated in stages with tolerable morbidity. Small (up to 0.4 cm) basal cell epitheliomas involving the eyelid margin can easily be shelled with minimal scarring.

Contraindications

Large diffuse basal cell or squamous cell carcinomas are not suitable for treatment by electrodesiccation and curettage. Likewise, fibrotic basal cell carcinomas and lesions that have recurred following properly performed electrodesiccation and curettage should not be treated by this method.

Advantages

In most resident training programs, students acquire the degree of manual dexterity that is necessary for removal and biopsy of small benign skin tumors. With a little extra supervised training and experience, the technique of biopsy, electrodesiccation, and curettage can be learned. No new or special equipment is necessary. The technique is surgically clean, but not sterile. Gloves, needle holders, needles, sutures, scissors to remove sutures, sterilizing equipment, thermocouples, special containers to hold and administer liquid nitrogen, and so forth are not required. Almost every dermatologist's office has a local anesthetic, curets, a Hyfrecator, and biopsy bottles.

Electrodesiccation and curettage is ideal for elderly and infirm patients. Examination, biopsy, and treatment can all be accomplished in one brief visit. The gear that is necessary can easily be carried in a small briefcase, and the technique can be performed in nursing homes or chronic disease hospitals. The patient who has a deathly fear of hospitals can be treated in the office. In the rare case in which the lesion obviously cannot be successfully treated, the procedure can be stopped, and further treatment can be arranged when the results of the biopsy report are known. A biopsy should be obtained in every case in order to avoid the necessity of another visit and the delay that results while the biopsy report is evaluated.

Disadvantages

The dermatologist must be able to select the appropriate cases. He must have been adequately trained under supervision in performing the technique. Occasionally, an irritable hypertrophic scar forms, but usually nothing need be done. One or two intralesional injections of triamcinolone acetonide will relieve the symptoms and will help flatten the scar. In 25 years I have never produced a keloid. Rarely, a localized coccal infection can occur in the submammary or retroauricular folds. An antibiotic ointment applied twice daily will prevent this. Once in a while, unsightly round white scars are produced on brown or red telangiectatic sun-damaged skin.

Hazards

One hazard is secondary infection. Once or twice a year I prescribe an oral antibiotic for an infection that has spread beyond the treated site. Once every 2 years I encounter a late hemorrhage from a wound on the vermilion border of the lip or the forehead. Patients receiving anticoagulant therapy have not presented a problem. I have never seen a systemic reaction to lidocaine. Flammable antiseptics should be avoided. In my experience, the risk of interference with pacemakers is more theoretic than real. If I am in doubt, I replace the Hyfrecator with the hot cautery.

Results

When the lesions are properly selected and the techniques properly performed, the results are excellent. The failures are more a fault of the operator than of the method.

Costs

Because neither training nor special equipment is necessary, and because the procedure takes only a short time, electrodesiccation and curettage is the cheapest way to treat skin cancers. At our skin cancer clinic, we have timed the technique of biopsy, electrodesiccation, and curettage and the surgical excision method. The former takes 5 minutes and the latter requires 20 minutes. No return visit to remove sutures is necessary with electrodesiccation and curettage.

References

1. Williamson, G. S., and Jackson, R.: The treatment of basal cell carcinoma by electrodesiccation and curettage. Can. Med. Assoc. J. 86:855, 1962.
2. Williamson, G. S., and Jackson, R.: The treatment of squamous cell carcinoma of the skin by electrodesiccation and curettage. Can. Med. Assoc. J. 90:408, 1964.
3. Jackson, R.: The treatment of basal cell carcinomas. Cutis 5:1231, 1969.
4. Freeman, R. C., Knox, J. M., and Heaton, C. L.: The treatment of skin cancer. A statistical study of 1,341 skin tumours comparing results obtained with irradiation, surgery and curettage followed by electrodesiccation. Cancer 17:535, 1964.
5. Knox, J. M., Freeman, R. C., Duncan, W. C., and Heaton, C. L.: Treatment of skin cancer. South. Med. J. 60:241, 1967.
6. Sweet, R. D.: The treatment of basal cell carcinoma by curettage. Br. J. Dermatol. 75:137, 1963.
7. Whelan, C. S., and Deckers, P. J.: Electrocoagulation for skin cancer. Cancer 47:2280, 1981.

EXCISIONAL ELECTROSURGERY (ENDOTHERMY)

Eugene P. Schoch, Jr., M. D.

Excisional electrosurgery has been defined and described elsewhere.[1,2] Briefly, this method entails the process of surgical excision of tissue by means of a bipolar cutting current rather than a scalpel.

When excisional electrosurgery is compared with conventional monopolar electrosurgery, some similarities and considerable differences are found. Both methods are rapid office procedures. In the process of curettage and electrodesiccation, the lesion may or may not have been diagnosed by biopsy before removal. A common verruca would not normally be examined histopathologically, but a suspected carcinoma would. Curettage must be performed carefully. Although "feeling" the diseased tissue through the curet may not sound very scientific, it yields remarkable results. The base of the lesion is then electrodesiccated to produce an eschar. Depending on the nature of the lesion, several separate curettages and desiccations may be performed on the same site.

There are several points of concern regarding the procedure of electrodesiccation and curettage. Aside from the original diagnostic biopsy, there is no secondary laboratory verification that all of a tumor has been removed. In addition, the final electrodesiccation of the site produces considerable tissue destruction, which may result in large, hypertrophic scars or even keloids.

Electrosurgical excision is a different procedure. It uses the energy generated by a bipolar current to actually cut tissue, as would a scalpel. By adjusting the quality of the current from pure cutting, which has very little hemostatic ability, to a blended cutting-coagulating type, one can control bleeding more satisfactorily, especially in a very vascular area.

The wound resulting from endothermy is different from that which occurs after curettage and desiccation. The tissues lining the surgical defect are essentially undamaged. There is a microscopic zone of electronecrosis surrounding the excised specimen and the remaining skin defect. Spotty areas of coagulum are present at sites of coagulated blood vessels. The wound then heals by secondary intention without the impediment of a large eschar. Healing is slow following this procedure compared with the sutured excisional method. Hemorrhage during convalescence does not present a major problem. Occasionally, the scar that results from the secondary intention healing is hypertrophic, but this occurs far less often than after electrodesiccation. Usually, the scar is soft and cosmetically acceptable to most patients.

Why, then, do we use electrosurgical excision rather than scalpel excision? The procedure is quick and requires a minimum of surgical equipment; it is an office procedure. We should exclude from consideration the small, elite group of dermatologic surgeons who consider themselves as technically capable as plastic surgeons. The average dermatologist will use both scalpel and electrosurgery for selected problems. For the *average* uncomplicated benign growth, such as a simple nevus, careful shave excision and light electrodesiccation is just as satisfactory as excision and suturing. This is more appropriate than electrosurgical excision.

Malignant tumor removal is a different problem. Electrosurgical excision more closely resembles Mohs microscopically controlled excision (fresh tissue technique) than conventional excision and suturing. The tumor is electroexcised in a manner conforming to the configuration of the tumor (with an appropriate border), such as is performed in Mohs surgery, rather than in the very large elliptic patterns that are necessary at times in excision and suture techniques. If the general surgical method is performed and an assessment of adequacy is desired immediately, then a special environment is necessary. The procedure must be performed in a general hospital operating room or the equivalent in a surgicenter that has frozen tissue examination capability.

Re-excision following excision and frozen study may be necessary because of inadequate extirpation of a malignant tumor resulting from overemphasis of cosmesis. Re-excision is expensive: The cost of operating room usage, charges for special services of the pathology department, anesthesiologists' fees, recovery room and, sometimes, overnight full hospital room charges, plus the surgical fee amount to a very substantial financial burden. It is illogical to brush off this cost factor by assuming that the patient's insurance will cover these expenses.

Electrosurgical excision may be performed in the office setting. The minimal surgical facility usually available in the average dermatologist's office is adequate. Even large malignant tumors that could be treated by the Mohs microscopically controlled excision method may be similarly excised by endothermy. The specimen is carefully mapped by colored dyes and submitted in formalin to a cooperative pathology laboratory that can provide a turn-around time of 24 hours. Should the tumor be inadequately excised, then re-excision is performed on the second visit. With this method, a great deal of hospital expense is spared. Most patients would opt for this choice.

The essential argument for office-based electrosurgical management of malignant tumors is cost-effectiveness. We believe that the results, i.e., the adequacy of removal and the scar that remains, are comparable with those obtained with Mohs chemosurgery excision. Of course, elaborate plastic surgical repair can usually produce better cosmetic results. The choice between practical, acceptable, adequate, lower-cost management and expensive plastic surgery is a decision to be made jointly by the patient and his physician. All factors, including time, convalescence, the patient's occupation and temperament, and cost, must be evaluated.

When all things are considered, we feel that properly performed electrosurgical excision compares favorably with other surgical modalities.

References

1. Schoch, E. P.: Excisional electrosurgery (endothermy) in dermatology. J. Dermatol. Surg. 2:240, June 1976.
2. Schoch, E. P.: Electrosurgical excision. In Epstein, E. (ed.): Skin Surgery, 5th ed.. Springfield, IL, Charles C Thomas, 1982, pp. 414–418.

MICROSCOPIC CONTROL OF SKIN CANCER: CHEMOSURGICAL METHOD

Rex A. Amonette, M.D.

The essence of chemosurgery is serial excision and microscopic study of chemically fixed tissue known to harbor malignancy. This allows the physician to identify the extent of the malignant process precisely and to excise the entire neoplasm under microscopic control.

Since 1936, this method of obtaining tissue specimens for frozen sections and microscopic control has existed. Dr. Frederic Mohs developed chemosurgery, a procedure that is unique in that the tissue to be removed for examination is prepared for excision by a fixative chemical—zinc chloride paste.

Methods of Obtaining Tissue Specimens

In order to discuss fixed tissue chemosurgery and its application to excision of skin cancers, it is necessary to understand the method of obtaining tissue specimens for frozen section surgery. After a brief description of the method of fixation, the "case for paste" will be presented.

Preparation and Fixation of Tissue for Excision

An anesthetic is needed only for initial application of the chemicals; the anesthesia is administered by local infiltration, regional block, or both. The first step consists of the application of dichloroacetic acid to the area of skin that is to be removed. This keratolytic agent coagulates epidermal proteins and renders the tissue permeable to the fixative that is applied in the second step.

The keratolytic acid is applied until the skin turns white, which indicates the penetration of the stratum corneum with coagulation of the protein in the cells of the stratum spinosum. The amount of keratolytic dichloracetic acid used depends upon the thickness and the hardness of the keratin layer. Some ulcerative skin cancers will require no acid applications, whereas thickened areas of the skin and heavily keratinized tumor surfaces may require that some of the keratin be scraped away before acid application.

Step 2 is the application of the zinc chloride paste for fixation of the tissue in situ. A layer of the fixative chemical is applied in a thickness ranging from a fraction of a millimeter to 4 mm or more, depending on the size of the tumor, the depth of penetration desired, and the thickness of the cornified layer. If the main mass has been excised prior to application of the zinc chloride paste, the thickness of application need be only 1 mm. Ordinarily, this provides the desired depth of penetration of approximately 2 mm.

Precise applications of the paste come with experience; the chemosurgeon has to consider the type of tissues involved, the vascularity and moistness of the surrounding skin, the environmental humidity, and the duration of exposure to the paste.

Step 3 involves application of an occlusive dressing, which is applied over the treated area to limit liquefaction or desiccation, either of which will affect the action of the fixative. The dressing is also necessary to hold the paste in place, thus avoiding fixation of uninvolved skin. The dressing consists of a layer of cotton covered by an overlapping petrolatum-coated cotton pad sealed in place with Micropore paper tape (3M Company).

Excision of Tissue Specimens for Frozen Sections

The fixative is allowed to penetrate for 4 to 24 hours. When adequate fixation has been achieved, as judgment dictates, sections of tissue approximately 1 cm^2 in area (or less) and 2 mm in thickness are surgically excised in a saucer-like shape. There is no pain or bleeding if the excision is made within the fixed tissue.

A map of the lesion site, with a number assigned to each section, is drawn at the time of excision. Each section, as it is removed, is identified by its corresponding number. Two intersecting edges are then colored with red and blue dyes. These indelible marks are preserved during the histochemical staining process and, when visualized microscopically, allow the chemosurgeon to locate the exact position of remaining malignancy—if present—within the particular sections obtained from precisely known areas.

Microscopic Examination

Microscopic survey is performed on frozen sections that have been cut horizontally from the undersurface of each excised tissue section and stained by hematoxylin and eosin or toluidine blue. Recognition of pathologic elements becomes rather easy for the experienced physician, and the location of the malignancy is marked on the original map of numbered sections and oriented exactly by the red and blue color coding. Zinc chloride paste is reapplied only to those areas of the previously treated site in which tumor is found by microscopic survey. All the aforementioned steps are then repeated.

Advantages of Chemosurgery

There are many advantages of fixed tissue chemosurgery when this technique is compared with other methods of therapy, including fresh tissue microscopically controlled excision. Some of these advantages are as follows:

1. Specimens of tissue that have been fixed in situ are easier to excise and to section. The tissue is firm and form-retaining and is easier to handle than fresh tissue.

2. Chemosurgery is essentially a bloodless procedure because of the tissue fixation.

3. This method avoids sacrifice of normal tissue, since only cancer-bearing tissues and a very small amount of surrounding tumor-free tissue in the form of a postoperative separation are removed.

4. Chemosurgery offers the advantage of tracing a cancer through soft tissue and through cartilage and bone, because the fixative also prepares bone for excision and subsequent microscopic examination.

5. The mortality and morbidity with the procedure are extremely low.

6. Since zinc chloride paste fixes nerve endings as well as tumor cells, local anesthesia is rarely needed. Anesthetic and epinephrine reactions are thus avoided. General anesthesia is essentially never used; another risk is therefore eliminated.

7. Postoperative wounds are free of infection following separation of chemical layer. The resulting granulation bed epithelializes remarkably well or is perfectly prepared for reconstructive surgery when it is needed.

8. With fixed tissue, there is avoidance of injections and incision into fresh tissue of lesions with metastatic capability, such as squamous cell carcinoma and malignant mela-

noma. Animal experiments have shown that chemical fixation in situ does not increase metastatic spread and may even help prevent metastasis.

9. Chemosurgery can be performed on patients with bleeding disorders, those with known reactions to local anesthetics, and patients with extremely large lesions and advanced skin cancer that might otherwise be considered inoperable.

10. Hospitalization is often not necessary, and the patient remains ambulatory.

11. The cost of chemosurgery is always listed as a disadvantage, but I consider the procedure to be one of the best bargains in medicine when one considers the time spent by several skilled professionals. The expense is sometimes two to four times that of conventional methods, but this cost can be reduced if hospitalization is avoided. Also, when considering cost, we also have to consider the success of the procedure and the concomitant avoidance of future surgery and time lost from occupation.

12. The final, but most important, advantage of fixed-tissue chemosurgery is its reliability and its ability virtually to assure cure of all basal cell carcinomas and most of the other common skin cancers. No method of therapy can approach the successful cure rate of chemosurgery in treatment of difficult skin cancers.

Disadvantages of Chemosurgery

When one considers the nature of skin cancers that are treated with this method, the advantages of fixed tissue chemosurgery outnumber the disadvantages. The disadvantages of applying zinc chloride paste to the patient's skin are:

1. The patient develops mild to severe pain caused by the acute inflammatory reaction (edema and leukocytosis).

2. Microscopic examination of the excised fixed tissue is sometimes difficult to interpret because of the inflammatory reaction that obscures the smaller groups of cancer cells.

3. Patient waiting time is greatly increased, because 4 to 24 hours are required for the chemical to fix the tissue properly. The procedure is also time-consuming for the surgeon and the technicians, since multiple stages of surgery require several days of treatment.

4. Chemosurgery is not readily available in every medical center in the United States. Most hospitals, clinics, and offices in which skin cancers are routinely treated are not equipped to perform this surgery. Considerable experience by a professional team consisting of a surgeon, nurses, and technicians is required in treatment of advanced lesions, especially when vital structures (eye, ear canal, large arteries, dura) are involved. Advanced skill is necessary to apply dichloroacetic acid and zinc chloride paste. Likewise, extensive experience in surgery and in processing specimens is required, particularly when tissues include cartilage, bone, muscles, or glands.

5. Occasionally, underlying cartilage or bone is undesirably fixed and is destroyed. Also, a perforation (ala, ear surface, lip) may occur with the chemical layer separation.

6. A delay is required before reconstructive surgery following fixed tissue chemosurgery can be performed, so that the underlying layer of fixed tissue can separate from normal tissue. This seldom represents a problem or a disadvantage, however.

Hazards and Complications

In addition to the aforementioned disadvantages of chemosurgery, three problems consistently arise. These are more in the nature of side effects from the surgery than true complications.

1. *Pain.* Every patient has some pain during the surgery, but the degree is variable. The initial anesthetic produces more pain from the natural sting of the medicine than from

the 30-gauge needle. There is considerable pain with each application of zinc chloride fixative, and with advanced lesions the pain can be intense. Some patients are stoic and tolerate pain without complaint, whereas others need strong analgesics, even through the postoperative inflammatory phase.

2. *Hemorrhage*. Most patients do not bleed excessively. However, within fixed tissue, the zinc chloride will occasionally weaken a vessel wall, and as the last layer of fixative separates, arterial bleeding can occur. Large vessels known to cross the surgical wound are ligated as a precautionary measure. Every patient has to be instructed following surgery concerning how to apply pressure. Patients should be told to seek medical help should excessive bleeding occur.

3. *Scar, contraction, and deformity*. Although both the patient and the chemosurgeon are concerned about cosmetic results, the main purpose of chemosurgery is complete removal of the cancer. Often the lesion is so large and involves such vital structures that scarring and wound contraction lead to undesirable deformity. Sometimes reconstructive repair or a plastic prosthesis is needed for proper function or cosmetic appearance.

Indications for Chemosurgery

The microscopic control of chemosurgery is advantageous in the treatment of almost all skin cancers. In years past, because of time constraints and limited availability, fixed tissue chemosurgery was confined mostly to outsized primary lesions or to recurrent carcinomas for which both radiation therapy and conventional surgical techniques were inapplicable. Today, fixed tissue chemosurgery still does not compete with conventional therapy for the majority of primary skin cancers. It is reserved for cancers for which conventional therapy has already failed or would probably fail if used.

Fixed tissue chemosurgery remains the treatment of choice for far-advanced basal cell carcinomas that have become excessively large in surface area, are deeply invasive, and have extensively invaded bone and cartilage.

Moderately large squamous cell carcinomas, if recurrent or if arising in skin that is not sun-damaged, are best treated with fixed tissue. This is particularly true of areas around the ears, the preauricular surface, the temple, and the scalp. Smaller squamous cell carcinomas, especially of the upper extremities, can be safely treated by the fresh tissue technique. Squamous cell carcinomas of the nail bed are more easily treated with this method, and invasive squamous cell carcinomas of the penis also are treated with fixed tissue in order to control bleeding.

Those chemosurgeons treating malignant melanoma use only the fixed tissue method.

Contraindications for Fixed Tissue

Fixed tissue removal is contraindicated mainly when fresh tissue microscopically controlled excision is the treatment of choice. The latter procedure is preferable for most moderate to small cancers not involving bone because it is associated with less pain, greater conservation of normal tissue, reduced patient waiting time, and possible immediate closure or repair.

The procedure also is contraindicated if there is danger of the chemical's touching the globe of the eye in treatment of extremely large and far-advanced cancers. Also, occasionally fixation has to be avoided when the chemosurgeon suspects that a separation layer will lead to penetration of a vital structure. Examples are fixation over the external carotid artery, the cavernous sinus, and the cribriform plate.

Results

The cure rate with fixed tissue chemosurgery is well established and remains unsurpassed. Chemosurgeons continue to report cure rates of 99+ per cent for basal cell carcinoma and 91 to 95 per cent for squamous cell carcinoma, depending on the site of origin.

I predict that the reliability and success of the procedure in treatment of extensive and life-threatening cancers of the skin and related structures will continue to be superior.

References

1. Amonette, R., and Shereff, R. H.: Basal cell epithelioma treated by Mohs' chemosurgery. Arch. Dermatol. 110:655, 1974.
2. Epstein, E., and Epstein, E., Jr.: Techniques in Skin Surgery. Philadelphia, Lea & Febiger, 1979, pp. 140–148.
3. Goldwyn, R. M., and Rueckert, R.: The value of healing by secondary intention for sizeable defects of the face. Arch. Surg. 112:285, March 1977.
4. Menn, H., Robins, P., Kopf, A., and Bart, R.: The recurrent basal cell epitheliomas. Arch. Dermatol. 103:628, 1971.
5. Menn, H.: Current management of cancer of the skin. Postgrad. Med. 52:161, 1972.
6. Mikhail, G. R.: Chemosurgery in the treatment of skin cancer. Int. J. Dermatol. 14:33, 1975.
7. Mikhail, G. R.: Squamous cell carcinoma of the penis. J. Dermatol. Surg. 2:406, 1976.
8. Mohs, F. E., and Guyer, M. F.: Pre-excisional fixation of tissues in the treatment of cancer in rats. Cancer Res. 1:49, 1941.
9. Mohs, F. E.: Chemosurgery, a microscopically controlled method of cancer excision. Arch. Surg. 42:279, 1941.
10. Mohs, F. E.: The chemosurgical treatment of tumors of the parotid gland: A microscopically controlled method of excision. Acta Union Int. Contre Cancer 9:105, 1953.
11. Mohs, F. E.: Chemosurgery: Microscopically controlled surgery for skin cancer—past, present, and future. J. Dermatol. Surg. Oncol. 4:41, 1978.
12. Mohs, F. E.: Chemosurgery: Microscopically controlled surgery for skin cancer. Springfield, IL, Charles C Thomas, 1978.
13. Robins, P., Henkind, P., and Menn, H.: Chemosurgery in the treatment of cancer of the periorbital area. Trans. Am. Acad. Ophthalmol. Otolaryngol. 75:1228, 1971.
14. Robins, P., and Albom, M. J.: Recurrent basal cell carcinomas in young women. J. Dermatol. Surg. 1:49, 1975.
15. Tomsick, R., and Menn, H.: Chemosurgical excision of subunginal squamous cell carcinoma. Hand 13:177, 1981.
16. Tromovitch, T. A., Beirne, G. A., and Beirne, C. G.: Cancer chemosurgery (Mohs' technique). Arch. Dermatol. 92:291, 1965.
17. Tromovitch, T. A., and Stegman, S. J.: Microscopically controlled excision of skin tumors: Chemosurgery (Mohs): Fresh tissue technique. Arch. Dermatol. 110:231, 1974.

CRYOSURGERY OF MALIGNANT TUMORS OF THE SKIN

Setrag A. Zacarian, M.D.

Introduction

Cancer of the skin is the most common malignancy in man.[1] Its treatment is relatively simple and effective, and the cure rate is high. Metastases are rare in basal cell carcinoma (0.1 per cent of cases), an important factor in its differentiation from epidermoid carcinoma. Basal cell carcinoma is the most common neoplasm we observe; it occurs most often on the head and the neck. The single most important cause of cutaneous carcinomas is cumulative exposure to sunlight. This discussion of cryosurgery for malignant tumors of the skin will be confined to basal cell carcinomas, epidermoid carcinomas, and basosquamous cell carcinomas. It will not include melanomas, because to my knowledge this neoplasm has not been subjected to cryosurgery in the United States.

The procedures that have been used in the therapeutic management of skin cancers are surgical excision, curettage and electrodesiccation, irradiation, Mohs chemosurgery (for the more difficult and recurrent carcinomas) and, since the early 1960s, cryosurgery. The five-year cure rates with each method as reported by Crissey[2] in 13 published studies involving 14,114 carcinomas of the skin are as follows: Mohs chemosurgery, 99.1 per cent; surgical excision, 95.5 per cent; irradiation therapy, 94.7 per cent; and curettage and electrodesiccation, 92.6 per cent. Cryosurgery for malignant tumors of the skin was introduced in the early 1960s by Irving Cooper, the father of modern cryosurgery.[5]

Methodology

In preparing to freeze a skin cancer, one may use local anesthesia if desired. This is a matter of choice, but local anesthesia is absolutely necessary if a micro-thermocouple needle to monitor the depth of freezing is to be implanted. A safe margin is outlined with a skin pencil marker at least 3 to 5 mm outside the visible margin of the tumor. The flow of liquid nitrogen then is directed intermittently to the center of the malignant growth. My own technique is to freeze for three to four seconds, stop for one to two seconds, and freeze again. If freezing is uninterrupted, a rapid extension of the ice front is developed peripherally at the expense of the ice front below the tumor. Also, continuous freezing will produce droplets of liquid nitrogen, which will trickle down from the treatment site. This is uncomfortable for the patient.

After adequate freezing has been achieved both on the surface of the tumor and in depth, one should allow the tumor site to return to its normal state and then institute a second freeze. This is referred to as the double-freeze-thaw technique and will insure a higher cure rate. The second freeze-thaw cycle will be achieved in less time than the first, because the microvessels are still under partial vasoconstriction from the first freezing and will afford less resistance to the extension of the ice front the second time around.[4]

There appears to be some confusion among operators regarding freezing and thawing cycles. Freeze-time is controlled; the practitioner decides how long to freeze a given neoplasm. The decision is based on the size, depth, and location of the tumor and the clinical judgment of the operator. One has no control of the thaw period, which will vary from

Table 1. INDICATIONS FOR MONITORING
CUTANEOUS MALIGNANCIES DURING
CRYOSURGERY

Lack of experience in cryosurgical technique
Tumors in specific anatomic sites:
    tumors in the medial canthus of the eyelid
    tumors in the ala nasi
    tumors in the nasolabial fold
    postauricular neoplasms
    tumors anterior to the tragus of the ear

one and one half to two times the duration of the freezing period. Cryobiologists have demonstrated that rapid freezing is lethal to cells and even more lethal in the thawing period, during which ice particles recrystallize.

When monitoring a skin cancer with thermocouple needles, one should try to achieve a temperature between −45°C and −50°C within the tumor.

One should bear in mind that freezing a tumor on the forehead, the temple, or the scalp will cause the patient to have a transient headache that may last from several minutes to as long as an hour. I have no explanation for this phenomenon, and many inquiries of neurologists have produced no satisfactory answer.

For periorbital cancers I use a Styrofoam shield to avoid undue spraying of liquid nitrogen onto the eyeball. If the tumor involves the lids, after anesthetizing the eye with tetracaine hydrochloride (Pontocaine) I insert a plastic Jaegher-Belke lid retractor (Storz Instruments, St. Louis, MO) and freeze the cancer without any fear of injuring the eye. Metal shields or instruments should not be used, because they will conduct the cold to the eyeball and will injure the cornea.

I prefer to use a cone spray technique rather than a probe method. I find that freezing is more rapid and intense with the former technique, with a greater depth of the ice front, in comparison with open spray of liquid nitrogen or a probe method. I use probes only when I am freezing leukoplakia and benign growths of the oral and buccal mucosa.

Every patient with a neoplasm that I suspect to be malignant is subjected to a biopsy. The histologic confirmation of the type of carcinoma, once established, helps me to choose the method of ablation. Basal cell carcinomas are classified according to four broad categories: adenoid, cystic, multicentric, and sclerosing (or morphea-type). The final decision to employ cyrosurgery therefore is dependent upon not only the *histology* of the malignancy but also its *anatomic site, the size of the tumor, the age of the patient,* and the risks involved in extensive surgery if it is being considered as an alternative treatment.

One last word on methodology: I recommend that the cancer therapist monitor all tumors that are subjected to cryosurgery in the beginning in order to become adept in freezing techniques. Once experience is gained, selected tumors at specific anatomic sites, in my opinion, are worthy of monitoring (Table 1). One can monitor the temperature with thermocouple needles, and once an electrical current flow measuring device becomes approved by the Food and Drug Administration, I believe that it will be more accurate in establishing cryonecrosis.[5,6]

Indications for Cryosurgery of Malignant Tumors

I have outlined in Table 2 what I consider to be acceptable indications for cryosurgery of cutaneous malignancies. There may be some differences of opinion among other cryosurgeons. These criteria have evolved from my 17 years of cryosurgical experience and are based on observation and, most importantly, hindsight. The selection of patients

Table 2. INDICATIONS FOR CRYOSURGERY OF MALIGNANT CUTANEOUS TUMORS

Tumors with Definable Margins
Nodular or ulcerated lesions
Instrument delineation by means of a curet
Chemical delineation by means of 5-fluorouracil
Tumors overlying cartilage and bone
Lentigo maligna (Grade 1 invasion)

Tumors for Which Cryosurgery Is More Suitable Than Other Modalities
Anatomic Site
Selected neoplasms of the eyelid, the nose, and the ear (preserving lacrimal apparatus and avoiding chondrone-crosis)
Tumors of the chest and back (wherein hypertrophic scarring is minimal with cryosurgery and no grafts are required)
Tumors on the tip of the nose (wherein surgical resection produces marked defects)
Nature of the Neoplasm
Infected tumors
A recurrent tumor from previous radiotherapy in a site of radiodermatitis
Patient Idiosyncrasies
Patients with pacemakers (electrocautery is contraindicated)
Patients of advanced age who are poor surgical risks
Patients with adverse reactions to anesthesia
Inoperable Patients
For palliation
For removal of bulk vegetative lesions

with skin cancer and the decision to employ cryosurgery have already been discussed in the section on methodology. Tumors overlying cartilage and bone are better suited for cryosurgery than for irradiation. Chondronecrosis has been reported from the latter modality but is extremely uncommon with cryosurgery. Patients with cancers of the medial canthus of the eyelid, when properly selected for cryosurgery, seldom develop epiphora.[7] The lacrimal duct and canaliculi tolerate reasonable freezing temperatures. Epiphora is not an uncommon complication following irradiation therapy or surgical extirpation of a tumor at the medial canthus.

Patients who develop keloids following surgery are ideal candidates for cryosurgery, since to my knowledge, the development of keloids following freezing of tumors has not been reported. Hypertrophic scars do develop, but these are infrequent; they resolve spontaneously and respond to intralesional injection of triamcinolone. Recurrent carcinomas following irradiation therapy are very often amenable to cryosurgery, with excellent wound healing. In addition to the superior cosmetic result that is obtained with cryosurgery of malignant tumors, this procedure offers an economic advantage in that it is an office procedure and therefore does not require hospitalization or hospital outpatient surgery. I need not go into the spiraling cost of medical care and hospitalization. Cryosurgery, whenever available and indicated for cutaneous cancers, is far less costly than irradiation therapy or surgery.

Contraindications for Cryosurgery of Malignant Tumors

The types of neoplasms that may contraindicate cryosurgery and their anatomic sites are presented in Table 3. Once again I want to remind the reader that the absolute and relative contraindications that I have outlined are based upon my own experience. Some criteria are self-evident; others need some further explanation. Sclerosing, or morphea-type, basal cell carcinomas are treacherous. Morphologically, unlike a nodular or ulcerated carcinoma of the skin, the borders of this type of tumor are not clearly defined. Basaloid cancer cells travel considerable distances along the collagen fibers of the dermis, far from the site of origin. Cryosurgery for this type of tumor, in my opinion, should not be em-

Table 3. CONTRAINDICATIONS FOR CRYOSURGERY OF MALIGNANT CUTANEOUS
TUMORS

Absolute Contraindications
Morphea-type, or sclerosing, basal cell carcinoma
Patients with abnormal cold intolerance
    Cryoglobulinemia
    Cryofibrinogenemia
    Raynaud's disease
    Platelet deficiency disorders
Relative Contraindications
Neoplasms of the scalp
Neoplasms of the ala nasi and the nasolabial fold
Neoplasms situated anteriorly to the tragus of the ear
Postauricular neoplasms
Lesions on the free margin of the eyelid
Tumors of the upper lip near the vermilion margin
Tumors of the lower legs, particularly the shins
Tumors situated on the lateral margins of the fingers and the ulnar fossa of the elbow and lesions in other sites
    overlying superficial nerves
Lack of clinical experience and skill of the physician
Nodular or ulcerated lesions over 3.0 cm in dimension (except for palliation)
Carcinomas affixed to underlying cartilage or bone
Recurrent carcinomas (except for palliation)

ployed unless the patient is far advanced in age or if surgery presents an undue risk. I have
had patients with small sclerosing-type carcinomas that were clinically observed to be less
than 1.0 cm in size and have witnessed surgical excision wherein the plastic surgeon had
to excise 1.5 to 2 cm beyond the visible surface margin to be assured by the pathologist
(using the fresh or the frozen tissue technique) that the margins were clear! In a recent
study of 496 recurrent basal cell carcinomas, the sclerosing type constituted 27.4 per cent.[8]
The pathologist's report should be respected.

Carcinomas of the skin of the mid-face, as outlined in Table 1, present a challenge to
all cancer therapists. In my own experience, the cure rate of cryosurgery for tumors at
these anatomic sites, in addition to that for lesions located in the postauricular region and
in the scalp, has varied from 90 to 92 per cent. In comparison, the cure rate of cryosurgery
of malignant tumors of the skin in other parts of the body is as high as 97 per cent.[4]
Perhaps one of the reasons for this is that the anatomic embryologic fusion planes in the
middle third of the face are potential pathways for the spread of islands of basal cell
carcinoma. This concept may also be true of the pre- and postauricular region as well as
the sulcus of the ear.[9,10]

Neoplasms frozen at the free margin of the eyelids may result in notching that is
permanent. This also holds true of cancers of the upper lip that are frozen at the vermilion
border or near it. The result is tenting or uplifting of the pink mucosa of the lip. It is
interesting that this does not occur (or, at least, I have not observed it) in tumors of the
lower lip at the vermilion edge.

The immediate complication of cryosurgery is the swelling that follows treatment,
particularly around the periorbital areas when tumors of the forehead, the temples, and the
scalp are frozen. This edema may last for several days, and extensive serous exudation
from the frozen tumor site also may occur. The average healing time is approximately 4
weeks from the initial freeze. Inflammation or post-treatment bleeding from the frozen tumor site is extremely uncommon. A transient complication is hyperpigmentation at the
treated site, which may last for several months. A more prolonged complication that lasts
for years is hypopigmentation; for some, this is permanent. Hypopigmentation is particularly prominent in the darker-complexioned individual. Atrophy at the site does occur,
sometimes at the lobule of the nose or at the mid-forehead; however, this is not a common
complication. Hypertrophic scars infrequently occur and, when seen, may be present on

the forehead, chest, and back and on the upper lip. This complication is transient; the scars, as pointed out earlier, resolve by themselves. Neuropathy has been reported following cryosurgery, which is why freezing of the lateral margins of the fingers and the ulnar fossa must be performed with caution. With rare exceptions, neuropathy has resolved by itself in time without any intervention. Tumors frozen at the lower extremities are amenable to cryosurgery, but the healing time may be as long as two months; secondary infection is not uncommon, and atrophy is a strong possibility.

DISCUSSION AND SUMMARY

Cryosurgery for malignant tumors of the skin is a controversial issue among cancer therapists. The English essayist William Hazlitt remarked in 1830: ''When a thing ceases to be a subject of controversy, it ceases to be a subject of interest.'' It is natural for any new modality or therapeutic regimen in medicine to have its skeptics. Cryosurgery does not have a long history; it is still in its infancy. When I started performing the procedure 17 years ago, only a handful of dermatologists and cryosurgeons were using this method in the United States.

One of the arguments against freezing skin cancers is, How do you know that you have frozen adequately both in depth and in the margin of the tumor, since you have no specimen to submit to the pathologist for verification? This is a valid argument, but when the radiotherapist treats cutaneous malignancies with irradiation, he does not have a specimen, either. Radiotherapy has been performed since the discovery of x-rays at the turn of the century. The radiotherapist measures the target distance, determines the half-value layer of aluminum, adds proper filters, and directs his electron energy within the first 3 to 4 mm of skin. This is exactly what the cryosurgeon does: He directs cold energy particles to the same depth and the same margins and very often monitors the temperature at a specific depth below the skin and within the tumor, carefully measuring with a template.

In my own series of over 4200 carcinomas of the skin in the past 17 years I have achieved a cure rate of approximately 97 per cent. Well over two thirds of my patients have been followed for more than 5 years. The key to success in cryosurgery for cutaneous malignancies is proper selection based on the histology of the tumor and appreciation of its anatomic site. This is the ground rule for successful cryosurgery of malignant tumors of the skin. If this rule is followed, one can achieve a high cure rate with a superior cosmetic result. The procedure can be performed with operative facility, comfort on the part of the patient, and economic efficiency. Let me conclude with one of my favorite quotations from Alexander Pope: ''Be not the first by whom the new attract—nor yet be the last to leave the old aside.''

References

1. Urbach, F.: Geographic distribution of skin cancer. J. Surg. Oncol. 3:219, 1971.
2. Crissey, J. T.: Curettage and electrodesiccation as a method of treatment for epitheliomas of the skin. J. Surg. Oncol. 3:287, 1971.
3. Cooper, I. S.: Cryogenic surgery: New method of destruction of extirpation of benign or malignant tumors. N. Engl. J. Med. 268:747, 1963.
4. Zacarian, S. A.: Cryosurgical Advances in Dermatology and Tumors of the Head and Neck. Springfield, IL, Charles C Thomas, 1977, pp. 3–37.
5. Zacarian, S. A.: Monitoring of the cryolesion. J. Dermatol. Allergy, 41–44, June 1979.
6. Zacarian, S. A.: How accurate is temperature monitoring in cryosurgery and is there an alternative? J. Dermatol. Surg. Oncol. 6:627, 1980.
7. Fraunfelder, F. T., Zacarian, S. A., and Limmer, B. L.: Cryosurgery for malignancies of the eyelid. Ophthalmology, 87:461, June 1980.

8. Levine, J. L., and Bailin, P. L.: Basal cell carcinoma of the head and neck: Identification of the high risk patient. Laryngoscope 90:955, June 1980.
9. Mora, R. C., and Rubins, P.: Basal cell carcinoma in the center of the face: The special diagnostic, prognostic and therapeutic considerations. J. Dermatol. Surg. Oncol. 4:315, 1978.
10. Levine, H., et al.: Tissue conservation in the treatment of cutaneous neoplasms of the head and neck. Arch. Otolaryngol. 105:140, 1979.

X-RAY THERAPY OF SKIN CANCER

Herbert Goldschmidt, M.D.

Introduction

Cutaneous malignancies can be treated effectively with various therapeutic modalities. Most dermatologists prefer surgical methods (curettage and electrodesiccation, scalpel excision, cryosurgery, or chemosurgery) to eradicate cutaneous cancers. In certain anatomic regions, radiation therapy offers a valuable and unique therapeutic alternative.

The goal of all modalities is to achieve a cure of the skin cancer with a good cosmetic result. The selection of the most suitable modality depends on the type, the size, and the location of the tumor and on the age of the patient. The careless application of any method can produce a poor cosmetic effect or can result in a recurrence. If the sole criterion of success is eradication of the lesion, surgical methods and roentgen therapy will yield similar results. It is obvious, however, that the use of either of these methods to the point of exclusion of others is certain to produce less satisfying cosmetic and functional results than will the use of each in cases in which it is best suited.

In the early years of radiotherapy, x-rays and radium were used by some dermatologists and radiotherapists for all skin cancers, often without fractionation and with excessive doses. Unsightly radiation scars developed many years after inappropriate radiotherapy,[1] thus creating the impression that these sequelae were inherent in the method and were unavoidable.

Fortunately, the uncertainties and pitfalls encountered in the early years of x-ray therapy have been virtually eliminated with modern equipment and techniques. Most radiation sequelae can be avoided by better patient selection, lower dosage schedules, the use of less penetrating radiation qualities, and rigorous adherence to radiation protection standards.

Frequency of Usage

The important role of radiotherapy in the treatment of skin cancers was emphasized in a review by the American Academy of Dermatology in 1974,[2] which showed that 89 per cent of over 2000 respondents used x-ray treatment or referred patients for x-ray therapy for selected basal cell carcinomas. Ninety per cent of these dermatologists stated that radiation treatment is indicated for more than 20 per cent of their patients. The continuing usefulness of radiotherapy in the management of cutaneous neoplasms was also emphasized in statistics from large dermatologic centers at which all modern therapeutic modalities (including cryosurgery and chemosurgery) are available. Chernosky[3] reported his experiences with various modalities in the treatment of 3817 skin cancers; over 10 per cent of these were treated in his office with x-ray therapy (with recurrences in only 2.5 per cent of cases). At the New York Skin and Cancer Unit, 19.7 per cent of 1000 patients with skin cancer received radiation therapy.[4-6] The cure rate was reported as 93 per cent. In Houston, 10 per cent of 2288 skin tumors were treated with x-rays with a cure rate of 94.7 per cent.[7] These cure rates are similar to the results obtained with other therapeutic methods in large comparative statistics.

Modern Indications for Radiotherapy

Theoretically, nearly all skin cancers in all locations can be effectively treated with x-rays. Experience over the past five decades has shown, however, that cosmetic results of radiotherapy are less satisfactory in certain anatomic regions.

1. *Location of the lesions.* There is general agreement[4-10] that ionizing radiation is at least equal to, and often preferable to, other treatment methods in skin cancers of the eyelids, the medial and lateral canthus of the eyes, the nose, the ears, and the lips. In carcinomas of the nasolabial fold and in preauricular and retroauricular areas (often with a tendency to deep invasion), radiation therapy is also considered the treatment of choice by many dermatologists. Large skin cancers of the cheek (or in other skin areas in which surgical excision may leave unavoidable deformities) often respond to radiation therapy with minimal scarring. The skin of the trunk and the extremities has a greater tendency to develop unsightly radiation sequelae, particularly telangiectases and pigment changes. Hence, radiation therapy is rarely advisable in these locations. In exceptional cases (e. g., large multiple superficial basal cell tumors of the trunk, inoperable tumors in any other skin area, or in patients who refuse surgery), radiotherapy offers a therapeutic choice when other methods cannot be used.

2. *Size of the tumor.* We find office radiotherapy particularly valuable in medium-sized tumors 2 to 6 cm in diameter. Lesions smaller than 1 or 2 cm in diameter can be treated equally well or better with surgical methods. Tumors larger than 6 to 8 cm in diameter are rarely seen in private practice and are best referred to specialized clinics.

3. *Age of the patient.* The age of the patient is also an important consideration in the decision to use or not to use x-ray therapy. In order to minimize the potentiating or additive hazards of solar irradiation in later years, sun-exposed areas in patients under 40 years of age should not be irradiated if equally effective alternative methods are available. In elderly patients, irradiation may be a more favored option, because there is comparatively less danger of late radiation sequelae. In addition, x-ray therapy is psychologically a less traumatic procedure for elderly patients who often fear surgery of any type.

4. *Contraindications.* In general, we do *not* use x-ray therapy for skin cancers that are located in regions other than the head and the neck, are over 8 cm in diameter, occur intraorally, invade bone, extend from the upper lip into a nostril, are secondary to radiodermatitis, or occur in osteomyelitis, chronic ulcers, and burn scars.[4,6] Radiotherapy in the dermatologist's office is mainly indicated for medium-sized uncomplicated basal cell carcinomas, squamous cell carcinomas, and keratoacanthomas. There are no basic differences in radiation methods for any of these tumors.

Radiation Factors

1. *Radiation quality.* The penetration of an x-ray beam can be expressed by the half-value layer or the half-value depth of the radiation. In modern dermatologic radiotherapy, the basic rule in the treatment of skin cancer is to select a half-value depth that approximates the actual depth of the tumor.[11] Actual measurements have shown that 50 per cent of all basal cell and squamous cell carcinomas are not deeper than 2 mm and only 25 per cent deeper than 5 mm. Consequently, a half-value layer ranging from 0.3 to 1.0 mm is sufficient for most skin cancers. More penetrating radiation is rarely needed; cosmetic results are better with less penetrating radiation.

2. *Radiation dose.* Most authors recommend that the base of the tumor should receive at least 20 to 30 Gy (2000 to 3000 rads) during fractionated therapy. The total exposure

(surface dose) recommended by dermatologic radiation experts for the treatment of skin cancers ranges from 3900 to 6000 R. This total dose is usually given in 6 to 12 fractions, administered either daily or two to three times a week.

Advantages of X-Ray Therapy

1. *Preservation of tissue.* By far the most important advantage of radiotherapy over surgical methods is the preservation of uninvolved tissue. All methods of cancer therapy require that an adequate margin of normal-appearing skin be included. Most surgical experts recommend the excision of an area at least three to six times larger than the actual visible tumor. This offers special problems in difficult anatomic areas. Inclusion of a sufficiently wide uninvolved border poses no problem to the radiotherapist, since the radiation field can easily be adjusted to the required area of treatment. Tumor margins may be made as generous as necessary (usually extending at least 0.5 to 1 cm on each side of the tumor) without permanent sacrifice of normal tissue. Since complicated reconstructive methods are not necessary, the contours of the involved tissue and of the surrounding normal skin will not be changed markedly by radiotherapy. Only deeply ulcerated carcinomas may leave depressed central scars. Consequently, for carcinomas of the nose, the eyelids, the ears, or the lips, or those in other areas in which tissue cannot readily be sacrificed, radiotherapy is often considered the method of choice.

2. *Irregular or ill-defined carcinomas.* Since the radiation port may be easily adjusted to the shape of the tumor with lead cut-outs, radiotherapy is sometimes preferable to surgical methods for lesions with very irregular or ill-defined borders. Even in sclerosing basal cell carcinomas, radiotherapy can be effectively used, although it is not usually the therapy of choice.[6,12]

3. *Inadequately excised carcinomas.* Postoperative radiation therapy is a simple and useful alternative following histologically demonstrated inadequate surgical excision of skin cancers. A sufficiently wide border can be included to destroy residual carcinomatous tissue. In most of these cases, full-tumor doses are indicated.

4. *Recurrent skin cancers.* Recurrences of surgically treated cancers can be successfully irradiated in patients for whom chemosurgery is not considered the best choice of treatment.

Menn and coworkers[13] have emphasized the high incidence of recurrences following treatment of recurrent skin cancers; the overall rate was 27 per cent. The recurrence rates after excision, and especially after curettage and electrodesiccation, were higher still (40 and 59 per cent). Mohs surgery, with a cure rate of over 90 per cent for recurrent basal cell cancer, was the most effective therapeutic modality.

5. *Hospitalization versus office therapy.* Even large or complicated carcinomas can be irradiated in the office. Since hospitalization is not required, costs can be considerably reduced, and the patient does not have to interrupt his daily activities for long periods.

6. *Other health problems.* Patients in poor health can often be treated with ionizing radiation with fewer complications and less stress than result from surgical methods. This applies especially to patients receiving coagulant therapy or those with allergies to anesthetics.

7. *Elderly patients.* Patients who fear surgery or refuse surgical methods for other reasons, especially elderly patients, can usually be persuaded to undergo radiation therapy. There is also comparatively less danger of late radiation effects in patients of advanced age.

Disadvantages of Radiotherapy

1. *Multiple office visits.* The most important disadvantage of radiotherapy is the need for multiple office visits, usually varying from 5 to 12 treatments. Several follow-up visits are also required. This relative disadvantage is especially important for working patients but less so for retired individuals (who represent the majority of patients treated with ionizing radiation).

2. *Radiation sequelae.* Whereas surgical scars often improve over the years, cosmetic results after radiotherapy tend to worsen in some patients.[4] Undesirable late changes in the treated area may include atrophy and depigmentation. Hyperpigmentation also occurs in some cases, often associated with the appearance of telangiectases. These cosmetic changes were common in the past but now are seen less often with the advent of modern radiation techniques. Pigment changes can be camouflaged with cosmetics, and telangiectases can be electrodesiccated. Late cutaneous radiation changes are less problematic in elderly patients than in younger individuals, in whom additional damaging factors (such as excessive exposure to sun, wind, and cold) may aggravate pre-existing radiation damage.

3. *Alopecia.* In hairy skin areas, a tumoricidal dose of ionizing radiation will always result in permanent alopecia. It is best to avoid treatment of these areas, even though hair transplants can be used effectively in areas of radiodermatitis.

Recent Advances in Dermatologic Radiotherapy

1. *Soft x-ray qualities.* The most important technologic advance in radiotherapy of skin cancers has been the introduction of beryllium-windowed x-ray machines, which have made it possible to reduce unnecessary damage to underlying uninvolved tissue by limiting the penetration of x-rays to the depth of the tumor itself. Cosmetic side effects following soft x-ray therapy are much less pronounced than after the use of more penetrating x-rays. Beryllium-windowed x-ray machines have also facilitated the treatment of very large skin tumors and have considerably improved therapeutic and cosmetic results in curved and irregular anatomic areas (such as the nose, the eyelids, and the ears).

2. *Dosage.* It has long been recognized that many cosmetic side effects of older radiation techniques can also be related to excessive doses. The most severe changes have been observed following "intensive therapy" with only one massive x-ray dose. The one-exposure method should not be used in modern therapy; skin cancers can be eradicated with intensive doses, but the associated late cosmetic effects tend to be worse with this form of therapy than with any other method. Modern x-ray therapy requires fractionation of the total dose.

3. *Radiation protection.* The recognition of late radiation effects on other organs has resulted in the development of modern radiation protection standards. Somatic and genetic late effects (including radiocarcinogenesis in internal organs, especially thyroid and breast cancer) can be reduced to a minimum by proper lead shielding, the use of treatment cones, and other protection techniques.[11,14,15]

References

1. Epstein, E.: Radiodermatitis. Springfield, IL, Charles C Thomas, 1962.
2. Goldschmidt, H.: Dermatologic radiation therapy. Current use of ionizing radiation in the United States and Canada. Arch. Dermatol. 111:1511, 1975.

 3. Chernosky, M. E.: Squamous cell and basal cell carcinomas: Preliminary study of 3,817 primary skin cancers. South. Med. J. 71:802, 1978.
 4. Bart, R. S., Kopf, A. W., and Petratos, M. A.: X-ray therapy of skin cancer: Evaluation of a "standardized" method for treating basal cell epitheliomas. Proceedings of the Sixth National Cancer Conference. Philadelphia, J. B. Lippincott Co., 1968.
 5. Kopf, A. W.: Therapy of basal cell carcinoma. *In* Fitzpatrick, T. B., Arndt, K. A., Clark, W. H., Jr., et al. (eds.): Dermatology in General Medicine. New York, McGraw-Hill Co., 1971.
 6. Gladstein, A. H., Kopf, A. W., and Bart, R. S.: Radiotherapy of cutaneous malignancies. *In* Goldschmidt, H. (ed.): Physical Modalities in Dermatologic Therapy. New York, Springer-Verlag, 1978.
 7. Freeman, R. G., Knox, J. M., and Heaton, C. L.: The treatment of skin cancer. A statistical study of 1,341 skin tumors comparing results obtained with irradiation, surgery, and curettage followed with electrodesiccation. Cancer 17:535, 1964.
 8. Schirren, C. G.: Die Röntgentherapie gutartiger und bösartiger Geschwulste der Haut. *In* Jadassohns Handbuch der Haut und Geschlechtskrankheiten. Suppl. vol. V/2. Berlin, Springer-Verlag, 1959.
 9. Storck, H., Ott, F., and Schwartz, K.: Haut. Handbuch der medizinischen Radiologie. Heidelberg, Springer-Verlag, 1972, pp. 17–160.
10. Schnyder, V. W.: Vor- und Nachteile der Rontgenweichstrahltherapie der Basaliome. Therapeutische Umschau/Revue therapeutique 33:525, 1976.
11. Goldschmidt, H., and Sherwin, W. K.: Reactions to ionizing radiation. J. Am. Acad. Dermatol. 3:551, 1980.
12. Bart, R. S., Kopf, A. W., and Gladstein, A. H.: Treatment of morphea-type basal cell carcinomas with radiation therapy. Arch. Dermatol. 113:783, 1977.
13. Menn, H., Robins, P., Kopf, A. W., and Bart, R. S.: The recurrent basal cell epithelioma. Arch. Dermatol. 103:628, 1971.
14. Goldschmidt, H., and Sherwin, W. K.: Office radiotherapy of cutaneous carcinomas I. Radiation techniques, dose schedules, and radiation protection. J. Dermatol. Surg. Oncol. 9:31, 1983.
15. Goldschmidt, H., and Sherwin, W. K.: Office radiotherapy of cutaneous carcinomas II. Indications in specific anatomic regions. J. Dermatol. Surg. Oncol. 9:47, 1983.

Editorial Comment

Most cutaneous cancers can be cured by a variety of methods, as demonstrated by the contributors to this symposium. The choice of modality is more dependent on the skill and experience of the therapist than on the patient or the neoplasm. It is an axiom that the most skilled operator of the worst method (if we knew which technique was the worst) can do a better job than the worst practitioner of the best method (again, if we knew which procedure would qualify for this ranking). Statistics do not solve the controversy concerning the rating of the approaches, since the skill of the physician, the ratio of difficult to simple cases, and so forth, vary among different series.

However, some methods have specific indications. Microscopic control is particularly necessary in large or recurrent tumors or in those situated at the corners of the eyes or in the paranasal areas. In the latter two locations, the tumors may be of the ''iceberg'' variety, with the major portion of the growth hidden below the superficial portions of the skin. X-radiation may be preferred in locations in which surgical attacks might result in excessive scarring or difficulty in obtaining a good therapeutic result because of the anatomic structures or features involved. Electroexcision allows for the removal of large neoplasms without undue morbidity and often with surprisingly good cosmetic results. Electrodesiccation and curettage affords a cure in many cases and provides a diagnostic biopsy prior to the institution of definite treatment.

Experience has taught that it is better to rely on one method of eradicating a cutaneous tumor than to employ two or more approaches concurrently. The use of many methods discourages the therapist from performing each technique to its optimal degree. In addition, therapeutic failures may result from the use of electrodesiccation plus excision or surgery followed by x-radiation. This combination is illogical and has been demonstrated to be inferior in practice. However, I often treat epitheliomas by electrodesiccation and curettage followed by ionizing radiation if the histopathologic examination dictates the need for the second agent. Actually, the electrodesiccation and curettage is used as a biopsy (you could use a shave or a punch biopsy for this purpose), but with the former modality, the lesion will probably be cured if the neoplasm is benign. If it is malignant, then the x-rays are employed for curative purposes.

The field has been covered so well in the preceding articles that further editorial comment is unnecessary. However, this statement should not be interpreted as indicating that I agree with everything that the contributors have said, because I do not. Furthermore, statements that would have been helpful in the comparison of these methods were left unsaid. Throughout this book I have tried to let the contributor have his say . . . right or wrong. After all, it is up to the reader to judge each contribution: to assess each statement critically and to decide which articles are valuable and with which ones he disagrees. He cannot incorporate into his practice every piece of advice offered between the covers of this volume. The reader must think for himself and must make his own judgments based on his training, beliefs, and experience. This is how the contributors reached the conclusions that they are offering in this book. The profession of medicine has many opinionated practitioners, and there is room for the reader's opinions, too.

Think It Over.

CHAPTER 10

METASTASES FROM SQUAMOUS CELL EPITHELIOMAS OF THE SKIN

METASTATIC SQUAMOUS CELL CANCER FROM THE SKIN

Robert J. Morgan, M.D.

A pertinent controversy in dermatology concerns whether or not squamous cell carcinomas of the skin metastasize with significant frequency and, if so, which associated factors enhance the possibility of metastases. The controversy does not include those squamous cell cancers that arise from junctions of body orifices, such as the mouth, the lips, the nasopharynx, the nostrils, the anus, and the urethra. Furthermore, the controversy does not include those cancers that arise at sites of ionizing irradiation burns (x-ray, radium, and so forth), chemical burns, chronic osteomyelitis and Marjolin ulcers, chronic draining sinuses, scars, hidradenitis suppurativa, lupus erythematosus, lupus vulgaris, leprosy, or Bowen's disease—all of which are acknowledged as producing cancers that may invade aggressively or may metastasize to regional nodes and systemic organs.[1-9] Neither does the controversy include those squamous cell cancers that develop in nail beds, on the genitalia, or on the soles of the feet.[10,11] Except for the rather indolent verrucous squamous cell cancer of the sole, which grows and spreads slowly, these too are known to metastasize unless they are removed relatively early.

Finally, the controversy does not concern those cutaneous cancers arising in patients with xeroderma pigmentosum. These can be lethal early if left untreated, as can those squamous cell cancers developing in immunosuppressed patients.[12] It is common knowledge that patients receiving immunosuppressive treatment develop epitheliomas of the skin more frequently than do healthy individuals, and these tumors are believed to follow a more aggressive course, thus showing a higher than normal frequency of metastases.[13]

What the controversy does center on is those squamous cell cancers that arise from actinic keratoses and those that arise de novo. The de novo squamous cell carcinoma is not common. It arises from clinically normal skin, appears as a nodule or a raised indurated area with early erosion, crusting, and surrounding erythema, and is variably painful. It grows rapidly and frequently metastasizes.

In 1965, Lund[14] evaluated the potential for squamous cell cancer of the skin to metastasize and concluded that in a dermatologist's practice these lesions seldom metastasize. This did not start the controversy, but it did stimulate other dermatopathologists to reassess their experiences.

Graham and Helwig[3,15,16] state that most squamous cell cancers of the skin arise in senile keratoses and that these "seldom if ever metastasize." They also acknowledge that de novo squamous cell carcinoma is more aggressive and may metastasize. Rosai,[17] a professor of pathology at the University of Minnesota, wrote that squamous cell cancer developing in actinic keratoses is "of low grade malignancy." Jansen[18] has made similar assertions about the low-grade potential of actinic squamous cell carcinomas. His clinical expertise *and* pathologic confirmation make his opinion particularly pertinent.

Bickers,[19] citing Lund's survey and his own experience, states that "the incidence of aggressive behavior [metastatic potential] is quite low in lesions of actinic origin." He admits that caution and concern should be maintained for those patients treated with PUVA. This therapy should increase the incidence of actinic squamous cell cancer, but the response has not been of significance yet.[20]

Szymanski[21] discounts the belief that squamous cell carcinoma of the glabrous skin produces a highly malignant tumor. In his evaluation of 2517 cases, only 6 were found to have metastases, or 0.23 per cent. He cites Lund's later study that found an almost identical percentage (i.e., 2500 cases and only 6 with metastases).

Mysliborski[22] claims that origin from sun-damaged skin can be determined either clinically or histologically. "This is important because squamous cell carcinoma arising from actinic keratoses is estimated to metastasize in less than 0.5 per cent and if metastasis occurs, it is generally *only* to regional nodes."

Arnold,[23] who has worked for 40 years at the Straub Clinic in Honolulu, says that neither he nor the pathologists and five general surgeons at the clinic have seen squamous cell carcinomas of the skin metastasize (excluding those at body orifices, and probably also excluding those in burns, scars, and ulcers). This would include carcinomas that originally had been treated (or neglected) by therapists less talented than the practitioners at the Straub Clinic.

On the other hand, Epstein and coworkers,[24] who evaluated 6900 patients with squamous cell cancer of the skin (data that were provided by the California Tumor Registry), found that 142, or approximately 2 per cent, had spread beyond the dermis at the time of diagnosis of the primary tumor, i.e., to lymph nodes or more distant sites. Furthermore, 2.5 per cent of these had evidence of metastases within 1 month after the appearance of the primary tumor, 40 per cent within 6 months, and 70 per cent within 1 year. It was also found in this study that 67.6 per cent of the primary lesions occurred on exposed skin (face, ears, neck, hands) and that only 39 patients had nonactinic preceding lesions (chronic ulcers, burn scars, or irradiation damage). The remainder, we presume, arose de novo or from actinic keratoses.

Schrek,[25] in a statistical analysis performed in 1941, found that 14 per cent to 20 per cent of epidermoid carcinomas of the skin metastasized. Ackerman and del Gato,[26] in 1947, stated that at least 5 per cent of the epidermoid carcinomas of the skin metastasize to regional lymph nodes and that those from the trunk and the extremities metastasize even more frequently. Prior to these relatively early dates, texts[27,28] had indicated a significantly higher rate of metastasis, probably because patients in those days procrastinated more in having their cancers treated. Johnson and Helwig,[3] reporting on adenoid squamous cell carcinomas, found that 2 of 155 lesions of this variant, or 3.2 per cent, metastasized by direct extension and that 3 more metastasized to distant sites.

Moller and associates[29] cited 153 cases of actinic squamous cell cancers, finding that 3.3 per cent metastasized. They concluded, "Squamous cell cancer of the skin should be considered a malignant tumor with higher incidence of metastasis than previously assumed."

Ames and Hickey[30] evaluated 1208 patients with squamous cell carcinoma of the skin of the extremities seen as M. D. Anderson Hospital in Houston. Seventy-five patients (6 per cent) had regional lymph node metastases *on admission,* and 15 more (1 per cent) had distant metastases *when first seen.* One hundred six patients (8.7 per cent) developed regional lymph node metastases. Eighty per cent occurred on the exposed parts of the forearm, the hand, and the finger. However, 41 of these were associated with Marjolin thermal burn ulcers and irradiation burns. There was nothing else in the other histories to account for the development of squamous cell carcinoma other than sun exposure and (in 3 cases) chronic arsenic ingestion.

Cassisi and coworkers[31] evaluated 22 patients treated at the University of Florida for squamous cell carcinoma of the skin metastatic to parotid nodes. Of these, six cases came from primary lesions on the temple, four from the eyebrow, three each from the forehead and cheek, and one each from the pinna of the ear, the ear lobe, and the postauricular and paranasal areas. The origin of the other two cases was not mentioned. No case had associated lesions other than those resulting from sun exposure. There was only a 25 per cent survival among patients who received combinations of surgery and radiation therapy.

J. Leslie Smith[32] of M. D. Anderson Hospital has been quoted as saying, "Almost all tumors [speaking of squamous cell carcinomas] arising de novo can be attributed to prolonged actinic irradiation usually observed on exposed skin of elderly males."

Bourne,[33] reporting from Queensland, Australia, found 13 patients with squamous cell carcinomas that spread by way of the cranial nerves and implied that all arose in sun-exposed areas. Only one had a pre-existing lesion (lupus erythematosus) other than actinic keratoses.

What of my own beliefs and experiences? I do not agree with the common view that statements based on impressions are valueless. In my opinion, these hypotheses have much merit if they are weighed against all extenuating and circumstantial evidence. Even statistics can be fallacious and must be judged carefully. However, we never should let our impressions transcend evidence.

Between 1970 and 1980, biopsies were performed on 436 squamous cell cancers that were diagnosed in my office. These were without precursor lesions other than actinic exposure and keratoses. I personally observed eight of these patients with squamous cell carcinomas of actinically exposed skin who suffered metastases beyond the dermis to nodes or distant sites. Seven of these eight patients had significant actinic keratoses. The diagnosis of squamous cell carcinoma of the skin was confirmed by histologic examination. Therefore, 1.6 per cent of my patients had *known* metastases from actinic exposed skin.

Two of these eight whose primary lesions were treated by me had metastases that were diagnosed and treated by others—I learned about the spread only fortuitously. Therefore, only 75 per cent of those patients in whom I treated the primary lesion returned to me because of metastases. An additional two patients had their primary cancers diagnosed or treated elsewhere. I saw them with keratoses and with metastatic nodes. In six of this total of ten patients, the primary lesion was on skin near the ear. One of the patients originally seen elsewhere came to me for persistent skin cancer and metastatic nodes. The patient had asked his first dermatologist if his cancer therapy could wait 1 month, until after he went on a Caribbean cruise. Quoting a dermatology text, the first dermatologist answered that since the cancer had arisen as an actinic keratosis, it was not likely to metastasize, and therapy therefore could wait. The patient procrastinated for 3 months, and metastasis occurred.

Over a period of months or years, patients sometimes forget about an earlier skin cancer. I wonder how many other patients whom dermatologists have treated for skin cancer later have appeared at the office of some surgeon, radiologist, or oncologist with metastatic cancer about which the dermatologist was never informed.

DISCUSSION

Squamous cell carcinoma of the skin can originate from the epidermis, from the adnexal epithelium, and from keratinous cysts. The variants of cutaneous squamous cell cancer are of interest and are among the factors that can influence metastasis. In 1932, Broders[35] classified them based on the ability of the malignant cell to mature and to keratinize, i.e., from great ability to inability (Grades I to IV). It long has been felt that well-differentiated

(Grade I) cancer is less likely to metastasize than is poorly differentiated (Grade IV) cancer. Most de novo cancers are poorly differentiated.

Some de novo cancers are composed of spindle-shaped, sarcoma-like cells and are quite anaplastic. Most spindle-cell squamous cancers result from irradiation, thermal burns, or trauma but may occur in actinic keratoses. Another variant is the adenoid squamous cell cancer, usually from the adnexal epithelium, which can be found arising from actinic damage as well as de novo. Acantholytic squamous cell cancer, or adenoacanthoma, develops in alveolar structures or from hair follicles. The potential of adenoacanthomas for metastasis is higher than that of cancers arising from the epidermis.

There are three varieties of verrucous squamous cell cancer of the skin, all of which grow relatively slowly but may invade deeply and still metastasize relatively slowly: the Ackerman verrucous squamous cell cancer of the lip, the verrucous squamous cell carcinoma of the soles of the feet and the palms of the hands, and the giant condyloma acuminatum of Buschke (vegetating masses with deep invasion, which are the quickest to metastasize of the three verrucous types).

When squamous cell carcinoma metastasizes, it may invade the lymphatics or the blood vessels, be borne to remote capillary beds, overcome natural resistance, and thrive. More commonly, tumors of the skin first invade contiguously and destructively into the dermis as coherent strands and columns. They usually reproduce the same histologic patterns in their metastases.

Factors that influence metastasis other than the variant of squamous cell cancer include the depth of invasion, the location (cancers of preauricular cheek and aural sulci origin are more likely to metastasize), the age of the patient (the older the patient, the higher the incidence of squamous cell cancer and the higher the incidence of metastases), and immunologic deficiency. In the absence of all these influencing factors, squamous cell cancer of the skin can occur and can metastasize.

The patient with proven cancer in a lymph node or another accessible site that has arisen from an unknown primary presents a diagnostic challenge and a therapeutic problem. "In over half the patients the primary lesion will never be found—this even includes patients who are closely followed and those eventually autopsied." Krementz cites papers from other institutions (M. D. Anderson, Mayo Clinic, Charity Hospital, and others) describing a total of 536 cases of metastatic cancer of the neck. The primary sites were successfully detected in only 170 cases.[34] It is logical to assume that many of those cases in which the primary site was not found could have originated from the skin and could have been "cured" long ago by a dermatologist or other primary physician who convinced the patient that he could forget the skin lesion.

It is admitted that individuals with squamous cell cancers of the skin who are treated at a cancer referral center may well not be representative of the overall population of patients with squamous cell cancer. The initial success rate of therapy by dermatologists who use excisional surgery, electrodesiccation and curettage, irradiation, or Mohs chemosurgery is consistently above 90 per cent. Most of the failures (10 per cent of cases) are followed by the same physician, and recurrences are treated successfully.

The surgeon or family physician who finds metastatic nodes or visceral metastases traditionally refers the specimen to a general pathologist. The general pathologists admittedly do not know the origin in a high percentage of cases of metastatic squamous cell cancer. The likelihood that a pathologist who sees a neoplasm in a skin specimen and concentrates on its type will see an adjacent actinic keratosis is no greater than the likelihood that a man would see the cap of a bikini-clad beauty strolling by. A dermatopathologist is not sent many specimens of metastatic nodes or viscera, so both general pathologists and dermatopathologists have incomplete knowledge of the frequency of metastatic squamous cell cancer from the skin. Certainly dermatologists, surgeons, and clinical oncologists lack complete knowledge.

Ideally, a squamous cell cancer of the skin should be excised. The excision should include surrounding skin showing actinic degeneration, actinic keratosis, Bowen's disease, and so forth. A tumor biopsy usually is not adequate for the pathologist to determine if a cancer has arisen in an actinic keratosis. Also, wide excision is not always the best way to treat the human being, since a nonmutilating simple tumor biopsy may be the most expedient way to make a diagnosis and a plan of therapy for a large and deep lesion.

CONCLUSIONS

1. Actinic squamous cell cancers can and do metastasize with significant frequency.

2. If only 1 to 3 per cent metastasize and disable, deform, or kill, this is sufficient frequency for us to abolish such minimizing phrases as "low-grade" and "seldom if ever metastasizing."

3. A significant percentage of those patients treated by dermatologists for their primary lesion are not seen by these specialists for their metastases. Hence, the dermatologists may not have knowledge of the spread.

4. A dermatologist's "failure to cure" may be seen in a hospital setting. Therefore, it is understandable that the incidence of metastases in a hospital is greater than the incidence of metastases seen in a dermatologist's office, or even in a dermatopathologist's office.

5. Actinic squamous cell cancers should be treated aggressively and with dispatch.

References

1. Horton, J., and Hill, C. J. (eds.): Clinical Oncology. Philadelphia, W. B. Saunders Co., 1977, pp. 670–672.
2. Lever, W., and Schaumberg-Lever, G. (eds.): Histopathology of the Skin, 5th ed. Philadelphia, J. B. Lippincott, 1975.
3. Graham, J. H., Johnson, W. C., and Helwig, E. G. (eds.): Dermal Pathology. Hagerstown, MD, Harper & Row, 1972.
4. Pinkus, H., and Mehregan, A. (eds.): A Guide to Dermatohistopathology. New York, Appleton-Century-Crofts, 1969.
5. Rook, A., Wilkinson, D., and Ebling, F.: Textbook of Dermatology, 2nd ed. Philadelphia, F. A. Davis Co., 1968.
6. Rosen, T.: Squamous cell carcinoma in black patients. Ortho Letter 1:2, 1981.
7. Curry, S. S., Gaither, D. H. and King, L. E., Jr.: Squamous cell carcinoma arising in dissecting perifolliculitis (hidradenitis) of the scalp. J. Am. Acad. Dermatol. 4:6, June 1981.
8. Kao, G. F., and Graham, J. H.: Carcinoma arising in Bowen's disease. Paper presented at 19th Annual Meeting of the American Society of Dermatopathology, San Francisco, CA, Dec. 1981.
9. Wolf, W. B., and Cohen, L. S.: Intraepidermal squamous cell carcinoma (Bowen's disease) of the dorsum of the foot. J. Am. Podiatry Assoc. 68:688, 1978.
10. Demuth, R. J., and Snider, B. L.: Primary squamous cell carcinoma of the foot. Ann. Plast. Surg. 4:310, Apr. 1980.
11. Turk, L. L., and Winder, P. R.: Carcinomas of the skin and their treatment. Semin. Oncol. 7:4, Dec. 1980.
12. Maize, J. C.: Skin cancer in immunosuppressed patients. JAMA 237:1857, 1977.
13. Reymann, F.: Treatment of multiple squamous cell carcinomas of the skin in an immunosuppressed patient. Dermatologica 160:304, 1981.
14. Lund, H. Z.: How often does squamous cell carcinoma of the skin metastasize? Arch. Dermatol. 92:635, Dec. 1965.
15. Graham, J. H., Bendl, B. J., and Johnson, W. C.: Solar keratosis with squamous cell carcinoma: A new biologic concept. Am. J. Pathol. 55:26A, 1969.
16. Bendl, B. J., and Graham, J. H.: New concepts of the origin of squamous cell carcinoma of the skin: Solar (senile) keratoses with squamous cell carcinoma. A. Clinicopathologic and histochemical study. Proc. Natl. Cancer Conf. 6:471, 1970.
17. Rosai, J., and Ackerman, L. V.: The pathology of tumors—part I. CA-A Cancer Journal for Clinicians. 28:6, Nov.–Dec. 1978.
18. Jansen, T.: Clinical Recognition of Skin Neoplasms. Chicago, Year Book Medical Publishers, 1976, p. 57.
19. Bickers, D. R.: Reply to a letter to the editor from Ervin Epstein. J. Am. Acad. Dermatol. 4:6, June 1981.

20. Roenigk, H. H., Jr., and Caro, W. A.: Skin cancer in the PUVA-48 cooperative study. J. Am. Acad. Dermatol. 4:3, March 1981.
21. Szymanski, F.: Squamous cell carcinoma of the Skin. *In* Graham, J. H., et al. (eds.): Dermal Pathology. Hagerstown, MD, Harper & Row, 1972, p. 626.
22. Mysliborski, J. A.: Cutaneous neoplasms. N. Y. State J. Med. 1716, Oct. 1980.
23. Arnold, H.: Letter to this author, dated Jan. 29, 1981.
24. Epstein, E., Epstein, N. N., Bragg, K., and Linden, G.: Metastases from squamous cell carcinomas of the skin. Arch. Dermatol. 97:245, March 1968.
25. Schrek, R.: Cutaneous carcinoma: III. A statistical analysis with respect to site, sex and pre-existing scars. Arch. Pathol. 31:434, 1941.
26. Ackerman, L. V., and del Gato, J. A.: Cancer: Diagnosis, Treatment and Prognosis. St. Louis, C. V. Mosby Co., 1947.
27. Stelwagon, H.: Diseases of the Skin, 4th ed. Philadelphia, W. B. Saunders Co., 1906.
28. Hyde, J.N., and Montgomery, F.H.: Diseases of the Skin, 7th ed. Philadelphia, Lea Brothers and Co., 1904.
29. Moller, R., Reymann, F., and Hov-Jensen, K.: Metastases in dermatological patients with squamous cell carcinoma. Arch. Dermatol. 115:703, 1979.
30. Ames, F. C., and Hickey, R. C.: Squamous cell carcinoma of the skin of the extremities. Internatl. Advances in Surg. Oncol. 3:179, 1980.
31. Cassisi, N. J., Dickerson, D. R., and Million, R. R.: Squamous cell carcinoma of the skin metastatic to parotid nodes. J. Fla. Med. Assoc. 65:9, Sept. 1978.
32. Smith, J. L.: Spindle cell squamous cell carcinoma. *In* Graham, J. H., et al. (eds.): Dermal Pathology. Hagerstown, MD, Harper & Row, 1972.
33. Bourne, R. G.: The spread of squamous carcinoma of the skin via the cranial nerves. Australas. Radiol. 24:107, July 1980.
34. Krementz, E. T., Cerise, E. J., Ciaravella, J. M., and Morgan, L. R.: Metastases of undetermined source. CA-A Cancer Journal for Clinicians 27:5, Sept./Oct. 1977.
35. Broders, A. C.: Practical points on the microscopic grading of carcinoma. NY State J. Med. 32:667, 1932.

SQUAMOUS CELL CARCINOMAS OF ACTINIC ORIGIN RARELY METASTASIZE BEYOND THE SKIN

David R. Bickers, M.D.

It is generally agreed that more than 80 per cent of all human cancers are of environmental origin and that skin neoplasms are the most common type of malignancy occurring in the human population. Compelling epidemiologic data indicate that skin neoplasms occur as a result of chronic cutaneous exposure to solar radiation or to selected carcinogenic chemicals. Experimental studies have shown that the induction of cancer requires at least two major steps: (1) *initiation* and (2) *promotion*. Initiation causes a permanent change in a cell such that it undergoes a mutagenic alteration. Promotion requires repeated exposure to promoting agents at frequent intervals and is a reversible process if discontinued prior to tumor development. The ultraviolet-B (290 to 320 nm) component of solar radiation and polyaromatic hydrocarbons generated by incomplete combustion of fossil fuels are potent initiators and promoters. It is therefore not surprising that repeated cutaneous exposure to these agents can result in tumor formation in the skin. These nonmelanoma skin cancers are generally not aggressive and rarely tend to metastasize beyond the local area of involvement.

In this discussion I will attempt to buttress my contention that these lesions are not aggressive by reviewing the existing literature and by providing the results of a survey that I conducted in 1981.

Controversy can be defined as a difference marked by the expression of opposing views. In this discussion I will take the position that squamous cell carcinomas of the skin arising in areas of the head, the neck, and the hands (all of which are directly exposed to sunlight) have little, if any, tendency to spread beyond the local site of involvement except by direct extension. It is essential that careful definitions of terms be established and that specific criteria for metastasis be used in the context of this discussion.

The negligible risk of metastasis of squamous cell carcinoma of the skin applies only to lesions that fulfill the following criteria:

1. The tumors must originate on sun-exposed areas of the head, the neck, and the hands.

2. Lesions developing at the mucocutaneous border of the lip must not be included.

3. Prior exposure to other oncogens, such as arsenic and ionizing radiation, must be rigorously excluded.

4. Chronic infection, such as osteomyelitis and chronic irritation in burn scars, or blistering disorders, such as epidermolysis bullosa, must be excluded.

These criteria, then, leave a well-defined category of cutaneous neoplasms that are largely the result of *chronic actinic exposure*.

It is also imperative to verify that metastasis has occurred and that the metastatic lesion is secondary to a primary squamous cell carcinoma originating in the skin. The definition of metastasis that will be used for this discussion is based upon that given by Lattes and Kessler.[1]

1. The primary carcinoma must arise in the skin. This excludes *epidermoid* neoplasms that may originate in other sites and may spread secondarily to the skin.

2. Metastases must be demonstrated at a site distant from the primary lesion. Direct extension is not metastatic.

3. Histologic similarity must exist between the primary tumor and the metastatic lesion.

As I will demonstrate, the rigorous application of these criteria to existing published information sharply reduces the number of valid cases in which metastases of squamous cell carcinoma of the skin has occurred.

One of the first to appreciate the role of sunlight in causing squamous cell carcinoma of the skin was the German dermatopathologist Paul Unna.[2] He used the term "carcinoma of the sailor's skin" to describe a malady that he had observed mainly in sailors who were chronically exposed to sunlight while spending their lives at sea. Unna contrasted these warty growths with those of the rodent ulcer of basal cell carcinoma, but he made no mention of the proclivity of these lesions to metastasize.

In 1921, Broders described 256 patients with squamous cell epithelioma of the skin who were treated at the Mayo Clinic.[3] These represented 12.5 per cent of all epitheliomas seen at that institution between 1904 and 1915. Seventy-eight per cent of the lesions occurred above the clavicle. The average size of the primary lesion in patients with metastases was 6.3 cm. In 32 of 52 cases in which lymph nodes and salivary glands were removed, metastases were identified, but their relationship to the primary lesion was not defined. The report by Broders does not fulfill the first and third criteria of Lattes and Kessler. Furthermore, the experience at the Mayo Clinic would necessarily include patients with very advanced disease. More than half had been treated elsewhere prior to coming to the Mayo Clinic. The *average size* of the primary lesion in this series was 6.3 cm, indicating that the tumor was quite advanced at the time of treatment at the Mayo Clinic.

In 1954, Modlin reported his experience with skin cancer at the Ellis Fischel Cancer Hospital in Missouri.[4] Lymph node metastases occurred in 52 of 444 patients with epidermoid skin cancers followed at that hospital for 5 years. This was a metastatic rate of 11 per cent. In all but 10 of the 52 patients, the primary lesion was larger than 2 cm in diameter; in 30 of the 52 patients, treatment of the primary lesion had been attempted previously but had been unsuccessful. None of the criteria of Lattes and Kessler were fulfilled in Modlin's study.

Katz and coworkers reviewed the experience with squamous cell carcinoma of the skin between 1946 and 1950 at the Roswell Park Memorial Institute in Buffalo, New York.[5] Four hundred thirteen patients, with a total of 601 tumors, were *admitted* in this 5-year period. Of these, 241 had squamous cell carcinoma of the skin without other malignancy or metastases at the time of admission. Measured by a life table technique, the probability that metastases would develop in this group of patients at the end of 5 years ranged from 2.6 to 3.6 per cent. The body site of the primary lesion and the age at onset could not be associated with the risk of metastasis. The major weakness of this study was the failure to verify the relationship of the metastatic lesion to the primary squamous cell carcinoma of the skin.

In 1965, Dunn and associates attempted to define the number of individuals in California with nonmelanoma skin cancer who ultimately died of their disease each year. Vital statistics data showed that 125 deaths could be attributed to skin cancer *annually*.[6] Careful review of the cases showed that the true number of deaths was 39. Of these, 29 individuals had squamous cell carcinomas. From these data it could be estimated that of the 6000 new cases of skin cancer diagnosed annually in California, 39 patients would die of their disease. Since 29 of the 39 would have squamous cell carcinomas and since approximately 38 per cent of the 6000 reported cases were squamous cell carcinomas, the percentage of fatal squamous cell carcinomas of the skin would be 1.27 per cent $\left(\frac{29}{6000 \times 0.38}\right)$.

These data did not provide any information on the primary site of skin involvement, and it could be argued that at least some of the lesions developed in areas that had not been exposed to sun and in areas of chronic inflammation, which are known to have a higher metastatic risk. On this basis, the aggressiveness of lesions of actinic origin would almost certainly be less than the data suggest, particularly since the total number of skin cancers must be considerably higher than 6000.

In 1965, Lund reviewed his experience with squamous cell carcinoma as a practicing dermatopathologist.[7] Tumors of the lip, the anus, the penis, and the vulva were excluded. One thousand consecutive skin biopsies were tabulated, and 82 squamous cell tumors were identified. Of these, 16 were keratoacanthomas, 4 were keratoacanthomas in which early squamous cell carcinoma could not be excluded, 17 were precancerous keratoses in which early carcinoma could not be excluded, 7 were squamous cell carcinomas with incipient invasion, and 17 were aggressive squamous cell carcinomas. Of the 82 lesions examined histologically, less than 25 per cent appeared to be aggressive lesions.

Lund then sent a questionnaire to 45 dermatologists in practice in the southeastern United States who regularly sent biopsies to his laboratory to inquire about the risk of metastasis of squamous cell carcinoma. Forty-three of the dermatologists responded, and of these, 28 (or 65 per cent) had not seen a single case of metastatic squamous cell carcinoma. The remaining 15 dermatologists could recall a total of 17 cases in their own practices and four additional cases outside their own practices.

From these data, Lund extrapolated to his own laboratory experience and stated that of 46,000 biopsies read in his laboratory over a 12-year period, he would expect four metastases—an incidence of metastasis of 0.1 per cent of squamous cell tumors. He next attempted to define the nature of the squamous cell carcinomas of the skin in which metastasis does occur. He obtained data by requesting information from other (unspecified) institutions on any squamous cell carcinoma of the skin that had metastasized. Twelve such cases were identified. Of these, five occurred in association with primary lesions of actinic origin and seven in association with primary lesions of nonactinic origin. Despite these findings, I must point out that Lund's data also do not fulfill the criteria of Lattes and Kessler for verification of metastasis.

In 1968, Epstein and coworkers reviewed the data of the California Tumor Registry of the Department of Health of the State of California.[8] Data were obtained from cancer cases in 38 hospitals and, as stated by the authors, "they represent the experience of the average hospitalized cancer patient . . . ." Six thousand nine hundred patients developed squamous cell carcinoma between 1942 and 1962. In 93 per cent of the cases, the diagnosis was confirmed histopathologically. In 442 cases, the squamous cell carcinoma had spread beyond the dermis at the time of diagnosis, but detailed study indicated that 300 of these had spread by direct extension. The remaining 142 (2 per cent) represented metastasizing squamous cell cancer of the skin. In 67.6 per cent of the cases, the primary lesions occurred on the exposed portions of the body; however, preceding skin conditions were recorded for only 39 patients (27.5 per cent of the total 142). These included chronic ulcers in 32 (82.1 per cent), burn scars in 5 (12.8 per cent), and chronic radiodermatitis in 2 (5.1 per cent). No preceding skin conditions were identified in the remaining 72.5 per cent of patients. Since it is unclear how many of these individuals were seen by dermatologists who might have recorded the presence of actinic damage, there is no way of knowing whether these patients with squamous cell carcinoma had antecedent actinic damage. It is inappropriate to conclude from these data, as did the authors, that squamous cell carcinomas of actinic origin have the same risk of metastasis as do lesions originating secondarily to other causes. A further major difficulty with the data of Epstein and colleagues is that the number of cases identified with metastases (numerator) is almost certainly accurate, whereas the total number of cases of squamous cell carcinoma of the skin (denominator) is grossly underestimated. This would certainly reduce the fraction of squamous cell carcinomas that metastasize.

Szymanski has described his experience with squamous cell carcinoma of the skin at the Research and Education Hospital of the University of Illinois.[9] Over a 25-year period, 2517 cases of squamous cell carcinoma of the glabrous skin (lip, mouth, penis, and vulva were excluded) were diagnosed. Szymanski was able to find only six cases (0.24 per cent) with metastases from primary squamous cell carcinoma of the skin. None of the criteria of Lattes and Kessler were fulfilled by his data, however.

A more recent report by Moller and associates reviewed the experience at the Finsen Institute in Copenhagen, Denmark.[10] Two hundred sixty four patients in whom the diagnosis of squamous cell carcinoma was made between 1950 and 1959 were studied. In 1977, 253 histologic preparations were reviewed. Of these, 186 were found to have definite squamous cell carcinoma and 25 were found to have probable squamous cell carcinoma. Patients were traced through the population register, and only two could not be found. On January 1, 1976, 24 men and 21 women of the original 141 men and 70 women were alive. Out of the total number of 211 patients, metastases were found in 11 (5.2 per cent)— nine men (6.3 per cent) and two women (2.8 per cent). Of those tumors originating on light-exposed skin (133), four were said to have metastasized (3.0 per cent). However, no data were provided concerning the possibility that primary lesions in some of these patients originated in scars or areas of chronic infection. Furthermore, no histologic verification of the identity of the metastatic lesions to the primary squamous cell carcinoma of the skin was provided, and therefore the study fails to fulfill the criteria of Lattes and Kessler.

In conclusion, I wish to describe the results of a survey conducted in the summer of 1981, in which a questionnaire was sent to a number of dermatologists throughout the United States to determine their experience concerning this issue.[11] The results of the survey serve to confirm the impression that metastases of squamous cell carcinomas of the skin, particularly those on sun-exposed skin, have little tendency to metastasize. In fairness, it should be pointed out that these findings also do not fulfill the criteria of Lattes and Kessler and are clearly anecdotal.

On the basis of my analysis of existing published data and the experience of dermatologists in active practice throughout the United States, I must conclude that squamous cell carcinomas arising on glabrous skin regularly exposed to sunlight have little, if any, tendency to metastasize. However, just as with any biological dictum, it is certainly clear that exceptions can and do occur. Biological variation is a law of nature, and it is therefore not surprising to find scattered evidence to support the concept that such lesions may occasionally behave in a more aggressive manner.

This striking tendency for localization of skin cancer within the tissue of origin remains unexplained, but a fuller understanding of the factors that account for it would undoubtedly enhance our knowledge concerning the biological behavior of neoplasms.

References

1. Lattes, R., and Kessler, R. W.: Metastasizing basal cell carcinoma of the skin—report of two cases. Cancer 4:866, 1951.
2. Unna, P.: The Histopathology of the Diseases of the Skin. Edinburgh, William Clay, 1896, p. 719.
3. Broders, A. C.: Squamous cell epithelioma of the skin. Ann. Surg. 73:141, 1921.
4. Modlin, J. J.: Cancer of the skin. Mo. Med. 51:364, 1954.
5. Katz, A. D., et al.: The frequency and risk of metastases in squamous cell carcinoma of the skin. Cancer 10:1162, 1957.
6. Dunn, J. E., et al.: Skin cancer as a cause of death. Calif. Med. 102:361, 1965.
7. Lund, H. Z.: How often does squamous cell carcinoma of the skin metastasize? Arch. Dermatol. 92:635, 1965.
8. Epstein, E., et al.: Metastases from squamous cell carcinomas of the skin. Arch. Dermatol. 97:245, 1968.
9. Szymanski, F.: Keratoacanthoma. In Graham, J. H., et al. (eds.): Dermal Pathology. Hagerstown, MD, Harper and Row, 1972, p. 625.
10. Moller, R., et al.: Metastases in dermatological patients with squamous cell carcinoma. Arch. Dermatol. 115:703, 1979.
11. Task Force on Photobiology. Chicago, American Academy of Dermatology, 1981.

Editorial Comment

The pendulum seems to be swinging away from the concept that squamous cell carcinomas of the skin caused by sunshine do not metastasize. This belief concerning the benignity of such solar-induced neoplasms was based on the writings of Lund, Graham, and Freeman. However, it was emphasized by these authorities that this applied only to those squamous cell epitheliomas associated *histologically* with actinic keratoses. All three agree that such sun-produced carcinomas of the skin can and do metastasize frequently and widely. Perhaps Winkelmann's view that the cases described by Graham and others are not epitheliomas at all but merely ''penetrating keratoses'' is valid. The biological behavior of the lesions seems to confirm his belief.

Dr. Bickers makes a strong case for the theory that squamous cell epitheliomas of the skin are not aggresive tumors. Carefully studied large series contradict this. It might be mentioned that questionnaires based on memory are notoriously unreliable. The human mind is not a computer; it does not retain all the information that is fed into it. We tend to recall the outstanding cases that we encounter and to forget the rest. This tendency increases with age. Therefore, the results of such questionnaires can be ignored. As an example, how many squamous cell cancers have you seen metastasize? Yet, when charts are reviewed, it is obvious that this occurs with disturbing regularity. These figures cannot be ignored.

A minor point: Dr. Bickers has stated that patients were hospitalized in the cases that I reported (reference number 8 in Bickers' article). Dr. Bickers pointed out that such cases constitute a special group with an increased chance of metastatic involvement. Although Dr. Bickers has quoted the publication correctly, few of these patients actually were hospitalized. The cases were reported by hospitals and university clinics, but most of the patients were treated as outpatients.

Think It Over.

CHAPTER 11

CRYOTHERAPY: SPRAYS VERSUS APPLICATORS

ADVANTAGES AND DISADVANTAGES OF CRYOSURGERY AND CRYOSPRAY FOR MALIGNANCIES

Ronald R. Lubritz, M.D.

The purpose of this article is to discuss the advantages and disadvantages of treating malignances by cryosurgery in general and cryospray procedures in particular. In order for this to be accomplished lucidly, it is best to summarize the history of dermatocryosurgery briefly.

Many physicians look upon cryosurgery as a recent development in the field of dermatologic management of various nonmalignant and malignant conditions. In point of fact, cryosurgical techniques have been used since shortly before the turn of the century. In 1899, Dr. A. Campbell White of New York published an article outlining his use of liquid air in the treatment various conditions.[1] Several methods of cryogen application, still in use today in modified form, were first described by Dr. White. His swab method consisted of a cotton tip applicator dipped back and forth into liquid air. Like our liquid nitrogen dip-sticks of today, the swab was then applied to the lesion to be treated. He fashioned applicators of various sizes and shapes. In this way, many different types of lesions, depending upon dimensions and configurations, could be treated. In 1907, Whitehouse described the spray method originated by White.[2] This consisted basically of a wash bottle with two linings; in effect, a Dewar glass reservoir. By using the finger to occlude the opening of a glass tube inserted into the bottle, one created pressure by boiling off liquid air to produce a spray from the outlet of a second tube. Dr. White did not stop with these developments; he also designed the first cryoprobes. For treatment of other conditions, he used various probes fashioned from aluminum, brass, and glass. Although swabs and probes were used intermittently, the spray method was abandoned until the 1960s.

Although the use of liquid air had definite advantages, severe limitations precluded its widespread popularity. Liquid air evaporated in a very short time, usually within a few days. It was not generally available and, when it was, it was quite expensive. The opposite is true of carbon dioxide. Because of its wide availability, its relatively low cost, and its ability to be stored for prolonged periods, this cryogen, which was first described by Pusey in 1907, has been used frequently in dermatology.[3] Since Pusey's work, carbon dioxide has been used in a variety of shapes and forms. Various molds of carbon dioxide can be made from trapping the solid particles while allowing gas to escape. These compressed crystals can be used in the treatment of various benign conditions. Carbon dioxide may be used as a slush producing a conforming mold or as a solid in the shape of carved pieces. This cryogen has definite limitations, however. Its most serious drawback is its shallow depth of freezing. Because of this, it is now used primarily for treating hemangiomas and superficial benign lesions.

For a brief time, liquid oxygen was used by several investigators. A major pitfall was that liquid oxygen, although relatively inexpensive, was flammable and therefore unsafe in many instances.

Freons have been investigated for use in dermatology. They have been employed by many for topical analgesia and as the primary cryogen for dermabrasion since Luikart, Ayres, and Wilson reported on the use of freon 114 in 1955.[4]

With the availability of liquid nitrogen in the 1940s, a new era in cryosurgery was soon to commence. Using the swab, or dip-stick, method, Allington popularized this cryogen for treatment of various cutaneous conditions.[5] The dawn of modern cutaneous cryosurgery arose somewhat belatedly in the 1960s. It was a neurosurgeon, Dr. Irving Cooper, who first described a closed-system apparatus utilizing liquid nitrogen in 1961.[6] This closed system involved cryoprobes. Its main advantage was that it was able to destroy tissue at a greater depth and in a reproducible and consistent fashion. Modified cryoprobes for treating various skin lesions were devised by Cahan.[7]

In 1966, Zacarian and Adham reported the development of modified cryoprobes consisting of copper cylindrical discs that could be brought down to temperatures approaching that of liquid nitrogen ($-196°C$).[8] This fundamental work proved that malignancies could be treated with cryoprobe methods. Because of the limitations and inconsistencies of cryoprobes, however, Zacarian adopted spray methods as well.

The cornerstone for modern dermatocryosurgical techniques was laid by Torre around 1965.[9] His cryojet system represented a spray apparatus, which could provide techniques that were not only efficient but also reliable. It is this prototype that provided the basic plan for many of the units in current use. The systems and clinical techniques devised by Torre and Zacarian have provided the impetus for such widespread use of present-day cryosurgery.

Cryosurgery

Advantages

Cutaneous cryosurgical procedures for malignancies overcome the therapeutic shortcomings of surgical modalities. The converse is also true. Other procedures compensate for the disadvantages of cryosurgery, creating a happy pairing. As a pertinent example, certain anatomic sites, such as the eyelid, the nose, and the ear, do not respond well to excisional surgery or to curettage or x-ray. Cartilage, however, tolerates cold quite well. Usually, lesions in these areas respond well to cryosurgery. In fact, these are preferred sites for some of the better cryosurgical results. Lesions of the anterior chest and the mandibular line are further examples of those for which cryosurgery can be performed effectively. Surgical excisions may respond with hypertrophic scarring; this is not the general rule with cryosurgery.

Secondarily infected lesions are not necessarily a contraindication to cryosurgery. Cryosurgical wounds show a surprisingly small incidence of secondary infection. One might expect surgical procedures of this type, which heal with exudative reactions in many cases, to become infected frequently. The opposite is true, however. Lesions that are already infected at the time of surgery seldom show much aggravation of the infection after treatment. The exceptions to this are seen in areas of the country where humidity is a factor.

Large malignant tumors can be treated by cryosurgery. Frequently with these types of lesions, or in specific areas where reconstructive surgery might be indicated, cryosurgery is a viable alternative. Lesions can be treated segmentally in one session. An alternative that some employ is to treat one section of the tumor, wait for healing, and then return to treat the remaining portion.

Tumor recurrences in cases of radiodermatitis can be treated by cryosurgery in some instances. Although somewhat longer healing times may result if the lesions are surrounded by extensive scarring, cryosurgery should be a consideration in these tumors.

Some dermatocryosurgeons feel that morphea-type lesions can also be treated satisfactorily. Dr. Gloria Graham, in particular, has impressive statistics showing this.[10] I feel that the jury is still out on sclerosing basal cell carcinomas. My own experience has been somewhat dismal with these lesions. It is difficult, however, to ignore Dr. Graham's statistical results; hence, cryosurgery should be mentioned here as an alternative form of therapy for morphea-type carcinomas.

Special circumstances can dictate the use of cryosurgery.[11-13] Patients receiving anticoagulants generally have no problem when cryosurgical procedures are employed. Because cryosurgery is primarily a bloodless procedure, anticoagulants do not preclude these techniques.

Patients with pacemakers pose no problem for the cryosurgeon. Because instrumentation involves no electrical apparatus, no interference is created to jeopardize pacemakers.

Local anesthetics are optional in many cryosurgical cases involving malignancies. For this reason, patients who are hypersensitive to local anesthetics are good candidates for these procedures.

Palliation in otherwise inoperable cases can be obtained with cryosurgery. In other cases, odor from necrotic or infected tissue can be eliminated with the use of these techniques, which are relatively simple to perform. The procedures are short in duration and require uncomplicated setups.

One of the major advantages of cryosurgery is that it is an office procedure, even when used on larger lesions.[14] Compared with that of other modalities employed in treatment of large or complicated cases, the operative setup for cryosurgery is simple. The instrument itself and the tissue monitoring device, if used, are the main components. A local anesthetic is optional, and a modifying device, such as a cone, is sometimes used. The entire setup can be moved from room to room. The basic cryosurgery unit can be easily transported to nursing homes or hospitals for bedside treatment.

Cryosurgical techniques are all fast procedures. Although the time that is required to perform freezing on individual tumors is probably as long or longer than that required for desiccation and curettage or simple excisions, much time is saved in not having to change and re-do setups. The speed of cryosurgery is shown dramatically in the case of special types of lesions (for example, vascular lesions) in which no great time or effort is necessary to stop bleeding.

Speed is only one advantage to be gained from the fact that cryosurgery is virtually bloodless. Cold exerts a selective destruction on tissue. Cellular elements are more susceptible than are stromal elements. This accounts for healing of blood vessels without rupturing. During the procedure itself, blood vessels are usually not damaged to the point of bleeding. However, delayed bleeding can occasionally occur.[15] Bleeding can also occur if the tumor invades a blood vessel and is unplugged by the freezing process. In addition, if a biopsy is taken, one should be sure to stop the bleeding before finishing the procedure. After thawing, bleeding can occur if the biopsy site is not properly coagulated in some fashion.

Cryosurgery is also advantageous when multiple lesions are to be treated in a single visit.[16] Patients who have multiple carcinomas scattered on exposed areas are seen frequently in the southern United States. Because cryosurgery is fast, bloodless, and an office procedure, it follows that multiple lesions can be treated at one visit if this is desired. If properly done, cryosurgery can be advocated in treatment of multiple tumors arising on sun-damaged skin.

Disadvantages

Cryosurgery, like x-ray therapy, is a field therapy and therefore has the disadvantages of any field therapy modality. Perhaps the chief disadvantage is that the lesion is destroyed in situ. When an excisional method is used, the tissue can be sent to the laboratory to be examined; one can check for margins and adequacy of removal. This cannot be done easily with a field therapy technique. This disadvantage is not limited only to field therapies. Although electrodesiccation and curettage is not a field therapy, the same limitation is present; when curettage is used it is difficult for the pathologist to examine margins.

Another disadvantage of cryosurgery is that the procedure should not be used in treatment of lesions with ill-defined margins. With these types of tumors it is difficult to estimate the field necessary for destruction and to calculate the limits of the adequacy of freeze around the tumor. Many recurrences with cryosurgery can be attributed to improper technique. Perhaps the greatest number of mistakes are made in the incorrect selection of tumors with ill-defined margins.

With cryosurgery, healing is prolonged in certain areas. This is especially true of the lower legs. For this reason, many dermatologists utilizing this modality do not attempt to treat malignancies below the knee. Healing times of several weeks to several months occur when these malignancies are treated. Malignancies are much more common in the elderly, in whom healing times are the longest. Secondary infection also occurs much more commonly on the lower leg.

Certain areas are associated with relatively high recurrence rates, especially the scalp and the ala nasi crease. In the scalp this is possibly associated with the high degree of vascularity and the presence of the tumor in and around multiple follicles. Recently, some have reported that the scalp can be treated successfully with hard freezing. Still, it can be safely stated that at this time malignant lesions on the scalp are a relative contraindication.

Cryosurgery can be used in combination with other procedures for lesions of the ala nasi crease. One of the most common treatment combinations is curettage followed by freezing the base of the lesion. This usually brings the cure rate up to a more acceptable figure. Combination procedures are not at all uncommon in cryosurgery.[17] Exophytic lesions in any area can be treated in this way, as can certain ulcerative lesions.

Cryosurgery may not be the treatment of choice in areas where nerves lie superficially. Permanent nerve damage has been reported in cases in which freezing has been carried out over these areas. Particularly vulnerable are the posterior lateral aspects of the tongue, the ulnar fossa, and the sides of the fingers. This admonition would hold not only for malignancies but also for nonmalignant lesions. Damage has also been reported with relatively light freezing, although in most cases it is temporary.

It should be obvious to many (but it still should be mentioned) that cryosurgery should not be used in cases in which there is known abnormal cold intolerance. Excessive scarring is possible in these cases, and at least one report has been published citing abnormal reactions to cold as a possible link to an untoward degree of scarring in a treated patient.[18]

Cryosurgery Spray

Advantages

There are two basic methods of cryosurgery for cutaneous malignant lesions: spray and probe. Most procedures for both malignancies and nonmalignant lesions involve spray techniques. There are several reasons why cryosurgery spray techniques are used for the bulk of these procedures. There is a minimum of equipment involved in cryospray. Usually the necessary supplies are the basic cryosurgical instrument and a spray nozzle. If devices are used to measure the adequacy of freeze, they are easy to place with cryospray procedures. If the lesion is not deep it may not be necessary to use instruments to measure the adequacy of freeze; clinical measurements, e.g., thaw times, may suffice. This minimal setup typically results in a speedy procedure. Moreover, because the cryogen is applied directly to the target area, the depth of freeze and the minimum temperature desired can be reached faster with cryospray than with cryoprobes. Torre has devised a technique whereby neoprene or plastic cones can be employed in what is called the "cone-spray" method.[19] This in effect produces the speed of a cryospray with the depth configuration reached by cryoprobe, thus incorporating the advantages of both procedures.

Another important advantage to the cryosurgical spray is that it eliminates adverse interface factors, and therefore more consistently reproducible results can be obtained. It is important to remember that air is a poor conductor and water is a fair conductor. Thus, if one places a solid probe on an uneven, dry surface, air is between the hills and valleys, and the surface itself is dry. Therefore, it is probable that a poor interface contact will be produced. The interface, which is the junction between the heat sink and the target, can be important in producing consistently good results. By direct application of the cryogen to the surface, as is done in a cryospray procedure, good contact is obtained and the possible adverse interface factors are minimized.

With the fine control available with most currently produced liquid nitrogen units, spray techniques can be used quite effectively on lesions with irregular borders. Spray freeze can conform the frozen area to an irregular pattern necessary to treat the lesion adequately with a minimum of destruction to normal tissue. This is not so easily accomplished with cryoprobes.

Spray procedures can be used on difficult areas.[20,21] For example, one can treat around the eyelids or on the inner canthi relatively easily with cryosprays while protecting the conjunctiva and the sclera by proper shielding devices. Spray freezing can be used to treat areas around the external nares and near the auditory canal as well as the posterior ear creases.

Disadvantages

Probably the main disadvantage of spray freezing is that the procedure produces a smaller ratio of depth of freeze to lateral spread of freeze. Figures are available stating the ratio of lateral spread of freeze to depth of freeze for cryoprobes.[19] However, for purposes of this general discussion it is probably best to visualize the differences in the configurations of the resultant ice balls formed with the two procedures. With cryospray, the ice ball that is formed resembles a saucer with a relatively "shallow" ratio of depth of freeze to surface lateral spread of freeze. On the other hand, the cryoprobe procedure results in an ice ball more closely resembling a soup bowl, with the depth of freeze "deeper" in relation to the lateral spread of freeze on the surface. From this first disadvantage follows the second: It is difficult to treat small, deep lesions with cryosprays without modification of the technique. Fortunately, this can now be done by use of the cone-spray technique developed by Torre. This procedure consists, in general, of using the spray inside a constricting neoprene or plastic cone. The cone is placed around the lesion to be treated, and the cryogen is sprayed into the cone. The adequacy of freeze can be measured not only by instrumentation but also by the lateral spread of freeze occurring as a normal halo around the cone itself.

Because cryosprays tend to form vapors after hitting the target area, problems can arise in confined areas, such as the inside of the mouth. These vapors can form to the point of obscuring vision. The best way to solve this problem is with a dental suction device.

Liquid nitrogen spatter can occur not only as the vapor spray makes contact with the skin surface but also more frequently with certain types of instruments. This can be a potential hazard when one is working around certain areas, such as the eyes. Proper precautions for shielding should be taken when lesions in a vulnerable location are treated.

An attempt has been made in the preceding pages to present the advantages and disadvantages of cryosurgery in general and cryospray techniques in particular in the treatment of skin malignancies. It is important to learn proper techniques, including accurate selection of lesions to be treated. Cryosurgical spray is a relatively simple, easily learned modality that can be of great benefit to the practicing dermatologist when performed correctly.

References

1. White, A. C.: Liquid air in medicine and surgery. Med. Rec. 56:109, 1899.
2. Whitehouse, H. H.: Liquid air in dermatology: Its indications and limitations. JAMA 49:371, 1907.
3. Pusey, W. A.: The use of carbon dioxide snow in treatment of nevi and other skin lesions. JAMA 49:1354, 1907.
4. Wilson, J. W., Luikart, R., and Ayres, S., III: Dichlorotetrafluoroethane for surgical planing. Arch. Dermatol. 71:523, 1955.
5. Allington, H. V.: Liquid nitrogen in the treatment of skin diseases. Calif. Med. 72:153, 1950.
6. Cooper, I. S.: Cryogenic surgery: A new method of destruction or extirpation of benign or malignant tissues. N. Engl. J. Med. 268:743, 1963.
7. Cahan, W. G.: Cryosurgery of malignant and benign tumors. Fed. Proc. 24:241, March–April 1965.
8. Zacarian, S. A., and Adham, M. I.: Cryotherapy of cutaneous malignancy. Cryobiology 2:212, 1966.
9. Torre, D.: Cutaneous cryosurgery. J. Cryosurg. 1:202, 1968.
10. Graham, G.: Cryosurgery of skin tumors. N.C. Med. J. 32:81, 1971.
11. Zacarian, S. A.: Cancer of the eyelid: A cryosurgical approach. Ann. Ophthalmol. 4:473, 1972.
12. Torre, D.: Dermatological cryosurgery: A progress report. Cutis 11:782, June 1973.
13. Gage, A.: Cryosurgery for difficult problems in cutaneous cancer. Cutis 16:465, 1975.
14. Torre, D.: Cryosurgery. In Andrade, R., Gumport, S. L., Popkin, G. L., and Rees, T. D. (eds.): Cancer of the Skin, Vol. 2. Philadelphia, W. B. Saunders Co., 1976, pp. 1569–1587.
15. Elton, R.: The course of events following cryosurgery. J. Dermatol. Surg. Oncol. 3:448, July–Aug. 1977.
16. Lubritz, R. R.: Cryosurgical management of multiple skin carcinomas. J. Dermatol. Surg. Oncol. 3:414, July–Aug. 1977.
17. Spiller, W., and Spiller, R.: Treatment of basal cell carcinomas by a combination of curettage and cryosurgery. J. Dermatol. Surg. Oncol. 3:443, July–Aug. 1977.
18. Stewart, R., and Graham, G. A.: Complication of cryosurgery in a patient with cryofibrinogenemia. J. Dermatol. Surg. Oncol. 4:743, 1978.
19. Torre, D.: Cryosurgical treatment of epitheliomas using the cone-spray techniques. J. Dermatol. Surg. Oncol. 3:432, July–Aug. 1977.
20. Zacarian, S. A. (ed.): Cryosurgical Advances in Dermatology and Tumors of the Head and Neck. Springfield, IL, Charles C Thomas, 1977.
21. Fraunfelder, F. T., Farris, H. E., and Wallace, T. R.: Cryosurgery for ocular and periocular lesions. J. Dermatol. Surg. Oncol. 3:422, July–Aug. 1977.

CRYOSURGERY FOR SKIN DISEASE: VARIANTS IN TECHNIQUE

Andrew A. Gage, M.D.

The two principal basic techniques of cryosurgery are spray freezing, in which the cryogen is sprayed on the tissue to produce freezing, and probe freezing, in which the cryogen is used to cool the metal instrument that is held in contact with the tissue to produce freezing. There are variants of these techniques. Direct use of the cryogen also includes applying liquid nitrogen on a cotton swab[1] and confining the spray by appropriate hollow cylindric or conical devices[2] and pouring procedures.[3,4] It should be recognized that these spray-limiting devices have the effect of creating a semi-opened, or even a nearly closed, system, and they cannot be classified purely as components of a spray technique (Fig. 1). The systems are also varied by combination with curettement,[5] electrocoagulation, or excision, which extends the ability of cryosurgical methods to deal with certain difficult advanced lesions.[6] All these procedures are currently in use, and often more than one may produce satisfactory results. The choice in part is a matter of preference as the physician develops a familiarity with one or another. However, often there are other reasons why one system may be better. It is the purpose of this article to provide an evaluation of the advantages and disadvantages of the several cryosurgical techniques in order to assist in the formulation of a rational choice. The emphasis will be on the comparison of spray and probe freezing methods.

Diverse cryosurgical techniques have been in use for 150 years and only recently have evolved sufficiently to permit extensive freezing of tissue and wider use, especially in the treatment of tumors. It is pertinent to consider this evolution briefly. The original method of application, first used in the mid-nineteenth century for the treatment of advanced incurable carcinoma of the uterine cervix or carcinoma of the breast, featured irrigation of the tumor site with cold (approximately $-10°C$) saline solution.[7] Reduction of tumor bulk and amelioration of pain and malodorous discharge were achieved by these initial, cumbersome techniques. The early use of cryosurgery in the treatment of skin disease with liquid air or dry ice about the turn of the century has been described by Torre.[8] Liquid air

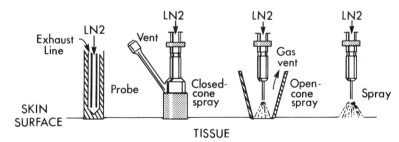

Figure 1. Differences and similarities in probe, closed-cone, open-cone, and spray devices. The probe (shown as a cutaway section) is closed entirely and, after change of phase, the gas is vented somewhere along the return line, perhaps even in the console. In both of the cone structures, the effect is to create an open probe (with some restriction of venting in the closed cone). The heat exchange surface is on the skin, instead of having metal interposed, and the venting is at the side or the top of the device. When cooled, the walls of the cone act as a circular probe. The open spray has nothing to confine dispersion.

administered as a spray or by swab and solidified carbon dioxide ($-78.5°C$) was used in the early 1900s to treat a variety of skin diseases, including lupus erythematosus, verrucae, nevi, and small skin cancers. The dry ice was easier to obtain and was more easily handled than the liquified gases. In later years, liquid oxygen was also used for the treatment of acne and other minor skin diseases.[9,10] After 1950, liquid nitrogen applied by a cotton swab became a conventional procedure in dermatologic practice. The freezing capability of this cryogen or similar agents, such as solidified carbon dioxide, was limited to a depth of freezing of no more than 2 mm.[11,12] Freezing by this cryosurgical technique is adequate only for minor conditions, but it is still useful today.[13]

Freezing with probes became possible following the development of cryosurgical apparatus by Cooper.[14,15] Subsequently, other types of cryosurgical apparatus employing liquid nitrogen and other cryogenic agents became available, and new uses were developed as techniques of freezing were adapted to the problems of treating disease. Equipment varied from simple, inexpensive, hand-held devices to sophisticated automated apparatus with probe heaters. In some apparatus, the cryogen was used in a closed system, so that it was never released on the tissue, whereas others permitted the direct application of the cryogenic agent; for example, by a spray. Additional information regarding the characteristics of cryogenic agents and the principles involved in the construction and operation of cryosurgical instruments may be found in general reference books on cryosurgery.[16,17]

Many liquid nitrogen devices, even the hand-held instruments, can be used for either spray or probe freezing. The hand-held devices are heavy, because the container filled with liquid nitrogen is kept in the hand, and therefore are somewhat more difficult to use with a probe than with a spray. It is cumbersome to hold a heavy weight steady in the hand, and therefore the bond between probe and tissue may fracture, and ineffective freezing may result. It is easier to spray with such devices, because the small movement caused by the weight in the hand is not important when there is no direct bond. I believe this accounts in part for the popularity of the spray techniques in dermatologic practice.

The choice of apparatus is related to the intended clinical use and must be made with some knowledge of the freezing capabilities of the cryogenic agents.[18,19] Commonly used cryogens are nitrous oxide ($-89.5°C$) and liquid nitrogen ($-196°C$). Freezing with nitrous oxide apparatus, which almost always is done with probes but may be done as a spray, is satisfactory for inflammatory disease or precancerous lesions with disease limited to the skin or the mucosa. It has proved useful in treatment of acne, for example.[20] Liquid nitrogen is the agent commonly used for the treatment of skin disease. Certainly the treatment of cancer requires the greater freezing capability of liquid nitrogen.

Freezing with Cryoprobes

In freezing with probes, the cryosurgical apparatus circulates the cryogen to the heat exchange surface applied to the tissue. As heat is withdrawn from the tissue, producing freezing, the liquid nitrogen changes to its gaseous phase, and the gas is exhausted either close to the heat exchange surface or at some point back along the line as far as in the console of the unit itself. Probes are available in diverse sizes and shapes, including flat, curved, or pointed freezing surfaces with straight or curved probe shafts (Fig. 2). The versatility of standard probes is increased by the use of metal end pieces or probe tip adapters, which increase or reduce the size of the freezing surface or change its shape to suit a particular need. The feed line that leads to the console may be vacuum-insulated or insulated with appropriate materials. Some apparatus permit disconnection of the probe assembly from the console so that it may be sterilized. This is advantageous in procedures that require sterile operations but ordinarily is not required for skin disease. Sophisticated units have automated flow controls and temperature controls that have special uses in cryo-

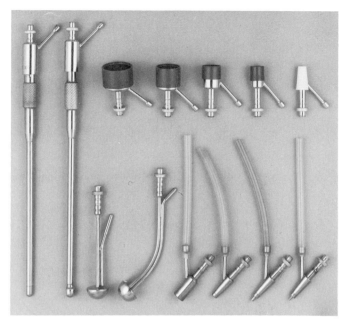

Figure 2. Assorted probe tips for a portable cryosurgical device that may be used with probe or spray. At the upper right is a grouping of open cones. The venting at the side is sufficiently small to cause it to function as a probe. In the open cone, there is no restriction of this venting. The remainder of the devices are closed probes of varying sizes and shapes for special functions. The long devices at the left may be used for the treatment of hemorrhoids, for example. The group of probes at the lower right have freezing surfaces that range in size from 1 to 5 mm to 1 cm. The smallest one has been used for the treatment of trichiasis.

surgery but ordinarily are not required in dermatologic practice. In these devices, the probe usually has a heater, which permits rapid warming of the probe for quick release from the tissues. Probes also may be used with portable self-pressuring apparatus and even with hand-held devices.

The operator chooses a probe appropriate to the lesion and applies it to the tissues. When the tissue is dry, such as the skin, a thin film of water-soluble hospital lubricating jelly should be applied to improve the contact beween the probe and the skin during freezing, because a good bond is necessary to facilitate heat transfer. When the probe becomes adherent to the tissue, careful attention must be paid to avoidance of movement, because any fracture of the bond between tissue and probe will interfere with heat transfer and will result in inadequate freezing. The cold probe acts as a heat sink and produces tissue freezing by removing heat from the tissue faster than blood supply can restore it. A large thermal gradient is needed to freeze tissue to some distance, so the probe should be as cold as possible. This also produces the most rapid freezing possible with the cryosurgical system being used.

The probe must be positioned carefully, because when freezing starts it can no longer be moved. As the temperature falls below zero, tissue adheres to the probe and becomes white and frosted in appearance. Tissue is frozen in increasing volume as heat is extracted, but the rate of extension of freezing slows as conditions at the periphery approach equilibrium between heat loss to the probe and heat supply by the circulation. Freezing is allowed to continue until the frosted appearance encompasses the entire lesion and, in the case of cancer, a margin of apparently normal tissue. Then the flow of liquid nitrogen is shut off and the probe is warmed with a heater or is allowed to thaw for removal. The probe heater, if present, is used only to speed release from the tissues, which then are allowed to thaw without assistance.

The amount of tissue frozen in a single application of the probe is related to the temperature of the probe, the duration of freezing, the area of contact between probe and tissue, and the blood supply to the tissue. It also depends on the quality of contact between probe and tissue, because any fracture of the bond interferes with heat transfer, which almost certainly causes insufficient freezing. This is a major technical point in probe freez-

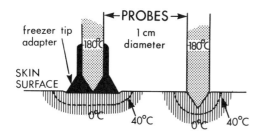

Figure 3. The effect of probe shape and area on the shape of the frozen tissue. In each instance, the standard 1-cm probe, bluntly pointed, is shown. When used alone, as on the right, with some pressure on the probe to cause indentation of the skin or other tissues, the frozen area is roughly hemispheric. When the freeze tip adapter is added to provide a wider freezing surface, the frozen area that results is broadened and less deep at a similar stage in freezing.

ing. The shape of the frozen area depends on the area of contact between probe and tissue, the blood supply to the area, and the pressure used in application. Small areas of contact produce roughly hemispheric lesions. A larger probe, obtained by adding a freeze tip adapter to the probe tip, will give a broader area with less depth penetration (Fig. 3). In general, the depth of freezing may be judged by the lateral spread of frost from the probe, and this is used as a guide in treatment.[21,22] Increased pressure on the skin by the probe will compress the tissue and will increase the depth of freezing. The increased probe pressure also has the benefit of decreasing the blood supply to the area, and this facilitates freezing.

Cryoprobes may be either applied to the surface of a lesion or inserted into the tissues to be frozen. Surface freezing, with slight pressure on the probe to improve tissue-probe contact, is used more commonly. As compared with insertion of the probe into the tissue, surface contact freezing has the following advantages: The need for anesthesia is lessened, no wound is caused, little or no bleeding occurs, and the danger of dissemination of tumor cells is minimized. On the other hand, some large, bulky tumors are penetrated rather easily. Insertion of the probe into the tissue increases the efficiency of freezing because of greater contact with the freezing surface and produces deep freezing proportionate to the extent of probe penetration. Penetration with pointed probes is not commonly used in skin cancers, with the exception of advanced protuberant or invasive lesions. Especially in vascular tumors, the penetration techniques are facilitated by the use of an apparatus that sequentially freezes the tissue with a cold probe and then heats the tissue sufficiently to prevent bleeding.[23,24]

The choice of technique and the selection of the appropriate probe are based on the kind of lesion to be treated. Non-neoplastic lesions warrant conservative treatment so that unnecessary tissue destruction does not produce a less favorable cosmetic result. Malignant lesions merit considerable attention to technique, including aggressive freezing to an appropriate tissue temperature,[25] and the cosmetic result is secondary to the need to cure the cancer. For example, probe freezing is the treatment of choice for small skin cancers that are less than 2 cm in surface diameter and only approximately 3 mm deep. Such lesions are the focal point of this discussion; both the spray and the probe techniques have been used successfully for treatment. In either the probe or the spray method, the border of the cancer is outlined with a skin-marking ink, because the spread of the white frost during freezing obscures easy determination of the extent of the lesion. A second circle is marked 5 mm outside of the cancer border. Freezing is done until the frost has spread to the outer circle. After thawing, the freezing process is repeated. This is a conservative technique without the use of thermocouples. Physicians with considerable experience in cryosurgery can achieve satisfactory results without thermocouples.[26] However, clinical judgment is sometimes misleading, and the use of thermocouples therefore often leads to a longer treatment period than does clnical judgment alone.

The use of thermocouples to monitor tissue temperature during freezing permits better control of treatment. These devices may be used in several ways. In one common technique, the thermocouple is inserted through normal tissue a few millimeters outside of the cancer and is passed to a subcutaneous position beneath the center of the cancer. The tissue

SITES OF THERMOCOUPLE INSERTION

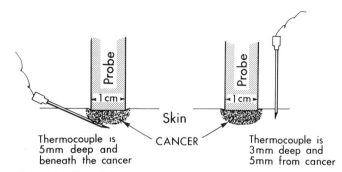

Figure 4. Typical sites of thermocouple insertion. Two useful methods of thermocouple insertion are shown. Either will yield satisfactory results when performed by an experienced practitioner. On the left is a thermocouple inserted at an angle from the side of the lesion through normal tissue. The thermocouple tip rests directly beneath the tumor at a depth of 5 mm. This thermocouple confirms the temperature at the depth of the tissue in the center of the lesion. It probably is the most common method of thermocouple usage in skin cancer. On the right is an alternative method of thermocouple usage. The thermocouple is inserted at the border of the tumor, 5 mm from the border and 3 mm deep. With this technique, the temperature registered at this thermocouple is interpreted as being the same temperature at the depth of the tissue beneath the tumor. This method assumes that the depth of freezing is approximately the same as the lateral spread of freezing from the probe. The advantage of this technique is that the thermocouple remains outside of the frozen area until the advancing ice front incorporates it. I believe it is relatively free of the error of conduction, which occurs with improper thermocouple usage. More than one thermocouple may be used, of course, and the two depicted techniques may be used jointly.

is frozen until the thermocouple registers −40°C. During the process, care is taken to freeze 5 mm beyond the cancer border.

My preference is to use probe freezing for such lesions and to modify the method of thermocouple usage. Skin cancers tend to grow by extension from their outer margins in the skin, so measurement of temperature at the border is advantageous. After the skin is marked in the usual manner, one or more thermocouples are placed perpendicularly 2 mm into the skin and 5 mm from the margin of the cancer (Fig. 4). A probe with a freezing surface as near as possible to the size of the cancer is used. Freezing is continued until the border temperature measures −40°C (Fig. 5). After thawing, freezing is repeated. This technique assures that the depth of freezing is approximately the same as the lateral spread from probe and that the temperature 5 mm deep in the cancer site is the same as that measured at the 5-mm border (the thermocouple site). As mentioned earlier, the amount of pressure used in the application of the probe may modify this relationship. This technique produces more extensive freezing than does the conservative probe method cited previously and will destroy more tissue, probably increasing the chance of a cure at a cost of a less favorable cosmetic effect.

The advantage of the probe technique is that it provides a more predictable area of necrosis than does a spray. In freezing from a single point or area, the gradients of temperature within the resulting frozen area are consistent and are subject to evaluation and interpretation from the single thermocouple. Depth penetration is much greater with the probe; since one is able to use pressure on the probe, the depth of penetration of freezing is increased because of compression of tissue. Pointed probes may be inserted into the tissue to produce deep freezing, which is generally needed only for advanced cancer that deeply invades the tissues. Probe freezing is safer because the cryogen is not released on

Degrees
Centigrade

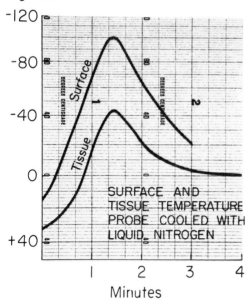

Figure 5.   Temperature record during the freezing of a small basal cell epithelioma with the probe technique. The surface temperature is recorded from a thermocouple placed between the probe and the tumor. This is useful because it quickly reveals any break in the bond between tissue and probe. The tissue temperature is recorded from a thermocouple placed 5 mm lateral to the border of the cancer, as shown in Figure 4. The freezing rate, measured along the steepest part of the cooling curve, is approximately 92° C per minute. Freezing was continued until the tissue temperature reached −40° C; then the tissue was allowed to thaw.

the tissues; therefore the agent cannot run off into undesired area and produce unwanted freezing. A probe is preferred when direct vision is not possible. Therefore, endoscopic freezing practically always will require the use of a probe, but in skin disease the device is not necessary.

Freezing with a probe is necessarily slower, because the cryogen must cool the probe before it freezes the tissue. Cryosurgical apparatus are sometimes engineered to work better at temperature of −160°C to −180°C, so the temperature gradient needed to extract heat is reduced in comparison with a spray. The principal disadvantage of probe freezing is related to the fact that the probe becomes adherent to the tissue, and careful attention must be paid to avoidance of movement. Any fracture of the bond between tissue and probe will interfere with heat exchange and will result in inadequate freezing. This bond is sometimes difficult to achieve over dry skin, especially skin over bony surfaces. The need to wait for thawing reduces the speed with which treatment can be given. This is particularly noticeable in the treatment of multiple skin cancers. In addition, the probe technique is more difficult to adapt to lesions with irregular shapes or uneven contours.

Freezing with Liquid Nitrogen Spray

The spray technique features direct application of liquid nitrogen to the tissues. This characteristically produces rapid superficial freezing of tissue, which easily can cover irregularly shaped or wide areas. The spray is produced by flowing liquid nitrogen under pressure through needles or small apertures in nozzles. Renewed interest in the use of spray techniques quickly followed Cooper's development of cryosurgical apparatus for probe freezing. The early Dewar flasks, which were large and which contained the cryogen for use as a spray or for probe cooling, were soon supplemented by hand-held spray devices, which included a small Dewar flask to hold the liquid nitrogen (250 to 500 ml). Most of these small units are self-pressurizing, and the liquid nitrogen is forced through the small feed lines to exit through small terminal apertures as a spray.[27,28] The design of the hand-held devices has improved to permit better control of the spray than was provided in some of the original apparatus. Adjustment of the spraying pressure, which is a major factor in good control of the spray, is accomplished by a small tabletop unit with a flexible feed line leading to a lightweight hand-held nozzle or probe. This is a self-pressurizing portable nonelectric system designed for use with spray cones, spray needles, or closed-end probes.[29]

Spray techniques for diverse skin diseases are varied according to the type of disease. The procedure required for the treatment of acne is different from that used for basal cell carcinoma, but some generalizations can be made. The operator directs the spray of liquid nitrogen from the nozzle of the apparatus over the tissues to produce freezing. If the diseased tissue is small, then spraying to a single point is satisfactory. If the diseased tissue covers several square centimeters, then the operator should use a spray pattern, moving the nozzle of the spraying device over the tissues in order to achieve even freezing.[26,30] The freezing ordinarily achieved in such patterns is wide but superficial. A nozzle of appropriate size for the lesion (usually a needle of 16 to 22 gauge) is selected. The smaller the needle aperture, the better the control (and the less the liquid nitrogen flow). The greatest problem is with small lesions, namely those 5 mm or less in diameter, because the spray naturally tends to disperse over a larger area. This problem is compounded by the use of excessive pressure in the Dewar flask or use of a needle that is too large. The techniques for diverse skin diseases are detailed in standard texts.[31-33] In the following paragraphs, I will deal with the procedures for focal areas of diseases such as skin cancers.

Several techniques are satisfactory for basal cell carcinoma. One method is to use an open spray of liquid nitrogen. After preliminary biopsy has established the nature of the disease, the margins of the tumor are traced with skin-marking ink, and a second marking is made 5 mm outside the tumor margin. A local anesthetic is injected beneath the tumor. This balloons the tissue, diminishes the blood supply to some extent, and facilitates freezing. This injection can be used to protect underlying strctures, such as cartilage or nerves, from freezing by displacing the skin from the deep tissue. A thermocouple is placed beneath the tumor in the manner already described, and the liquid nitrogen spray is directed intermittently over the entire tumor until the temperature reaches an appropriate level (Fig. 6). The spray pattern is planned to produce equal freezing in the entire area, including the 5-mm margin of normal tissue around the cancer. After thawing, the freeze-thaw cycle is repeated.

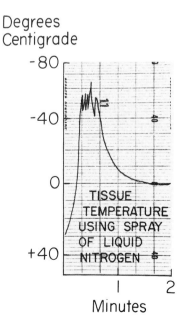

Figure 6. Temperature record during the freezing of a small basal cell epithelioma with the spray technique. The tissue temperature is recorded from a thermocouple placed immediately beneath the cancer, as shown in Figure 4. The rapid freezing is characteristic of the spray technique. Tissue temperature cools rapidly to less than −40° C (which was the goal in this treatment) and is held there for approximately 20 seconds—then the tissue is allowed to thaw. The rapidity of the thawing is noteworthy. The jagged appearance at the top of the temperature curve is characteristic of spray freezing.

In Torre's cone-spray technique,[2] a plastic cone is used to limit the run-off of liquid nitrogen during administration of the spray. The edge of the cone is moistened and is pressed firmly on the skin with the tumor in the central open area. Liquid nitrogen is sprayed into the cone until a frozen white rim spreads around its base and over an adequate margin of normal tissue. Thermocouples may be used to control this treatment; the procedures already have been described. This technique of confining the spray by the use of open or closed cylinders or cones offers a substantial advantage in dealing with small lesions, namely those approximately 2 cm or less in surface diameter. The spray-limiting device functions like a probe in many respects. The walls of the device provide some pressure on the skin and, when cooled by the spray, act as a probe. The tissue temperature changes produced by cone-spray freezing usually resemble those of probe freezing (Fig. 7).

The advantages of the spray technique are based on the easy and free movement of the spraying nozzle about the lesion and the use of the cryogenic agent at its coldest possible temperature. These two advantages result in quick, extensive, wide freezing. The physician does not have to wait for a probe to cool and is able to work from site to site or over a wide area without stopping for a thawing period, as is necessary with the probe method. The capability of freezing widely and superficially is ideal for many dermatologic uses, and the speed of the process is advantageous for the treatment of multiple skin carcinomas. The spray also has certain advantages in large cancers eroding the skin, especially if the treatment is combined with the use of other techniques, such as partial excision. Ordinarily, the depth of penetration of the open spray is too limited, and the tumor must first be debulked by some technique before the spray can be used.

The principal problem with the spray technique is that deep freezing is difficult to achieve. The spray produces no pressure on the tissue, so the pressure advantage of the probe is lost. Prolonged use of the spray in one area of tissue results in troublesome runoff of liquid nitrogen from the tissue, and undesired freezing of adjacent normal tissues may occur. These are major factors that limit the ability of the liquid nitrogen spray to achieve deep freezing quickly.

Use of the spray requires that the operator take precautions to protect important areas, such as the eye, against misdirection of the spray or dripping of liquid nitrogen from the nozzle. When using the spray in ulcerating lesions, the physician must be wary of insufflation of the tissues, which is especially likely in the loose tissues about the face or the neck. Insufflation is an avoidable complication and requires only careful observation of the tis-

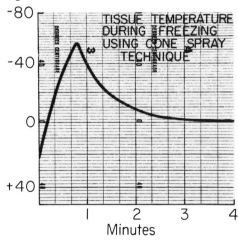

Figure 7. Temperature record during the freezing of a small basal cell epithelioma with a cone-spray technique. The tissue temperature is recorded from a thermocouple placed immediately beneath the cancer. The cooling curve closely resembles that of probe freezing. The tissue is cooled to a temperature colder than −40° C (which was the goal in this treatment) and is held there for approximately 20 seconds. Then the tissue is allowed to warm. The thawing curve is slightly slower than that of the spray technique, because the cooled cone acts as a heat sink and must be warmed by the tissue.

sues during freezing. The likelihood of its occurrence is reduced by the use of a cone with slight pressure about the area to be frozen. Ordinarily, insufflation will cause no problem, but fatal gas embolism has been described in dogs.[34] More likely is the possibility of infection, since liquid nitrogen may contain *Staphylococcus albus* and other organisms. Generally, infection is uncommon, but it may occur with either spray or probe techniques.

The Choice Between Probe and Spray

The physician must make a choice between probe and spray freezing based on certain basic differences in the procedures. The characteristic advantages and disadvantages of each technique result from the obvious difference that liquid nitrogen is confined to the apparatus in the probe method but is released on the tissues when used as a spray. The probe produces slightly slower, deeper freezing and a more predictable area of necrosis. The spray produces quick, superficial freezing. Both techniques must be used in accordance with the same basic principles of cryosurgery to insure tissue destruction; namely, rapid freezing to temperatures lethal for cells, slow thawing, and repetition of freeze-thaw cycles.

In part, the choice is determined by the equipment at the physician's disposal. Since the sophisticated automated instruments (including probe heaters) that are required for endoscopic freezing are not necessary for dermatologic practice, the available equipment is likely to be either a hand-held device or a tabletop unit with a flexible feed line terminating as a probe or spray nozzle. If only the hand-held device were available, I probably would use spray freezing more frequently, because the weight of the apparatus in the hand interferes with the motionless positioning required in probe freezing. On the other hand, if the tabletop device also were available (as it currently is), then probe freezing would be my preferred technique for almost all applications. My preference for the probe is based on its improved depth of penetration because of compression of the skin. In addition, the technique that I use freezes more extensively than is common in dermatologic practice.

The basic fact is that both spray freezing and probe freezing have been used with success. Special circumstances may indicate the choice of one technique over another. For superficial non-neoplastic disease of considerable extent, such as acne, the spray technique is probably the treatment of choice. For small skin cancers (up to 2 cm in surface diameter and with a depth of only 3 or 4 mm), my preference is probe freezing, because it is more predictable in my opinion. Most dermatologists use spray freezing techniques for small skin cancers, however, and certainly the cone freezing technique is highly satisfactory and has provided excellent results. For small lesions (that is, up to 2 cm in diameter), long-term cure rates of 98 per cent have been achieved.

For skin cancers that are moderate in size (namely, those over 2 cm in diameter), for which the depth of penetration be somewhat greater, I prefer the probe technique because of its greater depth of freezing capability. If a spray is used for such lesions, it is usually advisable to combine the spray with preliminary curettement of the lesion, a technique that has proved very useful in skilled hands. Long-term cure rates of 90 per cent have been reported. These results compare favorably with those of other methods of treatment.

Diverse techniques are needed to cope with the problem of large, advanced skin cancers. Bulky, protuberant lesions may be treated either with penetration probe freezing or by partial excision followed by either probe or spray freezing. Excision of most of the tumor by electrocoagulation followed by freezing of the base with a spray is an effective method of management of certain lesions. As the wound clears, histologic examination and treatment should be repeated as often as necessary in order to clear the wound of tumor before allowing it to heal. If the tumor is invasive rather than protuberant, then penetration techniques of freezing are often better. These procedures require the use of a probe. Fortunately, large, advanced skin cancers are relatively uncommon. Therefore, no large series is available to evaluate long-term results. In the small number of cases reported, it is clear that surprisingly good results can be achieved, even when the cases appear to present problems in management. In short, there is no clear-cut choice of one technique for the treatment of skin cancer. Either probe or spray methods may be used. The most important point is that whichever technique is employed, it is best to confirm clinical judgment during freezing by the use of monitoring devices, such as thermocouples. Careful application is essential to be certain that the desired result, a localized area of tissue necrosis, will be produced by freezing in situ. Whether the spray or the probe is used, the basic features of the cryosurgical technique are rapid freezing, slow thawing and, when thawing is complete, repetition of the freeze-thaw cycle.

References

1. Allington, H. V.: Liquid nitrogen in the treatment of skin disease. Calif. Med. 72:153, 1950.
2. Torre, D.: Cryosurgical treatment of epitheliomas using the cone-spray technique. J. Dermatol. Surg. Oncol. 3:432, 1977.
3. Marcove, R. C., Weis, L. D., Vaghaiwalla, M. R., Pearson, R., and Huvos, A. G.: Cryosurgery in the treatment of giant cell tumors of bone. A report of 52 consecutive cases. Cancer 41:957, 1978.
4. Dutta, P., Montes, M., and Gage, A. A.: Experimental hepatic cryosurgery. Cryobiology 14:598, 1977.
5. Spiller, W. F., and Spiller, R. F.: Treatment of basal cell carcinomas by a combination of curettage and cryosurgery. J. Dermatol. Surg. Oncol. 3:443, 1977.
6. Gage, A.: Cryosurgery for difficult problems in cutaneous cancer. Cutis 16:465, 1975.
7. Tytus, J.: Cryosurgery, its history and development. In Rand, R., Rinfret, A., and von Leden, H. (eds.): Cryosurgery. Springfield, IL, Charles C Thomas, 1968, pp. 3–18.
8. Torre, D.: Cradle of cryosurgery. N.Y. State J. Med. 67:465, 1967.
9. Irvine, H. G., and Turnacliff, D. D.: Liquid oxygen in dermatology. Arch. Dermatol. Syph. 19:270, 1929.
10. Kile, R. L., and Welsh, A. L.: Liquid oxygen in dermatologic practice. Arch. Dermatol. Syph. 57:57, 1949.
11. Grimmet, R.: Liquid nitrogen therapy. Histologic observations. Arch. Dermatol. 83:563, 1961.
12. Zacarian, S., and Adham, M.: Cryogenic temperature studies of human skin. Temperature recordings at 2 mm human skin depth following application with liquid nitrogen. J. Invest. Dermatol. 48:7, 1967.
13. Allington, H.: Cryosurgery. In Epstein, E., and Epstein, E., Jr. (eds.): Skin Surgery, 4th ed. Springfield, IL, Charles C Thomas, 1977, pp. 635–647.
14. Cooper, I. S., and Lee, A. J.: Cryostatic congelation: A system for producing a limited, controlled region of cooling or freezing of biologic tissues. J. Nerv. Ment. Dis. 133:259, 1961.
15. Cooper, I.: Cryogenic surgery. A new method of destruction or extirpation of benign or malignant tissues. N. Engl. J. Med. 268:743, 1963.
16. Garamy, G.: Engineering aspects of cryosurgery. In Rand, R., Rinfret, A., and von Leden, H. (eds.): Cryosurgery. Springfield, IL, Charles C Thomas, 1968, pp. 92–132.
17. Torre, D.: Cryosurgical instrumentation. In Zacarian, S. (ed.): Cryosurgical Advances in Dermatology and Tumors of the Head and Neck. Springfield, IL, Charles C Thomas, 1977, pp. 38–54.
18. Torre, D.: Alternate cryogens for cryosurgery. J. Dermatol. Surg. 1:56, 1975.
19. Torre, D.: Freezing with freons. Cutis 16:437, 1975.
20. Graham, G.: Cryotherapy in the treatment of acne. In Epstein, E., and Epstein, E., Jr. (eds.): Skin Surgery, 4th ed. Springfield, IL, Charles C Thomas, 1977, pp. 680–697.
21. Zacarian, S.: Is lateral spread of freeze a valid guide to depth of freeze?, J. Dermatol. Surg. Oncol. 4:561, 1978.
22. Torre, D.: Understanding the relationship between lateral spread of freeze and depth of freeze. J. Dermatol. Surg. Oncol. 5:51, 1979.
23. Keller, A., Volter, D., and Schubert, G.: Cryocautery of prostate. Urology 15:548, 1980.
24. Gage, A. M., Montes, M., and Gage, A. A.: Destruction of hepatic and splenic tissue by freezing and heating. Cryobiology 19:172, 1982.
25. Gage, A.: What temperature is lethal for cells? J. Dermatol. Surg. Oncol. 5:459, 1979.
26. Torre, D., Lubritz, R., and Graham, G.: Cryosurgical treatment of basal cell carcinomas. Prog. Dermatol. 12:11, 1978.
27. Tromovitch, T. A.: An intermediate cryosurgical unit: The TT 32. Cutis 16:502, September 1975.
28. Lubritz, R. R., and Johns, F.: A new simplified cryosurgical instrument: The Foster froster. J. Dermatol. Surg. 1:59, June 1975.
29. Zarcarian, S.: Benign and malignant cutaneous lesions. In Ablin, R. (ed.): Handbook of Cryosurgery, New York, Marcel Dekker, Inc., 1980, pp. 109–129.
30. Lubritz, R.: Cryosurgical spray patterns. J. Dermatol. Surg. Oncol. 4:138, 1978.

31. Zarcarian, S. A.: Cryosurgical Advances in Dermatology and Tumors of the Head and Neck. Springfield, IL, Charles C Thomas, 1977.
32. Epstein, E., and Epstein, E., Jr. (eds.): Skin Surgery, 4th ed. Springfield, IL, Charles C Thomas, 1977.
33. Ablin, R. (ed.): Handbook of Cryosurgery. New York, Marcel Dekker, Inc., 1980.
34. Harvey, H. J.: Fatal air embolization associated with cryosurgery in two dogs. J. Am. Vet. Med. 173:175, 1978.

Editorial Comment

It is impossible to state which of these two methods of applying cryotherapy is best. General acceptance favors the spray, and in Dr. Lubritz's hands it is probably the preferred method. On the other hand, I suspect that Dr. Gage can obtain superior results with applicators. Experience, training, and skill should dictate which method the practitioner adopts.

Although cryosurgery is an older method of eradicating various tumors, the newer approaches bear little resemblance to the procedures that were used in the past. The modality could not be used to treat malignancies if it were not for the availability of superior refrigerants and thermocouples that can be inserted into or under the tumor and the birth of a new generation of skilled cryotherapists.

Both contributors deserve credit for making important advancements in this field and for the training of others. Both are leaders in this area. Dr. Gage is a surgeon who applies cryotherapy to both superficial and deep neoplasms, and Dr. Lubritz is a dermatologist who uses his skills to cure cutaneous tumors.

I thank both of them for their contributions, which I believe add to the value of this volume.

Think It Over.

CHAPTER **12**

METHODS OF OBTAINING A SPECIMEN FOR MICROSCOPIC CONTROL

MICROCONTROLLED SURGERY (CHEMOSURGERY) FOR SKIN CANCER

Frederic E. Mohs, M.D.

Most dermatologists, and other physicians who are familiar with the tendency of many skin cancers to spread unpredictably into the surrounding tissues, recognize that complete microscopic control of excision provides maximal assurance of eradication of the neoplasms with minimal loss of surrounding normal tissues. Also, it is quite well known that complete microscopic control is achieved by excising the tissues of the cancerous area layer by layer and scanning the undersurface of each layer with the microscope by the systematic use of frozen sections.

During the 46 years since microcontrolled surgery was first used clinically and the 41 years since the first publications on the subject,[1,2] there have been some important innovations in the technique, but the essential idea of complete microscopic control has remained unchanged. However, as the changes in technique were being incorporated there was temporary diversity in the details of the technique that may have been viewed as controversy by those not active in the field.

The first major change in technique occurred in the early 1950s, when one of my trainees, R. R. Allington, M.D.,[3] suggested the use of dichloroacetic acid to secure prompt hemostasis after the main cancerous mass had been excised or cureted. Prior to that time, I had occasionally excised massive cancers before applying the zinc chloride fixative that was used to provide in situ fixation in order to facilitate the excision and handling of the tissue specimens. However, the time gained by the preliminary procedure usually did not counterbalance the time lost in securing hemostatis. After Allington's demonstration, the prompt control of capillary oozing permitted the frequent use of this time-saving and pain-reducing procedure.

Another major change in technique had its beginning in 1953, when I first excised tissues in the fresh, unfixed state to achieve the same complete microscopic control as that provided by the fixed tissue technique. I was having a movie made of the chemosurgical excision of a basal cell carcinoma of a lower eyelid when an unexpected lateral extension in the lid margin was encountered. In order to hasten the filming, I injected a local anesthetic and removed successive layers of unfixed tissues until a cancer-free level was reached. The process worked so well that after that time all eyelid margin cancers were excised with the fresh tissue technique, as were occasional relatively small cancers in other sites. In my first book on chemosurgery, published in 1956, this technique was described in a section titled ''Surgical Excision with Microscopic Control.'' It was pointed out that after a cancer-free level was reached, an immediate closure of the defect could be carried out.[4] However, I had doubts that the fresh tissue technique would be acceptable to many physicians, because with larger lesions not only was there more difficulty in excising and handling the tissue specimens, but also there was less accuracy in marking the source of the specimens, and the control of the bleeding required additional assistance.

These doubts were dispelled when T. A. Tromovitch, M.D., another of my trainees, presented a paper entitled "Microscopically Controlled Excision Using Fresh Specimens: A Review of 75 Cases" at the 1970 meeting of the American College of Chemosurgery (A.C.C.). In jest, he remarked that he supposed he would be expelled from the A.C.C. because he had omitted the chemical fixation, but I replied that if that were the case, I would also have to be expelled, since I had been forgoing in situ fixation in some cases since 1953. At any rate, I embarked on a program to use the fresh tissue technique in a large series of cases to compare its reliability with that of the fixed tissue technique and to delineate the cases in which the fresh and fixed tissue techniques were indicated. The excellent 4-year results of treatment with the fresh technique and the indications for the fresh and fixed techniques have been reported in my book published in 1978[5] and in other publications.[6-10] Similar high cure rates with the fresh tissue technique were reported by Tromovitch and Stegman.[11]

I have always emphasized that it was the complete microscopic control, and not the chemical fixation, that was the unique and important feature of chemosurgery. In 1936, the term *chemosurgery* was actually a second choice; the first choice was *microsurgery,* but since the latter term had already been used to designate microdissection it was not adopted. The term *chemosurgery* was chosen because at that time chemical fixation in situ was an integral part of the method. However, *chemosurgery* became a misnomer when the fresh tissue technique came along. Since chemosurgery had come to be synonymous with microscopically controlled surgery, the members of the American College of Chemosurgery decided in 1973 to use the terms *chemosurgery, fixed tissue technique* and *chemosurgery, fresh tissue technique* and to retain the name of American College of Chemosurgery.

Nonetheless, there is recurrent evidence of confusion with the term *chemosurgery* and, as a result, the possibility of changing the name has cropped up at intervals. I have been "test marketing" the term *microcontrolled surgery* as a fairly short and yet distinctive name that should not be confused with *microsurgery,* which now has a much more inclusive meaning than it did in 1936.

Microcontrolled surgery, fresh tissue technique currently is used for the removal of most cancers of the skin because it is fast and relatively painless and it often permits immediate repairs of defects. However, microcontrolled surgery, fixed tissue technique has three important indications. First, carcinomas that are extremely extensive, and particularly those that involve bony structures, are more reliably removed with the fixed tissue technique because of the bloodless field and because of the accuracy with which the specimens can be removed and oriented. Second, the fixed tissue technique is preferred for carcinomas of the penis[5] involving erectile tissue. Bleeding is difficult to control with the fresh tissue technique in this case, since the vascular spaces do not constrict and contract, as do vessels in other tissues. Avoiding erectile tissue, one can remove the main mass of the cancer surgically prior to applying dichloroacetic acid and zinc chloride; then one can carry out the rest of the procedure with the fixed tissue technique. There is no difficulty with bleeding either during excision of the layers of tissue or during separation of the final layer of fixed tissue several days later.

The third major use of the fixed tissue technique is for the excision of primary melanomas.[5,12,13] In this application, the technique is different from that used for basal and squamous cell carcinoma in two respects. First, there is no preliminary surgical removal of the main tumor mass; second, an extra margin of tissue is removed to encompass possible satellite deposits in the surrounding skin lymphatics. The width of the extra margin depends on the degree of malignancy of the primary melanoma, as determined by examination of sections cut with a cryostat. Standard surgical dissections of regional nodes are indicated as soon as there is deemed to be any question of possible involvement.

One benefit of the fixed tissue technique in the management of melanomas is that it provides a safe method for the biopsy of pigmented lesions. If the suspected lesion proves to be nonmelanomatous, the excisions can be terminated at an appropriately conservative level, but if the lesion is a melanoma, the excisions can safely be extended to an appropriately radical level. Although the safety of ordinary surgical biopsy of a suspected melanoma has been statistically documented[14] I nevertheless think that one should exercise care when performing this procedure, because melanoma often invades the walls of blood vessels and lymphatics and can hang precariously in the lumens of the vessels. Of course, I perform a biopsy with the chemosurgical technique, but if I were to take a surgical biopsy of a suspected melanoma, I would gently excise the specimen and would secure hemostasis by gentle application of a hemostatic, such as oxidized cellulose (Oxycel cotton), ferric subsulfate (Monsel's solution), or dichloroacetic acid. I would avoid sutures that might squeeze out malignant cells into the circulation, and I would avoid electrocoagulation, which can produce tissue steam that conceivably could propel clumps of melanoma cells into the vascular lumens.[15]

Besides providing a safe way to perform a biopsy of a suspected melanoma, chemosurgery has a number of other benefits for the management of melanoma, a few of which may be mentioned here. The microscopic control insures removal of all of the primary melanoma, including the unexpected outgrowths that can occur. Of course, the usual surgical excision with the wide extra margin also will assuredly eliminate such silent extensions, but on the face and near some important structures the motivation to save as much tissue as possible may cause transection of a slender outgrowth. Chemosurgical excision can be relatively conservative without danger that silent outgrowths will be missed. Another benefit of chemosurgical excision is that satellites do not develop as a result of the procedure. If satellites are present at the time of chemosurgical excision, they can be safely removed chemosurgically, even if they are some distance from the primary lesion. Because satellites develop by embolism and not by permeation of lymphatics, it is not always necessary to remove all of the tissues between the primary lesion and the satellite, especially if the latter is a considerable distance from the primary melanoma.

Both the fixed and the fresh tissue techniques should be available in chemosurgery clinics. In some cases, the fresh tissue technique may be used initially, but when the cancer extends so far around bony structures that the excisions become too difficult, the fixed tissue technique can be invoked. Conversely, if a structure is encountered during treatment with the fixed tissue technique in a site where conservation of important structures is important, the fresh tissue technique can be a welcome alternative. An example would be a cancer of the orbit skirting along the eyeball. In this case, it is possible to use the fresh tissue technique to dissect the cancer off the sclera in a conservative manner that avoids penetration and loss of the eye.

As with any new method, there are likely to be controversies as to the indications for use of microcontrolled surgery. For example, I have been told that using this procedure for small cancers of the skin "is like using a cannon to kill a fly." However, when facilities for microscopic control are available, the microcontrolled excision of small cancers is a simple and rapid procedure. Furthermore, even small cancers often extend much farther than their external appearance suggests. Probably the fact that I so often used illustrations of more advanced, complicated lesions in my publications gave rise to the false impression that the method was indicated only for such lesions.

Undoubtedly, the standard methods of treatment of cancers of the skin will continue to be used, but if routine follow-up examinations should reveal recurrence of the neoplasms, microcontrolled excision often can be a useful backup procedure.

References

1. Mohs, F. E., and Guyer, M. F.: Pre-excisional fixation of tissues in the treatment of cancer in rats. Cancer Res. 1:49, 1941.
2. Mohs, F. E.: Chemosurgery: A microscopically controlled method of cancer excision. Arch. Surg. 42:279, 1941.
3. Lunsford, C. J., Templeton, H. J., Allington, H. V., and Allington, R. R.: Use of chemosurgery in dermatologic practice. Arch. Dermatol. Syph. 68:148, 1953.
4. Mohs, F. E.: Chemosurgery in Cancer, Gangrene and Infections. Springfield, IL, Charles C Thomas, 1956.
5. Mohs, F. E.: Chemosurgery: Microscopically Controlled Surgery for Skin Cancer. Springfield, IL, Charles C Thomas, 1978.
6. Mohs, F. E.: Chemosurgery for skin cancer. Fixed tissue and fresh tissue techniques. Arch. Dermatol. 112:211, 1976.
7. Mohs, F. E.: Chemosurgery: Microscopically controlled surgery for skin cancer—past, present and future. J. Dermatol. Surg. Oncol. 4:41, 1978.
8. Mohs, F. E.: Chemosurgery for the microscopically controlled excision of skin cancer. Head Neck Surg. 1:150, 1978.
9. Mohs, F. E.: New aspects of microscopically controlled surgery for facial carcinoma and melanomas. In Bernstein, L. (ed.) Rehabilitative Surgery. New York, Grune & Stratton, 1981, pp. 46–59.
10. Mohs, F. E.: Chemosurgical techniques. Otolaryngol. Clin. North Am. 15:209, Feb. 1982.
11. Tromovitch, T. A., and Stegman, S. J.: Microscopically controlled excision of skin tumors: Chemosurgery (Mohs). Fresh tissue technique. Arch. Dermatol 110:231, 1974.
12. Mohs, F. E.: Chemosurgical treatment of melanoma: A microscopically controlled method of excision. Arch. Dermatol. Syph. 62:269, 1950.
13. Mohs, F. E.: Chemosurgery for melanoma. Arch. Dermatol. 113:285, 1977.
14. Epstein, E. H.: Biopsy and prognosis of malignant melanoma. In Epstein, E., and Epstein, E., Jr. (eds.), Skin Surgery. Springfield, IL, Charles C Thomas, 1977, pp. 783–788.
15. Amadon, P. D.: Electrocoagulation of melanoma and its dangers. Surg. Gynecol. Obstet., 56:943, 1933.

CHEMOSURGERY

Perry Robins, M.D.

Each year the number of skin cancers that are treated by Mohs surgery increases. The reasons for this are many. First, many more physicians today can expertly perform this procedure. Second, skin cancers treated with Mohs surgery have consistently higher cure rates than do those treated by other techniques. Third, the procedure has more practical advantages than do other techniques in eradicating skin cancers.

Chemosurgery was developed by Frederic E. Mohs more than 45 years ago. He combined the term "chemo-" (because the cancerous tissue was fixed in situ with the chemical zinc chloride) and the term "surgery" (because the procedure was followed by removal of the tissue by surgical excision and microscopic examination of the tissue). For the next 35 years, the procedure remained relatively unchanged. The tissue was treated with zinc chloride paste in situ, and 6 to 24 hours later the "fixed tissue" was surgically excised and examined microscopically for evidence of cancer cells. The procedure was repeated until the removed tissue was free of all evidence of neoplasm.

The fixed tissue technique, as it is now frequently called, required a considerable amount of time for each individual patient. On the initial visit, the tumor site was outlined. The area was first treated with dichloroacetic acid. This was followed immediately by administration of a very thin layer of zinc chloride paste to fix a thin layer of tissue in a 24-hour period. The tissue was immediately protected by an occlusive dressing made up of two layers of cotton containing a layer of petrolatum. The dressing prevented the zinc chloride paste from spreading, since its formulation was deliquescent. In a series of return visits, the fixed tissue was excised and was examined microscopically layer by layer until the area was shown to be free of neoplasm.

The effectiveness of the procedure became apparent. In the hands of qualified, trained individuals, consistently high cure rates were demonstrated.

Even though the worthiness of the technique had been demonstrated without doubt, it was slow to catch on. The zinc chloride paste was sometimes difficult to obtain. The formula had been published, but the fine stibinite powder and the *Sanguinaria canadensis* were not always readily available from commercial suppliers. The number of cases that a physician could treat in a given period was small, and the procedure was both time-consuming and demanding. Six cases were considered a full week's schedule. In addition, the patient experienced a great deal of discomfort and pain, and immediate repairs were not possible.

Fresh Tissue Technique Gains Acceptance

Exterior application of the paste followed by excision and histologic examination of the layers was performed at all sites except the periorbital area. It was feared that the paste might irritate the conjunctiva and might possibly damage the cornea. Consequently, for the area around the eyes, surgical excision and examination of the fresh tissues became the accepted practice. In the early 1970s, the fresh tissue technique was extended to treat cancers of the skin on every area of the body. Tromovitch and Stegman[1] were instrumental in promoting the fresh tissue concept. At the meeting of the American College of Chemosurgery in 1971, they reported that of 108 basal cell carcinomas treated by their method and followed for 3 to 8 years, only three recurred. Following this report, other physicians began to use the fresh tissue procedure on other areas of the body. Within 3 years, I had converted totally to the fresh tissue technique. Inasmuch as I achieved the same high cure rates with this method as with the fixed tissue technique, I rarely use fixative today and then only when confronted with extensive, well-defined squamous cell carcinomas.

Interest in the fresh tissue technique grew rapidly. Many more patients can be treated effectively in the same period with this method. Five to eight skin cancer patients can be treated in one morning, with several stages possible in one day. In addition, there is considerably less pain and swelling with the fresh tissue technique. Necessary repairs can be done immediately following the removal of the cancer.

With further refinement and improvement in tumor mapping and staining, the popularity of the Mohs technique has continued to grow. By now more than 50,000 cases of basal and squamous cell carcinomas are being treated by this method yearly in the United States alone. As stated earlier, acceptance of chemosurgery was not immediate, but as the technique has proved itself year after year with high cure rates, it has become almost universal.

Teamwork

Chemosurgery has bridged the gap separating different specialists—plastic surgeons, head and neck surgeons, tumor surgeons, ophthalmologists, and ophthalmologic plastic surgeons. The chemosurgeon is able to determine the limit of silent tumor extensions precisely by microscopic examination and thus does not remove excessive tissue unnecessarily. Other surgeons, in contrast, must approximate the boundaries of the neoplasm and must take an extra margin for safety. Knowing that the area is free of neoplasm allows the surgeon involved in reconstruction to concentrate solely on performing the most effective repair. For example, because of the difficulty in surgically repairing the lower and upper lids, an ophthalmologist will tend to be too conservative in the excision. Surgical specimens sent to the ophthalmologic laboratory for examination reveal that from 30 to 50 per cent of the surgical borders have not been adequately extirpated.

Cure Rate

Year after year, the chemosurgeon has consistently achieved the highest cure rate. For tumors near the eye and around the nose and the ears, for recurrent tumors at any location, and for tumors with ill-defined borders, chemosurgery is the treatment of choice.

Availability

Until several years ago, patients had to travel long distances to find Mohs surgery for skin cancer, if they found it at all. Today, most of the leading medical centers in the United States and abroad have functioning chemosurgical units. This in turn promotes the technique by allowing visitors and students to observe and train. Training in chemosurgery was very difficult to obtain. A physician could spend a few days or a few weeks observing Dr. Frederic Mohs in Madison, Wisconsin. This gave the trainee time to become familiar with the technique. The physician would then return home to perfect and master the procedure on his own.

Thirteen years ago, I began the first 1-year comprehensive training program in chemosurgery at New York University Medical Center, under the support of the dermatology and plastic surgery service. It was truly the first program in which qualified physicians could receive extensive training in all aspects of chemosurgery and general dermatologic surgery. On completion of the program, the chemosurgery trainees (19 to date) have started practices specializing in skin cancer in many of the leading medical centers throughout the world. Most of them have now established their own 1-year training programs. There are more than 150 members of the American College of Chemosurgery today, and the numbers increase substantially every year.

I anticipate that microscopically controlled surgery will increase in availability and popularity. We can anticipate that eventually nearly every surgeon will have the excised tissue processed and examined microscopically, thus affording the patient the ultimate in removal of skin cancers. In the years to come, most skin cancers will be treated in the physician's office, and frozen tissues will be prepared and examined while the patient is still on the surgical table.

Reference

1. Tromovitch, T. A., and Stegman, S.: Microscopically controlled excision of skin tumors: Chemosurgery (Mohs) fresh tissue technique. Arch Dermatol. 116:231, 1974.

USE OF THE CARBON DIOXIDE LASER IN MICROSCOPICALLY CONTROLLED EXCISION (MOHS SURGERY)

Philip L. Bailin, M.D.

In 1941, Dr. Frederic Mohs of the University of Wisconsin first described the microscopically controlled excision of skin cancer.[1,2] This method has undergone a remarkable evolution, as summarized by Swanson, Taylor, and Tromovitch.[3] In the 40 years since its initial description, this technique has gained remarkably widespread acceptance throughout the United States and many other countries as the most reliable and definitive method of treating cutaneous cancer (basal cell carcinoma and squamous cell carcinoma).

It is beyond the scope of this article to describe the Mohs surgical technique and all its ramifications fully. The reader is referred to Mohs' text[4] for a detailed description. It is important, however, to be aware that two forms of this technique now exist: the fixed tissue technique and the fresh tissue technique. The former utilizes the presurgical application of a zinc chloride chemical fixative paste, and the latter eliminates this presurgical fixative.

Each of these methods has advantages and disadvantages. The fixed tissue technique has been preferred for large complex lesions, because the fixative produces a dry wound base, allowing for more precise marking of the tissue for specimen orientation. The surgical excision of the tissue is easier with this method, because the fixative has a hemostatic action and the surgical field is virtually bloodless. Additionally, the fixative seals lymphatic vessels, which may prevent seeding of healthy tissue by malignant cells. Furthermore, if the tumor should invade bone, the fixative paste enables the Mohs surgeon to continue his excisional surgery into the bone following chemical fixation. The small segments of bone that are removed may be decalcified and examined by the same frozen section technique as is used for the soft tissue.

The fixed tissue technique, however, also has its disadvantages. It is extremely time-consuming, because the fixative paste must be given many hours prior to surgical excision to achieve its action. This technique is also extremely painful to the patient and, because of its chemical destruction, a significant amount of inflammation is produced that may damage surrounding normal tissues. This is particularly important on the eyelids and on the cartilaginous planes of the nose and the ears.

The fresh tissue technique of Mohs surgery likewise offers advantages and disadvantages. No period of chemical fixation is required, and sequential surgical excisions therefore can be done in a span of hours, rather than days. The excision is carried out under local anesthesia, making the procedure far more comfortable for the patient. The lack of chemical fixation means that there is essentially no inflammatory response and no damage to surrounding vital tissues such as that produced by the fixative paste. This further conservation of tissue is of utmost importance in critical anatomic areas, such as the nasal alae, the eyelids, and the ears. Since there is no chemical damage to the wound base and the surrounding tissues, it is possible to achieve immediate postoperative repair of fresh tissue wounds. This is in contradistinction to the mandatory waiting period following the fixed tissue Mohs technique, in which the final fixed layer must naturally separate prior to any plastic repair. It is evident that each of these methods offers advantages, but these should be balanced against relative disadvantages either to the surgeon or to the patient.

We have described another modification of the Mohs surgical technique for microscopically controlled excision.[5] In this variation, we have used the carbon dioxide laser to remove the tissue layers sequentially for horizontal frozen section examination. It is believed that this modification combines the best features of the fresh tissue technique and the fixed tissue technique while eliminating most of their individual disadvantages.

The Carbon Dioxide Laser

Laser is an acronym that stands for *l*ight *a*mplification by *s*timulated *e*mission of *r*adiation. The following is a highly simplified description of the function of a laser: Orbital electrons of atoms or molecules of a solid or gaseous material, excited by a pumping energy source (mechanical, chemical, or electrical), are thrown into unstable orbits. As the excited electrons fall back into their ground state, electromagnetic energy of a characteristic wavelength for each material is emitted. These beams then travel back and forth in the laser tube, reflected by mirrors at either end. The mirror at one end of the tube partially transmits, so that a portion of the energy produced in the tube passes through another series of mirrors and focusing devices to a handpiece that can be applied to tissue as a cutting or vaporizing tool. The power of the beam is determined by the mass of activated material, the size of the laser tube, and the power of the pumping energy applied.

Different types of laser energy have certain properties in common. The energy is monochromatic; that is, of a fixed characteristic wavelength. It is highly collimated, which is to say that the exiting rays are parallel. This enables them to be finely focused so that almost all of their energy can be brought to bear on a given target. In addition, laser light is coherent; that is, spatially and temporally in phase, a property that adds to the power exerted on the target.

The carbon dioxide laser is of the continuous type; i.e., the energy is produced and emitted steadily rather than in pulses, as it is with some other lasers. Nevertheless, the output at the handpiece can be delivered in single, timed pulses, if desired, by means of a shutter system. This makes the carbon dioxide laser more versatile than pulsed systems. Its output has a wavelength of 10,600 nm (far infrared).

Almost all the energy of a carbon dioxide laser is absorbed in water at a depth of 0.1 to 0.2 mm, and hardly any of that energy is scattered. Since soft tissues of the body are 80 to 90 per cent water, energy from a carbon dioxide laser causes instantaneous vaporization of that water (and tissue) at a temperature of 100°C, and heat is not conducted away from the site of impact. Tissue immediately adjacent to that destroyed is virtually unaffected. Thermal damage from the energy of a carbon dioxide laser has been shown to extend no more than 30 to 50 μm from the site of impact,[6] which means that a layer only one cell thick around the area vaporized may be damaged.

Another beneficial feature of the carbon dioxide laser is its hemostatic power. It seals vessels up to 0.5 mm in diameter on impact. This provides a dry operative field. Also, the beam is sterilizing, making the field less likely to become infected. Finally, although destruction of tissue by the carbon dioxide laser is based on heat, postoperative pain is virtually nil, in contrast with that produced by electrocautery or by cold-steel surgery. Research has shown that when tissue is destroyed by the carbon dioxide laser, nerve endings are sealed instantaneously,[7] whereas raw and frayed endings result from other forms of ablative surgery.

The carbon dioxide laser system is extremely versatile. If the beam is focused on the tissue surface, the impact spot is only 0.1 to 0.2 mm. The power density is in the range of 50,000 to 100,000 watts per cm^2. The beam thus focused incises tissue, acting as a laser scalpel. If the beam is defocused on the tissue surface, the impact spot size increases to 2 mm. In this mode, the power density is approximately 500 to 1000 watts per cm^2.

The beam then vaporizes the surface rather than incising it. Thus, the carbon dioxide laser can be used for incisional or excisional procedures as well as for vaporization.

Treatment Technique

We have used the Sharplan 733 carbon dioxide laser for our cases. Any carbon dioxide laser unit with a surgical handpiece mounted on an articulated arm system would be acceptable for this technique. The laser beam is generated in the laser tube and is delivered through a series of mirrors to the handpiece, which acts as a laser scalpel. Because it is in the far infrared portion of the spectrum, the carbon dioxide cutting beam is invisible to the naked eye. Therefore, these laser units have a coaxial helium-neon laser aiming beam of very low wattage. This visible red beam is aimed at the tissue and, when the laser is fired, the carbon dioxide cutting beam strikes the tissue at the exact point of focus of the aiming beam.

For this technique, the surgical site is prepared as it would be for standard fresh tissue Mohs surgery. The area is anesthetized by the local infiltration of an anesthetic agent, usually 1 per cent lidocaine. The inclusion of epinephrine in the anesthetic is not necessary for hemostasis, since the laser beam is hemostatic as it cuts. This allows the surgeon to perform surgery safely on patients with cardiovascular problems, in whom epinephrine could not be used without risk, or on patients receiving anticoagulant therapy.

The beam is focused to a 0.2-mm diameter on the tissue surface, and then the incision is made. As the beam is drawn across the tissue, it incises cleanly and hemostatically. The depth of the cut and the degree of hemostasis are inversely proportional to the speed with which the beam is drawn across the tissue surface. As the tissue is incised, both blood and lymph vessels are sealed.

With this beam, tissue can be cut precisely to variable depths and can be readily undermined. Thin tissue layers can be excised, much as would be performed with a scalpel. Extremely thin layers of tissue can be excised, if required, in certain anatomic areas, such as the eyelids, the lips, and the nasal alae.

The tissue layers excised with the carbon dioxide laser may be examined microscopically by means of horizontal frozen sections, as is done in the other forms of Mohs surgery. Sections taken with the carbon dioxide laser show remarkable preservation of tissue architecture. There is virtually no thermal distortion in the tissue, as there would be if the layers were to be excised with an electrosurgical apparatus. It is often impossible to differentiate under the microscope between sections that have been excised by a scalpel and those excised by the carbon dioxide laser. In fact, the preservation of the architecture may be even better with the carbon dioxide laser than with the fixed tissue method. This remarkable preservation results from the fact that the laser energy is totally dissipated in a very focal and localized way as the beam cuts. There is virtually no spread of thermal damage beyond 50 micra from the point of laser impact. This would be approximately a distance of only two epidermal basal cells.

The tissue bed that remains exposed after each layer is excised by the carbon dioxide laser is viable, yet totally dry. This hemostasis makes a precise orientation of tissue possible for subsequent mapping. Furthermore, there is no surface char (as there would be from an electrosurgical apparatus) and no subjacent layer of necrotic tissue (as there is with the chemical fixative paste). Additionally, the tissue bed is sterilized by the laser beam.

At the completion of the procedure, healing may be permitted to proceed by granulation, if this is the desire of the surgeon. It has been found that this granulation occurs at the same rate as does granulation following fresh tissue chemosurgery. It may be slightly slower than the rate of granulation following fixed tissue chemosurgery. The tissue bed is also immediately acceptable for primary repair either by direct closure or by flap or graft closure, if the surgeon so desires.

The carbon dioxide laser is also extremely useful when a cutaneous carcinoma has invaded cartilage, or even bone. The laser beam can be controlled so that even a delicate layer of perichondrium or periosteum may be stripped off for histologic evaluation. If this examination reveals invasion of the subjacent tissue, serial excisions of thin layers of cartilage or bone can be carried out with the laser beam until a tumor-free plane is reached. The remaining cartilage or bone is undamaged.

SUMMARY

We have found that the carbon dioxide laser modification of Mohs surgery can combine the advantages of both the fixed tissue and the fresh tissue techniques and, at the same time, can avoid their inherent disadvantages. As in the fixed tissue technique, hemostasis is inherent, the operative field remains dry and easily oriented for mapping, lymphatics are sealed, and cartilage and bone may be easily removed for sectioning. As in the fresh tissue technique, multiple layers may be taken in a single day, pain and inflammation are minimal, histologic detail is excellent, a minimum of normal surrounding tissue is sacrificed and, finally, immediate surgical repair may be undertaken.

Currently, the major disadvantages of the carbon dioxide laser modification are the cost and the size of the available instrumentation. Carbon dioxide laser systems are rather expensive at present, although smaller units that are more suited for office practice are now being offered at substantially reduced costs. As technology improves and demand increases, it may be expected that this instrumentation will be widely available. When this occurs, it seems likely that many Mohs surgeons will use the carbon dioxide laser modification in their practice.

References

1. Mohs, F. E., and Guyer, M. F.: Pre-excisional fixation of tissues in the treatment of cancer in rats. Cancer Res. 1:49, 1941.
2. Mohs, F. E.: Chemosurgery: A microscopically controlled method of cancer excision. Arch. Surg. 42:279, 1941.
3. Swanson, N. A., Taylor, W. B., and Tromovitch, T. A.: The evolution of Mohs' surgery. J. Dermatol. Surg. Oncol. 8:650, August 1982.
4. Mohs, F. E.: Chemosurgery. Springfield, IL, Charles C Thomas, 1978.
5. Bailin, P. L., Ratz, J. L., and Lutz-Nagey, L.: CO_2 laser modification of Mohs' surgery. J. Dermatol. Surg. Oncol. 7:621, August 1981.
6. Ben-Bassat, M., Ben-Bassat, M., and Kaplan, I.: An ultrastructural study of the cut edges of skin and mucous membrane specimens excised by carbon dioxide laser. *In* Kaplan, I. (ed.): Laser Surgery. Jerusalem, Academic Press, 1976, pp. 95–100.
7. Ascher, P., Ingolitsch, E., Walter, G., and Oberbauer, R. W.: Ultrastructural findings in CNS tissue with CO_2 laser. *In* Kaplan, I., (ed.): Laser Surgery II. Jerusalem, Academic Press, 1976, pp. 81–85.

MICROSCOPIC CONTROL OF SKIN CANCER EXCISION: MOHS CHEMOSURGERY VERSUS DOUBLE-BLADE SCALPEL

Henry H. Roenigk, Jr., M.D.
June K. Robinson, M.D.

Mohs[1] developed the technique of microscopically controlling his excision of skin cancer using the fixed tissue techniques on lesions. During the past decade, there has been a greater recognition of this procedure, and more physicians have been trained in the technique. It is now generally available in most major medical centers in the United States and in a few other countries. The technique was initially developed to treat recurrent basal cell and squamous cell carcinomas of the skin but has been extended to other tumors,[2,3] and to lesions with a potentially high rate of recurrence either because of their location or because of the morphology of the tumor. The fresh tissue technique[4] rather than the fixed tissue method is now generally used by most Mohs surgeons.

Cure rates for recurrent skin cancer, as reported by several authors,[2,4-6] approach 99 per cent with Mohs surgery. Very few other techniques (repeat excision, radiation therapy, cryosurgery, and electrodesiccation and curettage) can achieve such a high rate of success.

When used as the first treatment method, Mohs chemosurgery does afford adequate removal of all tumor and the avoidance of disfiguring recurrences. Mohs chemosurgery of recurrent tumors often leaves a large defect that must be treated by skin grafts or flaps or allowed to granulate in with less than a desirable cosmetic result in order to achieve a cure of the tumor. The use of Mohs chemosurgery as an initial treatment of all skin cancers is controversial, since other techniques, such as excision, cryosurgery, and electrodesiccation and curettage, give good cure rates with usually favorable cosmetic results.

Many dermatologists and most surgeons use the standard excisional method with primary closure for untreated basal cell carcinoma of reasonable size. Excellent cure rates can be predicted for most areas if the tumor is adequately excised. Two plastic surgeons reported a 5-year cure rate of over 98 per cent with the standard excision technique.[8]

Schultz and Roenigk[7] described the use of a double-blade scalpel and a double-edged punch to excise skin cancer and to provide a more thorough examination of surgical margins in an attempt to decrease the recurrence rate. In this method, the cosmetically superior primary surgical closure is used.

The purpose of this paper is to compare the double blade scalpel technique with Mohs chemosurgery and to point out the advantages and drawbacks of each technique.

Double-Blade Scalpel

With routine vertical sections of an elliptic excision specimen, the sample vertical sections that are taken to check for tumor invasion of surgical margins are only 7 micra in size. Any part of the surgical border not included in these sample sections could have undetected tumor invasion. The double-blade scalpel is used to take 2- to 3-mm sections representing a complete surgical border visualized histologically with flat sections.

Appropriate excision lines are drawn, as for routine excision. One performs excision with the outer blade of the double scalpel, following excision lines.

The central elliptic specimen is removed as usual and may be submitted for pathologic diagnosis and examination for any evidence of deep invasion of fat. The outer 2- to 3-mm strips are removed with fine forceps and a sharp scalpel; one should take care not to tear tissue. The sections may be removed in different segments if the excision is long. The specimens are coded with a map, which is placed in the patient's records.

The specimens are laid flat on moistened gauze, and the outer aspect is stained with India ink or silver nitrate to identify it as outer surgical margins. The specimen is clipped to a piece of strong cardboard and is put in 10 per cent formalin. These flat strips will represent the entire surgical border with epidermis at the top and fat at the bottom after the paraffin sections are cut.

The wound is closed with standard surgical technique. If frozen sections are used, closure may be delayed until the specimens are declared free of tumor.

DISCUSSION

The double-blade scalpel technique is an intriguing and innovative method of determining whether the margins of the excision are free of tumor. However, in practice it adds time to the surgical procedure and may not achieve its stated goal. For a number of reasons, the double-blade scalpel technique provides less reliable assurance than does Mohs chemosurgery that the entire tumor has been removed. Use of the double-blade scalpel will ordinarily entail removal of more healthy tissue than will Mohs surgery and may fail to remove all of the tumor in the initial procedures, thus requiring the patient to undergo a second operation after recovering from the first.

The most important reason that Mohs surgery is more reliable than the double-blade scalpel technique in assuring the physician that the entire tumor has been removed is the greater efficiency in having one physician excise the specimen, properly orient the tissue, map it, prepare the histopathologic specimens by frozen section technique, interpret these specimens, and locate the tumor, which may remain at the base of the wound. This is the key to achieving the high cure rates of the Mohs technique. With the double-blade scalpel method, the tissue is removed from the surgical field to be prepared for processing by a histopathology technician in a distant part of the hospital, or even across town. The technician must then orient and embed the tissue properly in paraffin. Later a pathologist scans a piece of tissue, looking for a tumor that he hopes is not present. Neither the histopathology technician nor the pathologist has any idea how the piece of tissue was oriented in the patient. The pathologist has not had the opportunity to examine the increasing cellular atypia of the carcinoma as it invades. The physician who removed the tissue waits for a report and only rarely examines the slides himself. In the course of this transaction, the specimen travels through many sets of hands, increasing the probability of loss of proper orientation.

Mohs surgery also affords technical superiority in the preparation of tissue sections for histopathologic evaluation. The surgeon who uses the double-blade scalpel technique must guess the proper depth for the central elliptic specimen. The base of the tumor must be examined by flat sections; otherwise, a deep extension of the tumor may be missed. Either technique is only as good as the pathologic specimen it provides. The Mohs fresh tissue technique provides rapid examination of frozen sections within 30 minutes to 1 hour of removal of the tissue from the patient. Every piece of tissue is examined on all edges, deep and superficial, with a cell-by-cell analysis.

The average histopathology laboratory technician is adroit in preparing small paraffin-embedded specimens for diagnosis. For this individual, cutting perfect sections along a curvilinear surface extending over 2 cm is very difficult. This type of skill must be used frequently in order to be maintained. The Mohs technician is trained to prepare frozen sections of large specimens swiftly and accurately and uses this skill daily, thereby maintaining his proficiency. The average surgeon or dermatologist does not have frozen sections available in his office.

Not only does the Mohs technique provide greater assurance of curing the patient by total removal of the tumor, but also it allows maximal conservation of healthy tissue. Whereas the Mohs surgeon need not guess at the proper margins for the excision, the surgeon using the double-blade scalpel almost inevitably must remove a margin of healthy tissue in order to reduce the likelihood that the tumor cells will be left unexcised. The resulting conservation of healthy tissue by the Mohs surgeon allows the use of less complicated methods of closure, thus facilitating superior cosmetic results.

Mohs surgery also insures that the tumor removal will be accomplished efficiently and in a single procedure. In contrast, use of the double-blade scalpel technique necessarily requires a second procedure if the pathology report indicates the presence of tumor in the margins. By the time the specimen has been read, the wound has been closed. If there is tumor beyond the edges of the excision performed by the double-blade scalpel, the surgeon is then faced with a second procedure in a patient who has some edema, some pain, and possibly even a hematoma. Under these circumstances, the second procedure carries more risk and is usually delayed for some months, making it even harder to find the remaining tumor in the midst of the contracted scar. In light of these difficulties, it may be necessary to refer patients for whom the initial procedure with the double-blade scalpel has failed to remove the tumor completely to a Mohs surgeon for the second operation.

The double-blade scalpel technique offers the previously unavailable option of examining the margins of an excised specimen of a primary tumor, but the physician must be careful, because the procedure can give a false sense of security about the accuracy of the diagnosis. When Mohs surgery is readily available, the double-blade scalpel is not advantageous to the patient, risks a second unnecessary procedure, and expends extra physician time. The Mohs technique is not meant to treat small primary tumors in noninvasive locations. These lesions are currently cured with electrodesiccation and curettage, excision without the double-blade scalpel, and cryosurgery. The double-blade scalpel technique may have some utility in treating such small primary tumors, although its superiority to alternate techniques has yet to be established.

The double-blade scalpel is not meant to take the place of Mohs microscopically controlled surgery. Mohs chemosurgery is ideally suited for recurrent tumors in which the margins for excision are uncertain and frozen section control of tumor removal is essential. For primary nodular basal cell carcinoma, squamous cell carcinoma, or malignant melanoma of reasonable size, most surgeons and many dermatologists prefer surgical excision. In most circumstances, primary closure is used with excellent cosmetic results. This method provides a better histopathologic check of such surgical specimens than is routinely available to the physician.

References

1. Mohs, F. E.: Chemosurgery: Microscopically Controlled Surgery for Skin Cancer. Springfield, IL, Charles C Thomas, 1978.
2. Tromovitch, T., and Stegman, S.: Microscopic-controlled excision of cutaneous tumors: Chemosurgery, fresh tissue technique. Cancer 41:653, 1978.
3. Menn, H., Robins, P., Kopf, A. W., and Bart, R. S.: The recurrent basal cell epithelioma. Arch. Dermatol. 103:628, 1971.
4. Mohs, F. E.: Chemosurgery for Microscopically Controlled Excision of Skin Cancer. J. Surg. Oncol. 3:257, 1971.

5. Cains, L. J., and Land, W. A.: Microscopically controlled excision of skin cancer in Australia: A report. Aust. J. Dermatol. 20:135, 1979.
6. Amonette, R. A.: Mohs' technique: Chemosurgery and fresh tissue surgery. *In* Epstein, E., and Epstein, E., Jr. (eds.): Techniques in Skin Surgery, Philadelphia, Lea & Febiger, 1979, pp. 140–148.
7. Schultz, B., and Roenigk, H. H. Jr.: Double blade scalpel excision of skin cancer. J. Am. Acad. Dermatol. 7:495, Oct. 1982.
8. Taylor, G. A., and Barisoni, D.: Ten years' experience in the surgical treatment of basal cell carcinoma. Br. J. Surg. 60:522, 1973.

LIQUID CRYSTAL THERMOGRAPHY IN THE PREOPERATIVE EVALUATION OF THE MARGINS OF BASAL CELL CARCINOMAS

Philip L. Bailin, M.D.
John L. Ratz, M.D.

The treatment of basal cell carcinomas, particularly by dermatologists, offers one of the widest choices of therapeutic modalities available for any neoplasm of man. Excision and closure, electrodesiccation and curettage, radiotherapy, topical chemotherapy, cryotherapy, laser therapy, and Mohs surgery are all available possibilities in most large medical communities. Many factors govern the physician's choice. Among these are the age and medical condition of the patient, the location of the tumor, the histologic pattern of the tumor, previous treatment history and, perhaps most importantly, size of the lesion. Of all these factors, the one that is often most difficult to ascertain clinically preoperatively is the true size of the tumor to be treated.

With the increasing use of Mohs surgery and its precise histologic tracking of skin tumors has come a more definitive way of measuring the true extent of such tumors. All practitioners of this method are repeatedly struck by the fact that they were often totally unable preoperatively to judge the true extent, both laterally and in depth, of the neoplasms they have been treating. The ability of basal cell carcinomas to extend deeply and widely as slender, finger-like projections and to follow tissue planes of minimal resistance frequently causes them to grow extensively in iceberg-like fashion under and away from the clinically visible lesion on the skin surface.

This propensity of basal cell carcinomas to progress deeply and widely away from their surface marker lesion often leads to a great deal of frustration and surprise on the part of both the patient and the clinician. All too commonly, a physician will initiate treatment with curettage and electrodesiccation and find, to his surprise, that a seemingly well localized lesion will involve a very large portion of the patient's face or scalp. With other methods (excluding Mohs surgery), the realization that the tumor has been more extensive than anticipated unfortunately may not come until much later, when a recurrence of the tumor is noted.

In an attempt to find a way of accurately determining the extent of basal cell carcinomas preoperatively we have used liquid crystal thermography.[1] We have found this to be helpful in ascertaining the lateral extent of tumors in many instances, but it is not a totally reliable method at present. However, because of its relatively low cost, safety, and ease of performance, this method may be used as an office adjunct to aid the clinician in his preoperative evaluation.

Liquid Crystal Thermography

Liquid crystal thermography was described initially by Fergason[2] in 1964. In that same year, the procedure was also reported in the dermatologic literature by Crissey and coworkers.[3]

Liquid crystal thermography involves esters of cholesterol that exhibit the mechanical properties of liquids and the optical properties of crystalline solids.[4,5] When they exist in the cholesteric phase (a state of matter with an ordered molecular arrangement intermediate between a true three-dimensional solid and a liquid), they are capable of displaying specific colors in response to temperature. Above a given temperature, these crystals exist purely as liquids, and below that given temperature they exist as three-dimensional solids. The crystals also exhibit the property of selective scattering of light: When they are illuminated by pure white light they selectively transmit specific wavelengths, reflect other wavelengths, and absorb none. Additionally, they are characterized by the phenomenon of circular dichromism, which is a selective scattering of right- and left-handed polarized light.

White light aimed at these crystals is separated into one component that has a clockwise rotational vector and another that rotates counterclockwise. One of these vectors will transmit light and the other will scatter light, both of specific determined wavelengths. This results in a maximal scattering of a specific wavelength of light as other wavelengths are transmitted through the material. When applied to a black surface, these crystals cause light reflected from them to appear as an irridescent color, whereas light transmitted by them is absorbed by the black surface. The color and intensity of the light that is reflected (scattered) depend on several factors, including the nature of the substance to which the light is applied, the angle of incidence of the light source, the observer's angle of view, and the temperature of the material to which the light is applied.

These properties give the esters of cholesterol the unique ability to demonstrate minute changes in temperature of a surface by displaying corresponding changes in color, the dominant wavelength of which is influenced by the temperature change of the surface being evaluated. These crystals are so highly sensitive to temperature that they respond with molecular rearrangements and resulting color changes to temperature fluctuations as small as 0.1°C and hence will transmit different colors that are displayed with spatial resolutions of 1000 lines per inch. This degree of sensitivity is far greater than that which can be achieved by other means (e.g., infrared thermography), yet the cost of this liquid crystal technique is far less than that of other, similar methods. One procedure currently can be done for approximately $2.00. The so-called thermogram that results from liquid crystal thermography occurs in colors that range from blue-violet at the warmest temperatures through intermediate colors to red at the coolest temperatures.

One can vary the temperature range being tested by using specifically prepared cholesterol esters with well-documented and specified given temperature ranges. Temperatures that are in the sensitivity range of the crystals fall into a respective ordering within the visible light spectrum. Temperatures that fall outside the range of the specific cholesterol crystals being used will appear black as a result of the presence of the black base coat that is necessary to prevent the backward reflection of light, which would obscure the selectively scattered colors. The actual display of color from the crystals is quite similar to the pattern seen from a film of oil atop still water in bright sunlight.

The temperature range of the cholesterol crystals is varied by altering the ratio of two components: cholesterol oleyl carbonate and cholesterol nonanoate. In addition to these ingredients, each commercially prepared liquid crystal contains 8 per cent cholesterol benzoate to maintain a 4° temperature sensitivity range. By varying the concentrations of the components of these crystals, one can evaluate temperature ranges from −20 to +250°C. However, each specific prepared liquid crystal will have only a 4°C temperature sensitivity range, and a given cholesteric liquid crystal will always exhibit the same color at a specific temperature. Therefore, many different commercially prepared crystals are available, each with a 4°C range. The most useful crystals for dermatologic surgical purposes fall within the following temperature sensitivity ranges: 30 to 33°C, 31 to 34°C, 32 to 35°C, 33 to 36°C, and 34 to 37°C. These have been the temperature ranges used most frequently in all cutaneous studies involving liquid crystal thermography.

Liquid crystal thermography had been used in many medical disciplines with a wide range of applications. It has been used in the detection of breast carcinoma,[5-8] for which it was found to be more reliable than either physical examination or mammography. It has also been employed successfully in the study of normal and abnormal venous patterns,[4] particularly the study of peripheral vascular diseases and the localization of incompetent perforator veins.[7] Other varied uses have been in placental localization,[7,9,10] prediction of the viability of pedicle flaps,[7,11] measurement of therapeutic responses to intra-arterially administered reserpine,[12] evaluation of the effectiveness of sympathetic blockade,[13] determination of the extent of pulmonary disease,[7] evaluation of exercise-induced cutaneous temperature changes,[7] elucidation of the pathophysiology of vitiligo,[7] and detection of the presence of primary or metastatic carcinomas in skin.[6]

In regard to detection of carcinomas, it has been found that skin is usually warmer over primary and metastatic carcinomas and sarcomas than over normal tissue.[6] The extent to which a malignant tumor in the skin can be identified depends upon the effective transfer of metabolic heat from the tumor cells to the skin surface. This is accomplished by the conduction of that heat through the overlying tissues, which of course is most effectively accomplished over short distances. The presence or absence of insulating substances, such as subcutaneous fat, also plays a role.[5] Liquid crystal thermographic measurement of skin temperatures over tumors can thus be useful in the measurement of tumor size, vascular physiology, and even response to treatment.[6] A hot spot over the tumor will be characteristic of the thermogram.[5] However, in some instances, marginal areas of a tumor may actually appear warmer than the center because of necrosis and tumor cell breakdown centrally.[6]

Patients have been studied with liquid crystal thermography for malignant melanoma, chondrosarcoma, bladder carcinoma, renal carcinoma, breast carcinoma, vulvar carcinoma, bronchogenic carcinoma, and malignant schwannoma.[6] In all of these, the cutaneous surface overlying the tumor mass was found to be warmer than the surrounding skin by a factor of 0.9 to 3.3°C. In Selawry's study, the thermographic outline of cutaneous tumors was found to exceed the palpable tumor mass by 0.5 to 4.0 cm, implying increased vascularization and tumor spread beyond the visible and palpable tumor margins.[6]

Method of Evaluating Basal Cell Carcinoma by Liquid Crystal Thermography

In 1981, we first reported the use of liquid crystal thermography to determine preoperatively the true margins of basal cell carcinoma.[1] Because the transfer of heat from the tumor to the skin surface results in a specific thermogram, and since the best results in other tumors have been obtained over short distances from areas not underlying an insulating layer of fat, we felt that application of this technique to basal cell carcinoma seemed most appropriate. Basal cell carcinoma is essentially localized to the dermis in most instances, although subcutaneous extension can certainly occur.

The method of obtaining the preoperative thermogram is really quite simple and can be done at minimal expense in any dermatologist's office. Cholesterol crystals with various temperature sensitivity ranges are commercially available. It was found that crystals with a range of 31 to 34°C are ideal for this type of endeavor. Skin temperature may vary between 30 and 35°C, depending upon the ambient room temperature, but the crystals with a 31 to 34° sensitivity range perform well when the skin surface is correctly prepared.

The first step in the procedure is to cleanse the skin surface properly with a lipid solvent material. Ethyl alcohol or isopropyl alcohol functions very well for this purpose. The reason for this initial cleansing is that the diffusion of skin lipids onto the thermographic field can shift the temperature sensitivity range of the liquid crystals that are employed.[4] It is important that a large area of skin (i.e., larger than the anticipated thermogram) be prepared before the procedure is undertaken.

Next, the entire field is brought to uniform temperature by cooling the skin surface with iced compresses for 15 to 20 minutes. When the skin is dried, the water-soluble black base coat is sprayed from an aerosol can over the field and then is dried using a hand-held hair dryer on a cool setting. This prevents premature warming of the iced skin surface. When this drying is completed, the cholesterol liquid crystals are sprayed over the field in a similar fashion and are also dried on a cool setting. The skin surface then begins to rewarm and, as it reaches the temperature sensitivity range of the crystals, a characteristic and reasonably persistent thermogram pattern results. This pattern can be measured with a caliper and photographed. Following this, as the thermogram begins to deteriorate, the skin surface is cleaned with soap and water. Surgical treatment of the area may then proceed immediately. The total thermography procedure takes only approximately 30 minutes and is totally safe and painless to the patient.

It was found that several technical difficulties may occur. One of these is the problem of finding the correct viewing angle of the thermogram as it forms. This results from the extreme shininess of the thermographic film on the skin surface. Skillful placement of the illuminating light source may correct this. The prime requirement is a constant light source, and, provided that its position and intensity are maintained, the color changes will accurately represent the proportional changes in temperature sensed by the crystals regardless of the angle of view of the observer.[4] A high-intensity, low-heat output light source, such as one used for surgery, will give excellent illumination for immediate evaluation of the thermogram.[5]

Photography of the resulting thermogram is a tricky proposition at best. Direct ocular observation is by far the best method for interpreting results. However, for recording purposes, Ektachrome-X color film, which is most sensitive to the blue-green range, is the best film available for the purpose. Some sharpness in the red-to-green area is lost with this film, as is spatial resolution.

It must be remembered that the actual temperatures measured are of virtually no importance for the purpose of measuring lateral tumor margins. Rather, it is the temperature differences that are of the utmost value. At times, it may be difficult to judge tumor margins by temperature variation with the basic technique of liquid crystal thermography. In these instances, it may be valuable to augment the regular thermogram by the technique of thermal stressing.

It has been found that temperatures of the skin overlying veins are 0.1 to 0.4°C warmer than the surrounding skin surface. The resultant thermograms exceeded the actual outline of the vein by 0.4 mm. When the skin tissue was "stressed" by hot or cold blowing air, one could induce temperature changes that were inversely proportional to the expected circulation of the skin, thus augmenting the aforementioned temperature gradient to a level of 0.9 to 2.2°C. At the same time, this allowed the thermographic distinction of the veins from the surrounding skin to be excellent.[6] Immersion of the tissue in hot or cold water can yield the same result. Such thermal stressing can also be used to augment the thermographic differentiation overlying tumor masses. This has been found to be a most valuable tool in performing liquid crystal thermography.

Clinical Results

Results of our preliminary study have been published.[1] In that study, patients with basal cell carcinoma of the skin were evaluated preoperatively by both clinical observation and liquid crystal thermography to determine lateral tumor margins. Following the thermographic procedure, Mohs surgery was performed on each patient and the tumor was removed in sequential stages until microscopic examination revealed no further tumor. The resultant defect, which represented total tumor extent, was then measured, and this measurement was compared with the preoperative clinical and thermographic evaluations.

It was found that, for basal cell carcinomas of heavy or moderate tumor density, such as solid or adenoid-cystic tumors, the thermographically measured tumor size exceeded the clinically determined tumor size substantially in almost every case. In several of these cases, the thermographic measurement was actually much closer to the true tumor size as determined by Mohs technique. However, for tumors of low tumor density, such as morphea basal cell carcinoma, thermography was of little help in determining accurate margins preoperatively.

We have stressed that several factors must be remembered. Measurement of the thermogram may be complicated by a relatively small amount of error because of observational factors and the somewhat transitory nature of the thermogram itself. More importantly, tissue relaxation resulting from elasticity following surgical removal of the basal cell carcinoma may distort the postoperative measurement size. Furthermore, every Mohs procedure involves the removal of a small but definite margin of normal tissue laterally, thus adding to a measurement that is possibly larger than true tumor warrants.

DISCUSSION

Techniques involving other than pure sensory means (observation, palpation) have been used to aid physicians in the preoperative determination of the lateral margins of skin tumors. Goldstein and associates[14] have studied ultraviolet photography for this purpose. This procedure has been found useful in highlighting or enhancing detection of inapparent skin tumors. With this technique, basal cell carcinomas appear darker (positive) on ultraviolet film than on black and white film. Benign lesions, conversely, appear lighter (negative) on ultraviolet film than on black and white photographic film. This technique, however, is not of much value in determining the true lateral extension of such tumors. Additionally, the procedure has been found to be time-consuming and quite expensive because of the special photographic equipment that is necessary.

Infrared thermography has also been extensively studied as an adjunct to clinical diagnosis.[15-17] It has been found useful in the evaluation of breast diseases, peripheral vascular diseases, cerebral circulation, bone and joint disorders, burn damage, thyroid disease, and placental localization. This form of thermography is based on the fact that every object emits infrared radiation, the extent of which relates to the temperature of that object. Skin temperature in these studies varied between 30 and 35°C, depending upon the ambient room temperature. To perform this technique adequately, a carefully controlled room environment is essential. Additionally, this technique, like ultraviolet photography, is time-consuming and quite expensive.

On the contrary, liquid crystal thermography is both a rapid and an inexpensive method for determining temperature variations. It may be conveniently performed in a dermatologist's office without the purchase of esoteric or expensive equipment. It is harmless to the patient and painless. In many instances, it is capable of demonstrating the lateral margins of basal cell carcinoma so that the surgeon may prepare both his patient and himself for the operative procedure and the likely postoperative result. The technique is still somewhat unreliable, however (particularly for low mass lesions), and is subject to a number of error-causing factors. Further refinements in the performance of the technique and in the liquid crystal products themselves may yield more reliable and more sensitive results. At this point, the potential seems great.

The major drawback, however, deals with the determination of the deep extent of the tumor. As was stated earlier, the closer the tumor to the skin surface, the greater the heat transfer and the more accurate the thermogram. Therefore, lateral margins may be relatively easily demarcated, but the depth of the tumor is not demonstrable by this technique at present. It may be that the combination of liquid crystal thermography with some form of ultrasonography may eventually prove to be a very reliable preoperative form of evaluation for basal cell carcinomas.

References

1. Ratz, J. L., and Bailin, P. L.: Liquid crystal thermography in determining the lateral extents of basal cell carcinomas. J. Dermatol. Surg. Oncol. 7:27, Jan. 1981.
2. Fergason, J. L.: Liquid crystal thermography. Sci. Am. 211:77, 1964.
3. Crissey, J. T., et al.: A new technique for the demonstration of skin temperature patterns. J. Invest. Dermatol. 43:89, 1964.
4. Crissey, J. T., Fergason, J. L., and Betterhausen, J. M.: Cutaneous thermography with liquid crystals. J. Invest. Dermatol. 45:329, 1965.
5. Davison, T. W., et al.: Detection of breast cancer by liquid crystal thermography, a preliminary report. Cancer 29:1123, May 1972.
6. Selawry, O. S., et al.: The use of liquid cholesteric crystals for thermographic measurement of skin temperature in man. Mol. Cryst. 1:495, 1966.
7. Davison, T. W.: Applications of liquid crystal thermography to clinical medicine and applied physiology. Doctoral dissertation, University of Michigan, 73–21, 089, 1973.
8. Logan, W. W., and Lind, B.: Improved liquid cholesterol ester crystal thermography of the breast. J. Surg. Oncol. 8:363, 1976.
9. Peterson, C. N., et al.: Placental localization by liquid crystal thermography. Obstet. Gynecol. 3:468, 1971.
10. Davison, T. W., et al.: Liquid crystal thermographic placental localization. Obstet. Gynecol. 42:574, 1973.
11. Freshwater, M. F., and Krijek, T. J.: Liquid crystallometry: A new technique for predicting the viability of pedicle flaps. Surg. Forum 21:497, 1970.
12. Chandler, C. Jr.: Liquid crystal thermography: A measure of therapeutic response to reserpine given intra-arterially. South. Med. J. 69:614, May 1976.
13. Diaz, P. M.: Use of liquid crystal thermography to evaluate sympathetic blocks. Anesthesiology 44:443, May 1976.
14. Goldstein, N., et al.: Ultraviolet photography of skin cancers and nevi. Cutis 16:858, Nov. 1975.
15. Aird, E.: Thermography. Nurs. Mirror 144:66, Feb. 1977.
16. Freundlich, I. M., et al.: Thermographic, radionuclide, and radiographic detection of bone metastases—a prospective comparison. Radiology 122:665, March 1977.
17. Monteyne, R., et al.: Diagnosis of bone metastases by thermography. J Belge Radiol. 59:9, 1976.

Editorial Comment

The history of this modality in the control of cutaneous cancer is of interest. In the early part of this century, "cancer quacks" used caustic pastes, usually containing arsenic, to treat these tumors. They often met with tragic results, since there was no method of determining whether or not the malignancy had been destroyed completely. Then Mohs discovered that his zinc paste fixed the tissues in vivo. He applied the paste, excised the fixed tissue, and then determined if the growth had been completely eradicated by examining the ingeniously marked undersurface of the specimen. R. R. Allington sped the process up by introducing dichloroacetic acid before therapy to remove the superficial portion of the tumor. Then certain plastic surgeons modified this by completely excising the tumor, marking the undersurface as Mohs did, and then checking the adequacy of the excision by a frozen tissue technique. Tromovitch further modified the procedure by returning to the piecemeal excisions advocated by Mohs and subjecting each slice of tissue to the use of frozen tissue sections—the so-called fresh tissue technique.

Since then, Roenigk has introduced his double-blade scalpel concept, and Bailin and Ratz have offered crystal thermography and laser surgery. Crystal thermography reveals invisible gross extensions of the tumor but cannot be considered a form of microscopic control. Laser surgery seems to produce superior sections for the crucial microscopic examinations, but its use is limited, because few are expert in this technique, and the cost of the equipment is considerable.

There is no question that Mohs and his followers have made a significant contribution to the control of skin cancer. Cases considered inoperable before the introduction of this technique are now salvageable. Improvements in technique can result only in the saving of more lives with less sacrifice of normal tissue; the morbidity and scarring will thereby be reduced There can be no controversy as to the value of this technique.

Think It Over.

SECTION 3

PSORIASIS

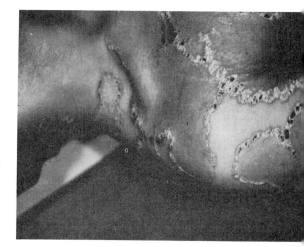

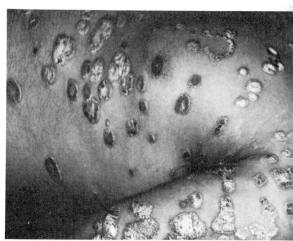

An unusual case of psoriasis of a marginated type.

CHAPTER 13

PUVA THERAPY

PUVA IN PERSPECTIVE

Thomas B. Fitzpatrick, M.D.
John A. Parrish, M.D.

Lusty, though we are loathsome to love. Keen-sighted, though we hate to look upon ourselves.
The name of the disease, spiritually speaking, is Humiliation.
Thus wrote John Updike about the plight of people with psoriasis*

PUVA Photochemotherapy Came at a Time When There Were Few Options for Treating Generalized Psoriasis

Methotrexate and PUVA are the most acceptable treatments for the control of severe generalized psoriasis. As with the management of many other chronic inflammatory diseases of unknown etiology, such as rheumatoid arthritis, control of psoriasis has been largely unsatisfactory. Systemic methotrexate was the first effective treatment for the clearing of psoriasis and for maintenance of a virtually disease-free state. Other therapies, such as ultraviolet-B phototherapy with or without tar, anthralin, or topical corticosteroids, might have achieved a temporary remission, but ideal protocols were unavailable, patient acceptance was less than complete, and maintenance was often not feasible with these methods. In 1974, the introduction of orally administered methoxsalen in combination with a newly developed, high-intensity artificial ultraviolet-A irradiator [1] provided a highly effective modality that, like methotrexate, not only induced a remission but also appeared practical for maintenance with infrequent treatments. This new technique, which came to be called PUVA (*p*soralen and *UVA*), became the first effective and convenient alternative therapy to methotrexate and the first demonstration of the concept of photochemotherapy.

Controlled clinical trials were required to establish safety and efficacy. Between 1975 and 1979, three multicenter clinical trials accumulated a large data base. A total of 5275 patients were treated in: (1) a 16-center American trial (1300 patients) sponsored by Sylvania Lighting Products, (2) a 12-center American trial (980 patients) sponsored by Westwood, and (3) a 17-center trial (2995 patients) involving most of the major European PUVA centers that was coordinated by Professor K. Wolff of Austria and Professor E. Christophers of Germany. As a result of these clinical trials, a detailed outline of the technique and effects of PUVA photochemotherapy was prepared in 1979. [2] The United States Food and Drug Administration's Bureau of Radiation Health then published specifications for the ultraviolet-A irradiator in the *Federal Register*. On May 20, 1982, after more than 7 years of extensive study, the Food and Drug Administration approved the use of PUVA to treat psoriasis.

---

*In a remarkably perceptive and poignant short story in *The New Yorker* (July 19, 1976) about a patient undergoing PUVA therapy.

Side Effects and Potential Risks of PUVA: Three Decades of Clinical Experience

PUVA is 36 years old. The PUVA discovery stimulated research concerning all aspects of psoralens; 790 publications appeared on psoralens in 1978 and 1979 alone. This burst of investigation can most accurately be termed a renaissance, since psoralens have been used for the treatment of vitiligo for over 30 years. A monograph on the chemistry, pharmacology, and toxicity of psoralens was published over 20 years ago.[3]

Several thousand patients have been treated for vitiligo with oral psoralens and with sunlight as the source of ultraviolet-A since the introduction of this technique in Egypt in 1947 by Dr. A. M. El Mofty. During this 36-year clinical experience, there have been virtually no reported side effects; however, infrequent side effects or common disorders, such as skin cancer, may have escaped attention, since there were no prospective studies and no follow-up reports. Moreover, the "new" PUVA involved the interaction of oral psoralen with an artificial high-intensity source emitting ultraviolet-A radiation. Eight years of experience with PUVA photochemotherapy using artificial ultraviolet-A irradiators have now been accumulated. Although the exposures are shorter with artificial irradiators than when sunlight is the source of ultraviolet-A, there is a larger number and greater frequency of treatments, and maintenance therapy may be continued the year around. These factors could change the incidence and type of side effects. Experience from the large clinical trials has shown that acute side effects can usually be avoided by careful dosimetry of drug and light.

The first 1380 patients treated in the mid-1970s are still being followed in the 16 centers, with physical examinations, serial eye examinations, and a variety of laboratory tests being performed. In the United States and Europe, over 5000 patients have been studied prospectively. PUVA is probably one of the most thoroughly monitored modalities ever introduced into dermatology.

The potential hazards of PUVA involve organ systems that are directly exposed to ultraviolet radiation and psoralen and diseases modulated by these systems. The organs directly exposed to PUVA include the skin, the eye, and circulating blood elements, including lymphocytes. The effect of PUVA on lymphocytes was first noted in a therapeutic setting; abnormal lymphocytes were cleared from the skin of patients with mycosis fungoides. In vitro acute exposures to PUVA result in decreased viability and function of lymphocytes. In vivo studies of the acute effects of PUVA on lymphocytes in humans have given conflicting results, but it is clear that circulating cells can be affected in normal persons and psoriatics. The largest study of PUVA-treated patients indicates no significant relationship between PUVA exposure and the risk of developing antinuclear antibodies.[4]

The potential adverse effects of PUVA on the skin can result from alterations in both epidermal and dermal components. PUVA alters all epidermal elements, e.g., keratinocytes, melanocytes, and Langerhans' cells. Dermal alterations occur in collagen, elastic tissue, and blood vessels. Many repeated exposures of skin to inflammatory doses of ultraviolet radiation from the sun or any other source lead to cumulative degenerative alterations in the tissue with accompanying histochemical changes and a clinical appearance described as "premature aging." Repeated phototoxic doses of PUVA over many years would be expected to add to these kinds of changes, which may not be completely reversible. This hazard must be considered when PUVA is chosen as a therapeutic option.

After 2.1 years of study, the 16-center American PUVA follow-up investigation, which enrolled 1380 patients, documented nearly a three-fold increase in the risk of cutaneous carcinoma in PUVA patients.[5] Now, after 5 years of prospective study, 85 of 1289 patients (7 per cent) have developed a total of 200 nonmelanoma skin cancers, including 65 basal cell and 135 squamous cell carcinomas—an average skin cancer incidence three times that expected in the general population. Squamous cell carcinomas, however, occur in a proportion that is significantly higher than expected in areas not normally exposed to sun, and the risk of squamous cell carcinoma is more than eight times that expected based on population rates. Further, the risk of squamous cell carcinoma after adjustment for age, geography, and skin type is higher in patients with greater exposure to PUVA. Also, the risk of squamous cell carcinoma is increased among patients with prior exposure to other carcinogens, including long-term ultraviolet-B radiation, ionizing radiation, and long-term tar therapy. This increase in risk among patients with prior exposure to other carcinogens is more marked in individuals with greater exposure to PUVA (more than 80 treatments) compared with similar patients with less exposure.[5] Honigsmann and collaborators also noted an increase in the risk of nonmelanoma skin tumors in PUVA-treated patients, but they observed that this increased risk was restricted to those individuals who had had prior exposure to arsenic, ionizing radiation, or methotrexate.[6] They failed to detect an increased risk among patients who had not been exposed to these agents. Moreover, other studies have failed to show an increase in cutaneous cancer in 2.1 years of follow-up.[7,8] Numerous case reports have documented the occurrence of multiple tumors and tumors in unusual locations following long-term PUVA therapy.

At this time, there is no evidence that PUVA-related tumors are more likely to metastasize than are tumors developing in association with exposure to solar radiation, but continued surveillance is required to insure that this will be the case for tumors developing after a longer latency period than has so far occurred. Cases of malignant melanoma in PUVA-treated patients have been reported, but the 16-center PUVA follow-up study has not documented a statistically significant increase in the risk of melanoma. Clinically striking pigmentary changes occur with prolonged therapy. In more than 20 per cent of patients enrolled in the 16-center study, the appearance of qualitatively moderate to severe densities of discrete macular hyperpigmentation on the buttocks (an area in which such changes are unusual in the absence of PUVA) has been noted. Studies of these lesions show that a PUVA lentigo has larger and more numerous melanocytes than does normal skin or a solar lentigo.[9]

Methoxsalen penetrates the lens of the eye after oral administration.[10] Unless the patient is adequately protected from ultraviolet-A during the 24 hours in which psoralens may be retained in the lens, the potential for photochemical interaction between psoralen and ultraviolet-A exists. Prolonged exposure or high intensities of ultraviolet-A alone can lead to cataract formation. When high doses sufficient to elicit striking cutaneous phototoxicity are used, PUVA can produce cataracts in animals. There are scattered observations that PUVA in therapeutic doses may carry long-term cataract risk in the unprotected eyes of patients. Lerman has noted enhanced fluorescence in the lenses of several long-term PUVA patients who did not use adequate eye protection.[11,12] The etiologic role of methoxsalen in the development of cataracts in PUVA-treated patients has not yet been defined. After 5 years, analyses of more than 5000 eye examinations have failed to reveal a substantial increase in the incidence of cataracts among PUVA-treated patients who used eye protection on the day of therapy. Ultraviolet-A–opaque sunglasses should be worn for a full day after ingestion of psoralens.

PUVA in Perspective

PUVA vis-à-vis ultraviolet-B. The place of ultraviolet-B phototherapy in the control of severe psoriasis has not yet been resolved. New high-intensity ultraviolet-B boxes, similar in size to PUVA boxes, have become available in the United States and Europe during the past few years. It is impossible to compare the efficacy and safety of high-intensity ultraviolet-B with those of PUVA or methotrexate for the control of psoriasis, because as yet there have not been large multicenter clinical trials using ultraviolet-B, and there are no published series involving more than a few patients in which there is adequate follow-up. It has been shown that for some patients with psoriasis, "aggressive" ultraviolet-B phototherapy (using frequent, high doses of UVB—up to 1.0 J per cm^2) is equal to PUVA for clearing; maintenance with ultraviolet-B using infrequent treatments, however, has not been possible thus far. Furthermore, the risks with high-intensity ultraviolet-B may be the same as with PUVA (e.g., sunburn cells, photocarcinogenesis, increase of sister-chromatid exchange, decrease in T lymphocytes, and so forth). The 50-year safety record of ultraviolet-B may not be valid because of the higher exposure doses being used at present. Also, there are inadequate follow-up data. Retrospective studies would indicate that ultraviolet-B phototherapy is also carcinogenic.[13]

PUVA vis-à-vis methotrexate. It is quite certain now that the hepatic fibrosis and cirrhosis that occur following weekly administration of oral methotrexate (2.5 to 5.0 mg at 12-hour intervals) are related to total cumulative dose.[14,15] In one series,[14] 11 of 43 patients receiving methotrexate, or 25 per cent, developed hepatic fibrosis that precluded further treatment with that drug. A liver biopsy is therefore mandatory in patients receiving over 2000 mg of methotrexate. (This dose is achieved in 33 months in a patient receiving three weekly doses of 5 mg.) Also, it is essential that patients abstain from alcohol, which appears to increase the risk of hepatic fibrosis or cirrhosis.[15] With these newly defined hazards of methotrexate, this therapy must be used only in disabling psoriasis and when there is no alternative therapy. One should be especially cautious in giving methotrexate therapy to patients under 40 years of age, who may require treatment for years.

No Technical Achievement or Scientific Advancement Will Ever Replace the Responsibility of the Physician

PUVA is effective in treating a growing number of dermatologic disorders (a partial list appears in Table 1). As with any successful therapy, it is not without side effects. Most short-term side effects are avoided by careful dosimetry. Each treatment adds, in small but finite measure, to the long-term risks listed previously. Continued prospective study of several thousand patients with severe disease gives us 5 years (and thousands of "PUVA joules") of "lead time" in discovering any additional unexpected long-term effects. These

Table 1. DISEASES RESPONDING TO PUVA

Disease	Number of Treatments to Clearing	Continued Treatment Requirements	Response Rate
Psoriasis	10–14	Yes, variable (0 to 60 per year)	90%
Mycosis fungoides	20–60	Yes, usually frequent; occasional remissions	80+% improvement; ? cures
Vitiligo	100–400	Not usually (if totally repigmented)	70% improvement
Eczema	20–60	Yes, frequent	<90% (aggressive therapy)
Lichen planus	10–20	Yes, variable	80+%
Urticaria pigmentosa	15–30	Yes	80+%
Polymorphous light eruption	10–20	Probably (each spring)	90+%
Actinic reticuloid	12	Yes	Several case reports
Palmar/plantar dermatitis	20–60	Usually	90+%

side effects would most likely be dose-related and could therefore be avoided in the more recently treated subjects.

The decision to use PUVA depends upon the benefit received and the number of treatments that will be required to achieve that benefit. If five exposures each year allow a person with polymorphous light eruption to resume a normal life, this is a small risk for a great benefit. Fifty treatments to induce clinical and histologic remission in early stages of mycosis fungoides seems a warrantable alternative to other forms of treatment. In many persons with disabling psoriasis, PUVA is far more effective than ultraviolet-B. PUVA is a logical alternative to methotrexate and, in many patients, requires little maintenance. Administration of hundreds of PUVA exposures for a period of years to treat a small area of psoriasis or vitiligo is not justified. There is no substitute for the judgment of an informed and concerned physician.

References

1. Parrish, J. A., Fitzpatrick, T. B., Tanenbaum, L., and Pathak, M. A.: Photochemotherapy of psoriasis with oral methoxsalen and longwave ultraviolet light. N. Engl. J. Med. 291:1207, 1974.
2. Epstein, J. H., et al.: Current status of oral PUVA therapy. J. Am. Acad. Dermatol. 1:106, 1979.
3. J. Invest. Dermatol. (Suppl.) 32:132, Feb. 1959.
4. Stern, R. A., Morison, W. L., Thibodeau, L. A., et al.: Antinuclear antibodies and oral methoxsalen photochemotherapy (PUVA) for psoriasis. Arch. Dermatol. 115:1320, 1979.
5. Stern, R. S., Thibodeau, L. A., Kleinerman, R. A., Parrish, J. A., and Fitzpatrick, T. B.: Risk factors and increased incidence of cutaneous carcinoma in patients treated with oral methoxsalen photochemotherapy for psoriasis. N. Engl. J. Med. 300:809, 1979.
6. Honigsmann, H., Wolff, K., Gschnait, F., Brenner, W., and Jaschke, E.: Keratoses and non-melanoma skin tumors in long term photochemotherapy (PUVA). J. Am. Acad. Dermatol. 3:406, 1980.
7. Lassus, A., Reunala, T., Idanpaa-Heikkila, J., Juvukoski, T., and Salo, O.: PUVA treatment and skin cancer: A follow-up study. Acta Derm. Venereol. (Stockh.) 61:141, 1981.
8. Roenigk, H. H., Jr., Caro, W. A., et al.: Skin cancer in the PUVA-48 cooperative study. J. Am. Acad. Dermatol. 4:319, 1981.
9. Rhodes, A. R., Harrist, T. J., Stern, R. S., et al.: The PUVA lentigo: Increased number of large, Dopa-positive melanocytes. J. Invest. Dermatol. 78:357, 1982.
10. Glew, W. B.: Determination of 8-methoxypsoralen in serum, aqueous, and lens: Relation to long-wave ultraviolet phototoxicity in experimental and clinical photochemotherapy. Trans. Am. Ophthalmol. Soc. 77:464, 1979.
11. Lerman, S.: Ocular side effects of psoriasis therapy. N. Engl. J. Med. 303:941, 1980.
12. Drake, L., Lerman, S., Megaw, J., and Gardner, K.: In vivo monitoring of ocular and cutaneous manifestations of PUVA therapy. J. Invest. Dermatol. 78:340, 1982.
13. Stern, R. S., Zierler, S., and Parrish, J. A.: Skin carcinoma in patients with psoriasis treated with topical tar and artificial ultraviolet radiation. Lancet 1:732, 1980.
14. Robinson, J. K., Baughman, R. D., Auerbach, R., and Cimis, R. J.: Methotrexate hepatotoxicity in psoriasis. Consideration of liver biopsies at regular intervals. Arch. Dermatol. 116:413, 1980.
15. Nyfors, A.: Methotrexate therapy of psoriasis: Effect and side effects with particular reference to hepatic changes. A Survey. Aarhus, Denmark, Laegeforeningens Forlag, 1980.

HAZARDS OF PUVA THERAPY

Elizabeth A. Abel, M.D.
Eugene M. Farber, M.D.

Photochemotherapy with psoralens and sunlight has been used for centuries in Egypt and India to treat certain pigmentary disorders. Photochemotherapy of vitiligo with artificial sources of nonionizing ultraviolet radiation has been available since the 1940s. However, it was not until the development of high-intensity long-wave ultraviolet (ultraviolet-A) irradiation sources that systemic PUVA treatment with 8-methoxypsoralen was introduced for psoriasis.[1]

There is no doubt that PUVA therapy is a highly effective treatment for psoriasis. This has been confirmed by several multicenter studies in the United States and in Europe.[2-4] Yet, we are also keenly aware that PUVA is a palliative form of treatment. Maintenance therapy is frequently administered in an attempt to prolong the remission; yet, despite continued treatment, psoriasis eventually recurs in most patients. At Stanford University, relapses occurred in 60 per cent of 130 patients in 1 to 6 months and in 93 per cent within 1 year; psoriasis developed on more than 5 per cent of the originally involved area of the body. For the young person, repeated intensive courses of PUVA therapy for flares of the disease would result in a high cumulative lifetime exposure to PUVA. As was true of x-ray therapy in its early stages, the safe upper limit of PUVA dosage is unknown. Major concerns with PUVA therapy are long-term side effects related to carcinogenicity, aging of the skin, pigmentary changes, immunologic alterations, and ocular toxicity (e.g., cataract production).

Although it has been almost 8 years since PUVA therapy was introduced for psoriasis, this treatment is in its infancy in many respects. There is still uncertainty regarding the exact mechanisms of action in psoriasis and other disorders, the most appropriate therapeutic schedule in terms of PUVA dosage and wave-band interactions and, most important, the full extent of long-term PUVA-related toxicity. It is well known that psoralen intercalates into cellular DNA and, with the absorption of a photon, forms monofunctional adducts to pyrimidine bases, which, with the adsorption of second photons, can form crosslinks with pyrimidine bases on opposite DNA strands.[5] Possible results of this sequence are DNA repair of the lesions, cell death, and mutation. DNA damage with resultant interference with cellular proliferation has been cited as a mechanism of action of PUVA therapy for psoriasis.[6] However, the extent to which other mechanisms play a role in the treatment effect is unknown. Such mechanisms might include cellular injury from phototoxicity, alteration of mediators of inflammation, immunologic events (e.g., lymphocytotoxicity), and melanogenesis.[5] Furthermore, the role of bifunctional and monofunctional adducts, in terms of efficacy as well as of mutagenicity and potential carcinogenicity, needs to be more fully defined.

There are important differences between the effects of psoralen photochemotherapy and those of ultraviolet-B phototherapy that may have relevance in terms of long-term toxicity. The melanogenic response from PUVA is deeper and longer-lasting than that from ultraviolet-B. This may be related to a change in distribution of melanosomes from a single to a dispersed pattern.[7] The time course of erythema following PUVA therapy shows a peak intensity at 48 to 72 hours. This may be delayed up to 96 hours, in contrast with 12 to 24 hours for the time of maximal erythema following ultraviolet-B exposure.[5] The time required for complete histologic response is also greater with PUVA than with ultraviolet-B.[8] Repair of ultraviolet-induced DNA damage differs with these two modalities. Ultraviolet-B–induced thymine dimers are repaired by classical excision mechanisms. PUVA-induced monofunctional adducts are subject to similar repair processes;[9] however, cross-links, which are rarely seen following ultraviolet-B exposure, may not be repaired by this system.[5] In a study in which the effects of single, equally erythemogenic doses of ultraviolet-B and PUVA were compared, the absence of thymidine incorporation caused by unscheduled DNA synthesis after PUVA treatment was unexpected. This might be explained by a prevalence of interstrand cross-links.[10]

Because the longer ultraviolet-A wavelengths penetrate more deeply into the skin, effects on the dermis are greater with PUVA than with ultraviolet-B. This may have relevance to the production of aging changes. Although the erythema dose response curve is much steeper with PUVA than with ultraviolet-B, acute toxicity can usually be controlled by appropriate dosimetry.[5] Chronic side effects, however, are a major concern, especially with regard to skin cancer.

There is considerable epidemiologic evidence implicating the role of solar radiation in the formation of skin cancer in humans. Artificial ultraviolet-B radiation and tar, which are components of the Goeckerman regimen, are known to be carcinogenic in laboratory animals. This treatment has been widely used for psoriasis since the early 1900s; there have been few reports of skin cancer associated with its administration for this purpose, however.[11] PUVA is also known to be mutagenic and carcinogenic in experimental systems.[12] Although PUVA therapy is a relatively new treatment, there is already clinical evidence of a significantly increased risk of skin cancer in certain predisposed PUVA-treated patients with psoriasis.[13,14] Squamous cell carcinomas predominate over basal cell carcinomas in such patients; the occurrence of these lesions on non–sun-exposed areas of the body adds to their significance. Stern and coauthors have pointed out the strong relationship between cumulative PUVA dose and the risk of nonmelanoma skin cancer. In patients with a prior history of exposure to cutaneous carcinogens, such as tar, light, and ionizing radiation, the frequency of squamous cell cancers is significantly higher after 80 PUVA treatments compared with less than 80 treatments.[15] Arsenic, which is carcinogenic per se, has been identified as an additional risk factor for skin cancer in PUVA-treated patients.[16] There are no reports of systemic metastases from PUVA-associated squamous cell carcinomas in patients with psoriasis;[15] however, Gilchrest has reported that a patient with mycosis fungoides who previously had been treated with electron beam died of metastatic squamous cell cancer following PUVA therapy.[17] Other investigators have not reported an increased incidence of squamous cell cancer following PUVA; however, their studies differ significantly from the 16-center study of Stern and coworkers in terms of PUVA dose, length of follow-up, and patient characteristics.[18,19] For example, in a study from Finland, patients with risk factors for skin cancer, such as a history of previous skin cancer or high sensitivity to sunlight, were eliminated from the PUVA trial.[19]

Stern's early data suggest that PUVA acts as a "promoter" of squamous cell cancer in patients previously exposed to carcinogens.[13,14] This view is further supported by findings of skin cancer or precancer in six of ten PUVA-treated patients with mycosis fungoides, most of whom had received prior treatment with ionizing radiation or topical nitrogen mustard.[20] The promoting effect of PUVA is thought to be a consequence of DNA damage, as evidenced by the rapid appearance of skin tumors in PUVA-treated patients with xeroderma pigmentosum who lack normal DNA repair capability.[21] Bridges postulated that suppression of immunologic surveillance in the skin may be a further mechanism for a "promoter" effect of PUVA. His concept is supported by studies in which transplanted ultraviolet-induced tumors grew in PUVA-treated mice but not in untreated animals.[22,23] Whether or not PUVA acts as a tumor initiator as well may not be known until a longer latent period has elapsed.

Premalignant lesions of actinic keratoses have been observed in PUVA-treated patients who had previously been exposed to arsenic.[16] In a study at Stanford University, actinic keratoses developed in 17 of 104 (16.3 per cent) PUVA-treated patients with psoriasis followed from 1 to 5 years.[24] In these patients, keratoses developed predominantly in sun-exposed areas, suggesting a possible acceleration by PUVA of actinically induced lesions. None of these patients had such lesions at the time of examination prior to PUVA therapy.

Histologic changes of the keratinocytes, termed epidermal dystrophy, have been observed by a number of investigators.[24-27] Epidermal dystrophy has been defined by Cox and Abel as any alternation in cell size or arrangement to a degree not seen in pretreatment control specimens from sunlight-exposed or sunlight-protected clinically uninvolved skin. In a follow-up report, epidermal dystrophy was observed in more than half of 70 patients 1 year or more following the onset of PUVA therapy.[24] Nuclear changes may represent evidence of disturbed chromosome replication, and focal disorientation of keratinocytes indicates disturbed maturation of cells. Because the minute foci of epidermal dystrophy histologically resemble actinic keratoses, there is concern for their premalignant potential. The fact that the dystrophic foci are small should not minimize their potential importance, since a clone of atypical cells that produces carcinoma probably arises from a single cell. Furthermore, the persistence of changes following discontinuation of PUVA therapy in some patients[24,26] suggests some basic alteration in the germinative population of keratinocytes that may continue to express itself over a long period.

In addition to changes in the epidermal keratinocytes, PUVA has been reported to have effects on other components of the epidermis and the dermis. Stimulation of melanogenesis is evidenced clinically by the deep, long-lasting tan of PUVA-treated patients. Ultrastructural abnormalities observed in the melanocytes of PUVA-exposed skin include altered mitochondria, swollen and distorted endoplasmic reticulum, and large lysosomes.[28] These changes were present in one patient 15 months after therapy had stopped.[28] Another pigmentary alteration is the frequent occurrence of lentigines on PUVA-treated sun-protected areas. Such lesions have not been reported following ultraviolet-B therapy. Melanocytic atypism, which has been observed in pigmented buttock macules following administration of PUVA, raises a concern that dysplastic nevi may be produced.[29]

Although PUVA may be effective for vitiligo,[30] paradoxically this treatment has been reported to cause pigmentary irregularity. A peculiar mottling with hyperpigmentation, depigmentation, and atrophy has been associated with previous overdosage of PUVA.[31] Irreversible hypopigmentation not related to phototoxicity has been observed by others.[32,33] A dual effect of PUVA on melanocytes in which overstimulation may occur is supported by the finding of increased intracellular lipid deposits, said to precede degeneration of cells, in melanocytes of biopsies from PUVA-treated patients obtained at the time of maximal tanning.[32] Neural factors may also play a role. Cutaneous nerve endings, which are not usually found in the epidermis, have been observed ultrastructurally to be in contact with melanocytes and keratinocytes.[7] Of interest clinically is the occurrence of a neuritic type of painful pruritus in certain PUVA-treated patients, some of whom were observed to have PUVA-related hypopigmentation.[34,35]

Changes related to Langerhans' cells following PUVA administration have suggested immunologic alterations. Studies have revealed either a depletion of Langerhans' cells in the epidermis[36] or an alteration of the structure of these cells,[37] depending on the histochemical (ATPase) or immunologic (Ia antigen) marker used. Langerhans' cells may be decreased following ultraviolet-B exposure as well.[38] An impaired dinitrochlorobenzene sensitization has been documented in PUVA-treated patients.[39] Altered cell-mediated immunity may be further evidenced by PUVA-induced inhibition of the epidermal cell–mixed lymphocyte reaction, which probably involves Langerhans' cells.[40]

Because ultraviolet-A penetrates more deeply into the skin than does ultraviolet-B, the effects of PUVA on the dermis may be considerable, including changes in circulating lymphocytes. Ultraviolet-B in addition to ultraviolet-A may cause a transient decrease in the proportion of T-lymphocytes, which is identified by the formation of E-rosettes.[38] Perhaps of greater immunologic significance are the studies of impaired mitogenic stimulation of lymphocytes from long-term PUVA-treated patients.[38] The possibility has been raised that the increased incidence of nonmelanoma skin cancer in certain PUVA-treated patients may in part be related to an immunosuppressive effect of PUVA.[38]

Dermal changes include a decrease in elastic fibers and subepidermal homogenization[31] in addition to irreversible compact fibrosis, or "pseudosclerosis," of the superficial dermis.[41] Dermal damage following PUVA administration is a frequent finding that has been confirmed by other investigators[7,42] and portends that premature aging of the skin is a risk of PUVA therapy. Focal amyloid deposits, which have been observed in the superficial dermis as an occasional complication of PUVA therapy, are of unknown significance.[43,44]

Ocular toxicity, especially cataract formation, has been cited as a possible major risk of PUVA therapy. There have been adequate studies demonstrating that the formation of cataracts in ultraviolet-exposed animals is augmented by the presence of large doses of psoralen.[45] Based on studies of Lerman and coworkers, psoralen may remain in the lens for 12 to 24 hours, with a risk of permanent binding to lens protein and chronic ocular toxicity, unless photic stimulation is avoided during this crucial period.[46] There are a few well-documented cases of PUVA-associated cataracts in which pre-PUVA eye examinations were performed. Kasick has reported bilateral punctate cortical opacities in two PUVA-treated patients who had had normal eye examinations prior to therapy.[47] Lerman has described additional cases.[48] In a group of 104 PUVA-treated patients with psoriasis who were followed at Stanford University for 1 year or more, nine developed lens opacities that had not been detected prior to therapy.[49] Anterior cortical lens changes were the most common type observed. In this group of patients, there were no cases of rapidly progressive cataracts or significant changes in visual acuity. It is recognized that because of the increased incidence of cataracts with age, it is difficult to attribute the onset of lens opacities in PUVA-treated patients specifically to their therapy. If cataracts are indeed a real risk of PUVA therapy, a significant increased incidence may not be apparent until after a long latent period has elapsed. Much attention has been devoted to the development of appropriate guidelines for eye protection during PUVA therapy. The revision of the original PUVA guidelines stresses the need for more stringent eye precautions.[50] According to the new recommendations, patients must wear ultraviolet-A–blocking wraparound spectacles on each day of PUVA treatment from the time of ingestion of the drug. It is strongly recommended that ultraviolet-A–blocking spectacles be worn on the following day of treatment as well.

Concern for long-term side effects of PUVA on the skin and the eye, initially based on in vitro and experimental studies, has been underscored by results of early clinical investigations. Data from the 16-center PUVA follow-up study in the United States support the hypothesis of a "promoter" effect of PUVA.[13,14] It is too soon to know whether or not PUVA acts as an initiator of skin cancer as well. Likewise, full effects of PUVA with regard to pigmentary changes, immunologic alterations, and eye toxicity may not be evident for many years. For this reason, PUVA is a more appropriate treatment for patients in the fifth to seventh decades of life than for those in the first two decades. However, Stern and Melski have noted that PUVA is less well accepted among elderly patients with severe psoriasis (greater than 70 per cent involvement), who are at lowest risk for the potential long-term toxic effects of PUVA.[51] Apparently, PUVA has not served as an alternative to hospitalization in this group.

The limited use of PUVA in selected patients according to established guidelines is of utmost importance.[50,52] It is essential to maintain careful records, to report any untoward side effects, and to monitor patients even after they have stopped receiving PUVA therapy. It is hoped that continued research in photochemotherapy and photobiology will result in PUVA modifications that will improve the risk/benefit ratio. The concept of combination therapy, such as PUVA plus retinoids or PUVA plus anthralin, is a significant advance that should increase total efficacy and decrease toxicity of each individual agent. Further areas of investigation include new psoralen derivatives, new irradiation sources, selected wave-band interactions, and new treatment protocols, such as split-dose PUVA.

References

1. Parrish, J. A., Fitzpatrick, T. B., Tanenbaum, L., et al.: Photochemotherapy of psoriasis with oral methoxsalen and long-wave ultraviolet light. N. Engl. J. Med. 291:1207, 1974.
2. Melski, J. W., Tanenbaum, L., Parrish, J. A., et al.: Oral methoxsalen photochemotherapy for the treatment of psoriasis: A cooperative clinical trial. J. Invest. Dermatol. 68:328, 1977.
3. Roenigk, H. H., Jr., Farber, E. M., Storrs, F., et al.: Photochemotherapy for psoriasis: A clinical cooperative study of PUVA-48 and PUVA-64. Arch. Dermatol. 115:576, 1979.
4. Wolff, K., Fitzpatrick, T. B., Parrish, J. A., et al.: Photochemotherapy for psoriasis with orally administered methoxsalen. Arch. Dermatol. 112:943, 1976.
5. Parrish, J. A.: Phototherapy and photochemotherapy of skin diseases. J. Invest. Dermatol. 77:167, 1981.
6. Walter, J. F., Voorhees, J. J., Kelsey, W. H., et al.: Psoralen plus black light inhibits epidermal DNA synthesis. Arch. Dermatol. 107:861, 1973.
7. Hashimoto, K., Kohda, H., Kumakiri, M., et al.: Psoralen-UVA-treated psoriatic lesions: Ultrastructural changes. Arch. Dermatol. 114:711, 1978.
8. Rosario, R., Mark, G. J., Parrish, J. A., et al.: Histologic changes produced in skin by equally erythemogenic doses of UVA, UVB, UVC and UVA with psoralens. Br. J. Dermatol. 101:299, 1979.
9. Kaye, J., Smith, C. A., and Hanawalt, P. C.: DNA repair in human cells containing photoadducts of 8-methoxypsoralen or angelecin. Cancer Res. 40:696, 1980.
10. Hönigsmann, H., Jaenicke, K. F., Brenner, W., et al.: Unscheduled DNA synthesis in normal human skin after single and combined doses of UV-A, UV-B, and UV-A with methoxsalen (PUVA). Br. J. Dermatol. 105:491, 1981.
11. Muller, S. A., Perry, H. O., Pittelkow, M. R., et al.: Coal tar, ultraviolet light and cancer. J. Am. Acad. Dermatol. 4:234, 1981.
12. Grekin, D. A., and Epstein, J. H.: Yearly review: Psoralens, UVA (PUVA) and photocarcinogenesis. Photochem. Photobiol. 33:957, 1981.
13. Stern, R. S., Thibodeau, L. A., Kleinerman, R. A., et al.: Risk of cutaneous carcinoma in patients treated with oral methoxsalen photochemotherapy for psoriasis. N. Engl. J. Med. 300:809, 1979.
14. Stern, R. S., Parrish, J. A., Bleich, H. L., et al.: PUVA (psoralen and ultraviolet A) and squamous cell carcinoma in patients with psoriasis. J. Invest. Dermatol. 76:311, 1981.
15. Stern, R. S.: Carcinogenic risk of psoriasis therapy. In Farber, E. M., and Cox, A. J. (eds.): Proceedings of the Third International Symposium on Psoriasis, Stanford, July 13–17, 1981. New York, Grune & Stratton, 1982, pp. 157–162.
16. Hönigsmann, H., Wolff, K., Gschnait, F., et al.: Keratoses and non-melanoma skin tumors in long-term photochemotherapy (PUVA). J. Am. Acad. Dermatol. 3:406, 1980.
17. Gilchrest, B. A.: Methoxsalen photochemotherapy for mycosis fungoides. Cancer Treat. Rep. 63:663, 1979.
18. Roenigk, H. H., Jr., Caro, W. A., et al.: Skin cancer in the PUVA-48 cooperative study. J. Am. Acad. Dermatol. 4:319, 1981.
19. Lassus, A., Reunala, T., Idanpaa-Heikkila, J., et al.: PUVA treatment and skin cancer: A follow-up study. Acta Derm. Venereol. (Stockh.) 61:141, 1981.
20. Abel, E. A., Deneau, D. G., Farber, E. M., et al.: PUVA treatment of erythrodermic and plaque type mycosis fungoides. J. Am. Acad. Dermatol. 4:423, 1981.
21. Reed, W. B., Sugarman, G. I., and Mathis, R. D.: DeSanctis-Cacchione syndrome: A case report with autopsy findings. Arch. Dermatol. 113:1561, 1977.
22. Bridges, B., and Strauss, G.: Possible hazards of photochemotherapy. Nature 283:523, 1980.
23. Spellman, C. W.: Skin cancer after PUVA treatment for psoriasis (letter to the editor). N. Engl. J. Med. 301:554, 1979.
24. Abel, E. A., Cox, A. J., and Farber, E. M.: Epidermal dystrophy and actinic keratoses in psoriasis patients following oral psoralen photochemotherapy (PUVA): Follow-up study. J. Am. Acad. Dermatol. 7:33, 1982.
25. Cox, A. J., and Abel, E. A.: Epidermal dystrophy. Occurrence after psoriasis therapy with psoralen and long-wave ultraviolet light. Arch. Dermatol. 115:567, 1979.
26. Ingraham, D., Bergfeld, W., Balin, P., et al.: Histopathologic changes in the skin after prolonged PUVA therapy and after discontinuance of PUVA therapy. In Farber, E. M., and Cox, A. J. (eds.): Proceedings of the Third International Symposium on Psoriasis, Stanford, July 13–17, 1981. New York, Grune & Stratton, 1982, pp. 457–458.
27. Niemi, K. M., Niemi, A. J., Juvakoski, T., et al.: Epidermal dystrophy in psoriasis patients with or without PUVA and with or without previous arsenic treatments. In Farber, E. M., and Cox, A. J. (eds.): Proceedings of the Third International Symposium on Psoriasis, Stanford, July 13–17, 1981. New York, Grune & Stratton, 1982, pp. 447–448.

28. Zelickson, A. S., Mottaz, J. H., and Muller, S. A.: Melanocyte changes following PUVA therapy. J. Am. Acad. Dermatol. 1:422, 1979.
29. Rhodes, A. R., and Harrist, T. J.: The PUVA lentigo: Increased number of large, dopa-positive melanocytes. J. Invest. Dermatol. 78:357, 1982.
30. Parrish, J. A., Fitzpatrick, T. B., Shea, C., et al.: Photochemotherapy of vitiligo. Arch. Dermatol. 112:1531, 1976.
31. Gschnait, F., Wolff, K., Hönigsmann, H., et al.: Long-term photochemotherapy: Histopathological and immunofluorescence observations in 243 patients. Br. J. Dermatol. 103:11, 1980.
32. Schuler, G., Hönigsmann, H., Jaschke, F., et al.: Selective accumulation of lipids in melanocytes during photochemotherapy. J. Invest. Dermatol. 76:427, 1981.
33. Todes-Taylor, N. R., and Abel, E. A.: Occurrence of vitiligo following PUVA therapy. Clin. Res. 30:161A, 1982.
34. Tegner, E.: Severe skin pain after PUVA treatment. Acta Derm. Venereol. (Stockh.) 59:467, 1979.
35. Miller J., Munro, D.: Severe skin pain following PUVA (letter to the editor). Acta Derm. Venereol. (Stockh.) 60:187, 1980.
36. Friedmann, P. S.: Disappearance of epidermal Langerhans cells during PUVA therapy. Br. J. Dermatol. 105:219, 1981.
37. Okamoto, H., and Horio, T.: The effect of 8-methoxypsoralen and long-wave ultraviolet light on Langerhans cell. J. Invest. Dermatol. 77:345, 1981.
38. Morison, W. L.: Photoimmunology. J. Invest. Dermatol. 77:71, 1981.
39. Moss, C., Friedmann, P. S., Shuster, S., et al.: Impaired contact hypersensitivity in untreated psoriasis and the effects of photochemotherapy and dithranol/UVB. Br. J. Dermatol. 77:377, 1981.
40. Morhenn, V. B., Benike, C. J., and Engleman, E. G.: Inhibition of cell mediated immune responses by 8-methoxypsoralen and long-wave ultraviolet light: A possible explanation for the clinical effects of photoactivated psoralen. J. Invest. Dermatol. 75:249, 1980.
41. Pierard, G. F., Franchimont, C., VanCauwenberge, D., et al.: PUVA and specific changes in the superficial dermis. In Farber, E. M., and Cox, A. J. (eds.): Proceedings of the Third International Symposium on Psoriasis, Stanford, July 13–17, 1981. New York, Grune & Stratton, 1982, pp. 459–460.
42. Zelickson, A. S., Mottaz, J. H., Zelickson, B. D., et al.: Elastic tissue changes in skin following PUVA therapy. J. Am. Acad. Dermatol. 3:186, 1980.
43. Greene, I., and Cox, A. J.: Amyloid deposition after psoriasis therapy with psoralen and long-wave ultraviolet light. Arch. Dermatol. 115:1200, 1979.
44. Hashimoto, K., and Kumakiri, M.: Colloid-amyloid bodies in PUVA-treated human psoriatic patients. J. Invest. Dermatol. 72:70, 1979.
45. Cloud, T. M., Hakim, R., and Griffin, A. C.: Photosensitization of the eye with methoxsalen. II. Chronic effects. Arch. Ophthalmol. 66:698, 1961.
46. Lerman, S., Megaw, J., and Willis, I.: Potential ocular complications from PUVA therapy and their prevention. J. Invest. Dermatol. 74:197, 1980.
47. Kasick, J. M., Berlin, A. J., Bergfeld, W., et al.: Development of cataracts with photochemotherapy. In Farber, E. M., and Cox, A. J. (eds.): Proceedings of the Third International Symposium on Psoriasis, Stanford, July 13–17, 1981. New York, Grune & Stratton, 1982, pp. 467–468.
48. Lerman, S.: Ocular phototoxicity and PUVA therapy: An experimental and clinical evaluation. Proceedings of the Seventh FDA Science Symposium – Photochemical Toxicity Symposium, March 16–17, 1981.
49. Abel, E. A., Haegerstrom-Portnoy, G., and Farber, E. M.: Ocular changes following 8-methoxypsoralen (PUVA) therapy for psoriasis. Presented at XVI International Congress of Dermatology, Tokyo, May 26, 1982.
50. Farber, E. M., Epstein, J. H., Nall, M. L., et al.: Current status of oral PUVA therapy for psoriasis: Eye protection revisions. J. Am. Acad. Dermatol. 6:851, 1982.
51. Stern, R. S., and Melski, J. W.: Long-term continuation of psoralen and ultraviolet-A treatment of psoriasis. Arch. Dermatol. 118:400, 1982.
52. Epstein, J. H., Farber, E. M., Nall, M. L., et al.: Current status of oral PUVA therapy for psoriasis. J. Am. Acad. Dermatol. 1:107, 1979.

Editorial Comment

Is PUVA the panacea for the "heartbreak" of psoriasis for which we have so diligently searched? Will this treatment enable us to wipe that dermatosis from the face of the world? Probably not, but it may be a step toward that goal. However, it should be remembered that PUVA is not an unmixed blessing. This treatment has been under investigation for a number of years; when its use becomes reasonably universal, new weaknesses and hazards may well become recognized. The high cost of the equipment may limit the spread of PUVA therapy from the armamentaria of the rank and file of practitioners.

The advocates of this modality announce happily that it has been accepted for use by the Food and Drug Administration, as if this acceptance indicates that PUVA is effective and safe. On the contrary, this sanction is not a guarantee. Furthermore, the FDA hesitated for years before granting its approval, which suggests that its blessing may have been given with a certain amount of reluctance.

The preceding articles have discussed the benefits and hazards of PUVA therapy. The really serious danger is the production of skin cancers. It is claimed that most of the subjects who develop such malignancies have had previous treatment with arsenic or radiotherapy or have had skin cancers in the past. In actuality, however, few people have been exposed to inorganic arsenicals. As far as radiotherapy is concerned, nothing is said in the available literature about the quality or quantity of the ionizing radiation nor the site to which it was administered in the unlucky individuals who subsequently developed cancers. It should be considered that before World War II, 40 to 50 per cent of patients consulting a dermatologist received radiotherapy. Furthermore, it is difficult to see how radiation therapy administered to the face would increase the risk of cancer on the trunk. Grenz rays are considered to be a form of ionizing radiation. Because of the lack of penetration of this type of radiation, its carcinogenic properties are minimal to none. Although the linear hypothesis presumes otherwise, it is doubtful that x-radiation is carcinogenic per se. (Too much radiation is admittedly carcinogenic, however.) This type of reasoning reminds me of the woman who was given x-ray therapy in New York and was afraid that her grandchildren in Seattle might develop genetic defects because of her exposure to the radiation.

There is another group who claim that skin cancers produced by PUVA therapy do not constitute much of a risk. It should be noted, however, that most of these cancers are of the squamous cell type and that they can metastasize and kill. Lund,[1] Graham,[2] and Freeman[3] have often been misquoted as stating that squamous cell cancers caused by sunshine do not metastasize. This has been denied by all three of these histopathologists. Rather, they say that skin cancers associated *histologically* with actinic keratoses do not metastasize. Winkelmann[4] goes even further, claiming that such sections should be classified only as "penetrating keratoses." Approximately 65 per cent of metastasizing squamous cell cancers occur on the face on the dorsa of the hands—areas of maximal sun exposure. I have seen one patient in whom PUVA therapy caused prickle cell cancers, which metastasized and probably caused his death. (Because an autopsy was not performed, however, this was not proved.)

A few papers have appeared that claim that skin cancer is more common in psoriatics than in other persons. They point to the large number of carcinoma-producing agents that are employed in the treatment of this disease, including tars, x-rays, and ultraviolet light. Traditionally, clinicians believed that the opposite was true . . . patients with psoriasis were *less* apt to develop such neoplasms. I have reviewed the records of 1000 patients in my practice with psoriasis and another 1000 with skin cancer. Only two names appear on both lists.

The proponents of PUVA hope to solve the problem of cancer production by decreasing the dose of ultraviolet light, adding methotrexate or systemic retinoids to their therapeutic regimen. Unfortunately, it is not well established that the production of skin cancer is dose-related. Further investigation should clarify this point.

Think It Over.

References

1. Lund, H. J.: How often does squamous cell carcinoma of the skin metastasize? Arch. Dermatol. 92:635, 1965.
2. Graham, J. H.: Precancerous lesions of the skin. Primary Care 2:699, 1975.
3. Freeman, R. G.: Histopathologic considerations in the management of skin cancer. J. Dermatol. Surg. 2:215, 1976.
4. Winkelmann, R. K.: Opinions. Schoch Letter 32:49, 1982.

CHAPTER **14**

ROLE OF PSYCHOSOMATIC INFLUENCES IN PSORIASIS

PSYCHOLOGICAL INFLUENCES ARE IMPORTANT IN PSORIASIS

Kenneth N. Epstein, Ph.D.

Documentation of the fact that psychological factors play an important role in determining the degree of disease or health in human beings has proliferated during the past 25 years. Investigators in this area are realizing that all states of health are related intimately to an individual's emotions, attitudes, lifestyle, and so forth.

Preliminary studies suggest that psychological factors may contribute to the exacerbation and the amelioration of psoriasis. Savin polled 48 patients with severe, chronic psoriasis and found that 50 per cent related worry to the occurrence of symptoms.[1] Farber and coworkers investigated 2144 patients; 40 per cent reported that their psoriasis occurred first during times of worry, and 37 per cent related exacerbations to worry.[2] Earlier, Epstein had noted that according to some clinicians, the disease commonly appears following a period of emotional upset, clears with a resumption of normal adjustment, and recurs during periods of stress.[3]

Unfortunately, most research efforts have failed to clarify the manner in which the mind and the body function together to produce the symptoms of psoriasis. Personality types have been studied in order to identify specific traits of people with psoriasis. Susskind and McGuire, using psychiatric interviews, found that psoriasis was not related to any single personality type. Also, they reported that psoriatics did not differ from the norm on the Maudsley Personality Inventory in terms of neuroticism.[4] Goldsmith and associates, using the Minnesota Multiphasic Personality Inventory, also failed to identify any one characteristic personality pattern for individuals with psoriasis.[5]

Another research methodology that has been unsuccessful in demonstrating the influence of psychological factors in psoriasis involves consideration of environmental stresses that intrude upon a patient. Baughman and Sobel[6] studied retrospectively the relationship of psoriasis to emotional upset over a 5-year period. To measure the degree of emotional trauma, they used the Social Readjustment Scale developed by Holmes and Rahe. This scale is based upon the occurrence of stressful life events, such as "death of a spouse," "taking a vacation," "losing a job," and so forth, which are reported by the patient to have occurred during each of the preceding 5 years. To measure the degree of psoriasis, Baughman and Sobel used their own Psoriasis Severity Scale,[7] which is based upon the occurrence of symptoms of psoriasis. The data obtained from each of these two questionnaires were analyzed to determine the degree of correlation between annual stress and severity of psoriasis. The mean degree of correlation for the entire sample was found to be of insignificant magnitude.

This study is fraught with methodologic problems. First, measures of the severity of

200

both stress and psoriasis depended upon the patient's ability to remember and report accurately for up to 5 years. Patients are notoriously unreliable in this regard. Furthermore, this methodology ignores the way in which the subject copes with stressful life events. It considers stress to be an independent entity existing outside of the individual and affecting everyone in the same manner, regardless of such variables as the significance of the event to the individual, his ego and coping style, and so forth. What may be more important than the simple occurrence of these global life events could be what happens hour by hour and day by day in the life of an individual as he interacts with his unique personality style in a variety of settings.[8]

In considering the effect of psychological factors on psoriasis, one must be aware that the cause and the effect are not noted simultaneously. As an example, alcohol can aggravate this cutaneous condition to an astounding degree, but the evidence of the exacerbation does not occur until as long as 6 weeks after the cessation of the alcohol consumption. The proof that this, or any other agent, is important in the etiology of the disease can be difficult to establish. However, when exposure to the etiologic agent occurs repeatedly, its importance becomes apparent.

To summarize, attempts to study the relationship between personality variables or stress and psoriasis have probably been unsuccessful because of methodologic difficulties. By artificially isolating the personality of an individual from its environmental influences and then studying either of these two variables in isolation, the investigators have failed to recognize the important interactional relationship. When one studies the role of personality and environmental factors in psoriasis, it is necessary to examine these variables as they relate both to each other and to physiologic factors existing in the individual with the disease. Similarly, researchers who try to identify precise steps along a chain of physiologic and biochemical events fail because they do not consider the many ways in which intervening psychological and social variables influence the pathway. Current treatments may alleviate symptoms but leave untouched the strains that produced the disease and those that continue to render the patient susceptible to it. Baughman and Sobel concluded their study of the role of stress and strain in psoriasis by emphasizing the need to delineate a measurable phenomenon that might mediate the pathway through which changes in emotional arousal influence the lesions of psoriasis.[6]

There are many ways by which psychological factors can influence the progression of a disease such as psoriasis at virtually any step in its etiology. The mind is influenced by and affects the endocrine system, the degree of sympathetic and parasympathetic arousal in the nervous system, the distribution of blood to the different parts of the body, the degree of tightness in the musculature, the effectiveness of the immunologic response, and so forth, all of which are linked to changes in the hypothalamus, the reticular formation, the limbic system, and the caudate nucleus. Indeed, there is an intimate association between the body and the mind, and the ways in which they interact upon each other are so numerous that it would be surprising to find any physical or psychological aspect of an organism that could exist without substantial antecedents from and effects upon the entire person as a holistic unit. Those who argue that either the mind or the body functions independently of the other or that pathologies in either area can exist without important changes in the other are becoming more and more isolated; many studies that contradict these theories have been conducted within interdisciplinary fields.

In an attempt to examine simultaneously both psychological and physiologic variables as an adjunct to standard medical treatments, I used biofeedback training and relaxation techniques to study psoriasis.[9] Biofeedback refers to the use of an electronic device to monitor a bodily process that is ordinarily outside the patient's awareness. When a person becomes aware of his own internal state through the aid of the biofeedback equipment, he can learn to modify it through voluntary means. Biofeedback is a potent new means of alleviating a wide range of psychosomatic symptoms. Using skin temperature biofeedback and relaxation techniques for 1 month, patients were able to reduce the severity of their psoriasis, as measured by the Psoriasis Severity Scale,[7] by 41 per cent, compared with only 7 per cent for a control group. Further, during the treatment period, skin temperature was monitored in order to investigate the role that it might play in mediating the course of the disease. It was found that the group instructed in relaxation and skin temperature biofeedback techniques increased their skin temperature in comparison with the control group. Also, those patients in whom psoriasis improved (whether or not they received biofeedback) experienced a greater increase in mean skin temperature than did the individuals in whom the psoriasis did not improve. Rises in skin temperature are accomplished by vasodilation of the arterioles of the skin. Although this study by itself does not prove that vascular changes truly contribute to the disease process, there is evidence from other studies to support this hypothesis.[10-14]

Vasoconstriction at the periphery can be regarded as part of the fight-or-flight response of the body to stress. There is an instinctive vasoconstriction at the periphery that is part of an overall psychophysiologic response whereby the organism builds up the energy necessary to battle with or to flee from a threatening event. However, the social pressures of modern societies frequently discourage behaviors that lead to the release of the built-up energy either through physical means or through the expression of emotion in other ways. Consequently, because of the individual's need to adapt to his environment, he may frequently not obtain a satisfactory discharge and may experience instead prolonged tension, which may include chronic vasoconstriction at the periphery. In people who are prone to develop psoriasis, chronic vasoconstriction at the periphery may lead to the signs and symptoms of this disease. "Diseases of adaptation" (a term coined by Hans Selye[15]) include those diseases that result when the body mobilizes to engage in fight-or-flight responses but is prevented from acting out these behaviors. If psoriasis is influenced by the prolonged constriction of the blood vessels of the skin, then it may be usefully regarded as a "disease of adaptation."

Vasoconstriction at the periphery prevents the free flowing of blood through the body. On one level, this infringement upon the movement of blood restricts the flow of oxygen and other metabolites to the tissues as well as the transportation of the waste products of local metabolism. However, on another level, blood is more than simply a medium that carries important biochemical products. Blood is also an energetically charged fluid that adds life, warmth, and excitement to parts of the body. Lowen[16] regards blood as the representative and carrier of Eros, since sexual excitement is accompanied by increased blood flow to the periphery, especially to the erogenous zones, such as the lips, the nipples, the genitalia, and so forth. For example, when these parts of the body become suffused with blood, an individual typically feels warm, loving, and excited. The flow of blood also can be viewed as accompanying other emotions when it follows different channels and excites different areas. For example, the feeling of anger is sometimes experienced in the body as an upsurge of heat that is carried by the blood into the regions of the abdomen, the chest, and the head. The well-known expression "hot under the collar" is possibly derived from this sensation.

The free movement of blood through the body as it carries (or is carried by) excitement is an important aspect of the quality of a person's emotional life.[17] Disturbances in this flow are accomplished by an inhibition of vegetative expansion at the peripheral blood vessels. Since the free flowing of blood is critical in transporting feelings through the body, its chronic blockage entails serious consequences from a psychological as well as a physiologic perspective. Psychologically, the chronic contraction of the smooth muscles surrounding the arterioles can be viewed as a suppression of feelings, since in the absence of movement there is nothing to sense or to feel. From a physiologic perspective, there is a restriction of the normal transporting of blood to the tissues and, consequently, in the nourishing and cleansing of these tissues. This aberration impairs the normal functioning of the skin, and this may be involved in the etiology of psoriasis.

The symptoms of psoriasis cannot be understood or analyzed individually; they should be examined only in connection with the overall functioning of the body and particularly in relation to the feelings of pleasure and pain as they are experienced or suppressed in the personality as a whole. A truly successful treatment of this disease therefore would need to address not only the chronic vasoconstriction in the arterioles but also the relationship of the individual to himself and to his environment. In other words, a complete cure would restore healthy functioning at both the psychological and the physical levels simultaneously.

Relaxation and skin temperature biofeedback training appears to reduce the symptoms of psoriasis by initiating changes in the organism that probably take place at many levels at the same time and include alterations in the peripheral vasculature. Since cortical, vascular, and muscular symptoms tend to operate in unity, the interventions affect all levels simultaneously. The changes that occur at the vascular level relieve the tension experienced by the individual. This may contribute to the alleviation of the disease process.

Individuals may be able to use stress reduction techniques, such as relaxation and skin temperature biofeedback training, in conjunction with routine medical treatments to help alleviate the symptoms of psoriasis. Since conventional treatment modalities can entail the risk of serious side effects and can be expensive, the introduction of these relaxation techniques could provide a significant contribution to the control and treatment of this prevalent disease.

References

1. Savin, J. A.: Patient beliefs about psoriasis. St. John's Hosp. Dermatol. Soc. 56:139, 1970.
2. Farber, E. M., Bright, R. D., and Nall, M. L.: Psoriasis. Arch. Dermatol. 98:248, 1968.
3. Epstein, E.: Self-produced dermatoses. Trauma 5:3, 1965.
4. Susskind, W., and McGuire, R. J.: The emotional factors in psoriasis. Scott. Med. J. 4:503, 1959.
5. Goldsmith, L. A., Fisher, M., and Wacks, J.: Psychological characteristics of psoriatics. Arch. Dermatol. 100:674, 1969.
6. Baughman, R., and Sobel, R.: Psoriasis, stress and strain. Arch. Dermatol. 103:599, 1971.
7. Baughman, R., and Sobel, R.: Psoriasis, a measure of severity. Arch. Dermatol. 101:390, 1970.
8. Lazarus, R. S.: A strategy for research on psychological and social factors in hypertension. J. Human Stress 4:35, 1978.
9. Epstein, K.: The Use of Skin Temperature Biofeedback in the Treatment of Psoriasis, Ph.D. dissertation, California School of Professional Psychology, Berkeley, 1979.
10. Ormsby, O., and Montgomery, H.: Diseases of the Skin. Philadelphia, Lea & Febiger, 1954.
11. Kulka, J. P.: Microcirculatory impairment as a factor in inflammatory tissue damage. Ann. N.Y. Acad. Sci. 116:1018, 1964.
12. Braverman, I. M.: Electron microscopic studies of the microcirculation in psoriasis. J. Invest. Dermatol. 59:91, 1972.
13. Braverman, I. M., and Yen, A.: Microcirculation in psoriatic skin. J. Invest. Dermatol. 62:493, 1974.
14. Braverman, I. M., and Yen, A.: Ultracirculation of the human dermal microcirculation. J. Invest. Dermatol. 68:44, 1977.
15. Selye, H.: The Stress of Life. New York, McGraw-Hill Book Co., 1956.
16. Lowen, A.: Physical Dynamics of Character Structure. New York, Grune & Stratton, 1958.
17. Lowen, A.: Bioenergetics. New York, Penguin Books, 1975.

EFFECT OF PSYCHOSOMATIC INFLUENCES ON PSORIASIS

Richard D. Baughman, M.D.

The dynamic interaction of psyche and soma in patients suffering from cutaneous disease confronts the physician regularly, especially in a process such as psoriasis, which is chronic, visible, genetically determined, and influenced by a variety of environmental, internal, and therapeutic factors. If emotional factors are related to psoriasis, do they represent cause, effect, or both in a vicious cycle? Like so many other clinicians, I had been taught that stress aggravates psoriasis, and patients are certainly conditioned to that attitude, as evidenced by such gratuitous comments as "It must be my nerves, isn't it?" Specific studies of patients' (subjective) attitudes reflect that 40 to 80 per cent consider worry, stress, disturbing life events, or emotionally charged events to be associated with the onset or flare-up of psoriasis. In the late 1960s, I began collaborative efforts with a psychoanalyst, Dr. Raymond Sobel, who was then demonstrating a positive correlation between stressful life events and the onset of a variety of somatic illnesses and events, such as motorcycle accidents. We tried to quantitate severity of psoriasis and to compare that score with standardized measures of life stress in a large population of patients whose psoriasis was severe enough to warrant hospitalization. Our work and a review of the subject were presented at the Second International Symposium on Psoriasis in 1976.[1]

We demonstrated that over a 5-year period there is a mild but statistically significant correlation between stress and psoriasis, and we identified those individuals with a high correlation as "stress reactors." We were unable to differentiate these "stress reactors" from those individuals with no correlation or those who seemed to thrive on stress according to any of the following: age, sex, religion, marital status, socioeconomic status, severity of psoriasis, or severity of stress. Furthermore, we were unable to identify any "psoriatic personality" according to Cattell's "Sixteen Personality Factor Questionnaire"; nor were we able to find any personality characteristic peculiar to a "stress reactor." If nothing else, I hope these studies will negate the existence of any pejorative and simplistic label, such as "psoriatic personality."

Since our initial unsuccessful attempts to characterize stress reactors had focused on intrapsychic factors, we turned our attention to interactive factors, such as family disorganization or disturbed parent-child relationships, which appeared to be the best predictors of accidental poisoning in toddlers and automobile accidents in teenagers. We employed three approaches to study an additional 48 patients: (1) a standardized questionnaire—the Structured and Scaled Interview to Assess Maladjustment (SSIAM), (2) a psychiatric interview, including a life history, with a specific emphasis on "coping style," and (3) in-depth, open-ended psychoanalytic interviews in a subgroup. Again, we found that a population with psoriasis, even including cases severe enough for hospitalization, did not appear to differ greatly from the normal population in these three measures of interactive factors.

We also encountered a lower incidence of alcoholism than expected among our patients, which led us to challenge another tenaciously held dogma; namely, that the severity of psoriasis is related to alcohol ingestion. By this time, a great deal of information had been accumulated concerning patients with cases of psoriasis that were severe enough to warrant inclusion in the early PUVA studies. Landeen, Maloney, Stern, and I[2] therefore examined laboratory and questionnaire data from the 16-center Oral Methoxsalen Photochemotherapy Cooperative Clinical Trial and a subgroup from that trial at the Dartmouth-Hitchcock Medical Center in an attempt to find any correlation between alcohol ingestion and severity of psoriasis in this group of closely followed, severely afflicted individuals. *No correlation* could be shown between alcohol use and (1) skin type, (2) age, (3) extent of psoriasis prior to administration of PUVA, (4) number of treatments or quantity of exposure to achieve clearing, (5) continuation in the study after 3 years, or (6) percentage of skin involved after 3 years. Determination of liver function correlated well with alcohol histories. The only way in which heavy alcohol users could be differentiated from nonusers was that the heavy users tended to have received a few more PUVA treatments over a long period.

What about the influence of psoriasis on the psyche? Other studies reviewed[1] indicated that people with psoriasis experience a bothersome incidence of disturbances, such as depression, contemplation of suicide, difficulty in establishment of social contacts and relationships, and difficulty in sexual adjustments. There is no more moving story of the meaning of psoriasis and its treatment than Updike's "Journal of a Leper,"[3] which is required reading in our program.

Do these negative or marginal studies of *populations* mean that there is no significant causal relationship between malfunctions in psyche and soma in *individuals* with psoriasis? The answer is no. In attempts to generalize from the specific we can lose track of the fact that psoriasis is a multifactorial heterogeneous disease with different determinants in different individuals at different times. Not *all* people with the genetic capacity for psoriasis respond to *each* episode of streptococcal pharyngitis with a guttate flare, but the relationship is frequent enough to establish causality. Similarly, not all people with the genetic capacity for psoriasis will respond to stress or alcohol abuse with a worsening of the disease. In fact, some thrive on stress and alcohol, whereas others clearly suffer.

We do not treat populations, we treat individuals. In those whom we identify as stress reactors, we should attempt to work out dynamics: Is the problem lack of compliance, secondary gain from attention, malingering, or a conversion reaction? In my own experience, severe events, such as automobile accidents or the death of a spouse, have most frequently been followed by significant flares, whereas low-grade chronic stress is poorly correlated with severity of psoriasis. Just as dynamics will not all be the same, the therapeutic approach must be tailored. For some, the relief of inpatient Goeckerman or Ingram treatment provides vitality for months or years until the next flare, whereas in others, the captivity negates the "clear skin" with which they leave. In yet another group, hospitalization fuels an anger-dependency cycle. Even when PUVA provides control, being "tied to it" engenders resentment when the patient becomes accustomed to normal skin but requires continuing treatment. Individual therapy, group therapy, hypnosis, and psychopharmaceuticals (including placebo) have been helpful for some (but beware lithium, in which the benefit in manic-depressive states can render the psoriasis unmanageable).

Perhaps most important is the recognition of the variety of ways in which this dermatosis can have a devastating impact on its host (how would each of us function differently with 30 per cent psoriasis?). Keeping that in mind, we may respond the next time to the query "Is it my nerves?" with an approach that is less pejorative than is allowing the patient the additional burden of thinking that his or her psyche is "to blame." A more appropriate response might be, "Of the many things that aggravate psoriasis, nerves may be one. Let us go through these factors and see how the psoriasis affects your life otherwise. Then we will see what we can do to improve your situation."

References

1. Baughman, R. D., and Sobel, R.: Emotional factors in psoriasis: Recent findings. *In* Farber, E. M., and Cox, A. J. (eds.): Psoriasis: Proceedings of the Second International Symposium. New York, Yorke Medical Books, 1977.
2. Baughman, R. D., Landeen, R. H., Maloney, M. E., and Stern, R. S.: Psoriasis and alcohol. *In* Farber, E. M., and Cox, A. J. (eds.): Psoriasis: Proceedings of the Third International Symposium. New York, Grune & Stratton, 1982.
3. Updike, J.: From the journal of a leper. New Yorker 52:28, July 1976.

Editorial Comment

The cause of psoriasis is unknown and, in fact, many etiologic factors may be capable of causing, precipitating, or exacerbating this dermatosis. In considering the importance of psychosomatic factors, one must keep in mind the different conclusions of the two previous articles. Certain problems exist that make it difficult to judge the importance of mental influences in the disease. Psoriasis is an erratic condition. This is particularly true with regard to its response or resistance to a given therapeutic approach. No treatment has been discovered that affects all psoriatics in the same manner. Furthermore, the eruption may clear spontaneously or may recur for no apparent reason.

Ingestion of alcohol may exacerbate the condition or may cause recurrences. Yet it is simple to demonstrate that there is an incubation period of approximately 6 weeks between the exposure to the liquor and the reappearance or worsening of the psoriasis. I have seen this occur in intermittent alcoholics. These individuals shun the drinks until someone forces them to have one or more cocktails. This results in a lessening of inhibitions, and the victim may drink continuously for as long as 6 weeks before "drying out." Then, after a hiatus of 6 weeks or less, the gross effect on the eruption can be seen. In all probability, there is an incubation period in those responding adversely to psychic influences. This interferes with the recognition of the effect of the mental stimulus.

Also, it should be remembered that the psoriatic need not be a psychotic; nor need he be a psychoneurotic or have the potential to become a neurotic. The type of psychic stimulus that often affects psoriasis is simple nervousness or unhappiness that we all feel. On the other hand, the incidence of psoriasis in mental institutions is high. Furthermore, one often sees severe eruptions of psoriasis developing suddenly and for the first time in elderly people who are in sanitaria, in contradistinction to the early appearance of this eruption in the "usual" patient.

The role of psychosomatic influences in psoriasis is still controversial. However, it seems likely that these factors are of importance in this disease.

Think It Over.

CHAPTER 15

THERAPY

TREATMENT OF PSORIASIS: USE OF CORTICOSTEROIDS

Herschel S. Zackheim, M.D.

Topical Corticosteroids

Topical corticosteroids continue to be the mainstay of treatment for ordinary plaque psoriasis. Vasoconstrictor assays indicate that ointment bases provide greater activity than do creams. However, patient preference largely dictates the choice of base. The use of plastic occlusion enhances the effectiveness of either form. A common misconception is that the plastic suit must be worn overnight in order to be effective. On the contrary, several hours are usually sufficient to achieve the desired hydration of the stratum corneum. Thus, the patient can put the suit on after supper and remove it and have a refreshing shower before retiring.

Solutions or gels are required for hairy areas, but even the most potent preparations may not budge thick plaques on the scalp. For this purpose, combination formulas with tar or keratolytics may be helpful, but intralesional steroids may be necessary. Pustular psoriasis of the palms of the hands and the soles of the feet and acute generalized pustular psoriasis are usually refractive to topical steroids. Similarly, nail involvement is influenced little by this therapy.

How Often Should Topical Steroids Be Applied?

Questions have arisen concerning the influence of the frequency of application of these agents on clinical efficacy and on the development of acquired resistance (tachyphylaxis). In view of the high cost of topical steroid preparations, this is a matter of no small concern. The concept of the stratum corneum as a reservoir for topically applied steroids that therefore favors slow absorption provides theoretical support for the possible effectiveness of infrequent applications.

Eaglstein and associates[1] reported that triamcinolone applied three times daily or six times daily was equally effective for various dermatoses. Similarly, Fredriksson and coworkers[2] found no substantial difference in results with halcinonide applied once or three times daily, although the onset of activity was more rapid with the more frequent schedule. Unfortunately, results with atopic dermatitis and psoriasis were lumped together in this study. On the other hand, Kaidbey and Kligman[3] found that three daily applications of betamethasone valerate were more effective than one daily application in a small series of induced *Rhus* dermatitis.

The suggestion has also been made that less frequent applications may diminish the tendency to acquire a resistance to the action of topical steroids. Thus, du Vivier and Stoughton[4] found that three daily applications of steroids for 4 days resulted in a diminution of the vasoconstrictor response. Following a rest period of 4 days, the response returned to its initial level. The acquired resistance to the vasoconstrictor effect may be related to the commonly observed acquired resistance to the therapeutic action of topical steroids (as well as other medications) following continuous usage. It is interesting to note that tachyphylaxis to vasoconstriction occurred more quickly with 0.5 per cent triamcinolone compared with 0.1 per cent. However, Harst and colleagues[5] found no better results in a small series of psoriasis patients when clobetasol was applied intermittently, as compared with continuously, over a 3-week period.

A recent study, by far the largest of its type, has attempted to come to grips with these questions.[6] Although some may view the conclusions with a jaundiced eye, since the report originates from one of the drug companies, this investigation appears to be excellently designed. In a double-blind, paired comparison involving 194 psoriasis patients, 0.1 per cent halcinonide cream applied three times daily gave significantly superior results to those obtained with one daily application over a 3-week period. However, the once-daily regimen was at least equal to the schedule of three daily applications in 47 per cent of cases. There was no statistically significant difference between the two schedules in the rate of development of satisfactory responses (e.g., development of tachyphylaxis).

Nevertheless, as was noted by the authors, nonequivalent doses (of necessity) were used. It is thus possible, as suggested by animal studies, that single applications of a higher concentration may provide as good a result as that obtained with more frequent applications of weaker strengths. Further clinical studies are needed.

Complications from Topical Steroids

When one considers the millions of patients and the tremendous amounts that have been used since the introduction of topical steroids some 30 years ago, one must regard these agents as the safest and most generally useful form of therapy in the history of dermatology. Nevertheless, a long list of complications has accumulated.[7,8]

The most serious side effects are ophthalmic, although fortunately these complications are rare. Ocular hypertension, glaucoma, and cataracts are known to occur following prolonged intraocular applications of steroids. Increased intraocular pressure and glaucoma have been reported in patients in whom topical steroids were applied to the eyelids and the periorbital region. Contamination of the conjunctival sac is the most likely mechanism, although absorption through the periorbital skin cannot be excluded.

The most common complication of topical steroids is cutaneous atrophy, and this is not limited to the fluorinated compounds. Intertriginous areas and those occluded for prolonged periods are particularly susceptible. Associated changes include purpura, telangiectasia, stellate pseudoscars, and even ulceration. Particularly distressing is perianal atrophy in patients treated for prolonged periods for pruritus ani. Overtreatment of diaper dermatitis has resulted in muscle as well as dermal atrophy.

Steroid rosacea is an iatrogenic disease secondary to administration of potent topical steroids. An initial favorable response in the patient with rosacea is followed by a papulopustular flare. Attempts to control the relapse with more potent steroids result in a more vicious rebound. Similarly, a high percentage of cases of perioral dermatitis are believed to have resulted from administration of fluorinated steroids. Topical, as well as systemic, steroids are acnegenic, and rebound pustular flares similar to those seen in steroid rosacea may follow the topical use of steroids for acne.

Miliaria and bacterial and yeast infections often occur in occluded areas. By suppressing inflammation, topical steroids may make superficial fungus infections unrecognizable ("tinea incognito"). Similar effects have been noted in yeast infections, and ordinary scabies has been converted to the Norwegian type. Prolongation of herpes simplex and molluscum contagiosum has been described. As a rule, pyodermas are not aggravated. Allergic contact dermatitis to topical steroids is rare but has been documented for triamcinolone and betamethasone.

Women are predisposed to develop hypertrichosis of the face from potent topical steroids. This may persist for many months after cessation of treatment. Hypopigmentation can also occur, although this is usually rapidly reversible.

With the advent of increasingly potent steroids, there is growing concern as to the possibility of pituitary-adrenal suppression from topical applications. Although in most instances this is detected only by laboratory abnormalities, clinical manifestations range from an impaired stress response to full-blown Cushing's syndrome. Such complications are most likely to occur with widespread use under occlusion. However, they have occurred without occlusion from some of the more potent compounds. Among those implicated are clobetasol propionate (not available in the United States), desoximetasone (Topicort), betamethasone valerate, triamcinolone acetonide, and others. Children are more susceptible to pituitary-adrenal suppression, and growth retardation may occur. Patients with hepatic or renal disease and hypothyroidism are also at increased risk.

The cost of potent topical steroids is high, but in view of some of the more serious complications from overuse, this may be a blessing in disguise.

Intralesional steroids are best regarded as an adjunct to topical therapy.[9] They are particularly useful for stubborn thick plaques of psoriasis on areas not particularly prone to atrophy, such as the scalp, the elbows, and the knees. A 1-ml syringe with a 30-gauge needle is preferred to the air-powered gun. The latter may cause unnecessary disruption of collagen and elastic fibers and has a higher risk of infection and serious accidents, including damage to the eye. The use of a syringe and a fine needle also permits more precise delivery of a defined dose. Triamcinolone, either acetonide or diacetate, is the drug of choice.

The same hazards that attend the use of topical steroids must be guarded against when intralesional preparations are used. The possibility of local atrophy from overdosage is great. Considerable caution should be used in areas where the skin is thin. The face, genitalia, lips, and buccal mucosa are particularly predisposed to atrophic change. The total dosage must be carefully monitored, because the possibility of pituitary adrenal suppression is as likely with intralesional as with topical therapy.

The controversy that surrounds the use of *oral versus parenteral steroids* is of little relevance to the treatment of psoriasis, inasmuch as the systemic use of steroids for this disease is generally frowned upon. Psoriasis is notoriously chronic, and any benefits that may accrue from systemic corticosteroids are short-lived. The patient soon becomes steroid-dependent and is at high risk for the development of all the well-known complications resulting from long-term use. Additionally, generalized pustular psoriasis occurs more often either in patients who are receiving systemic steroids or in those who have been recently taken off this medication. However, in life-threatening situations, administration of systemic steroids may be required.

References

1. Eaglstein, W. H., Farzad, A., and Capun, L.: Topical corticosteroid therapy: Efficacy of frequent applications. Arch. Dermatol. 110:955, 1974.
2. Fredriksson, T., Lassus, A., and Bleeker, J.: Treatment of psoriasis and atopic dermatitis with halcinonide cream applied once two-three times daily. Br. J. Dermatol. 102:575, 1980.
3. Kaidbey, K. H., and Kligman, A. M.: Assay of topical corticosteroids. Efficacy of suppression of experimental *Rhus* dermatitis in humans. Arch. Dermatol. 112:808, 1976.

4. du Vivier, A., and Stoughton, R. B.: Tachyphylaxis to the action of topically applied corticosteroids. Arch. Dermatol. 111:581, 1975.
5. Harst, L. C. A., de Jonge, H., Pot, F., et al.: Comparison of two application schedules for clobetasol 17 propionate. Acta Derm. Venereol. 62:270, 1982.
6. Sudilovsky, A., Muir, J. G., and Bocobo, F. C.: A comparison of single and multiple applications of halcinonide cream. Int. J. Dermatol. 20:609, 1981. (See also Commentary, Int. J. Dermatol. 20:594, 1981.)
7. Bondi, E. E., and Kligman, A. M.: Adverse effects of topical corticosteroids. Prog. Dermatol. 14:1, 1980.
8. Robertson, D. B., and Maibach, H. I.: Topical corticosteroids. Int. J. Dermatol. 21:59, 1982.
9. Callen, J. P.: Intralesional corticosteroids. J. Am. Acad. Dermatol. 4:149, 1981.

PSORIASIS AND THE SELECTION OF METHOTREXATE FOR THERAPY

Gerald D. Weinstein, M.D.

For patients with severe psoriasis, there are three major approaches to therapy: phototherapy with ultraviolet-B and tar (the Goeckerman treatment), photochemotherapy (PUVA therapy), and chemotherapy with methotrexate. The choice of which therapy to use in an individual case is based on many factors concerning the patient, the physician, and the availability of these and other less frequently used therapeutic modalities. Since all three of these modalities require extensive effort, great expense and, to varying degrees, risk to the patient, the extent or seriousness of the disease is an essential consideration in the selection of any of these therapies.

As a rule, most physicians will select the treatment with the *lowest risk/benefit ratio*. With currently available knowledge there is little doubt that the Goeckerman regimens involve the least medical risk to most patients. On the other hand, after 30 years of experience with methotrexate, we find that there is a significant hepatotoxic risk in certain patients, particularly those receiving high cumulative doses. This will be discussed in detail later. With PUVA the risk/benefit ratio is still an unresolved question. A significant incidence of skin cancers is being seen. This appears to be related to the cumulative PUVA dosage, but the long-term impact of this problem as well as the unknown possibility of any other side effects still requires one to have an open mind concerning the use of PUVA.

How does one decide which therapy of these three to recommend to a severe psoriatic? Some considerations are obvious. For a youthful patient, one would strongly lean toward Goeckerman therapy because of its long relatively safe history. In an older patient, there is a much lower risk for development of the long-term side effects that have been seen with methotrexate or PUVA. A past history of success or failure with any of the treatments will provide valuable help. The availability of any of the therapies either in the office of the community dermatologist or in a regional university or large medical center must be considered. The physical and psychological condition of the patient is important. The need for inpatient therapy versus the capability and desire for outpatient therapy will strongly influence both the patient and the physician. These and many other factors will lead to decisions made jointly by the physician and the patient after discussing the options. All three treatments are quite effective, at least initially, in a high percentage (75 to 85 per cent) of patients, but eventually some of the responders for unknown reasons become partial responders or even failures. It is then necessary to have good alternative treatments available for these patients.

With this background it is apparent that for the population of patients with severe psoriasis, these three therapeutic modalities should optimally be available. There is no best or first choice of these "big three" treatments for psoriasis. Each has a specific place in our armamentarium, and in many patients two, or all three, of these therapies can reasonably be used. This paper will highlight some of the principal considerations concerning methotrexate for psoriasis, but for specific details the articles cited in the references should be consulted.

Aside from methotrexate, several other "chemotherapeutic" drugs have been used for severe psoriasis. Most recently, mycophenolic acid and azarabine have had extensive clinical trials, but significant side effects prevented final approval by the Food and Drug Administration. Hydroxyurea is used occasionally in patients with liver disease who are unresponsive to other therapies. It has been suggested that this agent has a beneficial effect in pustular psoriasis, but this has not been adequately tested. Hydroxyurea, although available for treating various malignancies, is not approved by the Food and Drug Administration for psoriasis. The therapeutic index (benefits/side effects ratio) for hydroxyurea is much smaller than for methotrexate. The aromatic retinoid, etretinate, is currently being tested in several countries for potential use in psoriasis. Preliminary reports suggest clinical effectiveness in certain types of psoriasis, namely, erythrodermic psoriasis and pustular psoriasis. Because of significant toxicity it may well be several years before this drug is available for general use. At present, I am not aware of any other systemic chemotherapeutic drug in a clinical testing phase for psoriasis, and thus methotrexate appears to be the only such drug available for psoriasis in the foreseeable future.

Clinical Aspects

As indicated earlier, methotrexate is generally reserved for severe disease. A case of psoriasis is considered ''severe'' if one or more of the following characteristics are present: extensive recalcitrant skin involvement, physically or financially incapacitating disease, cosmetically disfiguring lesions, or severe psychological disturbance. Each of these criteria requires a judgment decision, for which there are no exact guidelines. The risk/benefit ratio of methotrexate must be weighed for each individual set of circumstances and must be compared with that of other available therapies.

After a patient has been selected as a candidate for methotrexate therapy, the pretreatment evaluation is of great importance. When taking the history and performing the physical examination and the laboratory evaluation, one should pay specific attention to the possibility of liver or renal disease. Since methotrexate is almost totally excreted through the kidneys, adequate renal function is essential in order for drug toxicity to be avoided. The blood urea nitrogen level and, particularly, the 24-hour creatinine clearance should be normal or near the normal level. Mildly impaired renal function, as frequently seen in older patients, can be offset by the careful use of lower drug doses.

After three decades of experience, researchers have found the liver to be the only significant site of chronic toxicity from long-term methotrexate usage. Within the patient's history, specific detailed information concerning alcohol consumption, past liver disease, arsenic intake, and diabetes should be evaluated. Although the standard liver function tests will sometimes elicit evidence of liver disease, too often (perhaps 50 per cent of the time) no laboratory evidence of hepatic fibrosis or cirrhosis will be found. Thus, a pretherapy liver biopsy has been necessary in most patients, since ''hidden'' cirrhosis is found in approximately 3 per cent of the population. In some situations, I will waive the liver biopsy requirement if there is no apparent evidence of liver disease (see Roenigk et al.[3]). These situations include anticipated short-term therapy of several months, medical contraindications to liver biopsy, patient refusal, and elderly patients in whom the long-term risk of hepatotoxicity is diminished by a limited life expectancy.

Methotrexate is used most frequently by the weekly triple dose[1] and the weekly single oral dose[2] schedules. In the triple dose schedule, methotrexate is given at 12-hour intervals for three doses, thereby providing a blood/tissue level for approximately 36 hours (the duration of the psoriatic proliferative cell cycle). Initially, a small test dose should be used for any schedule. We give one tablet (2.5 mg) followed by a second tablet 24 hours later as the initial dose. Each week thereafter, one tablet is added within the three 12-hour intervals, e.g., one tablet Monday night, Tuesday morning, and Tuesday night. The following week, two tablets, one tablet, and one tablet at 12-hour intervals will be given, assuming that no untoward side effects are present. In the average patient, by the time the dosage has reached two, two, and two tablets (5.0 mg every 12 hours for three doses), significant improvement is usually seen. I will generally maintain this dose for several weeks and then move the dose up or down according to the clinical response.

The single weekly oral dose is generally started with 5 to 10 mg and is increased by one tablet each week to a dosage range of 7.5 to 25 mg per week. If the intramuscular route of administration is used, the immediate blood level is higher but decreases more rapidly than that of the slowly absorbed oral doses. Therefore, the intramuscular doses are approximately 50 per cent higher than the oral doses for equivalent effects.

The triple dose and the single weekly dose schedules appear to produce equivalent clinical clearing, although no comparative study has been reported. Patient tolerance in side effects such as gastrointestinal distress or malaise may dictate a preference for one schedule or the other.

In the original study of the triple dose schedule,[1] it was noted that less drug is required with the triple dose schedule compared with the other schedules then in use. Thus, the triple dose schedule may result in a lower cumulative dose over a long period, thereby decreasing the risk of potential liver toxicity.

General guidelines for methotrexate doses are as follows:

1. Doses should be continually titrated for each *individual* patient.

2. One should try to reduce the dosage and to extend the off-drug intervals.

3. The goal of therapy should be *adequate* control with lowest dosages rather than complete clearing.

Methotrexate is effective not only in clearing psoriatic skin lesions but also in greatly helping the control of psoriatic arthritis. Most patients with psoriatic arthritis can be adequately treated with aspirin or nonsteroidal anti-inflammatory drugs. However, a small percentage of these patients have arthritis that is severe, progressive, and sometimes mutilating. Methotrexate, in the doses described earlier, is frequently effective for these patients and should be considered for treatment when the other usual antiarthritic drugs fail, even if there is only minimal skin disease.

Pustular psoriasis is a variant of psoriasis that is difficult to treat. For severe disease methotrexate is usually the treatment of choice, although unfortunately it does not work with the consistency seen when it is used to treat ordinary plaque-type psoriasis. Experience from several anecdotal reports suggests that for treatment of acute flares of pustular psoriasis, doses of methotrexate should be started on the low side and then gradually increased. In these reports, severe leukopenia was seen at "average" doses and when methotrexate was used in intervals of less than 1 week.

Long-Term Toxicity

Hepatotoxicity is the most significant long-term complication of methotrexate therapy for psoriasis. Both liver function tests and liver scans have been inadequate in predicting substantial changes in liver pathology. The accumulated experience has therefore made pre- and interim treatment liver biopsies necessary for the safest long-term use of methotrexate.

Recent studies indicate that the risk of fibrosis or cirrhosis increases with cumulative total doses as well as with other risk factors, including alcohol consumption, arsenic intake, previous liver disease, and diabetes. In patients *without risk factors,* the incidence of cirrhosis is quite low if the total cumulative dose is below 1.5 gm. Thus, in these patients the first repeat liver biopsy should be after a cumulative 1.5 gm, although in actual time this will vary greatly in different patients, depending on the weekly doses and the off-drug intervals during the year. In patients *with risk factors,* the liver biopsy should be repeated more often—after cumulative doses of approximately 1.0 gm. (Consult Roenigk et al.[3] for more specific details.)

In a study by Zachariae,[4] a group of patients who developed cirrhosis while receiving methotrexate were followed with repeated liver biopsies. Some of these patients continued to receive methotrexate. In general, the repeat biopsies showed no worsening of their disease and, in some cases, modest improvement. It appears that the clinical course of methotrexate-induced cirrhosis is, fortunately, not aggressive.

Other details relating to methotrexate usage are described in the listed references.[5,6] The evidence to date indicates that methotrexate is reasonably safe for use, at least within certain limitations. Thus, we can rightfully include it as an option in treating severe psoriasis, in addition to the alternatives of Goeckerman ultraviolet-B and PUVA. For some patients, we have advocated the periodic rotation of each of these modalities in order to decrease the exposure and the potential side effects of any one treatment for the individual patient. We are also fortunate that more effective therapies are available for severe psoriasis than for minimal psoriasis.

References

1. Weinstein, G. D., and Frost, P.: Methotrexate for psoriasis—a new therapeutic schedule. Arch. Dermatol. 103:33, 1971.
2. Roenigk, H. H., Jr., Fowler-Bergfeld, W., and Curtis, G. H.: Methotrexate for psoriasis in weekly oral doses. Arch. Dermatol. 99:86, 1969.
3. Roenigk, H. H., Jr., Auerbach, R., Maibach, H., and Weinstein, G. D.: Methotrexate guidelines—revised. J. Am. Acad. Dermatol. 6:145, Feb. 1982.
4. Zachariae, H., Kragbulle, K., and Sogaard, H.: Methotrexate induced liver cirrhosis. Br. J. Dermatol. 102:407, 1980.
5. Weinstein, G. D.: Methotrexate—diagnosis and treatment. Ann. Intern. Med. 86:199, 1977.
6. Weinstein, G. D.: Three decades of folic acid antagonists in dermatology. Arch. Dermatol. (in press).

PSORIASIS: THE GOECKERMAN TREATMENT

Harold O. Perry, M.D.

William H. Goeckerman outlined his treatment for psoriasis with the use of tar and ultraviolet light in *Northwest Medicine* in May 1925.[1] At that time, he indicated the salient features of the therapy: (1) Crude coal tar ointment is applied to the skin for 24 hours, (2) after 24 hours, most of the tar is removed by the use of an oil, (3) the patient is exposed to the ultraviolet light, (4) the patient is given a cleansing tub bath, and (5) the tar is reapplied. Goeckerman believed that the amount of ultraviolet light administered should be gauged by its effect on the skin. He advised producing a tan but avoiding severe sunburn. In his experience, patients could usually be relieved of their disease in 3 to 4 weeks.

Dr. Goeckerman recognized even then that the topical use of crude coal tar was more effective than was administration of other topical preparations. Moreover, he found that he could treat patients with acute psoriasis by this method without causing flaring of the skin. In his early studies, he compared the use of tar alone, the use of light alone, and the combination and found that the combination was more effective than was either component administered separately. This method of treatment has, of course, become known as the Goeckerman regimen. It has remained the mainstay of treatment for patients with severe psoriasis at the Mayo Clinic for more than six decades.

The method of therapy that we use has changed little from Dr. Goeckerman's original technique. However, we have made some modifications. If a patient presents with acute exfoliative psoriasis, it is our habit not to apply tar directly to the irritated skin. Rather, the patient is treated with wet dressings; topical steroid cream is applied before the wet dressings, which are then changed every 3 hours. Under most circumstances, 48 to 96 hours of such treatment reduces the acute flare of the psoriasis and permits progression to the use of the crude coal tar without irritation of the skin or flare-up of the psoriasis from the tar.

The tar preparations are applied to the skin two to three times a day, at least often enough to keep the skin continuously covered with tar. Although originally crude coal tar preparations were proposed by Goeckerman, over the years a variety of tars have been employed. Zetar, a modified crude coal tar, was popular for a time because of its better cosmetic acceptance. At times, various surfactants were applied with the crude coal tar as it was formulated in petrolatum in order to make it water-soluble and to permit easier cleansing of the skin. Various combinations of tar were applied for intertriginous use, such as 20 per cent liquor carbonis detergens in Nivea oil. A preparation consisting of 20 per cent oil of cade, 10 per cent sulfur, and 5 per cent salicylic acid in a water-soluble base is employed for therapy of psoriasis in the scalp. It is applied one to two times a day, and the hair is shampooed once daily. Rather than use the black tar if the psoriasis does not severely involve the face, we use a mild cream for lubrication. In other instances of very mild psoriasis, we use 1 per cent hydrocortisone cream. On still other occasions, we might use a steroid cream temporarily in an intertriginous area to reduce heavy plaques of psoriasis, and after this we use crude coal tar for at least 10 days. With this pattern of therapy, a rebound of the disease after the use of steroids alone is prevented.

At times, heavier and more resistant areas of psoriasis over the lower legs must be treated. A 3- to 4-day course of occlusive steroid therapy with Saran Wrap has been introduced into the program for localized areas in order to hasten the resolution of the heavier

Table 1.   AGE DISTRIBUTION OF
123 PSORIATIC PATIENTS TREATED
IN 1964 BY THE GOECKERMAN
REGIMEN*

Age	Male Patients	Female Patients
0–19	3	6
20–29	6	9
30–39	9	10
40–49	14	14
50–59	14	13
60–69	10	8
>70	4	3
Total	60	63

*From Perry, H.O., Soderstrom, C.W., and Schulze, R.W.: The Goeckerman treatment of psoriasis. Arch. Dermatol. 98:178, 1968. Used by permission of the American Medical Association.

plaques. The traditional tar and ultraviolet light therapy is administered for at least 10 days after the occlusive therapy so that the patient's skin is brought to a uniform degree of clearing.

The administration of ultraviolet light has really changed very little. The Hanovia alpine lamp is still used, and the entire body is exposed to minimal erythema doses of ultraviolet light, as originally recommended by Goeckerman. An additional measure that has been instituted is referred to as "spotting." This consists of outlining thicker and more resistant plaques of psoriasis wherever they might occur on the body with the use of paper or cloth toweling and exposing those thicker plaques to additional amounts of ultraviolet light. Areas commonly treated in this manner are the scalp, in which hair tends to filter out adequate light therapy, and the heavier plaques of psoriasis that usually occur over the elbows, the knees, and the lower legs. However, any area of the body might be managed in this way.

For initial therapy, patients are sometimes exposed to light in an ultraviolet light box for a few days before administration of the larger output of ultraviolet light from an alpine unit. This has been considered to represent only a time-saving feature of the therapy, and little consideration has been given to the alteration in the spectrum of light exposure that this involves.

In a study published in 1968,[2] we reviewed the medical records of psoriatic patients who were hospitalized during 1964 for treatment by the Goeckerman regimen. We found that treatment had been standardized as outlined previously. It was our goal from this study to determine the benefits of this therapy, the duration of hospital stay, the effectiveness in reducing remission, and the patient's satisfaction with the treatment. I am not aware of any similar study attempting to evaluate the Goeckerman program in this particular way. This study indicated that the therapy was indeed satisfactory, and this was true for patients of all ages, including the young and the very old (Table 1).

An effort was made to compare the remissions induced by the Goeckerman therapy with those that occurred spontaneously before the patients received the Goeckerman treatment. The average length of remission was increased by 1 year after the Goeckerman therapy. Similarly, the range in duration of remission increased as much as fourfold over that occurring spontaneously. We have always employed the median figure, however, in telling patients that they could reasonably expect a year's relief from their psoriasis after the Goeckerman therapy. This compares with one half year for the duration of spontaneous remissions (Table 2).

Table 2. REMISSIONS OF PSORIASIS BEFORE AND
AFTER GOECKERMAN THERAPY*

	Male Patients	Female Patients
Before Goeckerman therapy	21	33
Without remission	6	11
With remission	15	22
Length of remission (yrs)		
Average	0.6	0.5
Range	0.2–2.0	0.1–1.0
Median	0.5	0.5
After Goeckerman therapy	19	20
Without remission	0	1
With remission	19	19
Length of remission (yrs)		
Average	1.7	1.8
Range	0.2–8.0	0.5–5.0
Median	1.0	1.4

*From Perry, H.O., Soderstrom, C.W., and Schulze, R.W.: The Goeckerman treatment of psoriasis. Arch. Dermatol. 98:178, 1968. Used by permission of the American Medical Association.

The duration of hospitalization was correlated with the degree of cutaneous involvement (Table 3). The percentage of cutaneous involvement was estimated, and it was apparent that the greater the involvement, the longer the hospital stay. It also proved true that the longer the hospitalization, the greater the improvement (Table 4). Thus, there were direct correlations involving the severity of the psoriasis and the degree of improvement in relation to the duration of hospital care.

Patients' satisfaction with the therapy was assessed on the basis of their willingness to subject themselves to this period of hospital care for their disease. We have long recognized that some patients return every 1 or 2 years for therapy with the Goeckerman regimen. The remissions occurring with this treatment program are so satisfactory to patients that they are willing to spend the time and the money needed to obtain such a remission. Some who are in less favorable financial circumstances use their vacation time to obtain relief from their disease in this manner so that they can function with minimal attention to their skin in the intervening period. In this study, approximately 90 per cent of the patients traveled more than 100 miles for this care of their psoriasis. By comparison, in the general patient population registered in the Mayo Clinic Department of Dermatology, 60 per cent of the patients come from outside a 100-mile distance. Thus, in assessing the patient's desire for this therapy, we found a decided willingness to travel considerable distances to the Mayo Clinic for this purpose.

Table 3. DEGREE OF CUTANEOUS INVOLVEMENT AS COMPARED WITH DAYS OF
HOSPITALIZATION FOR 117 PSORIATIC PATIENTS TREATED IN 1964*

Cutaneous Involvement (%)	Hospitalization					
	Male Patients			Female Patients		
	No.	Days Average	Range	No.	Days Average	Range
<25	9	14.4	4–34	15	12.3	6–19
25–49	28	18.7	10–34	36	18.8	9–50
50–74	11	23.8	13–35	7	19.0	15–30
75 or more	9	24.0	13–51	2	42.5	21–64

*From Perry, H.O., Soderstrom, C.W., and Schulze, R.W.: The Goeckerman treatment of psoriasis. Arch. Dermatol. 98:178, 1968. Used by permission of the American Medical Association.

Table 4. DAYS OF HOSPITALIZATION REQUIRED FOR VARIOUS DEGREES OF
IMPROVEMENT IN TREATMENT OF PSORIASIS *

Improvement (%)	Hospitalization					
	Male Patients			*Female Patients*		
	No.	*Days*		No.	*Days*	
		AVERAGE	RANGE		AVERAGE	RANGE
<71	8	13.0	4–20	6	15.7	9–21
71–85	19	20.4	12–34	17	20.1	9–64
86–95	25	20.2	10–51	28	18.4	6–50
>95	5	24.2	16–35	10	16.1	8–29

*From Perry, H.O., Soderstrom, C.W., and Schulze, R.W.: The Goeckerman treatment of psoriasis. Arch. Dermatol. 98:178, 1968. Used by permission of the American Medical Association.

The question might be asked whether there are any complications from this treatment. I have earlier alluded to the possibility that a patient might be intolerant to tar and may react to its irritant effect. Some patients occasionally receive more than the minimal erythema dose of ultraviolet light and experience a sunburn. Those situations are uncommon and are not overwhelming contraindications to the continued use of the therapy.

A question is also often raised concerning the possibility of the development of cutaneous carcinoma in patients who receive the Goeckerman therapy.[3] Does tar or ultraviolet light (or both) cause an increased incidence of skin cancer in these patients? A recent survey by Pittelkow and coworkers[4] indicated after a 25-year follow-up period that the incidence of carcinoma in patients with psoriasis who had received the Goeckerman program was no greater than would be expected to occur in a normal population. A study by Maughan and associates[5] in a group of patients with atopic dermatitis who had received the Goeckerman therapy substantiated this finding.

The aforementioned findings contrast with statements made by others that an increased incidence of cancer has occurred with high exposure to tar and ultraviolet light.[3] These other authors, however, did not say whether such patients had previously received other carcinogenic modalities of therapy, such as x-ray, chemotherapeutic agents, or arsenic. Thus, the studies as reported may not be comparable.

Controversy has existed concerning the exact role of tar and of light in the Goeckerman program. Studies are available[6] indicating that the topical use of tar in the Goeckerman regimen does not seem to offer any particular benefit over the use of the petrolatum base alone. On the other hand, these same authors found that light therapy alone results in improvement of the psoriasis but not complete clearing. For clearing to be achieved, one has to combine moderately aggressive exposure to ultraviolet light with topical tar therapy.

The spectrum of ultraviolet light in the Goeckerman therapy has been studied.[7] The most effective therapeutic ranges are in the region of 296 to 313 nm. The use of less than 296 nm in the phototherapy of psoriasis is not very effective, even when the light is applied for increased exposure times.

The Goeckerman regimen continues to work effectively in clearing the skin and in providing a high degree of satisfaction among our patient population. Although we are aware of variations that have been proposed in the therapeutic use of this modality, our clinical success with the therapy has prompted us to continue to use it in the standard way. However, it becomes clear to us that many variations are used elsewhere when we study patients who have received the Goeckerman therapy in their local hospitals by their local physicians. When we discuss our approach with patients entering into our program, they tend to advise us how different our method is from the one they received elsewhere. Variations occur in the frequency with which the tar is applied to the skin, the color of the tar used and the extent of its application, and the degree of ultraviolet light that is administered. Thus, it is obvious that the administration of this therapy is far from standard.

Application of the Goeckerman regimen for outpatient management of psoriasis with the use of only a white petrolatum base and ultraviolet radiation has been proposed.[8] A recent summary of treatment programs by Cram[9] evaluates the standard Goeckerman program as described against the various modifications recommended. His belief substantiates ours, namely, that comparable results in therapy are not obtained unless the more standard program, including the use of crude coal tar and minimal erythema doses of ultraviolet light, is administered, as initially suggested. Like us, Cram believes that the Goeckerman program—whether carried out in the traditional manner in the hospital or on a modified outpatient basis—is consistently efficacious in most patients, for whom it provides long remissions with relative safety.

Over the years, numerous advances have been made in the therapy of psoriasis. There can be no doubt that the use of chemotherapeutic agents and the PUVA therapy (psoralen and long-wave ultraviolet light) are beneficial for selected patients. There are advantages and disadvantages to each of these methods. We are indeed fortunate to have all of them available for use.

Of all of the chemotherapeutic agents, methotrexate has been the single most effective drug and is the one that is employed most often for the management of very severe psoriasis.[10] Some 15 years ago, methotrexate was used almost indiscriminately, but sufficient guidelines for the use of this drug have been established to insure that relatively few patients now receive this potent drug as the primary therapeutic approach. Similarly, PUVA therapy, which enjoyed an initial burst of enthusiasm, continues to be used at our institution but at approximately 50 per cent of its level of use some 2 years ago.

In an effort to assess the frequency of use of the major modalities of therapy for severe psoriasis, namely, the Goeckerman regimen and PUVA therapy, we reviewed the records of patients seen at the Mayo Clinic for psoriasis during 1981. The medical record retrieval system permitted us to obtain statistics concerning approximately 96 per cent of the patients for that year. We saw 1230 patients with psoriasis during that period. About 220 of these patients were hospitalized for treatment by the Goeckerman program, and approximately 50 patients received PUVA therapy. These numbers exclude pustular psoriasis of the palms of the hands and the soles of the feet first described by Barber. The remaining patients were managed by other topical measures and did not require either of these more aggressive approaches. Thus, in our institution, the Goeckerman regimen remains the major therapeutic approach for the patient with severe psoriasis.

Again, these data emphasize that a substantial number of patients are willing to subject themselves to the isolation of hospitalization and the expense involved to obtain the beneficial results that are possible with the use of Goeckerman therapy. This is particularly true for patients with extensive psoriasis that disables them from performing their usual work or physical activity or those whose psoriasis represents a cosmetic disability. For such patients, the return to a productive life and a normal life style is worth the inconvenience and expense of hospitalization. Our studies indicate the absence of any significant long-term complications, including the development of skin cancer. Thus, we continue to use this treatment as a major therapeutic approach for selected psoriatic patients with severe and disabling disease.

References

1. Goeckerman, W. H.: The treatment of psoriasis. Northwest Med. 24:229, 1925.
2. Perry, H. O., Soderstrom, C. W., and Schulze, R. W.: The Goeckerman treatment of psoriasis. Arch. Dermatol. 98:178, 1968.

3. Stern, R. S., Zierler, S., and Parrish, J. A.: Skin carcinoma in patients with psoriasis treated with topical tar and artificial ultraviolet radiation. Lancet 1:732, 1980.
4. Pittelkow, M. R., Perry, H. O., Muller, S. A., Maughan, W. Z., and O'Brien, P. C.: Skin cancer in patients with psoriasis treated with coal tar: A 25-year follow-up study. Arch. Dermatol. 117:465, 1981.
5. Maughan, W. Z., Muller, S. A., Perry, H. O., Pittelkow, M. R., and O'Brien, P. C.: Incidence of skin cancers in patients with atopic dermatitis treated with coal tar: A 25-year follow-up study. J. Am. Acad. Dermatol. 3:612, 1980.
6. Le Vine, M. J., White, H. A. D., and Parrish, J. A.: Components of the Goeckerman regimen. J. Invest. Dermatol. 73:170, 1979.
7. Parrish, J. A., and Jaenicke, K. F.: Action spectrum for phototherapy of psoriasis. J. Invest. Dermatol. 76:359, 1981.
8. Le Vine, M. J., and Parrish, J. A.: Outpatient phototherapy of psoriasis. Arch. Dermatol. 116:552, 1980.
9. Cram, D. L.: Psoriasis: Current advances in etiology and treatment. J. Am. Acad. Dermatol. 4:1, 1981.
10. Roenigk, H. H., Jr., Auerbach, R., Maibach, H. I., and Weinstein, G. D.: Methotrexate guidelines—revised. J. Am. Acad. Dermatol. 6:145, 1982.

PSORIASIS: PUVA THERAPY

Charles Grupper, M.D.
Bruno Berretti, M.D.

The therapeutic association of psoralens and long-wave ultraviolet radiation (ultraviolet-A: 320 to 380 nm) is currently accepted in the treatment of psoriasis. This form of photochemotherapy is commonly referred to as PUVA. In clinical practice, the psoralen most frequently used is 8-methoxypsoralen administered orally. Topical psoralens in combination with ultraviolet-A irradiation are also used in a few European centers. The ultraviolet-A radiation source must incorporate a number of features: The source must provide a uniform dose on the entire surface of the patient's body, and the source output in the ultraviolet-A range must be continuously monitored by a dectector. 8-Methoxypsoralen is given orally at a starting dose of 0.6 mg per kg. Ultraviolet-A irradiation is delivered approximately 2 hours after drug administration. The frequency of sessions ranges from three to five a week during the initial phase. After the patient's skin has cleared, the frequency of treatments is reduced, or the therapy is discontinued.

Oral PUVA has proved highly effective in psoriasis.[1-3] Its acute clinical side effects (nausea, pruritus, phototoxic reactions and so forth) are clearly recognized. Long-term toxicity still remains controversial.

Since 1976 we have treated in our center in Aubervilliers, France more than 4000 patients suffering from severe chronic psoriasis involving more than 40 per cent of the body surface. We have performed the largest monocentric study, and we will compare our results with those of the more important groups in the literature in order to discuss the major controversial problems of this revolutionary method.

Method

We have described the standard PUVA protocol previously. Since we began using this form of treatment, we have made some changes in the original method.

Topical Medications. In the original treatment method, topical medications other than emollients were not used in PUVA patients.[4,5] The initial practitioners of this technique stressed the increase of relapses in PUVA patients treated at the same time with topical tar or steroids. In our center, on the contrary, we commonly add to the PUVA regimen topical "active" treatment of lesions by steroids, tar, salicylic acid, and so forth. The treated lesions have shown a more rapid improvement, and no increase of relapses has been noted with our combined therapy.

Reasons for Exclusion. We consider pregnancy, eye disorders, cutaneous premalignant or malignant lesions, previous therapy by ionizing radiation, and previous intake of arsenic to be reasons to exclude a patient from PUVA therapy (but these anamnestic data are often very difficult to establish). Systemic use of cytotoxic drugs must be discontinued before PUVA therapy is begun. However, some authors suppose the association of PUVA and methotrexate to be beneficial.[6] Youth of the patient is not for us an absolute contraindication to PUVA therapy; children are treated, but only in cases of severe disease.

Our PUVA Regimen. At the outset, our treatment followed the original protocol.[4] Both the same equipment (Waldmann-Sylvania) and the same psoralen (8-methoxypsoralen) were used. Nevertheless, some modifications were made, which we consider to be improvements over the original protocol: We adapted doses to the total body surface, instead of using the standard 0.6 mg per kg dosage. A per-session unit energy dose of 10 joules was never exceeded. (In slow responders, we increased the psoralen dose rather than the total energy dose.)

In a second phase, beginning in 1977, we made a major modification by replacing 8-methoxypsoralen with 5-methoxypsoralen. Considering the fact that, experimentally, 5-methoxypsoralen shows a photodynamic activity 20 per cent less than that of 8-methoxy-psoralen, we administered a minimum dose of 1 mg per kg. The upper limit of this dose was 1.2 or 1.5 mg per kg (according to the body surface). Like 8-methoxypsoralen, 5-methoxypsoralen was administered 2 hours before irradiation.

In the third phase, beginning at the end of 1977, we started using the combination of etretinate and PUVA (RE-PUVA) in the treatment of very severe psoriasis. These cases generally represented initial 5-methoxypsoralen or 8-methoxypsoralen PUVA failures or the classically resistant forms of psoriasis, including generalized or palmoplantar pustular psoriasis and psoriatic erythroderma. Initially, administration of RE-PUVA was carried out using 8-methoxypsoralen, but this was quickly replaced with RE-PUVA using 5-methoxy-psoralen. We have adopted the following protocol as current routine and standard treatment for RE-PUVA therapy: Etretinate is given at a dose of 1 mg per kg per day for 15 days, followed by a standard course of PUVA with a concurrent decrease in the daily etretinate dosage.

The clearing phase of PUVA or RE-PUVA consists of four sessions per week. After clearing, maintenance treatment is begun in some patients at longer intervals (once or twice weekly) for a limit of 50 sessions a year. Relapses involving more than 40 per cent of the body surface are re-treated by a new clearing phase.

Efficacy and Acute Side Effects

The results of our different PUVA protocols have been computerized. In all cases, there was a follow-up period of more than 6 months from the end of all PUVA treatment. Some patients have been followed for as long as 3 years. Our overall patient population includes 1259 patients treated with PUVA using 8-methoxypsoralen, 198 patients treated with PUVA using 5-methoxypsoralen, 80 patients treated with RE-PUVA using 8-me-thoxypsoralen, and 75 patients treated with RE-PUVA using 5-methoxypsoralen.

Tables 1 and 2 summarize the results and the incidence of side effects at the end of the clearing phase. Tables 3 and 4 summarize the results of the follow-up study. Considering the results for these various treatments, we do confirm the high efficacy of PUVA in psoriasis.

The replacement of 8-methoxypsoralen with 5-methoxypsoralen provides an undeniable improvement in the safety and efficacy of standard PUVA therapy, but we do not find the large decrease in clearing parameters that Hönigsmann reported in his study.[7] The

Table 1. CLEARING PHASE: COMPARISON OF FOUR PROTOCOLS

	PUVA–5-MOP*	PUVA–8-MOP*	RE-PUVA–5-MOP*	RE-PUVA–8-MOP*
Number of patients	198	1259	75	80
% of clearing (>75%)	82.3%	84%	92.1%	82.4%
Number of treatments	20.6	21.1	13.6	16.5
Total dose (J/cm²)	148	131	78.1	97.6
Duration (days)	44.6	42	25.9	38.9

*PUVA–5-MOP = PUVA using 5-methoxypsoralen; *PUVA–8-MOP* = PUVA using 8-methoxypsoralen; *RE-PUVA–5-MOP* = Etretinate plus PUVA using 5-methoxypsoralen; *RE-PUVA–8-MOP* = Etretinate plus PUVA using 8-methoxypsoralen.

Table 2. COMPARISON OF TOLERANCE AND SIDE EFFECTS WITH PUVA–5-MOP AND PUVA–8-MOP*

	Number of Patients	No Side Effects	Nausea	Sunburn	Pruritus	Headache
PUVA–5-MOP	198 (100%)	167 (84.34%)	2 (1.01%)	26 (13.18%)	8 (4.04%)	2 (1.01%)
PUVA–8-MOP	1199 (100%)	619 (51.62%)	133 (11.09%)	282 (23.51%)	134 (11.17%)	13 (1.08%)

*PUVA–5-MOP = PUVA using 5-methoxypsoralen; PUVA–8-MOP = PUVA using 8-methoxypsoralen.

major advantage of 5-methoxypsoralen is the far lower incidence of acute clinical side effects. 8-Methoxypsoralen and 5-methoxypsoralen PUVA studies cast serious doubt on the utility of a maintenance treatment for the prevention of subsequent relapses. Six months after the end of the PUVA therapy, we saw the same percentage of relapses, regardless of whether maintenance treatment had been instituted and regardless of the intensity of such maintenance treatment. Therefore, we are in agreement with the results and the conclusions of the European Clinical Cooperative Trial on Photochemotherapy.[3] This contradicts the results of the American Cooperative Trial.[1]

The association of etretinate with PUVA is superior to standard PUVA therapy. Therefore, we are in agreement with the results published by the other groups.[8-12] RE-PUVA affords a decrease in all parameters for clearing and a salvage of standard PUVA failures as well as successful treatment of the most refractory types of psoriasis (pustular and erythrodermic). Our study on the long-term population, which is unfortunately somewhat limited, shows a major decrease in the incidence of relapses after RE-PUVA therapy in comparison with standard PUVA therapy using 8-methoxypsoralen or 5-methoxypsoralen. Finally, the use of 5-methoxypsoralen instead of 8-methoxypsoralen in the RE-PUVA protocol presents the most advantages: It decreases even more PUVA parameters for clearing and increases even more the percentage of patients whose skin has cleared. In addition, it improves clinical acute safety remarkably, as exemplified by a major decrease in acute side effects.

Potential Long-Term Hazards of PUVA

Because PUVA is a new treatment used to treat chronic diseases requiring long-term therapy, there is concern over its possible long-term side effects. Principal current concern regarding long-term PUVA toxicity includes actinic damage of the skin, cutaneous cancers, and ocular damage (keratitis and cataract). The concern expressed frequently with regard to hepatotoxicity has begun to diminish as more data are accumulated.

Table 3. FOLLOW-UP STUDY (SIXTH MONTH): PROPORTION OF PATIENTS REMAINING CLEARED

	With Maintenance Treatment	Without Maintenance Treatment
PUVA–8-MOP*	157/502 (36.18%)	23/68 (33.82%)
PUVA–5-MOP*	22/67 (33%)	2/11 (19%)

*PUVA–8-MOP = PUVA using 8-methoxypsoralen; PUVA–5-MOP = PUVA using 5-methoxypsoralen.

Table 4. FOLLOW-UP STUDY
(SIXTH MONTH): PROPORTION
OF PATIENTS REMAINING
CLEARED

PUVA (8- and 5-MOP)* = 204/648 (32%)
RE-PUVA (8- and 5-MOP)* = 53/87 (61%)

*8-MOP = 8-Methoxypsoralen; 5-MOP = 5-Methoxypsoralen; RE-PUVA = Etretinate plus PUVA.

Actinic Damage. Epidermal and dermal changes have been reported in patients receiving long-term therapy.[13] Various authors have reported differences in the extent and the frequency of these changes. It is not known whether the histologic alterations seen with PUVA are reversible. We studied more than 500 skin samples before, during, and after PUVA therapy, and we found only a few reversible alterations without any relation to a build-up effect of PUVA. However, the degree of such changes with PUVA, the cumulative doses needed to cause such alterations, and their clinical relevance remain important research questions.

Carcinogenesis. Some experimental studies have suggested that PUVA may be carcinogenic.[13] Clinical and epidemiologic studies at present are controversial.[14-18] One of the two American cooperative studies found after a follow-up period of 4 years that the incidence of cutaneous carcinoma in PUVA-treated patients is more than 2.5 times that expected on the basis of the Fourth National Cancer Survey.[14] This relative risk is even worse in patients who had previously been exposed to other carcinogens (ionizing radiation, arsenic) or in those who have a higher innate risk of cutaneous cancer. In addition, these studies have established a relative excess of squamous cell carcinoma, the occurrence of squamous cell carcinoma on normally unexposed areas, and the association of higher cumulative exposure to PUVA with a higher risk of such tumors. The other large prospective studies that have been published since 1979[15-18] failed to demonstrate an overall increase in the risk of skin cancer. Nevertheless, two of the four[15-17] did detect an increased risk of cutaneous carcinoma among patients who had been exposed to other known carcinogens, i.e., ionizing radiation and arsenic, before PUVA therapy. Between 1975 and 1981, we studied more than 4000 patients with psoriasis who underwent PUVA therapy in our center. Thus, in 1981, we followed 2500 patients for 4 years. We noted only 8 premalignant or malignant cutaneous disorders. A recent examination of 300 patients who had received more than 2000 joules revealed no cases of precancer or cancer. No cases of squamous cell carcinoma were seen. Therefore, it is very difficult at present to say whether PUVA is carcinogenic or not. Some data seem to suggest that PUVA is a promoter of some well-known carcinogens, such as arsenic or ionizing radiation. Any hypothetical effect of PUVA as an initiator may not be clinically evident for a long time to come.[19]

When one decides to treat a patient with PUVA, one should weigh this potential risk carefully and should take special care in judging the hazards and benefits of PUVA in patients with known risk factors for cutaneous carcinogenesis, especially preceding arsenic or ionizing radiation exposure.

Ophthalmologic Risks. Several experimental studies have stressed the possibility of ocular damage when psoralens are combined with ultraviolet-A.[13] However, until now there has been no convincing evidence of eye damage in PUVA-treated patients.[13] Because of the serious nature of cataracts and the relative ease of using adequate eye protection, it seems prudent to insist on the use of ultraviolet-A–opaque eyewear from the time of ingestion of the psoralens for at least the remainder of the treatment day.

CONCLUSIONS _____

PUVA has been proved highly effective in treatment of chronic, severe, and refractory psoriasis. This form of therapy is accepted gladly by patients. The original regimen, which constituted a therapeutic revolution in 1974, should be modified to improve the risk/benefit ratio. One should pay attention to risk factors when selecting patients. The replacement of 8-methoxypsoralen with 5-methoxypsoralen and the combination of PUVA with etretinate does allow an improvement of the efficacy of treatment with the salvage of the more refractory clinical forms and a decrease of clinical acute side effects. In addition, RE-PUVA using 5-methoxypsoralen produces a significant decrease in clearing parameters. In comparison with standard PUVA, it seems to result in a lowering of the frequency of relapses after the cessation of treatment. On the contrary, maintenance treatment is not as essential as previously assumed and thus may not be necessary in the majority of patients. We feel that the clearing protocol of RE-PUVA with 5-methoxypsoralen is now the best PUVA regimen. It will provide the best opportunity for the reduction of the total cumulative ultraviolet-A energy dose, thus reducing the hypothetic danger of long-term hazards.

References

1. Melski, J. W., Tanenbaum, L., Parrish, J. A., et al.: Oral methoxsalen photochemotherapy for the treatment of psoriasis: A cooperative clinical trial. J. Invest. Dermatol. 68:328, 1977.
2. Grupper, C., Berretti, B., and Forlot, P.: Bilan de la PUVAthérapie à propos de 1400 cas personnels. Résultats et progrès récents en 1979. *In* Ichtyoses, Peau et Lumière. Actes du XVI Congrès de l'Association des Dermatologistes de Langue Française. Tunis, Sagep, 1980, p. 303.
3. Henseler, T., Wolff, K., Hönigsmann, H., and Christophers, E.: Oral 8-methoxypsoralen photochemotherapy of psoriasis. Lancet 1:853, 1981.
4. Parrish, J. A., Fitzpatrick, T. B., Tanenbaum, L., and Pathak, M. A.: Photochemotherapy of psoriasis with oral methoxsalen and long-wave ultraviolet light. N. Engl. J. Med. 291:1207, 1974.
5. Wolff, K., Hönigsmann, H., Gschnait, F., and Konrad, K.: Photochemotherapie bei Psoriasis. Klinische Erfahrungen bei 152 Patienten. Dtsch. Med. Wochenschr. 100:2471, 1975.
6. Morison, W. L., Momtaz, K., Parrish, J. A., and Fitzpatrick, T. B.: Combined methotrexate-PUVA therapy in the treatment of psoriasis. J. Am. Acad. Dermatol. 6:46, 1982.
7. Hönigsmann, H., Jaschke, E., Gschnait, F., Brenner, W., Fritsch, P., and Wolff, K.: 5-Methoxypsoralen (Bergapten) in photochemotherapy of psoriasis. Br. J. Dermatol. 101:369, 1979.
8. Fritsch, P. O., Honigsmann, H., Jaschke, E., and Wolff, K.: Augmentation of oral methoxsalen photochemotherapy with an oral retinoid acid derivative. J. Invest. Dermatol. 70:178, 1978.
9. Orfanos, C. E., Pulmann, H., Sterry, W., and Kunzig, M.: Retinoid–PUVA–RE-PUVA: Systemische Kombinations—Behandlung bei Psoriasis. S. Hautkr. 53:494, 1978.
10. Heidbreder, G., and Christophers, E.: Therapy of psoriasis with retinoid plus PUVA: Clinical and histological data. Arch. Dermatol. Res. 264:331, 1979.
11. Grupper, C., and Berretti, B.: Treatment of psoriasis by oral PUVA therapy combined with aromatic retinoid. Dermatologica 162:404, 1980.
12. Orfanos, C. E., Braun-Falco, O., Farber, E. M., Grupper, C., Polano, M. K., and Schuppli, R. (eds.): Retinoids—Advances in Basic Research and Therapy. Berlin, Springer-Verlag, 1981.
13. Parrish, J. A., Stern, R. S., and Fitzpatrick, T. B.: Evaluation of PUVA 1980: Its basic nature and toxicity. *In* Moschella, S. L. (ed.): Dermatology Update 1980. New York, Elsevier, 1980, pp. 313–337.
14. Stern, R. S., Thibodeau, L. A., Kleinerman, R. A., Parrish, J. A., Fitzpatrick, T. B., et al.: Risk of cutaneous carcinoma in patients treated with oral methoxsalen photochemotherapy for psoriasis. N. Engl. J. Med. 300:809, 1979.
15. Hönigsmann, H., Wolff, K., Gschnait, F., Brenner, W., and Jaschke, E.: Keratoses and nonmelanoma skin tumors in long-term photochemotherapy. J. Am. Acad. Dermatol. 3:406, 1980.
16. Grupper, C., and Berretti, B.: Tar, ultraviolet light, PUVA and cancer. J. Am. Acad. Dermatol. 3:643, 1980.
17. Roenigk, H. H., Jr., et al.: Skin cancer in the PUVA-48 cooperative study of psoriasis. J. Invest. Dermatol. 74:250, 1980.
18. Lassus, A., Reunala, T., Udanpaa-Heikkila, J., Juvakoski, T., and Salo, O.: PUVA treatment and skin cancer follow-up study. Acta Derm. Venereol. (Stockh.) 61:141, 1981.
19. Halprin, K.: Psoriasis and cancer. A.A.D. Annual Meeting, Symposium 336: Therapeutics. New York, December 11, 1980.

AN APPRAISAL OF THE RETINOIDS IN THE TREATMENT OF PSORIASIS

William D. Stewart, M.D.

There are now three generations of retinoids that are therapeutically useful in dermatology. This family of compounds has been moved quickly from development in the 1960s into position for striking against proliferative disorders. It behooves us to follow developments closely in order to be able to tend to our patients' needs responsibly. As clinical discoveries increase, past publications describing meetings to disseminate information concerning these important clinical agents are being left behind quickly in favor of an immense, rapidly growing body of investigative literature about the fine points of the biological activity of retinoids.[1-6]

The three generations of compounds are classified according to increasing potency. Various examples can be used to describe them; we will use the anti–mouse papilloma effect. The anti–mouse papilloma effect has been categorized by Bollag,[7] who developed this technique of studying antikeratinizing compounds. It is identified by a median effective dose (i.e., a dose that causes regression of 50 per cent of mouse papilloma tumors). The median effective dose of 13-*cis*-retinoic acid (a first-generation retinoid) is 800 mg per kg; that of etretinate (a second-generation retinoid) is 25 mg per kg; and that of the arotinoids (the new third generation) is 0.05 mg per kg. These last are potent antitumor compounds, but they also have strong vitamin A–like cellular effects. Their increasing potency is apparent.

The success of current dermatologic management of disease has been a result of our knowledge of a number of pharmacologic factors. Corticosteroid (and now, retinoid) influence on cutaneous cellular function is a major part of this dermatologic therapeutic armamentarium. The way in which we continue to use these new, immensely powerful compounds is of paramount importance. The two separate families, corticosteroids and retinoids, have intriguing similarities. Cytosol receptor proteins have been identified in a wide variety of tissues for retinoids, just as they were previously for corticosteroids.[8] The intracellular activities of physiologic concentrations of these compounds relate to cytosol binding, movement into an intranuclear position, combination with DNA, effect on RNA, and synthesis of new protein. These steps apply to both compounds.[9,10] Both have pharmacologic actions in larger concentrations but cellular regulatory function in normal concentrations. They interact with other regulatory compounds, such as polyamines and catecholamines,[11] and demonstrate both stimulatory and inhibitory (pleiotropic) influences on cell growth. Ornithine decarboxylase is a ubiquitous intracellular enzyme that initiates production of putrescine from ornithine, thus commencing the synthesis of a series of growth regulators.[12] In cases of psoriasis, there are abnormalities in this system—retinoids inhibit the enzyme. It is not known how early this inhibition occurs in the proliferative process, but it seems to precede some other markers.[13] Corticosteroids and other antipsoriatic agents inhibit ornithine decarboxylase as well. Retinoids within the cell have far-reaching effects on monosaccharide participation for protein synthesis[3,14] in proliferative cellular activity.

Cutaneous Benefit Versus Hazards

The keratinizing disorders, for which retinoids are beneficial because of their keratolytic effect, are well recognized. They demonstrate a variety of mechanisms, but all affect the final keratin product as a result.[2,15-17] One can assess the usefulness of these compounds in keratinizing diseases by considering the extent and duration of their action and the severity of unwanted effects. Retinoids promote epidermal cell proliferation and differentiation, secretion of intercellular mucus-like material, thinning of the stratum corneum, and some loss of integrity of this barrier in addition to the thinning. Keratolysis affects the outer compact layer for the most part.

These keratolytic changes are desirable in cutaneous disorders in which the pathologic process rests in the keratinized layer. The benefit in hyperkeratinizing disorders and dyskeratoses, lamellar and vulgar ichthyosis, bullous and nonbullous ichthyosiform erythroderma, keratosis pilaris, erythrokeratodermia variabilis, keratosis follicularis, pityriasis rubra pilaris, keratodermas, psoriasis, and the like can be judged easily, since it is seen promptly over the initial 6 to 10 weeks of treatment. Improvement in other disorders may be more subtle, either because the end point is less well defined or because it takes longer to achieve. Vesicular or spongiotic disorders of the palms of the hands and nail disorders may be placed in these categories.[18,19] Other keratinizing disorders, such as epidermolysis bullosa and Hailey-Hailey disease, may be minimally helped by retinoids or may not be clearly altered.[2,4]

Retinoids can set the stage for beneficial effects by other modalities, such as PUVA, ultraviolet-B, steroids, and other topical applications.[17] This is a mixed blessing, however. Thinning of the protective corneum not only increases heat transfer and lessens the ability of the individual to touch hot objects but also allows greater penetration of ultraviolet light for therapeutic effect in psoriasis and other diseases benefitted by ultraviolet light. Patients with Darier's disease are even more sun-sensitive than expected as a result of the retinoid action. In other patients also, the effect of ultraviolet light exposure is enhanced, and these individuals sunburn more readily than they expect. Their skin is softer and more delicate and is traumatized easily on hard, rough, or sharp surfaces. It is unknown whether this thinning of the outer layer will hasten aging or carcinogenesis from ultraviolet light, especially since one must consider that retinoids possess anticancer activity. Degenerative disorders arising from exposure to ultraviolet light enhanced with PUVA include aging, collagen effects, and amyloid deposits.[20,21] Whether retinoids taken over time will encourage these changes is controversial. In mucous membranes, which have minimal keratinization already, thickness of the outer layers becomes insufficient, and the membranes crack and bleed.[22] Some nail and hair growth also suffers in excess of the therapeutic advantage obtained. Nails soften and thin, often becoming easily traumatized, and hair may cease adequate growth.

Cutaneous side effects tend to appear in the first month of therapy but may occur much later and can vary with patient and drug. They include lip and mucous membrane dryness and fragility; epistaxis; skin sensitivity to heat, trauma, and pressure; "sticky" skin or thin skin; palm and sole exfoliation or sensitive palms and soles; nail changes; hair loss that is usually mild but is sometimes severe and can be total; retinoid dermatitis; scaling and red cutaneous changes, usually on the face; conjunctivitis or balanitis; pruritus; and paronychia.

The therapeutic benefits so far outweigh the obvious adverse effects of the retinoids on the skin. However, potential hidden hazards may alter our assessment. The chief beneficiaries of the future will be children with keratinizing disorders, which frequently produce real hardship. Nevertheless, the hampering effect of these agents on life style is not generally appreciated. Dependable therapy for these disorders will outweigh some of the hazard, but not all of it.

Noncutaneous Effect

Although the primary clinical effect of retinoid activity is on epithelial cells, these agents also influence nonepithelial cellular tissue in a number of ways. Dermal alterations from retinoids include actions on blood vessels, cellular infiltrates of mononuclear cells, eosinophils, Langerhans' cells, and lymphocytes.[23] Changes in collagen, ground substance, and anchoring fibrils by retinoids are well-defined effects. Retinoids also have demonstrated a modulating influence on immunologic functions in humans that occurs chiefly in connection with tumors but also is present in psoriasis[6,24] and inflammatory disorders, e.g., acne.[1,2] Stimulation and transformation of macrophages, monocytes, and lymphocytes have been observed under the influence of oral retinoids.[23]

Another action of the retinoids that is of great interest is their inhibitory effect on virus antigen induction. In China, research is in progress concerning causative factors in nasopharyngeal carcinoma.[25] Early induction of antigens of Epstein-Barr virus, signifying virus presence and activity, was inhibited by several retinoids, including Ro 10-9359. Antivirucidal activity is connected with damage to the capsid of the virus, preventing adsorption to host cells.[26] Herpes simplex type 2 is an example of a virus that is readily inactivated under controlled circumstances by retinoids.[26]

Multiple observations of patients on retinoid regimens for psoriasis have indicated that these drugs alleviate symptoms and signs of psoriatic arthritis particularly early in the inflammatory course of the disease.[27-29] This may be connected to the effect on rabbit synovial cell cultures reported by Brinckerhoff, in which retinoids were able to inhibit secretion of collagenase induced by phorbol esters on synovial fibroblast culture.[30] Retinoids also potentiate plasminogen activator levels in these fibroblast cultures and affect prostaglandin production.[30] The relationship of these cellular actions to the clinical antiarthritic action of etretinate is not clear. The results of studies of animal models have often been misleading when extrapolated to humans. This may be true with some retinoid work.

In our clinical experience, etretinate had an effect on six patients who demonstrated severe, painful, acute inflammatory signs at distal interphalangeal joints. The joints in one patient were adjacent to recent acute psoriasis of the fingers and toes—the only site of psoriasis he experienced. He was severely incapacitated by the joint symptoms, and treatment by etretinate alone over a 6-month period was sufficient to restore complete function of all ten joints and to clear signs of psoriasis from the skin. Five other patients have reported freedom from acute joint pain, motion limitation, heat, and swelling by etretinate prescribed for psoriasis. As a result, we have embarked on a study of the effect of these compounds on early inflammatory psoriatic arthritis. However, bone and joint symptoms of pain, tenderness, motion discomfort, and even swelling of joints have been reported in patients who have taken either etretinate or isotretinate.[1-4] There appears, therefore, to be an unexplained effect on joints and, perhaps, on bones by these compounds. Earlier reports on effects of vitamin A described bone and joint changes,[31] and retinoids in the subchronic toxicity studies reported by Kamm[42] discussed bone and joint effects in animals.

Thivolet[28] examined nine patients with psoriatic arthritis and described 5 good or very good results, but he did not enlarge on the duration of their symptoms or signs. He also mentioned favorable responses from other countries in the retinoid treatment of this disorder.

Stollenwerk[27] reported 24 patients with psoriasis and psoriatic arthritis treated with 1 mg per kg of etretinate. Eighty-three per cent showed definite joint improvement. Recurrences under treatment took place, as they do in the management of keratinizing disorders, particularly psoriasis. More than 50 per cent of patients were able to reduce or stop therapy with anti-inflammatory drugs, because they experienced a decrease in stiffness, swelling, or pain. Seventy-one per cent were able to maintain therapy after an average of 9 months. It is interesting to note that maximal recovery appears to take at least twice as long to manifest itself as does initial skin improvement. Most cases took 2 to 3 months to show improvement and 4 to 6 months for maximal benefit.

A satisfactory clinical study of adequate proportions remains to be performed in order to provide answers for questions concerning the efficacy of retinoids in early psoriatic arthritis. Kaplan[44] described improvement in four of seven patients with long-standing arthritis.

Anticarcinogenic Effect

It seems to me that a major area of interest concerning these compounds lies in the field of carcinogenicity. The retinoids have the potential to stave off predictable malignant alterations in cells exposed to carcinogens of various types. They inhibit carcinogen-induced hyperplasia, metaplasia, and proliferation of cells in cultures. They also inhibit induction of transformation of cultured cells and alter evidence of transformation by various growth stimulators. This was described by Sporn[32] and by many others,[33,34] following on the knowledge that naturally occurring vitamin A controls epithelial cell differentiation and inhibits development of squamous metaplasia in cells of epithelial origin by simple deficiency. This effect is described as ''physiologic'' because metaplasia in epithelial tissues can be prevented by the use of the vitamin A family of drugs.[32,35] Thus, physiologic defense mechanisms against the formation of epithelial cell cancer are called into play by the use of retinoids. The response of these mechanisms to topical retinoids may be different from their response to systemic retinoids.[36] This may reflect an influence on several growth factors that compete for cellular membrane receptors.[37] There are two phases—prevention of cancer and treatment of precancer—and it has not yet been defined for which the retinoids are useful. Evidence abounds to support their value in preventing early induced changes leading to cancer in the skin, the bladder, the gastrointestinal tract, and the bronchial epithelium of laboratory animals.[3,4]

Epithelia that are exposed to carcinogenic agents may become neoplastic or may retain their normal differentiation by a process of repair, preventing development of malignancy. Retinoids enhance the repair capability. The doses of naturally occurring retinoids that are required to accomplish this are larger than those of the more potent synthetic compounds. Vitamin A–deficient animals are more susceptible to carcinogenic agents and the development of epithelial cancer than are normally fed animals. Synthetic retinoids clearly demonstrate abilities for prevention of epithelial cancers, including those involving skin, the respiratory tract, the mammary gland, and the bladder, without being affected by diet. Bollag's mouse papilloma studies demonstrated that synthetic retinoids prevent carcinomas produced by topical anthracene and croton oil in mice that have a normal diet.[7] Further laboratory studies have indicated that these agents have strong tendencies to prevent cancer formed by the action of carcinogens in rat epithelial organs. In cultures, retinoids are anticarcinogenic when added to a culture at or after placement of the carcinogen. Mammary cancer induced by an oral anthracene compound in rats can be shown to be prevented or postponed by a retinoid compound, ostensibly through enhancement of intrinsic physiologic cellular defense mechanisms. Furthermore, retinoids, both synthetic and natural, can inhibit growth and transformation of selected epithelial and nonepithelial cell lines. Some retinoids are clearly effective inhibitors of carcinogenesis under specific circumstances,[38,39] and studies currently in progress seem to indicate that they have an ability to halt the progress of selected neoplastic diseases.[37] There is even some indication that established tumors may be inhibited by some retinoids.[35] Some of this inhibition is by cytotoxic activity.[40]

Some 10 per cent of basal cell carcinomas regress with oral and topical retinoids, and some regress completely.[35] Prophylaxis appears at present to be the most promising retinoid action in cancer treatment, since chronic maintenance therapy reduces predicted new lesion formation in basal cell nevus syndrome, xeroderma pigmentosum, actinic keratoses, porokeratosis, multiple keratoacanthomas, and tumors of epidermodysplasia verruciformis.[35]

The physiologic anticancer capabilities of these compounds have led to reconsideration of the concepts of carcinogenesis. Researchers are currently investigating the role of transforming cellular growth factors in some malignant processes to ascertain the effect of retinoids on these polypeptide compounds.[37] The potential of this activity may go far beyond single disease processes.[37]

Noncutaneous Benefit Versus Hazards

Cutaneous hazards from retinoid use have yet to be completely assessed, but unwelcome noncutaneous effects may be more significant. These include:

1. *Teratogenicity,* which makes contraceptive measures for women in the child-bearing age a necessity. Etretinate may be detectable in the plasma up to 140 days after treatment. Some effect has been seen on the gonadal epithelium of male guinea pigs at high dosage, but this has not been observed in sperm examinations in humans. Extrapolation of the effects of three compounds—tretinoin, etretinate, and isotretinoin—on more than one animal species is fraught with difficulty. Experiments indicate that these drugs are teratogenic, and the clinician should be alerted to this hazard. These studies, however, do not indicate the dose or level of retinoids that is hazardous to human fetal development. Isotretinoin in the rabbit and the rat is tolerated at higher doses than is tretinoin or etretinate. In the studies reported, isotretinoin has shown no adverse effects on postnatal development at doses that produce no intolerable maternal toxicity.[2,3,42] The effects of these agents involve the eye and the craniofacial and skeletal structures.

2. *Mutagenesis* does not seem to be a problem with the retinoids, which are nonmutagenic.

3. *Carcinogenesis.* The retinoids are probably not carcinogenic; on the contrary, they are even more likely to be anticarcinogenic.

4. *Hepatotoxicity.* Retinol is stored in Kupffer cells in the liver, and some is found in the parenchymal cells. Varying proportions of the oral dose have been measured in animal liver, and there is significant species variability. Liver biopsies taken after 6 months of administration of oral etretinate do not show a consistent microscopic effect on the liver in humans. Tests of liver function have, in general, remained within normal limits. However, there has been a significant number of undesirable abnormalities reported in patients during therapy with these drugs, including elevations in sedimentation rate.

Elevation of serum transaminase, alkaline phosphatase, lactate dehydrogenase, and bilirubin levels occurs during oral treatment with retinoids in regular clinical doses. These may return to normal while the drug therapy is continued; however, some isolated reports indicate a continued upward trend or maintained elevation until the drug is stopped. One case of toxic hepatic damage has been reported.[43] The rise in these determinants of liver function does not seem to be related to specific factors, although we have seen initial moderate elevations followed by a continued rise until the drug was stopped. The levels remained elevated until ingestion of alcohol was also stopped; then the concentrations slowly returned to normal. We feel that consumption of alcohol even in minimal amounts and ingestion of other hepatotoxic substances have no place in patients who are taking retinoids and who show any disturbances of liver function.

5. *Elevation of triglyceride and cholesterol levels* is seen with fluctuations that are probably related to dietary carbohydrate and fat intake. There is a quite marked variability of triglyceride concentrations in patients that is usually below upper normal levels. These changes are significant because elevated triglyceride and very low-density lipoprotein levels might possibly be related to coronary artery disease. We have found elevations in most of our patients (male and female, old and young) but have been more concerned if the elevation is high (above 300 mg per dl), if there is a history of family cardiovascular disease,

or if the levels continue to rise. Higher elevations can usually be promptly reduced by modification of diet. We decrease calorie intake in our patients by reducing their consumption of cholesterol and animal fat to less than one third of the total calories. There is controversy about carbohydrate restrictions; nevertheless, we also have our patients reduce carbohydrate consumption. Our perception is that triglyceride levels are frequently elevated in our patients at some stage, often after several months of therapy with etretinate. These elevations respond to diet promptly and tend to plateau around 300 mg per dl (the upper normal limit is 200). They may shoot up to 600 mg per dl or more in some patients but drop quickly when the drug is discontinued. Alcohol tends to enhance the elevation. If a patient persists in showing high elevations, we discontinue administration of the retinoid.

6. *Arthralgia* and muscle or bone pains occur at unpredictable periods and are apparently unrelated to previous or current disease, activity, trauma, or laboratory abnormalities. They are most often subjective but debilitating and are often persistent over days. They can be very severe and are not affected by dose alteration.

7. *Dose*. We begin all patients with 25 mg per day or less, and we find that often there is no need to go higher.

References

1. Orfanos, C. E., and Schuppli, R.: Workshop: Oral retinoids in dermatology. Dermatologica 157 Suppl. 1:1, 1978.
   The first European meeting.
2. Orfanos, C. E., Braun-Falco, O., Farber, E. M., Grupper, C., Polano, M., and Schuppli, R.: Retinoids. Proceeding of the International Dermatology Symposium. Advances in Basic Research and Therapy. Berlin, Springer-Verlag, 1981.
   The second European meeting.
3. Strauss, J. E., Windhorst, D. B., and Weinstein, G. D.: Oral retinoids—a workshop. J. Am. Acad. Dermatol. 6:4, 1981.
   The first American meeting.
4. Elias, P. M., and Williams, M. L.: Retinoids, cancer and the skin. Arch. Dermatol. 117:160, 1981.
   There are 355 references and a general update on all aspects.
5. Bollag, W., and Matter, A.: From vitamin A to retinoids in experimental and clinical oncology: Achievements, failures and outlook. Ann. N.Y. Acad. Sci. 359:9, 1981.
6. Farber, E. M., Cox, A. J., Nael, L., and Jacobs, P. H.: Psoriasis. New York, Grune & Stratton, 1982.
   Special section on retinoids, pp. 144 to 515.
7. Bollag, W.: Arotinoids. Cancer Chemother. Pharmacol. 7:27, 1981.
   A new retinoid class with particular properties.
8. Sakamoto, M., and Puhvel, S. M.: Cytosolic retinoic acid binding proteins in human skin. Clin. Res. 30:29A, 1982.
   In addition to a wide variety of animal tissues.
9. Lotan, R., Ong, D. E., and Chytil, F.: Comparison of the level of cellular retinoid binding proteins and susceptibility to retinoid induced inhibition of various neoplastic cell lines. J. Natl. Cancer Inst. 64:1259, 1980.
   Presence of retinoid binding proteins in tumor lines.
10. Lotan, R.: Effects of vitamin A and its analogs (retinoids) on normal and neoplastic cells. Biochim. Biophys. Acta 605:33, 1980.
    Intracellular events similar to corticosteroid actions.
11. Voorhees, J. J.: Polyamines and psoriasis. Arch. Dermatol. 115:943, 1979.
    Polyamine pharmacology in perspective. Editorial.
12. Lowe, N. J.: Epidermal ornithine decarboxylase, polyamines, cell proliferation, and tumor promotion. Arch. Dermatol. 116:822, 1980.
    Important perspective for the retinoids.
13. Laurahanta, J., et al.: Reduction of increased polyamine levels in psoriatic lesions by retinoid and PUVA treatments. Br. J. Dermatol. 105:267, 1981.
    Putrescine and spermidine/spermine ratio fell abruptly.
14. De Luca, L. M., Sasak, W., Adamo, S., et al.: Retinoid metabolism and mode of action. Environ. Health Perspect. 35:147, 1980.
    Intranuclear chemistry.
15. Marks, R., Finlay, A.Y., and Holt, P. J. A.: Severe disorders of keratinization: Effects of treatment with Tigason (etretinate). Br. J. Dermatol. 104:667, 1981.
    Drug seems to act at a late stage of epidermal differentiation.

16. Ehmann, C. S., and Voorhees, J. J: International studies of the efficacy of etretinate in the treatment of psoriasis. J. Am. Acad. Dermatol. 6 Suppl. 2:695, 1982.
    Over 1000 patients in double-blind studies. The addition of ultraviolet-A and ultraviolet-B is also reported.
17. Elias, P., et al.: Retinoid effects on epidermal structure differentiation and permeability. Lab. Invest. 44:531, 1981.
18. Thune, P.: Treatment of pustulosa plantaris et palmaris with Tigason. Dermatologica 164:67, 1982.
    Seven of 42 cleared completely.
19. Reymann, F.: Two years' experience with Tigason in the treatment of pustulosis palmoplantaris and eczema keratoticum manuum. Dermatologica 164:209, 1982.
    Total clearing not impressive; side effects significant in relation to disease.
20. Gschnait, F., Wolff, K., Hönigsmann, H., Stingl, G., et al.: Long-term photochemotherapy: Histopathologic and immunofluorescence observations in 243 patients. Br. J. Dermatol. 103:11, 1980.
    Identification of degenerative changes most likely due to ultraviolet light.
21. Greene, I., and Cox, A. J.: Amyloid deposition after psoriasis therapy with psoralen and long-wave ultraviolet light. Arch. Dermatol. 115:1200, 1979.
    Possible complication of PUVA proportionate to duration of treatment.
22. Williams, M. L., and Elias, P. M.: The pathogenesis of skin fragility from systemic retinoids is epidermal in origin. Abstract. Clin. Res. 28:585, 1980.
23. Tsambaos, T., and Orfanos, C. E.: Ultrastructural evidence suggesting an immunomodulatory activity of oral retinoid. Br. J. Dermatol. 104:37, 1981.
    Lymphocytes and monocytes replaced in subsequent biopsies by Sézary-like cells, activated macrophages, and L cells.
24. Wrba, H.: Stimulation of immune response in lung cancer patients by vitamin A therapy. Oncology 34:234, 1977.
    Immune potentiating effects against tumor.
25. Zeng, Y., Zhou, H. M., and Xu, S. P.: Inhibitory effect of retinoids on Epstein-Barr virus induction in Raji cells. Intervirology 16:29, 1981.
    Induction of Epstein-Barr virus antigen inhibited by retinoids. Very significant for possible treatment of nasopharyngeal cancer.
26. Reinhardt, A., Auperin, D., and Sands, J.: Mechanism of virucidal activity of retinoids: Protein removal from bacteriophage Φ6 envelope. Antimicrob. Agents Chemother. 17:1034, 1980.
    Various vitamin A derivatives are capable of this activity.
27. Stollenwerk, R., Fischer-Hoinkes, H., Komenda, K., and Schilling, F.: Clinical observations on oral retinoid therapy of psoriatic arthropathy. In Orfanos, C. E., et al. (eds.): Retinoids. Berlin, Springer-Verlag, 1981, p. 205.
    Impressive.
28. Thivolet, J., Robart, S., and Vignon, E.: Le rétinoïde aromatique associé à la photochimiothérapie pour le traitement du psoriasis et du rhumatisme psoriasique. Ann. Dermatol. Venereol. 108:131, 1981.
    One hundred of 107 cases cleared with combined PUVA and retinoids. Better than PUVA alone in eight of nine cases; arthritis improved.
29. Viglioglia, P. S., and Barclay, A.: Oral retinoids and psoriasis. Dermatologica 157 Suppl. 1:32, 1978.
    Proceedings of workshop held October 19, 1977 in Mexico City. Eight of nine cases of psoriatic arthritis improved.
30. Brinckerhoff, C. E., et al.: Effects of all trans-retinoic acid (retinoic acid) and 4-hydroxy phenylretinamide on synovial cells and articular cartilage. J. Am. Acad. Dermatol. 6:591, 1982.
    Inhibition of collagenase.
31. Oliver, T. K.: Chronic vitamin A intoxication. Report of a case in an older child and a review of the literature. Am. J. Dis. Child 95:57, 1958.
    Bone pain prominent.
32. Sporn, M. B.: Retinoids and carcinogenesis. NHI Reviews 35:65, 1977.
    Use of synthetic compounds to enhance physiologic mechanisms.
33. Lutzner, M. A., and Blanchet-Bardon, C.: Oral retinoid treatment of human papillomavirus type 5–induced epidermodysplasia verruciformis. N. Engl. J. Med. 302:1091, 1980.
    No evidence of remaining virus histologically or by immunofluorescence; 100 × reduction in viral DNA.
34. Matter, A., and Bollag, W.: A fine structural study on the effect of an aromatic retinoid on chemically induced skin papillomas of the mouse. Eur. J. Cancer 13:831, 1977.
    Subcellular observations but no explanations for the effect.
35. Peck, G. L.: Chemoprevention of cancer with retinoids. Gynecol. Oncol. 12:S331, 1981.
    Chronic maintenance therapy required.
36. Elias, P. M., et al.: Influence of topical and systemic retinoids on basal cell carcinoma cell membranes. Cancer 48:932, 1981.
    Topical and systemic effects differed on gap junction and desmosomes.
37. Sporn, M. B., and Harris, E. D., Jr.: Proliferative diseases. Am. J. Med. 70:1231, 1981.
    Retinoids and cellular transforming growth factors in an imaginative examination of current knowledge.
38. Nettesheim, P.: Inhibition of carcinogenesis by retinoids. Can. Med. Assoc. J. 122:757, 1980.
    Synthetics have a greater effect than do natural retinoids. Some tumors halted.
39. Freeman, H. J.: Retinoids and carcinogenesis. In Spiller, G. A. (ed.): Nutritional Pharmacology. New York, Alan R. Liss, Inc., 1981, pp. 203–216.
    A critical review.

40. Lotan, R., and Dennert, G.: Stimulatory effects of vitamin A analogs on induction of cell-mediated cytotoxicity in vivo. Cancer Res. 39:55, 1979.
   Probably an immunologic effect, but high concentrations were used.
41. Tsambaos, D., and Orfanos, C. E.: Chemotherapy of psoriasis and other skin disorders with oral retinoids. Pharmacol. Ther. 14:355, 1981.
   History, chemistry, mechanisms, application, and side effects of retinoids.
42. Kamm, J.: Toxicology, carcinogenicity and teratogenicity of some orally administered retinoids. J. Am. Acad. Dermatol. 6:652, 1982.
   Review.
43. Thune, P.: A case of centrolobular toxic necrosis of liver due to Tigason. Dermatologica 160:405, 1980.
   Alcohol not mentioned.
44. Kaplan, R. P., Russell, D. H., and Lowe, N. J.: Etretinate therapy for psoriasis: Clinical responses, remission times, epidermal DNA, and polyamine responses. J. Am. Acad. Dermatol. 95:8, 1983.
   Twenty patients, 6 months of treatment; slow relapses.

PERITONEAL DIALYSIS

Philip Anderson, M.D.

Introduction

Dialysis is not a possession solely of nephrology. Dialysis machines are not merely "artificial kidneys," as the newspapers and television imply. These common ideas are obstacles to our discussion. In order to understand dialysis, we should recognize that organs in the human body other than kidneys also may correct imbalances or eliminate impurities in blood by natural dialysis, as, for instance, the liver, the reticuloendothelial system, and even the skin itself, may do naturally. Mechanical dialysis is unnatural and may be therapeutic in many additional ways. Some of the effects on the blood of mechanical dialysis are approximately equal to some functions of normal organs and may be substituted (for example, peritoneal dialysis improves end-stage renal disease). Some effects of dialysis may grossly exceed any action of normal organs. For instance, peritoneal dialysis removes an enormous variety of small and large molecules and even whole cells, which the normal kidney leaves neatly in the body, undisturbed. One term for therapeutic dialysis is "blood scrubbing." The word "dialysis" sounds almost too gentle.

A common misunderstanding even among physicians is that the physiology and biochemistry of dialysis in humans are simple and already well known. In fact, much remains unknown. Some of the distortions induced by dialysis are transient and possibly trivial, but some may trigger other, more lasting, physiologic mechanisms, which, in turn, may modify diseases. Imaginative physicians hope to block a disease by dialyzing from the blood some component that is a necessary link in the chain of events causing the disease. For example, removing thyroglobulin from blood by peritoneal dialysis helps patients to survive a hyperthyroid storm until further therapy can be applied. A list is developing of such medical situations in which dialysis may help.

Often we speak of "the" cause of a disease. The "one and only" cause is only an artifact of conversation. Physicians are directing attention to that point in the chain of causative events at which they can intervene reliably to help the patient. For most systemic diseases, at some point in the causative chain, an important mediator probably circulates in the blood. Blood scrubbing, if we only knew how to do it more selectively and more gently, probably would be a valuable adjunctive therapy. The study of dialysis is promising as a source for new therapies.

Origins of Peritoneal Dialysis

Medical interest in peritoneal lavage is approximately one century old. In 1877, Wegner explored it as a means of controlling fever and hypothermia. The technique was used in the early decades of this century as means of giving parenteral fluids quickly and safely, especially to infants. Clark (1921), Putman (1923), and Donnan (1924) all displayed the physiologist's scientific interest in describing the lavage process, but Ganter (1923) first emphasized practical medical possibilities of using peritoneal dialysis to control uremia by "washing the blood." He was not able to achieve practical medical success, of course, but his plan and his enthusiasm were contagious.[6]

Practical success with peritoneal dialysis in humans depended on antibiotics, improved techniques for sterilization, design of new equipment, and, most important, an understanding of the true physiologic dynamics of the peritoneal dialysis system. By the 1950s all the pieces were available, and only a center for action was needed. When S. T. Boen moved from Holland to Seattle in the early 1960s, he started such a center at the University of Washington. Within 15 years, the worth of peritoneal dialysis had been well proved in Seattle. This was the result of a combination of research, clinical effort, and the education of nephrologists.[6]

Various techniques are used to treat uremia. Nolph, at Missouri, has become known for using continuous ambulatory peritoneal dialysis.[6] Recently, peritoneal dialysis also has been used for a wider range of acute dangerous diseases, particularly acute intoxications, envenomations, and poisonings. The new peritoneal dialysis techniques represent great practical improvements over the procedures of only 5 to 10 years ago, and physicians may need to reacquaint themselves with modern peritoneal dialysis.

What Is Dialysis Technically?

Peritoneal dialysis uses nature's version of a backup capillary kidney and at the same time is a means of restoring fluids and metabolites to the body. The solute and fluid exchange occurs between peritoneal capillaries and the dialysis solution. The precise anatomy and function of this complex membrane will be important as further basic improvements are made in the peritoneal dialysis technique.

Traditional hemodialysis is much more efficient than peritoneal dialysis in removing low–molecular weight substances from blood but does not restore fluids. Continuous ambulatory peritoneal dialysis also is able to control uremia and is better for removing middle-weight molecules (1200 to 10,000 daltons). Peritoneal dialysis also removes cellular exudates, large lipids, proteins, colloids, glycoproteins, and anything else that may enter the peritoneal cavity. It has the advantage of no connections directly into the vascular space, and therefore it does not initiate platelet pooling, extensive intravascular hemolysis, or other effects of more direct manipulation of the blood cells. Applications are facilitated further by the modern equipment.

Hemofiltration is a nondialytic technique that uses hydraulic pressure to filter rapidly middle- and large-weight substances from blood. Hemofiltration is more similar to peritoneal dialysis in this regard and less like routine hemodialysis. All of the hemodialysis variations require a special machine and, usually, reliance on a hospital and skilled technicians.

Peritoneal dialysis can be done more simply. It can be performed as an outpatient office procedure or, if the patient is trained, it can even be done at home with a minimum of costs and equipment. One future possibility is to influence the course and content of peritoneal dialysis pharmacologically, with vasodilators or specific chelators, intraperitoneally.

Complications of Dialysis: Total Experience

Many complications of peritoneal dialysis are known (Table 1). Some occur almost exclusively with the immunologic and metabolic damage of end-stage renal disease. Peritonitis is the most important complication of peritoneal dialysis, especially in persons with normal kidneys, who tend to have very few other problems with the procedure. Peritonitis is the major obstacle to wider use and acceptance of the technique.

Table 1. COMPLICATIONS OF PERITONEAL DIALYSIS

Peritonitis

Mechanical Complications
Abdominal pain, shoulder pain
Bleeding
Dialysate leak
Poor drainage through the catheter
   Loss of siphon effect
   One-way obstruction
   Wrong placement of catheter
   Fluid loculation
Perforation or laceration of internal organs
Intraperitoneal loss of peritoneal catheter

Dialysis Machine–Related Complications
Tube separation
Contamination
Faulty bag, tube, or adapter
Fibrin clot formation in tubes
Pump failure
Heat control failure
Loss of ultrafiltration capacity
Electrical or timer failures

Skin Catheter–Related Problems
Exit site infections
Skin discomfort
Scar, hyperpigmentation
Köbner effect

Medical Complications
Persistent ascites
Cardiovascular complications
   Hypovolemia
   Fluid overload, heart failure, and pulmonary edema
   Arrhythmia and hypokalemia
   Ischemic heart disease
   Myocardial infarction
   Pericarditis
   Hypotension
   Peripheral vascular disease

Gastrointestinal Complications
Hernia
Nausea
Vomiting
Constipation

Pulmonary Complications
Usually atelectasis

Metabolic Complications
Hyperglycemia or hypoglycemia
Hypernatremia
Alkalosis
Persistent metabolic acidosis
Hyperkalemia
Calcium disorders, osteodystrophy

Neurologic Complications
Peripheral neuropathy
Dialysis disequilibrium
Electroencephalogram abnormalities, convulsions
Sleep disorders
Neuropsychiatric problems

Nutritional Complications
Depletion of protein, amino acids, vitamins
Appetite suppression

Musculoskeletal Complications
Shoulder pain
Intrascapular pain
Lower back pain
Intravertebral disk pain
Neck pain, positional
Other muscle strains

Other Complications
Increased platelet counts
Polycythemia
Leg cramps
Kidney stones, renal colic
Reactive intraperitoneal mesothelial cells
Striae

Clinically, the peritonitis that commonly arises during peritoneal dialysis is unlike the peritonitis of ruptured bowels or gunshot wounds. The bacterial contamination in peritoneal dialysis is usually the spread of common flora from the skin into an intact cavity. The infection is then treated promptly by further dialysis and antibiotics. We suggest reporting the event more realistically as "half days with symptoms of peritonitis" per week of dialysis. During some episodes of peritonitis, the patient may have no symptoms. Only the physician becomes aware of turbidity in the peritoneal dialysis drainage and, after making cultures, treats the infection. Antibiotics can be given both in the dialysate and systemically. The site at which the catheter meets the skin is the source of most infections. The catheter should be removed if the infection persists. Quick success is usual after the "skin-to-catheter" site is clean.

Unusual infections from the bowel or those that come from within the dialysis equipment or solutions are much more threatening but have been increasingly rare in recent years. A successful dialysis program has few emergencies. A consulting nephrologist who is an expert in the management of rare peritonitis in dialysis patients is a valuable associate on these occasions. No such infections have happened in our series.

Historical Review of Dialysis Used for the Treatment of Psoriasis

Circulating among nephrologists in the 1970s was talk of the sudden recurring and vanishing of psoriasis in certain patients during dialysis of end-stage renal disease. Various explanations of these events were believable. For instance, large variations in protein synthesis during exacerbations and remissions in uremia would be likely to affect psoriasis. McEvory and Kelly provided the first detailed description in print of the clearing of psoriasis during hemodialysis in Ireland in 1976.[1] In Poland, Twardowski had seen the same good clinical response in several uremic patients and independently published his own report in 1977, in which he liberally hypothesized a specific "antipsoriatic" effect of dialysis.[2] Other clinicians before and since have noted similar clearing of psoriasis during and after various operations and serious illnesses and, of course, in severe end-stage renal disease. No presumptions that the situation is simplistic should be tolerated.

Twardowski, visiting the United States, joined with an established dermatology-nephrology group that had already been interested in the problem of psoriasis and interested in using peritoneal dialysis.[3,5,11] These techniques have been explained and studied by the nephrologist Karl Nolph.[6] Twardowski and this group immediately began to dialyze patients who had disabling psoriasis but no renal disease. The investigators did only a simple efficacy study without matched controls. The initial report of the group in 1978 described the first nephrologically normal psoriatic patients with severe persisting skin disease to be treated by dialysis and evaluated in a clinical research center.

Dialysis was performed on other nephrologically normal psoriatic patients, and discussions of the technique followed quickly internationally. In the United States, our group at Missouri used peritoneal dialysis mainly, whereas at the Cleveland Clinic Bailin's group used hemofiltration.[12] In Poland, Glinski achieved reliable results with peritoneal dialysis.[13,14] Glinski has suggested that removing white blood cells in large numbers and continuing the dialysis over 8 weeks may be crucial to success. In Israel, Halevy successfully treated all patients with doses of peritoneal dialysis that were larger than any used before.[15,16] Most communications about dialysis and psoriasis during 1978 through 1980 took place at meetings and through the mail; they were compiled with added opinions by Anderson.[17-19] The first conference on "Dialysis for Psoriasis" held at the National Institutes of Health in April 1979 was a stimulus to progress.[7-10, 20]

In Germany, Japan, Eastern Europe, Canada, and elsewhere, clinical anecdotes were published concerning the responsiveness to dialysis of some nephrologically normal psoriatic patients with exceptionally severe psoriasis. Failures were reported, but severe complications were few. Increasingly, dialysis is being used in centers of dermatology as one final resource of treatment of disabled persons who have not responded to other medications or who flare terribly after they must stop using methotrexate. Evaluating the use of dialysis in this context, I suggest that the "salvage index" of seemingly hopeless cases of psoriasis has been very encouraging.

We have no well-accepted explanation of how dialysis might work for psoriasis. No "antipsoriatic action" has been demonstrated biochemically. Clinical research concerning the many effects of dialysis on skin is ongoing, and some studies have been published. For a century the emphasis in research has been the anatomy of the cutaneous psoriatic lesions, epidermal kinetics, or biological mechanisms within psoriatic plaques. It seems refreshing to consider the possibility that psoriasis is induced in the skin by disorders in the systemic regulation system. A discussion of our own experience, logical analysis, and double-blind study follows.

Peritoneal Dialysis for Psoriasis Today: Logical Analysis and Double-Blind Trial

Psoriasis is a common disease that typically is mild. Occasionally, cases of psoriasis are severe, primarily as regards involvement of most all of the skin but also in terms of the depth to which the skin is damaged, the chronicity, and various other systemic features, which may include a terrible arthritis. No suitable system exists for measuring the severity of psoriasis. Of each 1000 persons with psoriasis, only a few patients are disabled severely. About these disabled patients we know extremely little. Medically documented details of the natural course are lacking. Much of what is accepted knowledge is anecdotal, partially documented, rooted in mere hearsay, or fanciful. Unassisted recall or questionnaires are useless in the determination of factual issues about these patients without verification.

No concepts about the etiology of psoriasis have been well accepted. When physicians treat ordinary psoriasis, they discover enormous and unexplained variations in response. Many patients recover seasonally, spontaneously, or with very little treatment. Some may respond only to methotrexate, only to retinoids, or only to some other difficult combinations of treatment. Some patients do not improve at all on any therapy. Some improve at first but relapse almost immediately. Overall, most mild psoriasis can be improved by the usual therapy, whereas very severe prolonged psoriasis may not often improve spontaneously and may be resistant even to the most skillful treatment.

Decisive studies of the systemic therapy of psoriasis in large matched and balanced populations that are well-designed and "controlled and blinded" are almost nonexistent. Controlled studies of any kind are uncommon. One valid design for tests of therapy without sham controls is the "flip-flop" study, which aims to show that psoriasis will remain in remission only while the treatment is sustained and will recur promptly when the treatment is stopped. The erratic natural course of psoriasis may disturb even a well-planned flip-flop study, although if sufficient clinical trials of equal duration are used and repeated often enough, some useful and even reliable facts may be gained.

Our initial interest was to apply a medium dose of dialysis in a flip-flop study to a few cases of severe psoriasis. The cases would be as similar as possible, and the patients would have no renal failure. The theoretic analysis is simple:

1. Psoriasis seems to be a systemic rather than a local disease.

2. Some systemic diseases have a mediator in the blood that, if removed, might cause improvement during dialysis (flip-flop study).

3. Present-day dialysis can remove some mediators to achieve improvement during dialysis.

Would cases of severe psoriasis exhibit clearing and recurrence when dialyzed? In such a simple study, the possible main outcomes are:

1. No patient improves despite vigorous treatment.

2. All patients improve dramatically and relapse when dialysis is stopped.

3. Some ambiguous mixture of the first two possibilities.

We found that the third possibility was correct but that the first possibility could be discarded. The unresponsive group is approximately one third to one half of all patients and includes many patients with pustular psoriasis and most elderly persons. However, some patients respond dramatically to peritoneal dialysis. Approximately 10 per cent respond fully and maintain their remission, some for years. Some patients respond at first and later relapse. Approximately 40 per cent of trials of vigorous dialysis, either peritoneal dialysis or hemofiltration, seem to achieve temporary improvement. In some of these, the flip-flop response is seen when dialysis is stopped and restarted. Not unexpectedly, in these early trials of dialysis in very ill, heterogeneous patients, the data could not be assembled into a tidy experimental design. Many technical problems occurred, some unexpectedly.

Most remissions from psoriasis have occurred within 6 to 12 weeks after peritoneal dialysis in persons whose prolonged disability had showed no improvement previously as a result of extensive topical care, rest, Goeckerman therapy, PUVA, and methotrexate. In older patients who have had unremitting generalized psoriasis and arthritis for 5 years, what are the true changes of a "spontaneous remission"? We suspect that they are very small. Our design presumes this conclusion in interpreting the remissions, but our placebo series sustains that presumption. The accurate observed data about the natural course are needed to improve experimental designs.

In response to our first published report, medical peers complained that the therapy was too aggressive, because, in their view, peritoneal dialysis was only a powerful placebo that acted somehow through the patient's mind to secure remissions of psoriasis. I do not agree with this. No evidence suggests to me that the seat of psoriasis is in the brain in the same sense as that of epilepsy or acute anxiety states. I considered the suggestion of a mysterious spirit in the brain activated by placebo to be even more imaginative than the hypothesis of some mysterious mediator in the blood. At least my mediator was chemical and not mythical. Both concepts could be tested further in a double-blind study.

In 1980, Fred Whittier devised the workable sham-dialysis unit. The Whittier unit actually does not accomplish a perfect sham but instead performs a tiny dialysis. Details are available elsewhere. Our double-blind design stipulated that the course of actual dialysis would be as uniform as possible and the patients would be as similar as possible clinically. We found that the sham dialysis could be wholly concealed, and we hoped that when the sequence of treatment was random the other variables would distribute themselves evenly in the two groups. When the double-blind study was decoded, we found that four of five patients receiving real dialysis had responded well, whereas none of five of the sham series patients had improved. One purpose of this design was to use the fewest patients, thereby including those that were most alike with regard to their disease, and to treat patients who were most likely to benefit from the therapy with the least risk overall. For purposes of the design, we presumed that the sham might be as effective as true dialysis therapy. The sampling was intended to reduce all variables among these cases. However, these individuals do not constitute a fair sample of all psoriatic patients or of all dermatologic patients.

This double-blind study demolished the "powerful placebo" theory. By 1981, reports of excellent responses to dialysis were commonplace,[21-28] and we can conclude from our study that the effect results from actual treatment. A few incurable psoriatics do achieve complete and amazing remissions after dialysis. What is the analysis? What does it mean? What possible explanations of our accumulated experiences are logically believable? The following possibilities should be considered:

1. Dialysis removes a distinct and specific blood-borne mediator of psoriasis to achieve a remission. Only one subtype of psoriasis responds fully, however. This subtype represents approximately 10 per cent of all cases of severe psoriasis.

2. Dialysis confers some general benefit to all ill persons, including those with severe psoriasis, but this benefit is wholly a nonspecific "homeostatic assist." Somehow, this small "assist" tips the balance in the body, and some natural remission occurs. The sham dialysis did not assist enough.

3. Some special immune defense system can implement a quick remission in psoriasis, and this system is activated by all noxious stimulations (or equivalent trigger) inside the peritoneal space. The effect is nonspecific and does not result from the removal of any mediator from blood or from any other action on blood. The sham dialysis was too gentle to trigger the defense.

4. The reported remissions are caused by adding lactate (or some equivalent chemical trigger) to the body fluids. The effect is not specific and does not depend on peritoneal access or dialysis. The sham did not add enough lactate to activate the defense.

5. Some combination of the four aforementioned possible explanations.

6. There is an entirely different explanation that takes into account that the remissions are a consequence of the treatments.

7. An exceptional run of coincidences involving no connection whatever between remissions and the treatments is in operation. This is expected to happen in less than 1 in over 100 comparable trials.

How To Do It

When it has been decided that a patient with psoriasis is a proper candidate for dialysis, one should take the following steps to insure safety in therapy:

1. Decide that no unusual risks prevail that make instilling fluid into the peritoneum unacceptable (prior surgery, peptic ulcer, diverticulitis, hernia, and so forth).

2. Decide that the cardiovascular stress will be within safe limits.

3. Decide that defenses against infections are at some acceptable minimum.

4. Assure good hydration and normal elimination from the bladder and the bowel.

Therapy should consist of:

1. Two days of continuous peritoneal dialysis with an exchange of approximately 2 liters per hour, or approximately 40 to 48 liters total per day.

2. Treatment each week for 4 to 6 weeks, depending on the severity of the disease.

3. Normal lubrication of skin and ordinary treatment of other medical problems.

4. Free intake of food and fluids.

SUMMARY

A theoretic but reasonable basis exists for attempting to resolve psoriasis by dialysis. Dialysis is a well-developed, safe, and modern technique. A small double-blind study has suggested that dialysis is effective per se (not as a placebo) in treatment of psoriasis. In the salvage of seemingly hopeless cases, the physician should expect 10 per cent remissions and 40 per cent useful improvement. The procedure remains experimental, and full verification depends on further experience.

References

1. McEvoy, J., and Kelly, A.: Psoriatic clearance during dialysis. Ulster Med. J. 45:76, 1976.
2. Twardowski, Z.: Abatement of psoriasis and repeated dialysis (letter). Ann. Intern. Med. 86:509, 1977.
3. Wei-Tzuok, C., Chung, H., Schitz, J., and Nakamoto, S.: In search of Psoriasis factors: A new approach by extracorporeal treatment. Artif. Organs 2:203, 1978.
4. Rubin, J., Rust, P., Brown, P., Popovitch, R., and Nolph, K.: A comparison of peritoneal transport in patients with psoriasis and uremia. Nephron 29:185, 1981.
5. Twardowski, Z., Nolph, K., Rubin, J., and Anderson, P.: Peritoneal dialysis for psoriasis. Ann. Intern. Med. 88:349, 1978.
6. Nolph, K. (ed.): Peritoneal Dialysis, vol. 2. Boston, Martinus Nyhoff, 1981.
7. Nissenson, A., Rapaport, M., Gordon, A., and Norins, R.: Hemodialysis in the treatment of psoriasis: A controlled study. Ann. Intern. Med. 91:218, 1979.
8. Nissenson, A., Rapaport, M., and Norins, R.: Dialysis and psoriasis (letter). Ann. Intern. Med. 92:709, 1980.
9. Buselmeier, T., Kjellstrand, C., Dahl, M., Cantieri, J., Nelson, R., Burgdorf, W., Bentley, C., Najarian, J., and Goltz, R.: Treatment of psoriasis with dialysis. Proc. Eur. Dial. Transplant Assoc. 15:171, 1978.
10. Buselmeier, T., Dahl, M., Kjellstrand, C., and Goltz, R.: Dialysis therapy for psoriasis. JAMA 240:1270, 1978.
11. Twardowski, Z.: Dialysis treatment in psoriasis also. Prezegl. Dermatol. 66:99, 1979.
12. Steck, W., Nakamoto, S., Bailin, P., Paganini, E., Cheng, K., Becker, J., Matkalak, R., and Vidt, D.: Hemofiltration treatment of psoriasis. J. Am. Acad. Dermatol. 6:346, 1982.

13. Glinski, W., Jablonska, S., Imiela, J., Nosarjewski, J., Jarzabek-Chorzelska, M., Haftek, M., and Obalek, S.: Continuous peritoneal dialysis for treatment of psoriasis. Arch. Dermatol. Res. 265:337, 1979.
14. Glinski, W., Jablonska, S., Jarzabuk-Chorzelska, M., Zarebska, Z., Imiela, J., and Nosarzewski, J.: Continuous peritoneal dialysis for treatment of psoriasis. Arch. Dermatol. Res. 266:83, 1979.
15. Halevy, J., Halevy, S., Feverman, E., and Rosenfeld, J.: Cases of remissions of psoriasis on hemodialysis with three month recurrence. Br. Med. J. 1:1490, 1979.
16. Halevy, S., Halevy, J., Boner, G., Rosenfeld, J., and Feverman, E.: Dialysis therapy for psoriasis. Arch. Dermatol. 117:69, 1981.
17. Anderson, P.: Dialysis for psoriasis. Artif. Organs 2:202, 1978.
18. Anderson, P.: Progress concerning dialysis of psoriatics. Artif. Organs 3:282, 1979.
19. Anderson, P.: Dialysis treatment of psoriasis (editorial). Arch. Dermatol. 117:67, 1981.
20. Anderson, P.: Report: National Institutes of Health conference on psoriasis and dialysis. J. Am. Acad. Dermatol. 1:565, 1979.
21. Sprenser-Klasen, L., Franz, H., and Rodermund, D.: Improvement in psoriasis by hemodialysis. Dtsch. Med. Wochenschr. 105:925, 1980.
22. Goring, H., Thieler, H., Guldner, G., and Schmidt, U.: Peritoneal dialysis therapy in psoriasis. Hautarzt 32:173, 1981.
23. Maeda, K., Kawaguchi, S., Niwa, T., Ohki, T., and Kobayashi, K.: Identification of some abnormal metabolites in psoriatic nail using gas chromatography and mass spectrometry. J. Chromatogr. 221:199, 1980.
24. Muston, H., and Concucas, S.: Remission of psoriasis during hemodialysis. Br. Med. J. 1:48, 1978.
25. Buselmeier, T., Cantieri, J., Dahl, M., Nelson, R., Baumgaertner, J., Bentley, C., and Gottz, R.: Clearing of psoriasis after cardiac surgery requiring cardiopulmonary bypass oxygenation: A corollary to clearance after dialysis? Br. J. Dermatol. 100:311, 1979.
26. Llewellyn, M., Nethercott, J., and Bear, R.: Peritoneal dialysis in the treatment of psoriasis (letter). Can. Med. Assoc. J. 122:13, 1980.
27. Rose, I.: Dialysis for psoriasis (letter). Can. Med. Assoc. J. 120:1209, 1979.
28. Lamperi, S., Buoncris, U., Carozzi, S., Cozzari, M., Icardi, A., and Transfori, D.: Gel filtration studies on uremic and psoriatic serum and dialysis fluid. Artif. Organs 4:338, 1980.

TREATMENT OF PSORIASIS AT THE DEAD SEA

Harold M. Schneidman, M.D.

Most physicians have knowledge of psoriasis therapy at the Dead Sea, but details of treatment and response are vague. Seeing cases of psoriasis and evaluating the Dead Sea program is a unique experience in several ways. One approaches this evaluation in both a spiritual and a scientific manner. Many believe that the Bible covers all aspects of human life and experience, past and present, and psoriasis is no exception. Reference is made in the Bible to a Persian general who sought treatment for leprosy from the prophet Elijah. The general spent 6 weeks at the Dead Sea under care of the prophet and was cured of his skin problem. It is likely that the general had psoriasis. In this modern era, one must remain a scientist and must assess this program at the Dead Sea critically and scientifically.

The program was initiated by Professor Dostrovsky of Hadassah University in the late 1950s. In 1971, management was taken over by Willie Avrick, a dermatologist from Denmark.

The treatment is classified as climate therapy; this includes sun, salt bathing, and rest. Petrolatum is used freely for dryness. Other medications, such as topical steroids, are permitted only on the request of the referring physician; this occurs only in a few cases. Most of the patients using topical steroids are able to stop within 2 weeks.

The patients spend 28 days undergoing treatment at the Dead Sea. The first day, they arrive at the airport and spend the night in a hotel in Tel Aviv. The next morning, the patients are transported by bus from Tel Aviv to a spa at the Dead Sea. Within this first 24 hours, a general medical checkup is performed. Any requests from the family physician are reviewed and are usually heeded. Any serious complications, such as cardiac, diabetic, or rheumatic problems, are evaluated critically, and the physicians decide whether these will interfere with the program. The personal physician in the home country is usually alerted in order to screen out such problem cases. Following this examination, the patients are assigned to their rooms; an orientation lecture is then given. After the lecture, the patients are allowed to go to the beach for sunbathing.

Patients can usually tolerate 2 hours of sun on the first day of exposure and 6 hours on subsequent days. During my visit, all patients were questioned critically regarding sunburn. A few developed a minimal erythema after the first day, and some suffered a mild erythema within 3 days. All patients spent several hours each day swimming in the Dead Sea. The minerals left a greasy film on the skin that could be washed off in showers located on the beach. There has been discussion concerning the role of the minerals in the water. The impression of the Dead Sea physicians is that the minerals play a minor role in the clearing. The mineral content of the Dead Sea water is listed in Table 1. A controversial question concerns the effect of radioactive elements on psoriasis; it is felt by the Dead Sea physicians and chemists that this effect is negligible.

Psychological factors have been discussed; I feel, as did the other physicians that I questioned, that these are significant. Living in a hotel environment rather than a hospital was considered to be important. It is obvious to one who hospitalizes many psoriatic patients that, after 7 days in a hospital room, the individual is "climbing the walls." There is little opportunity for walking, conversation, and freedom. At the Dead Sea Spa, on the other hand, the patient has a room of his own with cable television and air conditioning, and he is free to move throughout the spa. Meals are eaten in a dining room with other

Table 1. MINERAL CONTENT
OF DEAD SEA WATER

Fluoride	Calcium
Chloride	Magnesium
Bromide	Iron
Nitrate	Metasilic acid
Bicarbonate	Carbon dioxide
Sulfate	Hydrogen sulfide
Sodium	Radon: RN 222
Potassium	Radium: RA 226

people. The meals are lavish, and quantities are enormous compared with those of hospital meals. In the evening, there is an opportunity to attend a lecture, to see a movie, or to talk with other patients in the cocktail lounge. Mingling with other people who suffer from the same condition allows patients with widespread psoriasis to gain confidence as they compare their response with that of other patients. The degree of improvement becomes a contest.

Why does the treatment work? The Dead Sea is 1300 feet below sea level. A layer of air fills this gap and filters out short waves of the sun, leaving predominantly long waves above 320 nanometers. Short waves contribute less than 10 per cent of the spectrum. The remaining long waves are the type that is used in the PUVA regimen. I asked the physicians at the Dead Sea, "Why not give oral psoralens, since this might improve the results and might cut down on the treatment time?" The Israeli physicians were reluctant to do this; they prefer to adhere to natural treatment and pure climate therapy.

I was impressed with the conservatism shown by the physicians at the Dead Sea in evaluating treatment. Scientifically, their results have to be critically compared with those of currently available treatment modalities. The forms of therapy that can be compared with the Dead Sea program include hospitalization, treatment at day care centers, outpatient care, other varieties of climate therapy (such as traveling to Hawaii or to sunny resorts in the Mediterranean area), and PUVA. Retinoids, alone or in conjunction with PUVA, constitute a current development and are too new in the United States to compare with the Dead Sea program.

Comment

Indications

Climatotherapy at the Dead Sea is indicated for most types of psoriasis. The guttate variety, the plaque type, and generalized erythroderma respond well. Inverse psoriasis responds more slowly and less effectively. Pustular psoriasis responds poorly. Arthritis in patients with minimal or extensive skin involvement improves remarkably with climatotherapy.

The original protocol established the following criteria for inclusion of patients in the Dead Sea regimen: (1) widespread disease, (2) resistant disease, (3) history of repeated hospital admissions, and (4) refusal to enter the hospital after numerous admissions. These criteria continue to be valid. Contraindications for therapy include (1) medical problems, such as chronic alcoholism; (2) psychiatric problems; and (3) a history of photosensitivity.

Advantages of the Dead Sea Regimen

The Dead Sea program is a natural approach to treatment of psoriasis, utilizing sun, bathing, and rest (physical and psychological). It avoids drugs, topical steroids, topical tars, and psoralens. Patients are placed in an environment in which they are not embarrassed to sunbathe in public, and they compete with one another with regard to progress and clearing of their psoriasis. The recurrence rate within 1 month is slightly lower with this regimen than with other forms of therapy. Complete clearing for a period of 1 year is experienced by 20 per cent of the patients. In patients who come back to the Dead Sea for the second and third time, the duration of clearing grows longer and longer. Physicians who have managed the program at the Dead Sea and those who have visited and observed the program place great importance on the psychological benefits.

The treatment of chronic skin disease in a hotel resort environment offers unusual advantages. This single aspect of the Dead Sea program may cause it to gain greater acceptance in the future in the treatment not only of psoriasis but also of other chronic skin diseases. The cost of treatment in a hotel resort environment is less than the cost of therapy in a hospital.

Disadvantages of the Dead Sea Program

The program involves a trip to Israel with the expense of air travel and land arrangements. Insurance programs in the United States will not pay for this; however, insurance programs in other countries, such as Holland, Belgium, Denmark, Sweden, and Germany, will pay for the trip and the treatment at the Dead Sea. The government insurance programs have come to the conclusion that the trip is less expensive than hospitalization and that the remissions are longer-lasting than those obtained with hospitalization and other forms of therapy.

Tables

Tables 2 through 5 show the results in 562 patients treated up to the time of my visit. Over 3000 patients have been treated up to the present, and the accumulated statistics do not vary appreciably from those presented in the tables. The recurrence rate within 1 month is 35 per cent. Although this may seem high it compares favorably with the recurrence rate within 1 month following the Goeckerman regimen (45 per cent recurrence), anthralin therapy (53 per cent), and treatment with topical steroids (95 per cent). It is noteworthy that no recurrence was reported in approximately 20 per cent of patients. One hundred

Table 2. PERCENTAGE OF SKIN INVOLVEMENT IN 562 PATIENTS

Number of Patients	Percentage of Involvement
10	75%
217	30–75%
306	5–30%
29	15%

Table 3. RESULTS AFTER 4 WEEKS

Cleared	25%
Improved	70%
Unchanged	5%
Worse	0.5%
Not indicated	1%

Table 4.   RECURRENCES

In 1 month	35%
In 3 months	25%
No recurrence	20%
Unknown	20%

Table 5.   RESULTS CONCERNING
ARTHRITIS SYMPTOMS

155 patients—118 improved (75%)

fifty-five of 562 patients had arthritis. The majority of these patients attained complete clearing or great improvement of the arthritis.

Compared with the usual treatment modalities in the United States and Europe, the Dead Sea program has proved equal to all available therapies and, in my evaluation, safer and better.

Editorial Comment

Probably no dermatosis is as erratic in its response to therapeutic measures as is psoriasis. The old cliché, "One man's poison is another's nectar" is applicable in the management of this disease. A remedy may work like a miracle in one case (or in many cases) and yet may prove completely ineffective in the next individual with an identical eruption. A remedy may work like magic in a patient during one attack but may fail completely during a recurrence in the same patient. This makes judgment of therapies for this condition difficult.

I visited the National Institutes of Health a few years ago and was shown a patient with a severe bilaterally symmetric eruption of psoriasis on the elbows. One elbow had been treated topically with a placebo; the other had been treated with a solution of nitrogen mustard. The elbow treated with the nitrogen mustard had cleared completely, and the other was unchanged. Inspired, I returned home and tested this procedure on a man with a severe generalized eruption whom I had treated for years without being able to eradicate the cutaneous manifestations completely. Within 6 weeks his skin had cleared for the first time. I then tried the identical approach on ten other patients, but none of them showed any improvement at all. In the meantime, the original patient suffered a recurrence. Resumption of the nitrogen mustard therapy did not have any effect.

According to the literature, dialysis is one of the more promising procedures for treatment of severe psoriasis at this time. Its use is limited, however, because the scarcity of artificial kidneys makes dialysis impractical for a "frivolous disease," such as psoriasis. The need to keep kidney sufferers alive far outweighs the indication for dialysis in treatment of an eruption. On the other hand, in my experience some of the worst and most therapeutically resistant examples of psoriasis have occurred in patients receiving dialysis for renal dysfunctions. Furthermore, the condition cleared completely in at least one of these patients when the individual received a successful kidney transplant. Of course, it must be admitted that the effect of dialysis in a patient with normal kidney functions may be different with regard to psoriasis from the effect in a patient with little or no renal function.

As this is written, 13-*cis*-retinoic acid has not been released for general use. Its value in this disease may rest in its use as an adjunct to PUVA. Reports suggest that its administration may reduce the amount of PUVA required to obtain the desired effect, therefore reducing the adverse reactions that occur with PUVA—especially squamous cell cancers. The experience of Grupper and Berretti in France is noteworthy because of the large number of patients they have treated, most of them successfully. Their finding that PUVA does not prevent recurrences even if the cleared patient receives so-called prophylactic treatments is very important and may indicate that therapists employing such preventative measures are merely fooling themselves as well as their patients. The Goeckerman treatment as practiced at the Mayo Clinic is considered to be one of the safest and most effective therapeutic approaches, and I concur with this judgment.

Methotrexate, and aminopterin before that, have exerted a beneficial therapeutic effect in a significant number of patients with psoriasis. Having used these agents for many years in many hundreds of patients before the hysteria regarding hepatotoxicity surfaced, I encountered very few side effects and no evidence of liver damage. However, the strict guidelines promulgated by the Food and Drug Administration and the American Academy of Dermatology discouraged practitioners from continuing to use these agents. The need for pretreatment and follow-up liver biopsies should cause the clinician to hesitate before using this approach in his practice. The need for repeated blood counts and liver tests seems to be excessive. So, for practical purposes, the patient with psoriasis consulting a private practitioner is denied these effective, relatively safe agents because of unreasonable blocks put in the way of the physician who might elect to use them. The greatest hazard is a medicolegal one. If you have not conformed to all of the excessive requirements for use of methotrexate and aminopterin, it may be very difficult to defend a malpractice action connected with the administration of these chemotherapeutic agents, regardless of the actual merits of the case.

Think It Over.

SECTION 4

ACNE

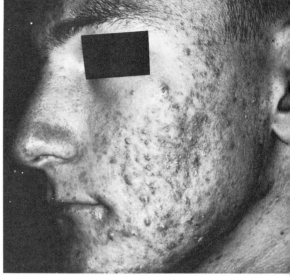

A typical severe example of acne.

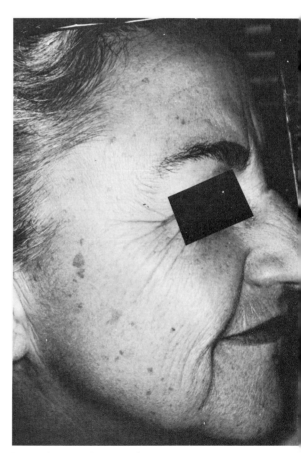

Rhytids that could be treated with collagen injections.

CHAPTER 16

PATHOGENESIS

ACNE: THE ASHES OF A BURNT-OUT CONTROVERSY

Sam Shuster, M.B.

In one of his more cynical moments, de Selby said, "the academic sieves the ashes of life." What he meant by that is obvious when one considers his later analysis of historical theory and the infamous quip that "serious debate takes over from relevance." In other words, serious debate can begin only when it is sufficiently detached, and that occurs only when it is no longer relevant because the problem has been solved. That is precisely the present situation of adolescent acne. The appalling pseudoetiologic nonsense that has been discussed for years has all been washed away by the indisputable evidence that the primary factor is sebum production, out of which all else springs. But that is not to say that these old ideas will retire gracefully. We accept new facts, but we do not like to trade in the ideas into which we have grown and that therefore give comfort. Ideas disappear only as the intellectual warriors, who bear them as a coat of arms, die and are buried with them, just as the fighting apparel was buried with the more physical warriors of the past. Beliefs about acne will change only with the passing of a generation, as the old ideas are encoffined and laid to rest, with a short, silent moment in which we remember the fun of old, irrelevant battles.

This essay, therefore, is not so much a contribution to a living debate as the celebration of a wake, albeit a little before its time. As such, it will vary stylistically from the light-hearted to the light-headed. I will not load the argument with distracting footnotes (though I will stamp on a number of feet-of-note that might be found there); this I hope will bring pleasure to the reader as well as leavening to the task of the writer, both of whom are renowned for laziness. It will also please those whom I propose to insult, because by failing to document my arguments fully they will have a ready-made escape route. I offer this to them with magnanimity and good will, but not without deviousness, because I would have them escape cleanly; the field has been cluttered with their idle chatter for too long.

What is the controversy about? On one side is my reductionist theory, which explains adolescent acne by an increase in sebum excretion—bacterial colonization and inflammation are secondary events. The other is not so much a theory as a doss house of half-awake pretenders—sebum composition, lipases, bacteria, food, sex, psychodrama and, above all, duct blockage. The last is the current mistress of the Acne Barons (Kligman, Strauss, Plewig, and Cunliffe—I suspect Peter Pochi is really a double agent).

Despite an occasional lapse from etiologic grace, exploitation of which I will defer to Peter Pochi, I have been as obsessed as any Texan by the dominance of the rate of production of (sebaceous) oil and have long professed surprise with the intellectual layabouts and academic mystery men who have so confused a simple subject. The evidence for the primary role of sebum excretion is that it correlates better with the severity of acne than does any other characteristic (Cunliffe and Shuster, 1969). Pochi and Strauss (1964) were the first to record this relationship, but they failed to realize its importance as they took up the curious North American obsession with sebum composition and duct blockage. So it was left to me to carry the torch for sebum excretion when Cunliffe deserted the cause and joined them. The illogicality of their argument for excluding seborrea as the primary factor is simply illustrated. *"There is considerable variation* in sebum production *within the group of patients with* acne, *indicating that the disease is not related solely* to sebaceous gland activity"* (Strauss, 1979). Substitute: *"There is considerable variation* in porphyrin production *within the group of patients with* porphyria, *indicating that the disease is not related solely* to porphyrin metabolism"* (Shuster, now).

Overlap is a ubiquitous biological phenomenon. In acne, this is partly caused by an incorrect experimental paradigm, because you cannot control a variable by reference to a normal subject without acne. The equation of controls with normality is one of the most common errors made in medical research. Depending upon what problem you wish to resolve, a control may be an entirely normal person (a few such still exist), or it may be a one-legged heterosexual male standing on his contralateral arm. (Perhaps the Boards should try the question: "In what experimental study would a one-legged . . . [etc.] . . . be a suitable control?") Because acne is almost universal (Fellowes et al., 1981), a "normal control" without acne is a younger person in whom acne has not developed, an older one in whom acne has burnt out, or one of the few teen-aged individuals who never develop acne. None of these "controls" is relevant. The essential paradigm in acne research relates defects to severity, and inappropriate use of normal subjects as controls means that much acne research is invalid.

In addition to the relationship of sebum excretion rate to acne severity, Cunliffe and I found (1969) that when the acne regressed, the increased rate of sebum excretion persisted and therefore suggested a second factor. That deduction was logically unsound (Shuster, 1980). Because the rash of chicken pox does not persist when the virus can still be found does not exclude its viral cause; the explanation is immunologic resistance. The question could therefore be: What other factor causes acne to disappear? It could be that acne is terminated immunologically or, more likely, that as the structure of the hair follicle changes over the years it can no longer sustain the condition. The point is that increased sebum production is an adequate explanation by itself, and the simple fact that ends doubt is that its reduction will *by itself* improve acne, and the degree of cure depends only upon the degree of reduction, regardless of whether this is achieved by blocking lipid synthesis with a metabolic inhibitor, endocrinologically by an antiandrogen, or with that magnificent therapeutic accident, 13-*cis*-retinoic acid. Forget primary changes in microbes, lipases, and sebum composition; forget the psyche, the fried food, and blocked ducts. Remove sebum and you remove acne.

So what has the debate been about? Why, despite the evidence for seborrhea, do dermatologic journals still carry advertisements for agents alleged to act by relief of duct blockage? This returns us to the Four Knights of the Blackhead and their magic mottos: "Acne is strictly a follicular dermatosis"; "the primary event is ductal obstruction"; "the prime defect is abnormal keratinization"; and "the comedo is the initial primary lesion of acne." Let us now examine this comedo of errors. I suspect that the idea of duct obstruction took hold more by the sociality of science than by its content—that the enduhring engospelation by acne cosmetica, detergica, mechanica, and other kligmania led on to the "central role of the comedo" when the only evidence of its centrality was its position in the duct.

In Plewig and Kligman's book (1975), the power of the argument is laid out (in both senses) by the motivating quotation (confucianly attributed to a man called Confucious [sic]) that "one picture is worth a thousand words." Having read some of the words used, I cannot say I disagree. The power of a myth is inversely related to the factual force of an argument: "Acne pustules arise from comedones." Of course they do not, as every dermatologist with half an eye knows, and as their photographs show, the blackhead is a modest individual sitting quietly in the duct minding its own business (until it is inexpertly squeezed). The simple observer must therefore conclude either that blackheads are acne-protective (more a wedge than a plug?) or, as the pictures show, that they are associated with spent, inactive glands. But the plumbing school of acne has observed the obvious with the eye of the devious, because its members go on to say that although "acne pustules arise from comedones, the latter are usually invisible." That is like a medieval proof of witchcraft in an innocent old crone, because the very absence of its signs shows unnatural aid in their concealment! In any case, if the small, "invisible" ones cause trouble, why should the bigger ones not cause even bigger trouble—at least sometimes? Then what about "comedogenicity"? My fourth law of science is: Phenomena are more easily created by names than by evidence. I suspect that the comedogenic response of the rabbit ear occurs even to a smile, especially Philadelphic, and it is just as nonspecific.

Apart from the quiet and irrelevant backwater of the comedo, there is excellent evidence of lipid deposition and keratinization of the follicles in acne, but neither their cause nor their functional consequences are known. In particular, the idea that they precipitate a sequence of duct blockage onward to rupture of a follicular time bomb can be taken only as a literary artifact, as an aesthetic appreciation of one aspect of the histology of acne, and as one of the many stories of the whodunit of acne written at the fireside for the bedside. Nor should the folliculitis induced by environmental agents confuse the issue; it does not allow the inference that duct obstruction is involved in adolescent acne.

My main objection to the duct blockage theory is its poor experimental base. There has been no attempt to establish whether or not the changes in the follicle do in fact constitute a barrier by correlating the size of the assumed "plug" with impairment of sebum excretion. But there is indirect evidence: Cunliffe's group (1975) has shown that what they consider to be follicular "plugs" correlate with severity of acne and decrease in size when the acne is improved with tetracycline. Yet tetracycline does not lead to an increase in sebum excretion rate, which it should, since most follicles have these "plugs." Why has this functional evidence that the "plugs" do not block the ducts been ignored, as has Cunliffe's less critical evidence that cellophane tape stripping does not increase sebum excretion? And why do the very people who reject the etiologic significance of the quantitative correlation of sebum excretion rate and acne severity nevertheless accept duct blockage on its eyeball recognition without any functional evidence of a quantitative relationship between "plug" size and blockage? Belief in duct blockage has all the perverse characteristics of a myth: It persists in spite of reality. One has therefore to conclude that it fills an emotional need; whether this relates to early problems with potty training or whether it is a simple phallic extension of a castration complex or a belated meow in an arrested Oedipus are topics for conjecture with as much future as the theory of duct obstruction itself.

Since the plumbing school of acne continues to exist without evidence, let us join them in the game. Consider for the sake of argument (and surely, for the sake of argument, that is what the argument is about) that duct obstruction and an increased rate of sebum excretion had both been shown to occur in acne. Then the possibilities are that neither, one, or both factors are causally related to acne.

1. If neither is related, there is no debate.

2. If just one factor is related etiologically, then the other is neutral and is associated either (a) secondarily or (b) fortuitously. If one considers that it is related secondarily, since duct blockage would immediately and necessarily exacerbate the effect of a particular rate of sebum excretion (whereas the converse is not inevitable), duct blockage logically excludes itself. If only one factor is etiologically involved, it has to be seborrhea. A fortuitous association can be dismissed, as will be explained later.

3. If both factors are etiologically involved, they may be (a) independent, (b) related by a common mechanism, or (c) related causally.

If they are independent, then the association must be random, and the same degree of acne will result from a high rate of sebum excretion with little blockage and vice versa (and all grades between). This is not the case for sebum excretion or for the keratin "plugs" studied by Cunliffe's group, both of which correspond to the severity of acne. We can exclude this possibility; the same argument applies to the aforementioned fortuitous association.

If the two factors are related indirectly by a common mechanism (e.g., if the same sebotrophic stimulus acts on the gland to produce lipid and on the duct to produce lipid and keratin), then the magnitude of one will correspond to the magnitude of the other, and either could be taken to represent the other. The correct experimental procedure is to use the most measurable factor and to reject its validity only when the evidence of prediction proves it inadequate. Thus, until duct blockage is measurable, the mechanism should be taken to be indistinguishable from the rate of sebum excretion.

Finally, the major, and yet the simplest, logical knot in the "debate": does the increased sebum production cause a blocked duct, or does a blocked duct cause an increase in sebum production? It is self-evident that, whereas there are countless ways in which an increased rate of sebum excretion *could* cause secondary changes in the duct, the notion that a blocked duct could increase sebum production is nonsense.

So, if you prefer to believe that acne is primarily a disorder of duct blockage, the logical consequences you face are either (1) the seborrhea is secondarily provoked by the blockage or (2) the seborrhea is an unrelated finding, even though its quantitative relationship to acne has been proved. If you believe the first, you will believe anything, and if you believe the second, you are willing to disbelieve anything. I suspect that the reason the plumbing school of acne has refused to consider its logical position is that the analysis leads to such clear conclusions: On purely theoretic grounds, duct obstruction can be dismissed as ignorable or untenable.

The weakness of both fact and theory that we have seen in the duct-gland debate characterizes the whole of the acne field. This field is marked by the still-undefined areas of endocrine control (Shuster, 1981); the obsession with androgen and the erroneous attribution of its action to conversion to dihydrotestosterone (Shuster, 1982); the dollars and man-hours wasted demonstrating that changes in surface lipid composition are secondary and the failure to look at sebum in the individual sickening glands, where it might matter; the hideously irrelevant work on lipases; the sterile studies of bacteria, the obvious role of which was doubted because their enzyme activity was found to be decreased before they died (can you imagine the converse?) and because the number of organisms in the duct was unchanged by antibiotics (you could as well expect the volume of water in the pipe between tank and faucet to change with flow); the attempt to win a Nobel Prize in the back kitchen by establishing how a possibly novel proinflammatory cascade functions. (This approach was described in an article about the Schitz Test [Shuster, 1979], which was named after its inventor, Dr. Schitz, who, despite the fortuitous onomatopoeia, achieved fame from studies based on the intradermal injection of feces); and, finally, the suggestion that widespread persistence of a socially disadvantageous condition should lead us to consider that acne might have a biological purpose (Shuster, 1976). I could continue but for editorial impatience, reader boredom, and writer's cramp.

The problem with opening a badly overfilled cupboard is that you can never get the stuff back in again. Let me share a now equally open secret: That was my intention, because I believe that before any new useful questions can be posed, it is first necessary for us old acne warriors to leave the battlefield. There is no longer any intellectual interest in the subject for us, and we have no new ideas worth the fight. Without these we will simply inhibit the young, and if nothing else blocks their thought ducts it will be us and our dated battles. The elimination of acne by drugs that simply impair sebum production answers the major etiologic question. We should be content with that; there is nothing more to be gained by raking over the ashes of a burnt-out past.

References

Cunliffe, W. J., and Cotterill, J. A.: The Acnes: Clinical Features, Pathogenesis, and Treatment. London, W. B. Saunders Co., Ltd., 1975.

Cunliffe, W. J., and Shuster, S.: Pathogenesis of acne. Lancet 1:685, 1969.

Fellowes, H. M., Billewic, W. Z., and Thompson, A. M.: Is acne a sign of normal puberty? A longitudinal study. J. Biosoc. Sci. 13:401, 1981.

Plewig, G., and Kligman, A. M.: Acne: Morphogenesis and Treatment. Berlin, Springer-Verlag, 1975.

Pochi, P. E., and Strauss, J. S.: Sebum production, casual sebum levels, titratable acidity of sebum, and urinary fractional 17-ketosteroid excretion in males with acne. J. Invest. Dermatol. 43:383, 1964.

Shuster, S.: Biological purpose of acne. Lancet 1:1328, 1976.

Shuster, S.: All my eye and intradermal faeces. World Med. 14:93, 1979.

Shuster, S.: Acne: Possibilities and probabilities. Acta Dermatol. 5(Suppl. 89):33, 1980.

Shuster, S.: Reason and the rash. Proc. R. Inst. Gt. Britain 53:136, 1981.

Shuster, S.: The sebaceous glands and primary cutaneous virilism. In Jeffcoate (ed.): Androgens and Anti-androgen Therapy. Chichester, John Wiley & Sons, Ltd., 1982.

Strauss, J.S.: Sebaceous glands. In Fitzpatrick, T. B., et al. (eds.): Dermatology in Internal Medicine. New York, McGraw-Hill, 1979, p. 442.

PATHOGENESIS OF ACNE: IMPORTANCE OF FOLLICULAR EPITHELIAL CHANGES

Peter E. Pochi, M.D.

The pathogenesis of acne vulgaris is complex. Several factors are known to be important, namely, sebum, the microbial flora, and abnormal follicular epithelial differentiation.[1-3] Of these etiologic influences, follicular occlusion was the first to be recognized as an adverse factor for the simple reason that it could be appreciated clinically—that is, as the visible presence of comedones.

An unsettled issue, however, has revolved around the question of what is the primary abnormal event in the development of the acne lesion. In a sense, such an argument is perhaps less deserving than is warranted. If, for example, follicular retention hyperkeratosis in acne could be stimulated to develop as a result of the presence of sebum, the apparent primacy of sebum would not necessarily mean that sebum is *more* important than follicular hyperkeratosis in the formation of the acne lesion. On the other hand, if follicular obstruction were indeed the "first thing" to occur in acne, this fact would not necessarily supersede or diminish the importance of other factors, such as sebum, bacteria, and so forth. Put another way, what comes first is not necessarily worst. As the interrelationships among the various factors become better understood, it is likely that what will emerge is a picture in which pathologic events occur in concert and not merely in a linear sequence. As such, interpretations as to what is most significant may lead to specious conclusions.

Nonetheless, the role of the aberrant development of the follicle in acne is the least readily dismissible. Admittedly, sebum is indeed a central factor in the pathogenesis of the disease. This lipid material is comedogenic,[4] an irritant,[5] and a substrate for *Propionibacterium acnes*.[6,7] Worse cases of acne tend to have higher sebum levels, and treatments that result in a significant decrease in sebum usually lead to an improvement in the disease. Individuals without acne, however, have sebum that qualitatively differs little, if at all, from acne sebum.[8] The same can be said of the presence of *P. acnes*. The only clearly distinctive pathophysiologic alteration of the pilosebaceous system in individuals with and without acne is the abnormal epithelial differentiation that results in the formation of comedones.

Knutson[9] and Wolff and associates[10] have described in considerable detail the ultrastructural features of the formation of acne comedones. These lesions develop in specialized pilosebaceous structures, termed sebaceous follicles, that have a large follicular channel but a small vellus hair. Associated with the follicle are large, multiacinar sebaceous glands. In acne, the initial morphologic changes occur in the follicular epithelium of these sebaceous follicles. The most prominent alteration is in the horny layer of the follicular epithelium. Normally, the stratum corneum here is thin, and the horny cells formed are often fragmented and fail to form coherent layers of cells, as is seen in the epidermis or even in the upper reaches of the follicle. Keratohyaline granules are small and sparse, but lamellar granules are quite numerous.

In the development of the acne comedo, the follicular epithelium undergoes striking alterations. The horny layer becomes very much thicker, with the retention of several to many layers of fully keratinized cells, often containing numerous intracellular lipid inclusions. Also, the granular layer becomes thickened with abundant and large keratohyaline granules. At the same time, the lamellar granules become greatly reduced in number. No information is at hand concerning morphometric measurements of the thickness of the viable epithelium in comedones as compared with uninvolved follicles. It has been shown with the use of tritiated thymidine, however, that there is increased labeling of the epithelial cells of the comedo as compared with noncomedonal epithelium.[11] Thus, one may conclude that the pathology of acne is the overproduction of adherent horny cells of the follicular epithelium.

There is general agreement that comedones are requisite precursors of the inflammatory lesions of acne vulgaris.[1] In early reported histologic studies at the light microscopic level, it was shown that inflammation could occur in normal-appearing sebaceous follicles in the apparently normal skin of subjects with acne.[12] However, no evidence has ever been demonstrated that these microscopic inflammatory foci progress to clinical inflammatory lesions. It has been subsequently conceded that these lesions are infrequent and microscopic only and resolve spontaneously rather than progress to clinically apparent inflammatory lesions.[1] Thus, the comedo, which results from the abnormal follicular process of keratinization that has been described previously, is the precursor lesion for the subsequent formation of the inflammatory acne lesion.

The central question remains, then, as to what leads to the formation of comedones. Knutson has speculated that the horny abnormalities are somehow linked to the lamellar granules, which are lysosomal in nature.[9] Their large numbers in the normal sebaceous follicular epithelium may indicate increased activity, resulting in dysadhesion of horny cells. A decrease in their activity would therefore allow the horny cells to "stick" to one another more readily. Others have postulated that these granules produce a cementing substance, and therefore their depletion during comedo formation is an indication that they are being used for intercellular adhesion and consequent retention of horny cells.

However, these postulated mechanisms afford no insight into the stimulus or stimuli responsible for these changes in the first place. Few clues are currently available, although it has been suggested that sebum itself, as mentioned earlier, may be the stimulus for their formation. Sebaceous lipids, such as free fatty acids and squalene, are comedogenic when applied topically to the inner surface of the rabbit ear.[4,13] Also, it is known that comedones appear early in the prepubertal period, when sebaceous gland activity is reawakening.[14] Sebarche generally occurs earlier than is usually appreciated, namely, at the age of 6 years in girls and 7 years in boys.[15] It is not known for certain whether acne comedones, which can be detected only by electron microscopic examination, can occur prior to an increase in sebum production.[16] Since there are no known family pedigrees in which asebia is a feature, the determination of which comes first is at present difficult to ascertain. One way in which the matter might be settled is to observe whether a significant and prolonged reduction of sebaceous gland activity leads unequivocally to a diminution in comedo formation. Even if this were not to occur, however, it might be hard to draw any positive conclusion, since the reversibility of the previously sebum-stimulated lesion remains to be demonstrated. In the rabbit ear, artificially-induced comedones decrease in size slowly over several months.[4] Although it has been reported that the marked reduction of sebum secretion induced by orally administered isotretinoin is also attended by a decrease in comedones,[17] the latter is not necessarily dependent on the former because of the direct antikeratinizing property of the drug.

On the basis, then, of the information that is currently available, it is evident that abnormal keratinization of the follicular epithelium in the sebaceous follicle is the pathologic hallmark of acne vulgaris and the proximate event leading to the inflammatory phase of the disease. Whether sebum functions to aggravate this pathologic process or whether it does much more, as suggested earlier, still needs to be demonstrated. The precise interrelationships of sebum, bacteria, and other factors remain to be elucidated in order for an accurate view of the evolution of the acne lesion to be provided.

References

1. Plewig, G., and Kligman, A. M.: Acne: Morphogenesis and Treatment. Berlin, Springer-Verlag, 1975.
2. Cunliffe, W. J., and Cotterill, J. A.: The Acnes: Clinical Features, Pathogenesis, and Treatment. London, W. B. Saunders Co., Ltd., 1975.
3. Pochi, P. E., Leyden, J. J., Shalita, A. R., and Strauss, J. S.: Acne. Current Concepts, The Upjohn Company, Dec. 1981.
4. Kligman, A. M., and Katz, A. G.: Pathogenesis of acne vulgaris. I. Comedogenic properties of human sebum in the external ear of the rabbit. Arch. Dermatol. 98:53, 1968.
5. Kellum, R. E.: Acne vulgaris. Studies in pathogenesis: Relative irritancy of free fatty acids from C_2 to C_{16}. Arch. Dermatol. 97:722, 1968.
6. Rebello, T., and Hawk, J. L. M.: Skin surface glycerol levels in acne vulgaris. J. Invest. Dermatol. 70:352, 1978.
7. McGinley, K. J., Webster, G. F., Ruggieri, M. R., and Leyden, J. J.: Regional variations in density of cutaneous propionibacteria: Correlation of *Propionibacterium acnes* populations with sebaceous secretion. J. Clin. Microbiol. 12:672, 1980.
8. Strauss, J. S., Pochi, P. E., and Downing, D. T.: Skin lipids and acne. Annu. Rev. Med. 26:27, 1975.
9. Knutson, D. D.: Ultrastructural observations in acne vulgaris: The normal sebaceous follicle and acne lesions. J. Invest. Dermatol. 62:288, 1974.
10. Wolff, H. H., Plewig, G., and Braun-Falco, O.: Ultrastructure of human sebaceous follicles and comedones following treatment with vitamin A acid. Acta Derm. Venereol. (Stockh.) 55(Suppl 74):99, 1975.
11. Plewig, G., Fulton, J. E., and Kligman, A. M.: Cellular dynamics of comedo formation in acne vulgaris. Arch. Dermatol. Forsch. 242:12, 1971.
12. Strauss, J. S., and Kligman, A. M.: The pathologic dynamics of acne vulgaris. Arch. Dermatol. 82:779, 1960.
13. Kligman, A. M., and Kwong, T.: An improved rabbit ear model for assessing comedogenic substances. Br. J. Dermatol. 100:699, 1979.
14. Bloch, B.: Metabolism, endocrine glands and skin-diseases, with special reference to acne vulgaris and xanthoma. Br. J. Dermatol. 43:61, 1931.
15. Pochi, P. E., Strauss, J. S., and Downing, D. T.: Skin surface lipid composition, acne, pubertal development, and urinary excretion of testosterone and 17-ketosteroids in children. J. Invest. Dermatol. 69:485, 1977.
16. Lavker, R. M., Leyden, J. J., and McGinley, K. J.: The relationship between bacteria and the abnormal follicular keratinization in acne vulgaris. J. Invest. Dermatol. 77:325, 1981.
17. Plewig, G., Nikolowski, J., and Wolff, H. H.: Action of isotretinoin in acne rosacea and gram-negative folliculitis. J. Am. Acad. Dermatol. 6:766, 1982.

CHAPTER **17**

IMPORTANCE OF DIETARY CONTROL

DIET IN ACNE
Morris Waisman, M.D.

The view that dietary restrictions are important in the management of acne was until recent times an article of faith with dermatologists. Up to the 1950s, authors traditionally recommended that a variety of supposedly harmful foods be eliminated from the diet of patients with acne. Subsequently, it became fashionable to be less dogmatic about the role of foods or to deny outright that foods have anything to do with the disease. Most modern textbooks adopt a "straddling" position and suggest that diet is probably of little or no consequence but that if a patient harbors the notion of an adverse effect, the physician should tolerantly sanction the withdrawal of the suspected foods.

Dermatologists are aware that acne flares conspicuously during the high-living, gluttonous diversions of the festive holiday seasons. Although a scientifically acceptable explanation for the phenomenon is lacking, the reputed scarcity of acne during famine may provide some insight. It has been postulated that milk aggravates acne because of its content of androgenic steroids, but this is unconvincing. If it were true, formula-fed babies would be frequent victims of acne. Admittedly, the incrimination of acnegenic foods is empirical and arbitrary, and rigid diets have too often been imposed on patients exploitatively, without good reason or mercy.

Despite the academically distinguished array of dietary nay-sayers and disprovers, I contend that some foods are a cause of significant aggravation of acne in some patients. The fact that many, or perhaps even most, acne patients may not suffer unequivocal adverse reactions to foods does not exclude foods from suspicion. Analogously, not all acne patients are inevitably made worse by iodide or bromide medication, either.

The manifesto by Fulton and associates[1] is supposed to have laid to rest once and for all the notion that chocolate exacerbates acne. Many of my patients know better. Experimental "proofs" by lesion counts are often demonstrably unreliable and represent only the execution of a self-fulfilling prophecy. For example, numerous highly lauded and widely used but therapeutically deficient topical medications for acne carry the certification of investigators who conveniently recorded reductions in lesion counts.[2] The procedure may be valid, but the counters are not always to be trusted. (Incidentally, most of these virtuoso acneologists are also hopelessly unaware of the Latin reality that the spurious word "comedone" is not the singular of "comedones.")

As a practical reminder, whatever the dietary opinions of the physician, acne patients *expect* to be given a diet. For many it represents a precautionary expedient—a safety net that is psychologically supportive if not scientifically founded.

The shortcoming of the dietary taboos of the past was their sometimes brutal assault on the patients with such a profusion of prohibitions as to make compliance unlikely. The inordinate numbers of purportedly detrimental foods seemed to be based on the criterion that anything cherished by the teen-aged palate must be forbidden. Also, a high rate of noncompliance obviously accomplishes the trick of transferring blame for treatment failure from the physician to the patient.

What foods should be eliminated? The prohibitions are few, and they affect only a minority of patients,[3] but initially they should be observed by all. Routinely I exclude chocolate, nuts, cola drinks, and spicy foods, and I advise that dairy products and citrus juices be taken in moderation (not more than one glass of milk and one glass of orange juice per day). Teen-agers can live with a diet like this. As an exercise requiring self-discipline, it also provides a measure of how dependably the patients will adhere to the rest of the prescribed treatment regimen for acne.

Sweets and fatty foods need not be restricted, except in overweight patients and those with nutritional imbalances. These foods probably do not exacerbate acne. Patients should be encouraged to relate their own experiences and beliefs concerning diet and to call attention to other foods that they consider harmful.

The diet I offer is neither bleak nor permanent. After a month or two, a trial of tapering down starts; one excluded item at a time is added at 2-week intervals. The patient may thereby learn which foods, if any, are indisputable or doubtful offenders. It also may be discovered that small amounts of some foods may be taken safely, whereas larger portions spell trouble. Usually, clear-cut decisions do not emerge, because other, peripheral factors also act to influence the course of acne. Most of my patients elect to continue to follow the diet after a fashion.

In a comfortable relationship between patient and physician, the teen-ager with acne is passably cooperative or at least is honest in admitting departures from righteousness. The goldbricks, rebels, and resisters are quickly identified. The judgments of teen-agers about the effectiveness (or lack thereof) of their treatment for acne, including diet, are by and large credible. They deserve listening to.

References

1. Fulton, J. E., Jr., Plewig, G., and Kligman, A. M.: Effect of chocolate on acne vulgaris. JAMA 210:2071, Dec. 1969.
2. Waisman, M.: Present-day treatment of acne: Doubts, disappointments and discontent. Int. J. Dermatol. 16:493, July/Aug. 1977.
3. Minkin, W., and Cohen, H. J.: Effect of chocolate on acne vulgaris (letters). JAMA 211:1856, March 1970.

THE ETIOLOGIC IRRELEVANCE OF DIET IN ACNE VULGARIS

David R. Bickers, M.D.

Diet is a word derived from the Greek *diaita,* which literally means a manner of living. This is diet in its broadest sense, but in the context of health, diet has come to refer to the food, drink, and medications ingested each day. In the most general sense, nutrition is the study of food and the body's utilization of chemicals in food. The physician must be concerned with the effect of nutrition and diet upon health, although not all dietary items have nutritional value. The word "nutrition" originates from the Latin word *nutire,* to nourish, and can be defined as the sum of the processes whereby food is ingested and utilized by living things.

The role of diet and nutrition in human health has been a major preoccupation of physicians for centuries. The most obvious manifestations of radical change in the amount of food ingested are the amount and distribution of body weight of a human subject. An individual starved of calories loses body fat and then lean body mass, whereas overindulgence leads to accumulation of fat as a stored form of energy resulting from the excessive caloric intake.

Certain organic substances contained in the diet are essential nutrients that are required in minute amounts as prosthetic groups of enzymes and are critical for a variety of catalytic activities. These substances are vitamins; the word is derived from the Latin *vita,* meaning life, and amine, since early discoveries suggested that these substances were amines.

The study of the role of vitamins in human disease has largely focused upon syndromes that result from deficiency of one or another of these substances. As shown in Table 1, several of the vitamin deficiency syndromes have dermatologic manifestations that are, in some instances, highly characteristic. It is therefore apparent that the skin and changes in its appearance and consistency may offer valuable clues to the existence of vitamin deficiency. Furthermore, this demonstrates that most diseases of the human population for which a specific dietary element has been identified usually relate to a deficiency of the substance in the diet or in its absorption into the body. The number of human diseases that can be directly attributed to the excessive ingestion of dietary food and drink is relatively small if we ignore natural substances that have toxic effects in biological systems. On the other hand, it is well known that the administration of certain drugs, either in normal doses or in excessive amounts, may be associated with a variety of toxic syndromes.

Acne vulgaris is one of the most common dermatologic disorders afflicting the human population. Typically the disease begins at, or shortly after, puberty, affects both sexes, and persists intermittently until early adulthood. The disease varies in severity from a few small comedones to large numbers of cysts that heal slowly, leaving considerable scarring. Acne is currently thought to be a disease of the sebaceous gland in which changes in keratinization in the wall of the follicle lead to a sequence of pathologic changes that culminate in comedo formation with subsequent inflammatory change.

The role of diet in acne vulgaris remains highly controversial.[1-3] However, a random survey of current editions of several leading textbooks of dermatology reveals that nearly all minimize the role of diet in this disease, although this unanimity is based upon no scientific data whatever aside from a smattering of controlled studies.[4] Rather, the opinions expressed are the result of the collective experience of numerous dermatologists over many years.

Table 1.   VITAMIN DEFICIENCY
DISEASES

Vitamin	Disease
A	Xerophthalmia, phrynoderma
B_1	Beriberi
B_2	Stomatitis, glossitis, seborrheic dermatitis
Niacin	Pellagra
B_6	Stomatitis, seborrheic dermatitis, peripheral neuropathy
B_{12} and folate	Anemia
C	Scurvy
D	Rickets and osteomalacia

It must be considered that the development of acne, like that of all diseases, is influenced by multiple factors. In searching for the cause of any disease, one must seek to identify genetic and environmental factors. The genetic factors that predispose to the development of acne are poorly understood. One might hypothesize that inherited characteristics that influence sebum production and constitution as well as the secretion of sex steroid hormones could be important determinants for the development of acne.

Environmental factors that could potentially influence acne include diet, physical and chemical exposures, and so forth, all of which constitute a "life style."

Careful studies have shown that sebum production is a necessary, but not a sufficient, condition for the development of acne vulgaris.[5] Yet there is no real agreement that patients with acne secrete substantially larger amounts of sebum than do appropriately matched control populations without acne. Furthermore, even when one supposes that there are substantial differences in sebum production among individuals with and without acne, there is little evidence to indicate that normal dietary manipulations appreciably alter the chemical composition of sebum. Thus, it is known that even in the face of total calorie deprivation, sebum production is maintained at 40 to 50 per cent of normal levels. Even starvation may not cure acne! It is clear that androgenic hormones in addition to sebum production play an important role in the development of acne vulgaris. The role is a permissive one, although their mechanism of action is unclear, aside from their ability to bring about maturational changes in the sebaceous follicle at puberty, which results in increased sebum production.

Since acne is an almost universal disease among postpubertal teen-agers, the incrimination of any particular foodstuff would require that it be ingested in "excessive" amounts by virtually everyone in the affected population, but in "normal" or deficient amounts by those who are not affected. In fact, it could be argued with equal justification from the data that are currently available that acne is a deficiency disease that results from the inadequate ingestion of a substance that precludes the development of the pathologic process resulting in the acne lesion. The disappearance of acne in the post–teen-age years could then be explained by the repletion of this unknown inhibitor of the "acne factor." Since most adults continue many of the dietary habits acquired during earlier growth and development, it is difficult to see how the same diet could be pathologic at one stage but without effect at another.

It has been said that the primary factor in a disease is not one in whose presence the disease always occurs but rather is one in whose absence the disease never occurs. By this criterion, the elimination of certain foods or the alteration of the existing diet must clearly be shown to prevent development or to reverse the disease. The burden of proof rests with those who advocate a significant role for diet in acne.

Table 2. REPUTED DIETARY
EXACERBATORS OF ACNE VULGARIS

Chocolate
Nuts
Candy
Soft drinks
Shellfish
Cheeses

Dietary deficiencies of vitamin A and zinc are postulated by some to be important causes of acne vulgaris, and oral supplements of these substances have been used in the treatment of the disease. Controlled studies, when they have been done, have never provided one shred of evidence to verify the efficacy of these approaches. It is important to point out that a major impediment to ascribing cause and effect in acne vulgaris relates to the imprecise methods currently available to evaluate change in activity of the disease. These may include lesion counts and weighed severity, in which the clearing of the inflammatory lesions is given greater weight than the disappearance of noninflammatory lesions, such as comedones. Since in the natural history of acne vulgaris comedones may persist for varying periods and then intermittently but unpredictably evolve into inflammatory papules and pustules, a change in the numbers of comedones may be the most accurate measurement for evaluation of changes in acne. This becomes particularly evident when one considers that inflammatory papules and pustules are actually "late" lesions of acne that tend to evolve and remit rather quickly. Thus, acne does not consist of one type of lesion but rather multiple types of lesions, each of which may evolve at a different rate. This makes evaluation of the disease extremely difficult.

The available literature regarding dietary excess in acne is almost completely anecdotal. Furthermore, the foods that have been incriminated are among those most widely ingested at one time or another by the majority of the human population of all ages. Table 2 lists several that appear in most texts. As pointed out by Plewig and Kligman,[1] all of the blacklisted items are delicious and delectable for the adolescent palate, and the suggestion that these items exacerbate acne is largely punitive. As mentioned earlier, it is impossible to understand how the ingestion of these foods between the ages of 12 and 20 years is acnegenic but in adulthood is without such effect.

Since a broad definition of diet refers to more than ingested food and drink, it is important to consider other elements of an individual's life style that could influence the development of acneiform eruptions.[6] Here the evidence is more compelling. It is clear from a variety of sources that excessive ingestion of or exposure to halogens, such as bromine, iodine, and chlorine, can exacerbate an acne-like condition characterized by comedones, papules, and pustules in sebaceous-rich areas of the skin. Acneiform eruptions can occur in association with the ingestion of, or the exposure to, a number of drugs and chemicals, some of which are listed in Table 3.

If a broader view of diet is taken to include environmental exposure to toxic chemi-

Table 3. DRUGS AND CHEMICALS
ASSOCIATED WITH ACNEIFORM ERUPTIONS

Iodides	Bromides
Isonicotinic acid hydrazide	Corticosteroids, androgens
Phenytoin	Trimethadione
Phenobarbitone	Polyhalogenated hydrocarbons
	Polychlorinated biphenyls
	Polybrominated biphenyls
	Tetrachlorodibenzo[p]-
	dioxin

cals, then the role of halogenated hydrocarbons must be included in this discussion. In contrast with the lack of any reliable data supporting the role of dietary food and drink as etiologic factors in acne vulgaris, ample evidence exists for the effect of the halogenated hydrocarbons on this disorder. The general term "chloracne" has been used for this condition, and the offending agents are largely encountered by direct cutaneous exposure to the chemicals.[7] However, the ingestion of these compounds can also evoke an acne-like eruption. This was demonstrated by an incident that occurred in Japan in 1968. A large number of individuals accidentally ingested large quantities of polychlorinated biphenyls that had leaked into rice oil during processing. This resulted in the development of Yusho, or oil disease, in which there were acneiform eruptions in association with cystic swelling and hypersecretion of the meibomian glands.

Numerous reports in the literature attest to the risk of developing chloracne in occupational settings in which there is heavy exposure to various halogenated hydrocarbons, including the polyhalogenated naphthalenes, biphenyls, dibenzofurans, dioxins, and azoxybenzenes. It is of considerable interest that these compounds are among the most potent porphyrinogenic substances yet identified for the liver. The relationship, if any, between their ability to stimulate hepatic porphyrin synthesis and to cause chloracne is unknown.

Chloracne differs from acne vulgaris in that almost any exposed area may be affected, although this is most prominent in body areas that are rich in sebaceous glands. There may be associated cutaneous hyperpigmentation. In fact, some believe that the cutaneous manifestations of chloracne provide one of the most sensitive indicators of excessive human exposure to the halogenated hydrocarbons.

In summary, there is currently no verifiable information to indicate that intake of food and drink appreciably influences the development of acne vulgaris. On the other hand, certain drugs and toxic environmental chemicals, such as the halogenated hydrocarbons, are clearly capable of eliciting an acneiform disorder, suggesting that some exogenous substances can trigger the disease.

References

1. Plewig, G., and Kligman, A. M.: Acne: Morphogenesis and Treatment. Berlin, Springer-Verlag, 1975.
2. Frank, S. B.: Acne Vulgaris. Springfield, IL, Charles C Thomas, 1971.
3. Rasmussen, J. W.: Diet and acne. Int. J. Dermatol. 16:488, 1978.
4. Fulton, J. E., Plewig, G., and Kligman, A. M.: Effect of chocolate and acne vulgaris. JAMA 210:2071, 1969.
5. Strauss, J. S., Pochi, P. E., and Downing, D. T.: Skin lipids and acne. Annu. Rev. Med. 26:27, 1975.
6. Reisner, R. M.: Acne vulgaris. In Conn, H. F. (ed.): Current Therapy 1982. Philadelphia, W. B. Saunders Co., 1982, pp. 609–616.
7. Taylor, J. S.: Environmental chloracne: Update and review. Ann. N.Y. Acad. Sci. 320:295, 1979.

ACNE, DIET, AND THE CONVENTIONAL WISDOM

E. William Rosenberg, M.D.

There are at least three reasons why most dermatologists do not believe that diet has anything to do with acne:

1. Major textbooks say so.

2. Almost all the young people they see are on typical American diets, yet some have acne and some do not.

3. Many teen-agers with severe acne have on their own or at a parent's urging modified their diets with little or no favorable effect on the acne.

Common sense thus tells us that we are looking in the wrong place for a culprit. It is my belief, however, that this sensible consensus is wrong.

I will discuss the second reason first. If everyone eats much the same kind of food and only some people develop acne, does that prove that diet does not cause acne?

No, not at all. Whenever an environmental influence for a disorder is spread over an entire population that represents diverse gene pools, the determinant of who develops the disorder is genetic susceptibility. The fact that all are not affected by the environmental insult does not negate its essential role. It has been well put that a primary factor in disease is not one in whose presence disease will always occur but one in whose absence disease will not occur.[1]

The same principle is illustrated by another common, but much more serious, malady: heart disease. Epidemiologists have been at great pains in studying influences on this disease to sort out nature from nurture, to identify what cannot be changed from what can.

The gamut of genetic input is certainly well represented in a large population as heterogeneous as that of the United States, but the range of dietary input is not. Even given ethnic differences and even including the poor, the vast majority of Americans are on a high–saturated fat, high-cholesterol, high-salt diet.

To compare the effect of different diets on heart disease rates, American scientists have had to look outside their own country to countries where the diet is low in fat, such as Japan and parts of Africa, Central America, South America, and the Near East. In these cultures, the effects of very different diets on a whole range of genetic substrates can be demonstrated.

In Japan, which has highly industrialized urban centers like those in America but a traditional diet that is very low in fat, heart disease rates have been low. (With salt intakes that are even higher than those in America, however, Japanese stroke rates are among the highest in the world.)

Japanese migrant studies effectively dismiss the idea that some kind of genetic protection may be responsible for the low rates of heart disease in that country. Long-term studies reveal that Japanese migrants to Hawaii and California who change to western diets develop rates of heart disease approaching those of people who were born in the United States.[2]

Much evidence from around the world[3,4] supports the observation that on high-fat diets, some people will develop coronary heart disease and some will not; on a low-fat diet, no one will, whether genetically susceptible or not.

I believe that the same principle applies to acne. Unfortunately, we do not have international prevalence rates for acne, which would allow us to search out correlations. There are, however, some intriguing suggestions from various sources.

Surveys of disease in Kenya[5] and Zambia[6] report far less acne than is now found among young black people in the United States. A diabetologist and epidemiologist in South Africa is quoted as saying that acne became a problem for Zulus moving to cities.[7] The difference between having and not having acne may therefore be a western-type, high-fat diet.

Necropsies and observations of Okinawans during World War II revealed no acne among these people, who subsisted on a largely vegetarian diet.[8] Comments from other investigators have indicated that acne is rare among populations whose diets are low in saturated fats. Such countries include Korea, Peru, Ecuador, Spain, Turkey, and southern Italy.[9]

Also of interest is an account of medical problems emerging in groups of Eskimos after World War II. Concurrent with a change from traditional diets to western fare rich in processed foods, sweets, and salt came hypertension and heart disease, obesity and diabetes, dental caries, and acne.[10,11]

Similarities in the emergence of acne and coronary heart disease in populations can lead one to believe that the first, like the second, is not an acute response but a long-term chronic effect of a particular kind of diet. The mechanisms of atherosclerosis and heart disease are beginning to be understood. Those of acne are not, yet there are possibilities that can be considered.

But first, what of our third reason why dermatologists doubt the relationship of diet to acne: the failure of dietary manipulation to affect the course of acne?

There are many examples of diseases for which removal of the cause will not effect a cure. There is not much argument that cigarettes are causative in lung cancer. But the smoker who gives up his habit after he develops cancer of the lung has little hope of benefit. It has not been demonstrated that the condition of victims who continue to smoke becomes appreciably worse than does that of those who quit.

Hypertension is another example of a disorder that may continue its course after the cause has left the scene. There is a growing medical consensus that sodium is the primary factor in high blood pressure.[12] As yet, no cultures have been identified in which the people are on low-salt diets but have hypertension. Yet there are primitive, traditional cultures in which the people are on high-salt diets and have hypertension.[13] And in migrating or acculturating populations changing from low to high salt consumption, high blood pressure has been found to develop in sodium-susceptible people.[14,15]

Preponderant evidence ties sodium to hypertension etiologically, although there are other important factors, such as obesity. Cure is another matter, however. A Mayo Clinic study showed that half of all hypertensives became normotensive with salt restriction and weight reduction when needed.[16] But for some cases of established high blood pressure, particularly those of long duration and high levels, even severe salt restriction that is difficult for most people to tolerate is often unsuccessful. In these cases, medication coupled with a more moderate degree of salt restriction must be the answer.

The mechanisms by which smoking induces lung cancer and sodium produces hypertension have not been fully or satisfactorily elucidated. Obviously, however, biochemical changes can lead to structural changes in the lungs, the arteries, and the kidneys.

My feeling is that a comparable effect occurs in the skin with acne. One possibility is that this happens by way of a mechanism that is a function of accelerated maturation.

The most careful studies of the timing of puberty suggest that maturation is dependent on total body mass and is independent of height, relative weight (and, thus, leanness or obesity per se), and even age, within limits. Puberty is most likely to begin when the individual has reached 85 per cent of adult weight. In whites this is approximately 102 lbs for females and 121 lbs for males. In Orientals, the maturation weight is approximately 13 lbs less for females.[17,18]

Data collected over the last 140 years show a dramatic change in the age of menarche for young women in western Europe and the United States. In 1860 the typical age at first menstruation was 16.6 years.[19] Today in the United States it is 12.7 years.[20]

Some have attributed at least part of this decline in age at maturation to the stimulatory effect of artificial light on pineal function.[21] Many authorities, however, believe that the trend is a direct result of diets that are high in fats and sugar, which result in larger, heavier children.[22]

Skeletal growth and muscular development do not quite keep up with this early hormonal development. The 13-year-old mother will likely have a more difficult delivery than will the fully grown woman in her later teens or twenties.[23,24] In the same way, the anatomic and hormonal aspects of follicular function may be out of phase with each other. My own observations suggest that in many patients with acne the precipitating factor is not oversecretion of sebum but secretion through follicular openings that are not yet large and mature enough to provide adequate outlet.[25,26]

There are probably no records on the prevalence of acne in the 1840s, but it is still possible to survey more primitive populations in which children mature at 15 to 17 years of age. And a very good study could be undertaken that examines lean, exercising ballet dancers or athletes in whom menarche is "delayed" until 16 years of age or after because of their low body weights.[27,28]

The influence of diet on hormonal function is already being studied in relation to cancer of the breast. Hill and Wynder have provided women with a standard western diet and a strict vegetarian diet for 2 months at a time.[29] Measurement of overnight prolactin levels has shown that the women secrete far more prolactin on the high-fat diet.[29] The significance of this response is obvious because of the effect of prolactin on breast physiology. The study is also a good demonstration of the profound effect of diet on hormonal function.

Finally, it is possible to speculate that the amount and composition of sebum may vary somewhat, depending on the condition of the fatty substrate that travels to the functioning epithelial cells of the sebaceous gland. If this hypothesis is correct, diet would be implicated as the environmental factor that determines whether sebum would be thick and solidified or thin and free-flowing.

The fact remains that the conventional wisdom is, as stated in most textbooks, that diet has nothing to do with acne. There are two possibilities to consider with regard to this commonly held belief.

One possibility is that medical textbooks are naturally oriented toward cure rather than prevention, and diet will not cure acne. I believe that this may be the case. Acne may be the result of an acquired structural defect of the skin. If this is the explanation it may follow that, once established, acne cannot be cured or even much ameliorated by diet.

A second possibility is that I am wrong and acne can be cured by diet before it has run its course. The problem in this case may be that studies have not been of long enough duration or have not elicited enough compliance. Some trials may have focused too narrowly on restriction of or challenges with particular foods. If diet causes acne, it is probably the totality of the diet—the amount of fats, sweets, and refined carbohydrates—that is relevant, not specific foods, such as milk, eggs, or chocolate.

Acne is probably a multifactorial disease in the sense that influences other than diet are also at work, including mental and physical stresses, allergies, and weather conditions, some of which also affect the hormonal milieu. The presence of other variables that are difficult to identify and quantify makes the results of dietary trials even more difficult to assess.

Where does all this leave us? I believe the dermatologist is uniquely positioned to give advice that is bound to be helpful and cannot be harmful.

There are better reasons than treatment of acne for changing to a diet that is lower in fats and higher in unrefined carbohydrates. It seems evident that atherosclerosis, hypertension, maturity-onset diabetes, and bowel diseases in western societies are largely attributable to the western diet.[30] Increasing evidence implicates the same diet as the leading cause of certain major cancers in western people.[31,32]

The same diet that I believe would prevent acne if started early enough would also prevent major degenerative diseases. It may be prudent at this time to advise all who will listen to adopt such a diet.[33] Even if it will not cure acne, it can prevent or delay ills of much greater magnitude.

In addition, modification of diet may help to prevent acne in the patient's younger siblings and in the patient's own progeny in the future. We can also tell parents and parents-to-be that there is hope that a change in diet may result in a later age of sexual maturation for future children. Parents of teen-agers will understand when I say that this may turn out to be no small blessing in itself.

References

1. Burkitt, D. P.: Dietary fibre and "pressure diseases." J. R. Coll. Physicians Lond. 9:138, 1975.
2. Blackburn, H.: Workshop report: Epidemiological section. Conference on the health effects of blood lipids. Optimal distributions for populations. Prev. Med. 8:612, 1979.
3. Blackburn, H.: Progress in the epidemiology and prevention of coronary heart disease. In Yu, P., and Goodwin, J. (eds.): Progress in Cardiology. Philadelphia, Lea & Febiger, 1974, pp. 1–36.
4. Stamler, J.: Population studies. In Levy, R., Rifkind, B., Dennis, B., et al. (eds.): Nutrition, Lipids, and Coronary Heart Disease. A Global View. New York, Raven Press, 1979, pp. 25–88.
5. Verhagen, A.R.H.B.: Skin diseases. In Vogel, L. C., Muller, A. S., Odingo, R. S., et al. (eds.): Health and Diseases in Kenya. Nairobi, Kenya, East African Literature Bureau, 1974, pp. 499–507.
6. Ratnam, A. V., and Jayaraju, K.: Skin diseases in Zambia. Br. J. Dermatol. 101:449, 1979.
7. Cunliffe, W. J., and Cotterill, J. A.: The acnes: Clinical features, pathogenesis and treatment. In Rook, A. (ed.): Major Problems in Dermatology, vol. 6. Philadelphia, W. B. Saunders Co., 1975, pp. 13–14.
8. Steiner, P. E.: Necropsies on Okinawans. Anatomic and pathologic observations. Arch. Pathol. 42:359, 1946.
9. Hoehn, G. H.: Acne and diet. Cutis 2:389, 1966.
10. Bendiner, E.: Disastrous trade-off: Eskimo health for white "civilization." Hosp. Pract. 9:156, 1974.
11. Sinclair, H. M.: The diet of Canadian Indians and Eskimos. Proc. Nutr. Soc. 12:69, 1953.
12. Meneely, G. R., and Battarbee, H. D.: High sodium–low potassium environment and hypertension. Am. J. Cardiol. 38:768, 1976.
13. Page, L. B., Vandevert, D. E., Nader, K., et al.: Blood pressure of Qashqai pastoral nomads in Iran in relation to culture, diet, and body form. Am. J. Clin. Nutr. 34:527, 1981.
14. Trowell, H. C.: From normotension to hypertension in Kenyans and Ugandans 1928–1978. East Afr. Med. J. 57:167, 1980.
15. Page, L. B., Damon, A., and Moellering, R. C.: Antecedents of cardiovascular disease in six Solomon Islands societies. Circulation 49:1132, 1974.
16. Hunt, J. C., and Margie, J. D.: The influence of diet on hypertension management. In Hunt, J. C. (ed.): Hypertension Update, vol. 4. Bloomfield, NJ, Health Learning Systems, Inc., 1980, pp. 37–47.
17. Frisch, R. E.: Weight at menarche: Similarity for well-nourished and undernourished girls at differing ages, and evidence for historical constancy. Pediatrics 50:445, 1972.
18. Frisch, R. E., and Revelle, R.: Height and weight at menarche and a hypothesis of menarche. Arch. Dis. Child 46:695, 1971.
19. Mausner, U. S., and Bahn, A. K.: Epidemiology: An Introductory Text. Philadelphia, W. B. Saunders Co., 1974, p. 75.
20. Age at menarche: United States. In U.S. Department of Health, Education and Welfare: Vital and Health Statistics. Washington, D.C., U.S. Government Printing Office, 1973, series 11, no. 133.
21. Jafarey, N. A., Khan, M. Y., and Jafarey, S. N.: Role of artificial lighting in decreasing the age of menarche. Lancet 2:471, 1970.
22. Schaefer, O.: Pre- and post-natal growth acceleration and increased sugar consumption in Canadian Eskimos. Can. Med. Assoc. J. 103:1059, 1970.
23. Duenhoelter, J. H., Jiminez, J. M., and Baumann, G.: Pregnancy performance of patients under 15 years of age. Obstet. Gynecol. 46:49, 1975.
24. Hassan, H. M., and Falls, F. H.: The young primipara. A clinical study. Am. J. Obstet. Gynecol. 88:256, 1964.
25. Rosenberg, E. W.: Management of skin problems in the adolescent. South. Med. J. 58:1555, 1965.
26. Rosenberg, E. W.: Treatment of acne. Br. Med. J. 2:175, 1973.
27. Frisch, R. E., Wyshak, G., and Vincent, L.: Delayed menarche and amenorrhea in ballet dancers. N. Engl. J. Med. 303:17, 1980.

28. Frisch, R. E., Gotz-Welbergen, A. V., McArthur, J. W., et al.: Delayed menarche and amenorrhea of college athletes in relation to age of onset of training. JAMA 246:1559, 1981.
29. Hill, P., and Wynder, E.: Diet and prolactin release. Lancet 2:806, 1976.
30. Trowell, H. C., and Burkitt, D. P. (eds.): Western Diseases: Their Emergence and Prevention. Cambridge, MA, Harvard University Press, 1981.
31. Reddy, B. S., Cohen, L. A., McCoy, G. D., et al.: Nutrition and its relationship to cancer. Adv. Cancer Res. 32:237, 1980.
32. Doll, R., and Peto, R.: The Causes of Cancer. Quantitative Estimates of Avoidable Risks of Cancer in the United States Today. New York, Oxford University Press, 1981.
33. Select Committee on Nutrition and Human Needs, United States Senate: Dietary Goals for the United States, 2nd ed. Washington, D.C., U.S. Government Printing Office, 1977.

Editorial Comment

Controlled studies indicate that foods have no effect on acne. However, does this negate the years spent in building up empirical knowledge that certain foods do have a deleterious effect on this condition? For instance, I did not conquer my acne problem until I stopped eating chocolate. Recurrences were noted soon after I ingested some of that delicious stuff. My wife had the same experience, but the food that was critical in her cure was unboiled milk. It is certainly true that a disease can be precipitated or aggravated by a food that is not eaten in excess by the sufferers or avoided by those spared the ravages of the condition. Any experienced clinician can recall encountering instances of true acute food allergy or hypersensitivity in his practice.

Dr. Rosenberg's concept of avoiding or controlling acne by increasing the health of the victim is interesting and tantalizing. Yet, we must realize that the average teen-ager is in the best health of his life. I can remember some horrendous cases of acne in football players. Of course, if the patient is suffering from a deficiency state or a metabolic imbalance, such as diabetes, dietary correction may play an important role in the management of the acne. Fortunately, few patients with acne display such complications.

If other ingestants, such as drugs, may clearly exacerbate or precipitate acne or even produce an eruption that resembles acne, it is difficult to deny that certain foods could not do the same. After all, many medications are related to foods or are derived from them.

Our treatment of acne is not so successful that we can ignore any approach that may help us in managing this condition. Therefore, I believe that the patient should receive any assistance that dietary control may impart. Empirically, my routine is to exclude the following dietary elements: oranges, tomatoes, nuts, iodine (salt, fish, seafood, and so forth), unboiled milk and milk products, chocolate, spinach, and pork. For every food that is banned, there is an adequate substitute. The patient need not go hungry—it is necessary only for him to consume different foods. There is no reason for the patient to lose weight or develop any deficiencies while following the regimen. It probably would increase patient cooperation if the physician were to emphasize that this is an important facet of the therapy.

Perhaps some day we will have a treatment so specific that such adjunctive treatment as the annoyance of a diet will be unnecessary. However, today that possibility is only a faint glimmer of hope on a distant horizon.

Think It Over.

CHAPTER 18

THERAPY

SOME CONTROVERSIAL AREAS IN THE TOPICAL TREATMENT OF ACNE

Ronald M. Reisner, M.D.

The two most important therapeutic modalities that have been developed for the management of severe acne during the last quarter century are oral antibiotics and oral 13-*cis*-retinoic acid. Both are systemically administered drugs, and each has significant unwanted effects on other areas of the skin and on internal organs. The ideal dermatologic therapy, however, is still topical therapy, which is applied to the involved site and affects only the area to which it is applied. Fortunately, a number of useful and effective topical agents are now available, and investigators continue to study new areas that promise an eventual realization of the ideal of complete and exclusive topical management of acne. Such agents would include new or improved topical sebostatics, agents normalizing follicular keratinization, agents that are bactericidal for *Propionibacterium acnes,* and inhibitors of the host inflammatory response to follicular contents.

Until these ideal drugs appear in daily practice we shall have to continue to remain familiar with and weigh the advantages and disadvantages of the older and newer agents. We must select from among these substances to provide optimal care for our patients in the treatment of acne, which is the most common of all skin diseases in the practice of medicine.

I would like to review some of the pros and cons and the controversial aspects of a few selected topical modalities.

One of the oldest topical agents in acne therapy is sulfur. In 1972, Mills and Kligman set off a ripple of surprise and concern in the dermatologic world when they reported that sulfur-containing agents were comedogenic in the rabbit ear model and, when applied under occlusion for 6 weeks, in humans.[1] The earliest identifiable morphologic event in the evolution of acne is comedogenesis at the electron microscopic level. This leads, in some follicles, to inflammatory lesions, including pustules, papules, and nodules. Accordingly, Mills and Kligman suggested that therapy with sulfur might actually be aggravating acne— a subtle effect that might go unnoticed because of the lag time of several months or more between the initiation of microscopic comedogenesis and the appearance of clinically visible lesions.

Controversy was focused, among other things, on the validity of the rabbit ear model as an assay for clinically significant comedogenicity of topically applied compounds in humans as well as on the extrapolation of the findings (both rabbit and human) to the actual clinical situation in view of the long and apparently safe use of sulfur. Although sulfur was increasingly being displaced by more effective agents and its eﬃ﹍acy compared with that of newer agents, such as retinoic acid and benzoyl peroxide, was clearly low, it had never been viewed as naturally producing new disease. Sulfur, although it has been looked upon as an antiseptic agent, does not influence the follicular population of *P. acnes,*

271

and although it has long been regarded as a keratolytic, it acts instead as an irritant, thus producing the scaling that has been interpreted as keratolysis. It is this irritancy that has to a considerable extent served as a basis for the continued use of sulfur as a mild exfoliant to aid in the involution of pre-existing low-grade inflammatory lesions—pustules and papules—by hastening their resorption.

The controversy concerning the rabbit ear model remains unsettled to this day. The rabbit ear certainly has some strengths. It appears to be the best of the few available animal models for comedogenesis. The rabbit responds with comedo formation to administration of coal tar and chlorinated naphthalenes, as do humans, and responds with a comedolytic effect to administration of topical retinoic acid, as do humans. No other animal model does either. The rabbit produces comedones on exposure to a variety of cosmetic agents, which in some instances appears to have clinical relevance.

The rabbit ear model also certainly has weaknesses. Topical steroids are comedogenic in humans, but not in the rabbit ear. A variety of substances that appear not to be comedogenic to a clinically significant degree in the human are mildly to moderately comedogenic in the rabbit ear. The comedonal lesions in the rabbit ear do not progress and become inflammatory lesions, as they do at times in humans. Nor are the rabbit comedones themselves as tightly compacted as are human comedones. The model thus appears to be a useful stimulus to further examination of our clinical observations and conclusions and an inducement to new clinical insights rather than the source of final answers.

Concern about the comedogenicity of sulfur continued. In 1978, Strauss and coworkers re-examined the issue by repeating the experiments of Mills and Kligman in two separate studies of 12 and 40 subjects, respectively. The studies were performed in two different institutions with two different investigators.[2] In addition, controls of a sulfur preparation in another vehicle (Carbopol-934P) were added to evaluate the effect of sulfur without the Triton X-100 surfactant contained in the original preparation used by Mills and Kligman. The Triton X-100 vehicle used alone and a dry patch also were evaluated as controls. One of the two sulfur preparations (5 per cent sulfur in Triton X-100 or 5 per cent sulfur in Carbopol-934P) and one of the controls (Triton X-100 vehicle alone or a dry patch to evaluate the effect of occlusion only) were applied under occlusive patch in each subject for 6 weeks with changes three times weekly. Biopsies were taken before and after the 6-week period. In the interest of objectivity, Dr. Kligman read the biopsies as unknowns.

The results confirmed the hypothesis of those whose clinical experience had exonerated sulfur of the possibility of significant comedogenicity. Of 20 occlusive patches in each category, the following sites were positive for comedones:

5 per cent sulfur in Triton X-100—5/20
5 per cent sulfur in Carbopol-934P—4/20
Triton X-100 vehicle—7/20
Occlusion only—5/20

The most comedogenic substance—slightly exceeding occlusion alone—was the Triton X-100 vehicle itself.

It might be argued that a study conducted over a longer period, which would have been more comparable with the long use of sulfur in the treatment of acne, might have revealed effects not seen in the 6-week-long study. On the other hand, occlusion would certainly be expected to intensify the reaction, if a reaction were to occur at all. When a well-designed study and long clinical experience bring us to the same conclusions, we have used some of our best tools to resolve a vexing controversy and can reasonably feel that the matter is settled for practical purposes.

Not too long ago, an advertisement commonly seen in dermatologic journals depicted a little creature vigorously scrubbing the plugged orifice of a pilosebaceous follicle to release its dammed-up contents, to the advantage of the beleaguered patients with acne. Today, with appreciation of the fact that comedo formation starts deep in the infra-infundibular portion of the pilosebaceous follicle and extends upward to produce a firmly seated keratinous plug, which may be difficult to remove even with vigorous use of a comedo extractor, this seems a naïve view.

This advertisement was appealing in its day, in part because it suggested that rubbing and scrubbing can somehow hasten the disappearance of this "dirty, oily disease." This instinctive effort to cleanse has been carried to extreme in some patients, so that new lesions have been produced by a combination of mechanical rupture of follicles and induction of comedones by repeated applications of weakly comedogenic cleansing agents. But, when performed in moderation, is this rubbing and scrubbing helpful, harmful, or neither?

In a more elegantly presented form, this rubbing and scrubbing approach is used with such abrasive materials as pumice, graded particles of fused aluminum oxide, polyethylene, abradant pads, and so forth.

There has been a wide range of opinion concerning abrasives; some have been quite enthusiastic, whereas others feel that not only do they add little or nothing, but also they may be irritating to skin already damaged by acne and may induce follicular rupture and exacerbation. For example, in a study conducted by Mills and Kligman in 1979, five groups of ten patients each who had moderate acne with conspicuous comedones were evaluated.[3] The patients were treated with one of the following twice daily for 8 weeks without concomitant therapy: Brade-A-Foam, Brasivol Medium, Pernox, Buf-Puf, and a polystyrene pad with Ivory soap. Lesion counts were performed prior to and at the end of the study.

The authors concluded that none of the abrasives tested had a clinically significant effect in eliminating comedones. They found that closed comedones were completely unresponsive and that no more than a 20 per cent reduction occurred in open comedones. Papulopustules diminished by 17 to 32 per cent with the various forms of treatment. This appeared to be related to the dryness and peeling that occurred in most patients. In some patients, new crops of papulopustules were observed at an unspecified later time. It was implied that this might have been secondary to the use of the abrasive material. The investigators' overall assessment was that in skin with acne, which is vulnerable to chemical and physical trauma, the risks of abrasives outweigh the slight beneficial effects.

A more favorable view was presented by Millikan and Ameln in 1981 in their evaluation of benzoyl peroxide versus benzoyl peroxide plus Buf-Puf.[4] They treated 48 patients with mild to moderate acne for 12 weeks with 5 per cent benzoyl peroxide gel applied to the whole face once each evening. One side of the face was also scrubbed with the Buf-Puf pad, and the other was left untouched. No other topical or systemic therapy was used. The investigators evaluated the degree of acne by assessing the percentage of distribution of lesions by type (a measurement that is confusing to me) and the results of a special observational index. They concluded that both benzoyl peroxide and the combined Buf-Puf–benzoyl peroxide regimen produced clinically significant improvement, with the latter providing slightly better results.

Using their measurement of the percentage of distribution of lesions by type, Millikan and Ameln found that benzoyl peroxide produced statistically significant improvement in only two of six categories—pustular acne (left side) and open comedonal acne (right side). The side on which the pad was used was randomized. The categories were pustular (left side), pustular (right side), open comedones (left side), open comedones (right side), and closed comedones (right side and left side). The Buf-Puf–benzoyl peroxide regimen produced statistically significant improvement for all but the closed comedones on the right side. In contradistinction to the observations of Mills and Kligman, Millikan and Ameln found added beneficial effects on comedones with the use of an abrasive pad along with the benzoyl peroxide. Mills and Kligman, on the other hand, used only the abrasive and no other therapy. The Buf-Puf–benzoyl peroxide regimen was most effective for pustules and open comedones. It was felt that the overall enhancement of response observed with careful, nonexcessive use of skin abrasion as an adjunctive form of therapy was sufficient to recommend its use.

The controversy still remains unresolved, with anecdotal clinical experience and careful studies yielding conflicting results. My own summation is that careful use of abrasives can help induce more rapid resolution of papules and pustules, but it is an inefficient way to do so. It is difficult to imagine how abrasives could unseat comedones—open or closed. It is possible that excessive or overly vigorous use can produce flares through mechanical rupture of follicles. On balance, my own view at this time is that the small risks outweigh the even smaller benefits in most patients. The psychological impact might be useful in maintaining cooperation in some patients, however. As is so often the case, one must use clinical judgment and must evaluate the needs of each patient individually.

Another area in which a wide diversity of opinion and practice exists among dermatologists is acne surgery. By this I mean specifically the extraction of open and closed comedones and the incision and drainage of pustular or cystic lesions, or both. Some feel that acne surgery is an important part of patient management and do it themselves, some delegate it to trained assistants, others perform limited acne surgery on demand, and still others feel it is minimally useful or actually harmful and do not use it at all. The published literature tends to reflect this diversity of viewpoint.

Few studies have been published that address this issue. Lowney and coworkers in 1964 considered the value of comedo extraction on one half of the face versus no comedo extraction on the other.[5] They concluded that extraction was of value on the forehead but less advantageous on the cheeks. It is interesting to note that they also found a decrease in the number of inflamed lesions and observed that inflamed cystic acne was made worse. This suggests that the increased vulnerability of follicles to mechanical rupture and the intensification of the response from such rupture may be an underlying cause of the severe cases of cystic acne.

Of four recent major general dermatology texts, two specifically advocate comedo extraction and incision and drainage of pustules and cysts as an important part of the treatment of acne. The other two indicate that acne surgery is helpful and aids in the involution of individual lesions. It is emphasized that in order to be useful rather than harmful, the procedure must be performed properly. This includes correct placement of the instrument for open comedones and the addition of appropriate incision for closed comedones and pustules. This essentially precludes home use of the comedo extractor by the patient.

Since open comedones are largely quiescent lesions rarely leading to inflammatory sequelae, the main effect of their removal is an immediate cosmetic one. This can be valuable to patient morale. Removal of closed comedones is more difficult, requiring an enlarging of the opening to the surface with a knife or a needle. It has, however, the added potential benefit of reducing subsequent inflammatory lesions, although most closed comedones that lead to inflammatory lesions are probably too small to be seen and extracted. Pustules can be nicked very superficially and drained without increased risk of scarring. In my opinion, few but the ripest fluctuant cystic lesions are ever worth incision and drainage today with the availability of intralesional steroids and cryotherapy, although there remain a few who still advocate this procedure. The fear here, of course, is of adding to the scarring.

If acne surgery is performed, should the physician do it? Here, too, there is a diversity of opinion.

Baer and Kopf, in commenting on Lowney's article in the 1965 Year Book of Dermatology, asked ". . . is it worthwhile for persons who have had 4 years of college, 4 years at medical school, and a minimum of 4 years of subsequent training to devote what probably amounts to hundreds of thousands of man-hours a year to the removal of comedones?"[6]

The answer is probably not, if one performs only the sheer technical act of extracting the comedo. However, the time required for the physician to do all or some of the needed acne surgery may be well spent if it is used simultaneously as a time to review the patient's medications, to determine how the patient is feeling, and to maintain rapport. The importance of "staying in touch" psychologically and of "laying on of hands" should not be underestimated, particularly in the management of a long-term, chronic problem, such as acne. ,

My own view, then, is that acne surgery is a useful addition to the management of acne, especially in patients with multiple comedones, primarily because of its salutory immediate cosmetic effects. I feel that it is rarely indeed that one finds incision and drainage to be a useful treatment for cystic lesions. I also feel that the physician should perform all or part of the acne surgery, using it and the required time to enhance the important physician-patient relationship—that much-maligned cliché that remains a fundamental and powerful tool of the physician as healer.

References

1. Mills, O. H., and Kligman, A. M.: Is sulphur helpful or harmful in acne vulgaris? Br. J. Dermatol. 86:620, 1972.
2. Strauss, J. S., et al.: A re-examination of the potential comedogenicity of sulfur. Arch. Dermatol. 114:1340, 1978.
3. Mills, O. H., and Kligman, A. M.: Evaluation of abrasives in acne therapy. Cutis 23:704, 1979.
4. Millikan, L. E., and Ameln, R.: Use of Buf-Puf and benzoyl peroxide in the treatment of acne. Cutis 28:201, 1981.
5. Lowney, E. V., et al.: Value of comedo extraction in treatment of acne vulgaris. JAMA 189:1000, 1964.
6. Baer, R. L., and Kopf, A. W.: Editorial comments. In Baer, R. L., and Kopf, A. W. (eds.): The 1964–1965 Year Book of Dermatology. Chicago, Year Book Medical Publishers, 1965, p. 62.

SYSTEMIC AND TOPICAL ANTIBIOTICS IN ACNE

Alan R. Shalita, M.D.

The treatment of acne with broad-spectrum antibiotics has gained widespread acceptance during the past three decades. Although these therapeutic agents have been used principally by dermatologists, the combination of efficacy, dosage flexibility, and a relatively wide range of safety has led to widespread recognition of their usefulness in the management of inflammatory acne by pediatricians, internists, and other physicians. More recently, many of these broad-spectrum antibiotics have been incorporated into effective delivery systems for topical application to the skin, and their dosage flexibility has thus been augmented. Nevertheless, all of these compounds are associated with side effects and toxicity, which the prudent physician must consider in weighing the risk/benefit ratio for an individual patient.

Although a variety of antibiotics had been assayed for acne treatment, beginning with penicillin and the sulfa drugs in the immediate post–World War II period, the results of such treatment were, at best, mixed. With the introduction of tetracycline and erythromycin in the early 1950s, however, effective antibiotic therapy for acne was demonstrated clearly. Although the use of these drugs was, at first, empirical, there rapidly appeared a series of reports explaining the mechanism of action of broad-spectrum antibiotics in acne as well as establishing a clearer understanding of the pathogenesis of this troublesome disease. Indeed, the history of these investigations provides an excellent example of how empirical clinical judgment can provide the stimulus for basic research into the pathogenesis of a disease.

The observations that tetracycline and erythromycin reduced the titratable acidity of skin surface lipid suggested that these antibiotics were effective because of a reduction in the fatty acids of sebum. This led to investigation of the genesis of these free fatty acids, and it became apparent that the intrafollicular microflora, principally *Propionibacterium acnes,* were responsible for producing these fatty acids. Thus, it became evident that the principal mechanism of action of these antibiotics was their antibacterial effect on *P. acnes.* Further studies of this micro-organism demonstrated that it produces a variety of extracellular products, such as lipases and chemotactic factors. Broad-spectrum antibiotics inhibit lipase and neutrophil chemotaxis, and it is now believed that they may play an anti-inflammatory as well as an antibacterial role.

The systemic antibiotics used in acne treatment include tetracycline, minocycline, demeclocycline, erythromycin, clindamycin, and trimethroprim-sulfamethoxazole. Systemic antibiotics have the advantages of therapeutic efficacy, dosage flexibility, and relative safety. They are indicated primarily for the treatment of moderate to severe papulopustular and nodulocystic acne. They may all be used in combination with a variety of topical agents, thus enhancing their therapeutic efficacy.

The disadvantages of systemic antibiotics in acne treatment include the relatively long delay before a therapeutic effect may be observed and numerous unpleasant side effects that may occur with these drugs. In addition, recent experience suggests that *P. acnes,* the organism for which these drugs is targeted, may develop a resistance to broad-spectrum antibiotics. Finally, the emergence of resistant gram-negative organisms, although uncommon, is a stubborn problem that may occur.

Topical agents, on the other hand, offer the advantage of delivering broad-spectrum antibiotics directly to the target tissue and have a more rapid onset of therapeutic effect than do their systemic counterparts. They also offer the advantage of few, if any, systemic side effects and are easier for the patient to use.

The disadvantages of topical antibiotics are that they are less effective than orally administered antibiotics, have less dosage flexibility, and may produce local irritation. The last problem may be augmented when these agents are used in conjunction with other topically applied agents. The emergence of resistant organisms is also a problem with topical antibiotics.

Systemic Antibiotics

Tetracyclines

Tetracycline and its derivatives (demeclocycline, minocycline, and doxycycline) have been demonstrated to be effective in the treatment of inflammatory acne. They produce a significant reduction in the inflammatory lesions of acne in most patients when given in adequate dosage and decrease dramatically the follicular population of *P. acnes*. The optimum dose for initiation of therapy with tetracycline is 1 gm per day. This dose is then increased or decreased, depending upon the response of the individual patient. Some patients may respond to doses as low as 250 mg of tetracycline per day. On the other hand, it appears clear that many patients with more severe inflammatory acne may require doses of tetracycline as high as 3 gm per day.

The tetracycline derivatives—demeclocycline, minocycline, and doxycycline—are effective in lower doses than those of tetracycline, apparently because of their higher lipid solubility and ultimate tissue concentration.

The safety of the long-term administration of tetracycline, particularly in divided doses totaling 1 gm or less per day, is now well-established. There appear to be no significant deleterious effects on the hematopoietic, hepatic, or renal systems in the overwhelming majority of patients. Nevertheless, a number of unpleasant or troublesome side effects may be encountered. The earliest of these is the staining of the deciduous teeth. In addition, photosensitivity reactions may occur and may include photo-onycholysis. Vaginal candidiasis is relatively common in women, particularly in those also taking oral contraceptives. A variety of vague gastrointestinal disturbances, including nausea, esophagitis, gastritis, and diarrhea, have been reported, but colitis is rare. At higher doses, renal diabetes insipidus may occur, and a Fanconi-like syndrome has been reported with the administration of outdated tetracycline. Finally, a major disadvantage of tetracycline is the fact that it readily binds to polyvalent cations, such as calcium, iron, magnesium, and zinc. Thus, it must be taken on an empty stomach, either 1 hour before or 2 hours after meals.

Although they offer the advantage of improved efficacy at lower doses, the tetracycline derivatives also have greater side effects and costs. Demeclocycline is more phototoxic and causes a dose-related renal diabetes insipidus more readily than does tetracycline. Minocycline produces a dose-related vertigo. It does not appear to be phototoxic. Doxycycline may be used in patients with renal insufficiency but otherwise produces side effects similar to those of the other tetracyclines.

Erythromycin

Erythromycin base, as well as several of its salts, has been demonstrated to be effective in the treatment of inflammatory acne. The estolate salt appears to be the best absorbed and the most effective, but because of potential hepatotoxicity it is not widely used. All other forms of erythromycin appear to be roughly equivalent. In general, somewhat higher doses of erythromycin are required to achieve an effect comparable with that of tetracycline. Vaginal candidiasis and gastrointestinal disturbances occur with approximately the same frequency as with tetracycline. Photosensitivity is not a problem with the use of erythromycins. It is puzzling, therefore, that erythromycin has not achieved the popularity of tetracycline for use in the treatment of acne.

Clindamycin

Clindamycin is highly effective in reducing the follicular population of *P. acnes*. It produces an excellent clinical response when administered to patients with inflammatory acne in divided doses of 300 mg per day. A major problem with clindamycin, however, is the occurrence of pseudomembranous colitis, which is more frequent with this drug than with tetracycline or erythromycin. Although the etiology of this colitis is now known to be overgrowth of the *Clostridium* species, which can be treated with oral vancomycin, this side effect has precluded the more widespread use of oral clindamycin.

Trimethoprim-Sulfamethoxazole

Although trimethoprim-sulfa combinations have been shown to decrease fatty acids in skin surface lipids, there is little information concerning their clinical use in acne. My experience suggests that this drug combination is beneficial in patients with severe nodulocystic acne that has proved refractory to therapy with more conventional antibiotics. In addition, my preliminary experience suggests that it is a useful drug for treating gram-negative folliculitis. The major complication is the relatively frequent incidence of cutaneous side effects, notably erythema multiforme and, rarely, Stevens-Johnson syndrome. This precludes the routine use of this drug for acne therapy.

Topical Antibiotics

During the past few years, several manufacturers have designed vehicles for the incorporation of broad-spectrum antibiotics for topical application in acne patients. The first of these incorporated tetracycline in a highly sophisticated vehicle. Formal clinical investigation of this drug suggested clinical efficacy comparable with that of 500 mg of oral tetracycline. Subsequent clinical experience, however, suggests less activity of this drug. The yellow discoloration of the skin that occurred after topical application of this formulation appears to have been remedied by vehicle changes.

More recently, 1.5 per cent and 2 per cent formulations of erythromycin base as well as 1 per cent clindamycin phosphate have become available in commercial, hydroalcoholic forms. Prior to the release of these stabilized preparations, a variety of extemporaneous mixtures were compounded by dermatologists and pharmacists. These generally included 2 per cent erythromycin base or 1 to 2 per cent clindamycin hydrochloride in a variety of different vehicles. It would appear that in these formulations, clindamycin was superior to erythromycin in clinical efficacy, although no adequate controlled studies were reported.

The situation with the commercially formulated preparations of these antibiotics is less clear-cut. National cooperative studies of the clinical efficacy of the various erythromycin formulations and the one clindamycin formulation demonstrated roughly equal reductions in inflammatory lesions, in the range of 50 per cent to 60 per cent. Direct comparison of the 1.5 per cent erythromycin formulation and the 1 per cent clindamycin solution showed no significant difference between the two.

One other preparation recently made available is meclocycline in a cream base. Formal investigation of this compound suggests clinical improvement in approximately 55 per cent of the cases, but no direct comparisons with the other antibiotics have been published. The singular advantage of this product would appear to be the relatively nonirritating effect of the cream vehicle. This is particularly advantageous in cold, dry climates or when the antibiotic is to be used in conjunction with an irritating compound.

Of particular interest is the role of topical antibiotics in acne therapy when compared with systemic antibiotics as well as with other topical antibacterial agents. Certainly, topical antibiotics are associated with fewer side effects than are systemic preparations. The latter reactions are principally local and relate to dryness and peeling from the hydroalcoholic vehicles. There are infrequent reports of diarrhea following use of topical clindamycin. I am not aware of any reports of colitis associated with administration of commercially formulated clindamycin solutions. On the other hand, the relative lack of dosage flexibility makes topical antibiotics less effective than their systemic counterparts. Furthermore, there appears to be an increase in the development of strains of *P. acnes* that are resistant to these topical antibiotics. This resistance appears to cross-react among the different compounds in the group and also with the systemic counterparts.

Since none of these agents appears to be more effective than benzoyl peroxide applied topically, there arises the question of the relative value of these agents compared with benzoyl peroxide, to which resistance does not appear to occur. It has therefore been suggested that topical antibiotics be used only in those patients who do not tolerate benzoyl peroxide because of either allergic contact dermatitis or primary irritant reactions. Another approach has been the sequential or combined use of benzoyl peroxide and topical antibiotics. One study suggests clinical superiority of a benzoyl peroxide–erythromycin preparation when compared with either agent alone or with the vehicle alone. Adequate studies of bacterial resistance to these combined therapies have not been reported.

Finally, it should be mentioned that usually none of these therapeutic agents are used alone. The sequential use of tretinoin and topical antibacterial agents enhances the therapeutic efficacy of these agents and reduces the need for systemic antibiotics in patients with mild to moderate inflammatory acne. Thus, the final choice of systemic or topical antibiotic therapy should logically take into consideration the combined or sequential application of other therapeutic modalities. In the final analysis, when one selects the antibiotics or combination of drugs to be used, one should consider the risk/benefit ratio and should take into consideration the severity of the disease, the patient's response to prior therapy, and, ultimately, the particular response to a given therapeutic regimen.

13-*CIS*-RETINOIC ACID IN THE TREATMENT OF ACNE

Ronald M. Reisner, M.D.

The Food and Drug Administration released 13-*cis*-retinoic acid on September 13, 1982 for general prescription use for the treatment of severe cystic acne unresponsive to conventional therapy under the Hoffmann-La Roche trade name of Accutane.

Based on the carefully documented experience published to date, which involves over 300 patients who have completed treatment protocols plus approximately 500 additional patients evaluated in unpublished studies, this agent appears to be a remarkable addition to our therapeutic armamentarium.

Many important questions remain unanswered, however. The experience that the practicing clinician will help accumulate should provide answers to these questions in the months and years ahead.

The optimum duration and dose levels have yet to be completely established. I will review briefly the investigational experience to date, which provides some guidelines. Since the drug has not been used with concomitant therapy in any studies as yet, the effect of combined treatment with the usual topical and systemic agents on outcome or on the required dose and duration of therapy remains to be determined. Careful clinical observation by the thoughtful practitioner has much to contribute here.

The precise mechanism of action of 13-*cis*-retinoic acid remains unknown. Its short-term effects seem to be related to the enormous reductions in sebum production that it causes, with accompanying atrophy of sebaceous glands and, at times, their almost complete disappearance.[1,2] It also affects other presumptive etiologic factors in acne and has been associated with a reduction in numbers of *Propionibacterium acnes* organisms, a decrease in inflammatory response, and alterations in keratinization.

Whether these or other factors explain the currently mysterious long-term improvement, which in some cases has now been documented for durations of up to 4 years after courses of only 4 months of therapy, also remains to be explained.

Experience with a little over 300 patients both in Europe and in the United States has been published to date. I would like briefly to summarize some of the practical conclusions that might be drawn.

Dose.   The dose employed has usually varied from 0.5 to 2.0 mg per kg per day, commonly divided into two equal doses each day.

Duration.   The duration of most of the protocol studies has been between 8 and 16 weeks with variable periods of follow-up, some now extending as long as 4 years. Some patients have undergone a second course of therapy. In general, there should be a waiting period of at least 8 weeks between the first and second courses because of the continuing improvement that can be seen in the weeks and months after completion of the first course.

All investigators have observed dramatic improvement in nodulocystic acne. As you may recall, Peck and associates originally reported 100 per cent clearing in 13 of their 14 patients.[3] Other investigators have also noted excellent results, although generally with a lower percentage of clearing. This is probably related to the fact that most subsequent studies did not employ doses as large as Peck's (average of 2.0 mg per kg for 16 weeks). The duration of therapy is also important. Shorter studies do not fully reflect the very significant continuing improvement that has been observed even after discontinuation of therapy. Plewig and Nikolowski have noted similarly favorable responses in rosacea and gram-negative folliculitis.[4]

My initial assessment of our experience at UCLA and of the available data—balancing the sometimes faster response with higher doses against the concomitant increase in side effects—is that the commonly used dose will be between 0.5 and 1.0 mg per kg per day, divided into two daily doses and given for 16 weeks. The package insert suggests 1.0 to 2.0 mg per kg per day given in two divided daily doses for 15 to 20 weeks. With the addition of other treatment, it may be possible to decrease the daily dose and, possibly, the duration of therapy with 13-*cis*-retinoic acid.

Time Course of Patient Response. Sebum production is maximally suppressed at approximately 3 to 4 weeks after initiation of therapy. Clinical improvement is slower, since 13-*cis*-retinoic acid has the predominant effect of preventing new lesions; existing lesions still require time to undergo involution. As a rule of thumb, at about 6 weeks, decreases in numbers of lesions by approximately one third can be seen, and by the thirteenth or fourteenth week numbers of lesions have decreased by approximately two thirds, even if therapy has been discontinued at 12 weeks. By about 6 months, even if therapy has been discontinued at between 12 and 16 weeks, decreases in lesion numbers of 80 to 90 per cent can be seen.

It also appears that the length of the remission may be related in part to dose level and duration of therapy. Flares, when they occur, are generally mild and should be controllable with conventional methods without the necessity of instituting another course of 13-*cis*-retinoic acid therapy in many cases.

In general, facial lesions appear to respond more rapidly than do those on the back or the chest.

All types of lesions—comedones (both open and closed), papules, pustules, and nodulocystic lesions—have been shown to respond to therapy with systemic 13-*cis*-retinoic acid. However, issues of safety (both short-term and long-term), efficacy, and cost all enter into the decision regarding the use of 13-*cis*-retinoic acid for patients other than those with severe nodulocystic acne unresponsive to conventional therapy. There will probably be a great deal of pressure from patients to be given this new drug for mild acne. However, because of the significant adverse effects that may be seen with 13-*cis*-retinoic acid, it should be reserved for patients with significant cystic acne inadequately responsive to conventional therapy.

Among the side effects that have been observed to date are the following:

1. 13-*cis*-Retinoic acid has been shown to be teratogenic in animals, although no teratogenicity has yet been demonstrated in humans treated with this agent. However, the risk does exist. For this reason, patients who are pregnant or who are planning to become pregnant during the period of treatment should not receive 13-*cis*-retinoic acid. Women who have childbearing potential also should not be given 13-*cis*-retinoic acid until it is ascertained that an effective form of contraception is being used and that they fully understand the potential risks to the fetus should they become pregnant during treatment. If pregnancy does occur during treatment, the physician and the patient should promptly discuss the entire issue of continuing the pregnancy.

As a further precaution, it is recommended that contraception be continued for 1 month or until a normal menstrual period has occurred after completion of a course of therapy with 13-*cis*-retinoic acid. The 1-month contraception recommendation is probably on the conservative side, in view of the known terminal elimination half-life of 13-*cis*-retinoic acid of from 10 to 20 hours, but it would be wise to heed this advice.

2. Perhaps the next most significant side effect seen with 13-*cis*-retinoic acid is the elevation in plasma triglycerides observed in approximately one fourth of all patients treated. Other lipid abnormalities that have been observed are a decrease in high-density lipoproteins in approximately 15 per cent of patients and an increase in serum cholesterol in approximately 7 per cent. Although the significance of these changes with regard to cardiovascular risk is far from clear at this point, every effort should be made to control

significant triglyceride elevations by such measures as limitation of dietary fat and alcohol and weight reduction. Reduction of the dosage of 13-*cis*-retinoic acid also may permit continuation of therapy in individual patients. Another risk associated with marked elevations in serum triglycerides is the precipitation of acute pancreatitis. To date, all of the observed serum lipid abnormalities have been reversible with discontinuation of the 13-*cis*-retinoic acid.

3. Approximately 16 per cent of patients have developed musculoskeletal symptoms. Five patients who were being treated for disorders of keratinization, which, unlike acne, require continuing therapy, have developed skeletal abnormalities after treatment of 2 years or more. Three adults developed hyperostosis with degenerative changes in the spine, and two children developed x-ray changes suggestive of possible premature closure of the epiphyses. Although it appears that these are changes unlikely to occur in individuals receiving the short courses of therapy required for acne, it would nonetheless be desirable to be aware of them.

4. Approximately 90 per cent of patients receiving 1.5 mg per kg per day for 20 weeks developed dryness of the lips or cheilitis, or both. About half of these patients developed conjunctivitis or other eye irritation. A smaller percentage, 15 to 30 per cent, developed one or more of the following: xerosis and desquamation, dry mouth, pruritus, epistaxis, nausea, vomiting, and gastrointestinal disturbances. Another 10 per cent experienced thinning of the hair, lethargy, or fatigue, and 5 per cent developed palmar or plantar desquamation.

5. Hematologic changes have included decreases in red blood cells and white blood cells and increases in platelets in a small number of patients. White blood cells have also been seen in the urine, and some abnormalities of liver function tests have been observed.

Since Accutane is formulated with parabens as preservatives, it obviously should not be given to patients who are sensitive to parabens. Also, since it is a vitamin A derivative, patients should be advised against taking additional vitamin A to avoid an additive toxic effect.

6. Testicular atrophy has been observed in animal studies; however, human males have shown no significant abnormalities in sperm count or motility.

A number of other minor side effects have been reported, including many that are of very low incidence and may bear no causal relationship to 13-*cis*-retinoic acid therapy.

This catalog of side effects makes it clear that 13-*cis*-retinoic acid must be used with discrimination and knowledge in the management of acne. It is clearly not the first-line drug for the routine care of the majority of patients with acne. The physician using it should be fully conversant with the entire range of therapeutic agents used in acne and should be adept in their selection and use. In this way, indiscriminate use of this potent new agent with all its associated hazards will be avoided.

With the vast array of synthetic retinoids that are being prepared and that have yet to be studied, 13-*cis*-retinoic acid and its sister compound, etretinate, are only the tip of the iceberg. Based on the experience with these two drugs, it would appear that many of the new synthetic retinoids will have distinctive individual properties, profiles of therapeutic efficacy, and side effects. We may well yet see in the years to come even more effective and safer drugs in this group—not only for acne but also for the whole range of disorders of epithelial differentiation, including disorders of keratinization and neoplasms. Ultimately, we may even have the ideal dermatologic version of these drugs for topical application without systemic side effects.

Despite all the current sociopolitical and economic problems of medicine in general and dermatology in particular, this remains an exciting and satisfying time in which to be practicing our specialty.

References

1. Farrell, L. N., Strauss, J. S., and Stranieri, A.: The treatment of severe cystic acne with 13-*cis* retinoic acid: Evaluation of sebum production and the clinical response in a multiple-dose trial. J. Am. Acad. Dermatol. 6:602, 1980.
2. Goldstein, J. A., Socha-Szott, A., Thomsen, R. J., Pochi, P. E., Shalita, A. R., and Strauss, J. S.: Comparative effect of isotretinoin and etretinate on acne and sebaceous gland secretion. J. Am. Acad. Dermatol. 6:760, 1982.
3. Peck, G. L., Olsen, T. G., Butkus, D., Pandya, M., Arnaud-Battandier, J., Gross, E. G., Windhorst, D. B., and Cheripko, J.: Isotretinoin versus placebo in the treatment of cystic acne. J. Am. Acad. Dermatol. 6:735, 1982.
4. Plewig, G., Nikolowski, J., and Wolff, H. H.: Action of isotretinoin in acne rosacea and gram-negative folliculitis. J. Am. Acad. Dermatol. 6:766, 1982.

TREATMENT OF ACNE: CRYOTHERAPY

Ervin Epstein, M.D.

In my experience and in my hands, the treatment of acne with the local application of refrigerants has been one of the most effective modalities tried.[1] This therapy may be delivered in a variety of ways; the therapeutic benefits result from the freezing rather than from the choice of methods and the materials employed. The simplest and least expensive approach is to use carbon dioxide "slush," which is produced by fracturing Dry Ice with a hammer until it is transformed into a powder. Enough acetone is added so that it assumes the consistency of a sherbet. One can obtain the same mixture by procuring the powder from a commercial cylinder of carbon dioxide. Liquid nitrogen can be applied with a large ball of cotton on an applicator stick or, better yet, with a cryoroller. Liquid nitrogen also may be applied as a spray. Graham, who has written extensively on the subject, prefers to use nitrous oxide spray.[2] Experience, familiarity, and availability determine the approach chosen by the individual practitioner.

First let us consider the indications for this type of therapy. It can be used profitably in treatment of any type of acne. It is particularly effective in the presence of pustular lesions, including acne conglobata. Since adverse publicity has turned x-ray therapy into a "no-no," cryotherapy has become my number one modality for the management of acne. Of course, there are contraindications to its use, and it therefore cannot be employed in all cases. For instance, its use should be confined to whites. Heavily pigmented skin often responds by pigmentary alterations, especially hyperpigmentation, although depigmentation also may result. One should treat the chest, especially the breasts, carefully and with great restraint, since this area tends to scar if the treatment is applied with too much enthusiasm. If the patient is overly intolerant of discomfort, this form of therapy should be avoided. Application of these refrigerants causes a stinging sensation that may discourage the patient with little or no stoicism. However, after a few treatments, none of the patients complain about this discomfort. Perhaps those who cannot tolerate the sensation of cold are eliminated voluntarily after the first few applications. Actually, pain is not a serious problem.

This modality offers certain advantages for the treatment of acne. It can be used concurrently with local and systemic therapy. The necessary materials are readily available. The cost of the refrigerants varies but is not excessive. Since one can get results with a cotton applicator and crushed Dry Ice, the cost can be reduced to a minimum. Liquid nitrogen can be stored in the office for weeks and therefore can be quickly available whenever a patient requiring this therapy appears. As this is written, the copper cryoroller costs less than $20 and, as far as we can tell, lasts forever. It is singularly free of the need for repairs. Freezing therapy is also beneficial in the management of acne scarring.

Of course, there are disadvantages to this therapy as well as advantages. The possibility of pigmentary changes in dark-skinned races has been alluded to earlier. If the treatment is administered with too much vigor, burns may result. These may be painful and slow to heal. Undesirable scarring may eventuate. These unfortunate sequelae must be avoided at all costs. If one adopts a spray such as is used for liquid nitrogen or nitrous oxide, the equipment is costly, although minisprays have proved to be satisfactory and are comparatively inexpensive. Repeated treatments are necessary, usually at intervals of 1 or more weeks. Therefore, treatment may be prolonged for months or more.

Other than the few comparatively trivial hazards mentioned previously, cryotherapy is safe. There are no delayed or chronic complications. Systemic disturbances are absent. The treatment can be repeated as often as necessary. The therapeutic results are equal, and, in my experience, superior to those of any other physical modality. They are better than those obtained with any local applications that I have used. If I had a choice between cryotherapy and oral antibiotics for the control of acne, I would definitely choose the former. Best of all, cryotherapy can be combined with local therapy, dietary control, administration of antibiotics, *cis*-retinoic acid, and other treatment modalities. Try it . . . you'll like it.

In a cooperative patient, cryotherapy is one of the more successful forms of therapy at our disposal. From conversations with clinicians it is evident that this method of clearing the eruption of acne is not used as much by dermatologists as it should be. This can be explained only by a lack of familiarity on the part of the clinicians, which can be blamed on the lack of training in cryotherapy for the control of this dermatosis in many centers. The dermatologist should be conversant, and even expert, in the use of this method before he enters practice. Unfortunately, this is often not the case. Therefore, if you are one who knows little or nothing about the freezing treatment of acne, you are advised to gain more knowledge and experience in this approach to the management of this unfortunate and nearly universal derangement. It is simple and easy to learn, and its application will add to your therapeutic armamentarium and to patient satisfaction.

References

1. Epstein, E.: Acne surgery. *In* Epstein, E., and Epstein, E., Jr. (eds.): Skin Surgery, 4th ed. Springfield, IL, Charles C Thomas, 1977, pp. 821–822.
2. Graham, G.: Cyrosurgery in the treatment of acne. *In* Epstein, E., and Epstein, E., Jr. (eds.): Skin Surgery, 4th ed. Springfield, IL, Charles C Thomas, 1977, pp. 680–700.

ACNE SURGERY
Stuart Maddin, M.D.

It was more than 150 years ago that reports first appeared recommending the mechanical extraction of comedones. Such intervention was justified on the basis of reducing the subsequent development of inflamed lesions. By the turn of the century, it was recognized that comedo extraction was of most benefit when used in the treatment of superficial acne. A more recent study (1964)[1] concerning comedo extraction suggested that acne surgery was beneficial for superficial acne, especially over the forehead. When carried out on the cheeks or on cystic lesions, the procedure worsened acne. In the nearly 20 years since this report appeared, there has been a dearth of information that supports the need for carrying out acne surgery.

With the increasing availability of more effective anti-acne medications, the controversy that once was associated with the need for acne surgery has abated. There is no doubt that the availability of retinoic acid, benzoyl peroxide, intralesional corticosteroids, and topical and systemic antibiotics has greatly reduced the need to resort to mechanical emptying. The newest agent, 13-*cis*-retinoic acid (Accutane), will supply even further assistance to us in the management of the hitherto treatment-resistant forms of the nodulocystic and conglobate varieties of acne.

However, in spite of the therapeutic advances in the management of acne, there are still dermatologists who are of the opinion that active intervention, i.e., comedo removal, is necessary and should form part of the anti-acne treatment regimen.

The most persistent argument presented to justify acne surgery centers on the need to evacuate comedones or to incise and drain pustules and cysts. Such mechanical removal or drainage is thought to aid in the more rapid involution of individual acne lesions. It is implied that local surgical treatment removes the foreign bodies that are responsible for the occlusion of the follicular duct, which in turn causes the formation of comedones, pustules, and cysts.

Removal of Comedones

It has long been recognized that closed comedones eventually become pustules. The clinical benefit that follows the removal of the follicular plug is short-lived; recurrences are common. The removal of open comedones does not influence the clinical course of acne, since such lesions do not lead to inflammatory change. If comedones are not removed properly, i.e., with a minimum of trauma, more lesions may develop at or near the site of damage.

If the attending dermatologist elects to remove comedones, he should first achieve a certain degree of proficiency in order to cause as little tissue trauma as possible when carrying out the procedure. In some cases, this task is delegated to an office nurse because it is both time-consuming and tedious. Some dermatologists instruct the patient or the parent, so that this procedure can be carried out at home. A number of authorities (Moschella,[8] Strauss[9]) recommend that acne surgery not be carried out at home.

It should also be noted that "deep pore cleansing" that has long been popular in Europe as carried out by estheticians and cosmetologists is now gaining widespread acceptance in North America. There has been a proliferation of so-called skin salons that devote a good deal of their time to the management of superficial acne, using both manual and mechanical pore cleansers.

Following the favorable report in 1969 by Kligman[10] concerning the use of retinoic acid for altering epidermal hyperkeratosis and removing keratotic plugs, a major therapeutic advance was registered in terms of controlling comedo formation. The continued topical use of retinoic acid over 3 to 5 weeks will bring about a marked reduction in the formation of comedones.

Opening of Pustules

Although it has long been popular to incise and express the contents of pustules with the hope that such lesions will heal more quickly, it is the opinion of a number of authorities, including the editor of *Controversies in Dermatology*, that such surgical intervention (i.e., incision) not only increases scarring but also often leads to the formation of an "ice-pick" type of scar. Such a scar is peculiarly resistant to removal by dermabrasion (see the section on dermabrasion).

If the dermatologist wishes to perform acne surgical techniques, the judicious use of a Number 11 (Bard-Parker) surgical blade is recommended. The point should be gently inserted into the lesion, and the contents should be carefully expressed.

Since the mid-1970s, dermatologists have had an increasing array of antibiotic agents suitably formulated for topical use, and these are effective in controlling pustular acne. They include clindamycin phosphate lotion, erythromycin base, and tetracycline hydrochloride.

Removal of Milia

Milia occur not only in association with acne vulgaris but also as a postoperative complication following dermabrasion. These lesions are similar to comedones but are completely roofed over with a thin layer of skin. In other instances, they are made up of very small sebaceous cysts.

One can most easily accomplish the successful evacuation of such lesions by carefully piercing the overlying roof of skin with a needle and then gently expressing the contents.

Removal of Cysts

A variety of surgical approaches are recommended for the removal of several types of cysts that accompany acne. Such techniques include total excision and incision with drainage. The majority of surgical approaches will lead to the formation of permanent scars. In the past, it was argued that such surgical intervention helps reduce the size of the scar that inevitably occurs.

With the availability of systemic antibiotics and, if necessary, intralesional injection of corticosteroids, it is now seldom necessary to drain or incise cysts unless they are fluctuant and persistent.

CONCLUSION

Although dermatology, like other medical disciplines, encourages the expression of divergent opinions concerning the clinical management of patients, it is nevertheless important that all of us periodically review the usefulness of the treatment techniques that we apply. The ancient dictum that emphasized the need for surgical intervention to bring about drainage or removal of foreign material from the follicular orifice of individual acne lesions (i.e., inspissated sebum, epithelial debris) in the hope that such action would lead to more rapid healing is no longer as valid a concept as it once was. It has long been recognized that many patients with acne (even of the more severe variety) that are treated with routine topical and systemic anti-acne measures heal without scar formation.

It is well recognized that the majority of practicing dermatologists advise patients not to pick or excoriate acne lesions in order to reduce scarring. After such warning has been given to the patient, it is difficult for the physician to vindicate his routine use of acne surgery. It is even more difficult to justify surgical intervention that includes incision of pustules and cysts.

If on occasion a dermatologist is of the opinion that acne surgery is necessary, the following two considerations should be noted: (1) The operator should possess a degree of surgical skill. In addition, (2) it is essential to have the proper equipment available: a sharp, pointed Number 11 Bard-Parker scalpel blade, a Number 25 needle, and a comedo extractor. Many dermatologists restrict the performance of these techniques to their offices and discourage acne surgery at home.

For the majority of acne patients, however, the conservative (nonsurgical) approach will suffice.

References

1. Lowney, E. D., Witkowski, J., Simons, H. M., and Zagula, Z. W.: Value of comedo extraction in treatment of acne vulgaris. JAMA 189:108, 1964.
2. Epstein, E.: Acne surgery. In Epstein, E., and Epstein, E., Jr. (eds.): Skin Surgery, 4th ed. Springfield, IL, Charles C Thomas, 1977, pp. 456–460.
3. Strauss, J. S.: Dermatology. In Fitzpatrick, T. B., et al. (eds.): General Medicine, 2nd ed. New York, McGraw Hill Book Company, 1981, p. 448.
4. Stewart, W. D., Dauto, J. L., and Maddin, W. S.: Dermatology, 4th ed. St. Louis, C. V. Mosby Co., 1978, p. 88.
5. Tolman, E. L.: Dermatology, vol. 2. Philadelphia, W. B. Saunders Co., 1975, p. 1134.
6. Ebling, F. J., and Rook, A.: The sebaceous gland. In Rook, A., et al. (eds.): Textbook of Dermatology, vol. 2, 3rd ed. Oxford, Blackwell Scientific Publications, 1979, p. 1723.
7. Reisner, R. M.: Acne vulgaris. In Maddin, W. S. (ed.): Current Dermatologic Therapy. Philadelphia, W. B. Saunders Co., 1982, p. 5.
8. Moschella, S. L., Pillsbury, D. M., and Hurley, H. J., Jr.: Dermatology, vol. 2. Philadelphia. W. B. Saunders Co., 1975, p. 1134.
9. Strauss, J. S.: Diseases of sebaceous glands; acne vulgaris. In Fitzpatrick, T. B., Eisen, A. Z., Wolff, K., Freedberg, I. M.; and Austen, K. F. (eds.): Dermatology in General Medicine, 2nd ed. New York, McGraw-Hill, 1979, p. 448.
10. Kligman, A. M., et al.: Topical vitamin A acid in acne vulgaris. Arch. Dermatol. 99:469, 1969.

TREATMENT OF ACNE: DERMATOLOGIC RADIOTHERAPY

Ervin Epstein, M.D.

Any discussion of the use of ionizing radiation in the treatment of a benign dermatosis must address two issues: (1) the safety or hazards of the therapy, and (2) the therapeutic benefits to be obtained by its use.

Hazards of Dermatoradiotherapy

X-radiation therapy for benign conditions has fallen into disrepute because of the ignorant writings of lay authors and the misguided pontifical statements arising within governmental agencies. The latter has made the use of ionizing radiation for treatment especially hazardous from a medicolegal standpoint. There is no question that overdosage of such therapy is dangerous and even carcinogenic; however, there is no *proven* evidence that properly applied treatment with ionizing radiation is hazardous. Those who quarrel with this statement argue on the basis of a linear hypothesis, yet the linear hypothesis represents an exercise in illogic. It postulates that all x-radiation is carcinogenic and that the incidence of malignancies is related to the dose in a linear fashion. In other words, if 1000 rads produce 1000 cases of cancer, 1 rad will cause the development of one malignancy. This is as illogical as the statement that if a 100-mile-per-hour wind will blow the roof off a barn, a 10-mile-per-hour wind will blow off 10 per cent of the roof.

Even the prestigious BEIR (Biologic Effects of Ionizing Radiation) committee of the National Research Council admits that the linear hypothesis has never been proved and probably never will be proved but should be accepted for public health reasons.[1] This compares with the cries of the doom predictors that some day an earthquake will cause the state of California to fall into the sea. However, even they do not advocate evacuating California at this time. On the other hand, the foes of x-radiation tells us to abandon dermatologic radiotherapy because some day it may be found that such rays have dangers that are not obvious at this time. The following quotation from Teller should be of interest: "Our 'nuclearphobia' affects medicine directly. Since 1945, the number of people killed by radiation can be counted in the dozens; the number killed because of lack of radiation diagnosis and treatment in, say, cancer can be counted in the hundreds of thousands and maybe the millions. This is an example of how misinformation about radiation can scare. People are scared to use something that can save their lives."[2]

The only established dangers of x-radiation therapy as administered by competent dermatologists concern radiation burns—radiodermatitis. This is a manifestation of overdosage and can lead to many complications, including ulceration, necrosis, keratoses, cancers, and even fatalities. However, the knowledgeable dermatologist treating a benign condition such as acne limits his total dose to less than 1000 rads. When this schedule has been used (division of the dose into 12 equal treatments that total 660 to 900 rads), I have never seen a radiodermatitis develop or malignant degeneration ensue.

Many physicians feel that x-radiation is unnecessary because of the use of antibiotics, corticosteroids, 13-*cis*-retinoic acid, hormones, and other agents. This is illogical for two reasons. First, x-ray therapy does not replace these other agents; rather, it complements them. Ionizing radiation therapy is an adjunct to, not a replacement for, these modalities.

Secondly, the dangers of a radiodermatitis are much smaller than the aplastic anemia, the dissemination of a malignancy or tuberculosis, the rupture of a peptic ulcer, or the manifestation of a major psychosis that can occur with the use of drugs. No one ever received an x-ray burn from a dose of 75 rads or a cancer from this amount of ionizing radiation. The point is that drugs may cause severe and unpredictable damage. The hazards of x-radiation are known and are definitely dose-related. There is no explosive idiosyncrasy to these rays. I have seen two patients die from the ingestion of a single aspirin tablet as a result of hematologic reactions.

There is a second group of potential hazards—unproved but commonly described—that may manifest themselves some day. *Genetic damage* has been established in the *Drosophila* fly but has decreased in frequency and severity as scientists have begun working with higher orders of animals. *Leukemia* has not been established in acne patients. *Basal cell epitheliomas* have been reported in patients without radiodermatitis. Radiation therapy was used frequently in the past (up to 50 per cent of a dermatologist's practice), and basal cell epitheliomas (about 3 per cent of my practice) were a common occurrence. If this tumor did not develop in patients who received such treatment, it would have been established that x-radiation prevents the development of basal cell epitheliomas. *Thyroid cancer* occurs mainly in patients who received radiation therapy in infancy, especially for shrinkage of the tonsils, the adenoids, or the thymus gland. Radiotherapy was never performed for acne in patients under the age of 16.5 years. Many patients have called me to say that they had been warned about the possibility of developing a cancer of the thyroid gland because they had received x-ray therapy from me for their acne. I have reassured them that the possibility of such a relationship was remote but have told them that nothing would be lost by having a checkup of their thyroid gland. Also, I asked them to call me if anything amiss were to be found. No patient has ever called me back after having the recommended examinations. Two classmates of mine married and produced four children. The older boy and girl had severe acne and received a full course of radiation therapy from me. Thyroid neoplasms were never manifested in these children. The two younger children who did not have acne or x-radiation therapy did develop thyroid neoplastic disease at the ages of 18 and 19 years. One of these neoplasms was malignant. Why should this occurrence not be given as much credence as the reported instances in which a patient had x-ray therapy and later developed a thyroid cancer?

Only time will tell if we can connect cancer of the breast and other organs to the use of these rays. However, in the meantime the lawyers and insurance companies are playing a game. The lawyers claim that everything that happens to a patient who has had irradiation is due to the rays, and the insurance companies tremble when they consider the effect that the mention of x-radiation will have on the minds of the jurors. At present it is ridiculous to connect any damage other than radiodermatitis to dermatoradiotherapy.

Therapeutic Results of Dermatoradiotherapy in Acne

More than 1000 patients with acne treated with x-radiation in my practice were reviewed from a number of standpoints. I believe that the figures are significant and can be compared with statistics concerning the other approaches discussed in this section of the book. This study was reported, and the summary at the end of the article cited in the references presents the important conclusions drawn from this observation.[3] In addition, the statistical results of the investigation are included in this discussion (Tables 1 through 6), so that the student who wishes to evaluate the decisions made on the basis of this investigation and to form his own opinions will have the opportunity to do so. It should be noted that not all compilations add up to 100 per cent in the tables, since those causes listed as "not specified" are not included.

A total of 1051 patients with acne were treated with x-radiation (59.1 per cent of all

Table 1. THERAPEUTIC RESULTS IN
ACNE TREATED WITH X-RADIATION*

Degree of Improvement	Number of Patients
0 to 25%	100 (9.5%)
26% to 50%	88 (8.4%)
51% to 75%	125 (11.8%)
76% to 85%	162 (15.4%)
86% to 95%	324 (30.8%)
96% to 99%	53 (5.0%)
100%	146 (13.8%)
Not specified	53 (5.3%)

*From Epstein, E.: X-ray therapy in acne: Therapeutic
response and patient cooperation. Cutis 8:321, 1971. Used by
permission.

Table 2. PATIENT COOPERATION AS
INDICATED BY NUMBER OF TREATMENTS*

Number of Treatments	Number of Patients	Per Cent
1	30	2.8%
2 to 5	186	17.7%
6 to 9	202	18.2%
10 to 11	105	9.9%
12 to 14	526	50.5%
15 to 16	2	0.2%

*From Epstein, E.: X-ray therapy in acne: Therapeutic re-
sponse and patient cooperation. Cutis 8:321, 1971. Used by permission.

Table 3. EFFECT OF SEVERITY OF ERUPTION ON COOPERATION
(NUMBER OF TREATMENTS)*

	Number of Patients		
Number of Treatments	Mild	Moderate	Severe
1	3 (3.6%)	18 (3.5%)	9 (1.9%)
2 to 5	23 (28.0%)	110 (21.6%)	52 (11.3%)
6 to 9	12 (14.6%)	106 (20.8%)	84 (18.3%)
10 to 11	17 (20.7%)	49 (9.6%)	39 (8.5%)
12 to 14	27 (32.9%)	225 (44.2%)	274 (59.6%)
15 to 16	0	1 (0.2%)	1 (0.2%)

*From Epstein, E.: X-ray therapy in acne: Therapeutic response and patient cooperation. Cutis 8:321,
1971. Used by permission.

Table 4. EFFECT OF SEVERITY OF ERUPTION ON THERAPEUTIC
RESULTS*

	Number of Patients		
Degree of Improvement	Mild	Moderate	Severe
0 to 25%	11 (13.4%)	52 (10.2%)	37 (8.0%)
26% to 50%	8 (9.7%)	48 (9.4%)	31 (6.7%)
51% to 75%	14 (17.0%)	66 (12.9%)	45 (9.8%)
76% to 85%	11 (13.4%)	66 (12.9%)	85 (18.5%)
86% to 95%	23 (28.0%)	143 (28.0%)	158 (34.4%)
96% to 99%	2 (2.4%)	26 (5.1%)	25 (5.4%)
100%	8 (9.7%)	76 (14.9%)	62 (13.5%)
Total—86% to 100%	33 (39.1%)	245 (48.0%)	245 (53.3%)

*From Epstein, E.: X-ray therapy in acne: Therapeutic response and patient cooperation. Cutis 8:321, 1971.
Used by permission.

Table 5. EFFECT OF DOSAGE OF X-RADIATION ON THERAPEUTIC RESULTS*

Degree of Improvement	Number of Patients			
	Less Than 200 Rads	*201 to 500 Rads*	*501 to 700 Rads*	*701 to 980 Rads*
0 to 25%	70 (48.2%)	21 (10.1%)	9 (2.8%)	0
26% to 50%	18 (12.4%)	59 (28.6%)	7 (2.2%)	4 (1.0%)
51% to 75%	1 (0.6%)	63 (30.5%)	37 (11.7%)	24 (6.2%)
76% to 85%	1 (0.6%)	32 (15.5%)	79 (25.0%)	50 (13.0%)
86% to 95%	2 (1.2%)	23 (11.1%)	130 (41.1%)	169 (44.0%)
96% to 99%	0	1 (0.4%)	5 (1.5%)	47 (12.2%)
100%	0	7 (3.3%)	49 (15.5%)	90 (23.4%)

*From Epstein, E.: X-ray therapy in acne: Therapeutic response and patient cooperation. Cutis 8:321, 1971. Used by permission.

the patients with this dermatosis encountered in a private practice). Two dosage schedules were used: The total doses of each were approximately 660 rads and 900 rads, each given in 12 treatments over a period of approximately 4 months. There were no significant differences in therapeutic results obtained with the two schedules. This suggests that the usual recommended weekly dose of 75 rads could be reduced to 60 rads without sacrificing benefits.

The acne of nearly 14 per cent of the patients cleared completely, and more than 50 per cent obtained better than an 85 per cent improvement. Nearly 65 per cent of the patients receiving one half of the recommended therapy were in the highly benefited group (86 per cent improvement or better). More than one half completed the 12 treatments, and 80 per cent submitted to more than six treatments, which indicated good patient cooperation. These figures did not decrease during the 1946 to 1960 "maximum scare period," demonstrating that there was no real resistance to radiation therapy on the part of the patients.

Of the parameters studied, the most important were the number of treatments and the total dosage, followed by the severity of the eruption, the age of the patient, and the extent of involvement. The effects of age on the therapeutic results suggest that therapy should be withheld until the patient is between 16 and 17 years of age. Less important were sex of the patient, duration of the condition, and type of equipment used. It is felt that this study demonstrates that ionizing radiation exerts a beneficial effect on acne. No comparisons were drawn with systemic medications, which can and should be used concurrently with x-radiation. However, it should be stressed that x-ray treatments of the quantity and quality recommended here are safer than antibiotics, estrogens, corticosteroids, and other agents. Although the aforementioned figures indicate that x-rays have a therapeutic effect in acne, the cure rate is less than older studies would have led us to anticipate. Therefore, other measures should be added to the regimen of those receiving this form of therapy.

Table 6. EFFECT OF NUMBER OF TREATMENTS ON THERAPEUTIC RESULTS*

Degree of Improvement	Number of Treatments					
	1	*2 to 5*	*6 to 9*	*10 to 11*	*12 to 14*	*15 to 16*
0 to 25%	9 (9.0%)	72 (72.0%)	11 (11.0%)	6 (6.0%)	2 (2.0%)	0
26% to 50%	15 (17.0%)	37 (42.0%)	33 (37.5%)	0	3 (3.4%)	0
51% to 75%	3 (2.4%)	19 (15.2%)	55 (44.0%)	16 (12.8%)	32 (25.6%)	0
76% to 85%	1 (0.6%)	4 (2.4%)	57 (35.1%)	29 (17.9%)	71 (43.8%)	0
86% to 95%	2 (0.6%)	1 (0.3%)	37 (11.4%)	42 (12.9%)	240 (74.1%)	2 (0.6%)
96% to 99%	0	0	1 (1.9%)	2 (3.7%)	50 (94.3%)	0
100%	0	0	8 (5.5%)	10 (6.8%)	128 (87.7%)	0

*From Epstein, E.: X-ray therapy in acne: Therapeutic response and patient cooperation. Cutis 8:321, 1971. Used by permission.

References

1. The effects on populations of exposure to lower levels of ionizing radiation (BEIR report). Washington, D.C., National Research Council, National Academy of Sciences, 1972.
2. Teller, E.: Interview. AMA News, July 30, 1982, p. 18.
3. Epstein, E.: X-ray therapy in acne: Therapeutic response and patient cooperation. Cutis 8:321, Oct. 1971.

COLLAGEN FOR IMPLANTATION: PROBLEMS FOR CONSIDERATION

Richard G. Glogau, M.D.

The introduction of Zyderm into clinical practice has been an exciting development. There is no question that it has changed the way in which my associates and I approach the problems of scar repair. Despite all the positive aspects of Zyderm that have convinced us to use it, there remain a number of considerations on the negative side.

First and foremost, like most modalities in medicine, Zyderm rarely delivers the perfect result. The majority of scars for which the material is appropriate can be corrected to 80 per cent, or even 90 per cent, of their contour deformity at best. However, absolutely smooth contours are rarely achieved and even more rarely maintained.

Second, the cost of the material is substantial. An average adult with moderate acne scarring can count on spending over $1000 for a series of injections. Although this is not out of range compared with the cost of other cosmetic procedures, such as full-face dermabrasion or chemical peeling, and although it certainly is less than the cost of procedures such as the face lift, it is a significant amount of money.

The multiplicity of injections needed to correct the scars of an average patient must be taken into consideration. This is not a process that is done on one day and completed within the week. Adjustments and repeat evaluations are necessary for optimal use of the material. Four months' time to complete treatment is not unusual.

There are also problems with the basic application of the material in scar repair. The visual impact of a scar is largely, but not completely, the result of a contour defect. Such other qualities as the surface texture, the color, the contrast with the surrounding skin, the presence or absence of adnexal structures (such as hair and sweat glands) and the light-reflecting ability of the skin are significant factors that determine the visual appearance of any scar or wrinkle. Anyone who has seen a slightly depressed scar from a shave biopsy on the nose will appreciate that the prominence of the defect has little to do with contour and much to do with the other qualities mentioned.

Unfortunately, Zyderm can repair only the contour of the scar. I have not seen it make a significant difference in color, surface texture, or any of the other factors mentioned. The physician should analyze the patient's cosmetic scars carefully and should discuss these factors with the patient. Some patients will not be suitable candidates for Zyderm but may benefit from other modalities, such as dermabrasion, chemical peels, or even judicious use of makeup, which may produce a desired change in the factors that are unrelated to the contour deformity, such as color, texture, reflection of light, and so forth.

Another difficulty encountered with the use of Zyderm is the variability of response of different types of scars in different types of people. As more clinical experience is accumulated, there is no question that physicians are becoming more adept in selecting patients who are likely to respond to the material. However, certain types of scars, such as ice-pick scars and viral pox scars, fail to respond in almost all patients. Some defects, such as the very fine wrinkles on the upper lip, will respond well in some patients. In other individuals, however, the physician will be able to produce only a fullness or distortion of the angle between the vermilion and the skin above the upper lip without effecting much change in the wrinkling. In other cases, such as old, depressed acne scars on the upper back, good results can be obtained, but only with substantially larger volumes of material. There are no hard and fast ways to predict how the patient will respond and what total volume will be required to produce a given correction.

The most significant limitation of Zyderm has been realized only with long-term follow-up studies: A substantial number of patients will continue to require maintenance injections at intervals varying from 3 months to 1 year in order to maintain the optimum correction that was obtained with the initial series of injections. Corrections originally seen may approach 80 to 90 per cent of a contour defect. Typically, the patient may lose 15 to 25 per cent of that correction over time. The only significant contributing factor I have identified is the severe calorie and protein restriction seen in some fad dieters, in whom drastic reduction of food intake has correlated rather well with a rapid loss of correction in the Zyderm implant. I now routinely caution patients that they should achieve their desired maintenance weight level before undertaking Zyderm implantation.

The safety profile of Zyderm continues to be good. Three per cent of 9427 patients tested in a monitored program showed an untoward test response, which was defined as erythema, induration, tenderness, or swelling of the test site with or without pruritus that persisted for more than 6 hours or appeared more than 24 hours after implantation or the onset of rash, arthralgia, or myalgia. The majority of these patients showed reactions of the test site only. Pathologic examinations of biopsies of the site showed foreign body or necrobiotic granulomas typical of a chronic local inflammatory response (clinical data on file, Collagen Corp.). Pretreatment test implantation continues to be a wise and a necessary precaution prior to treating patients.

More significant problems have occurred in patients who have developed late sensitization reactions. Adverse treatment responses were seen in 1.3 per cent of the 5109 patients treated in the clinical verification program monitored by the Collagen Corporation. Forty per cent of these responses occurred in patients who had had unrecognized or unreported positive test implantation responses. All adverse treatment responses to date have been at the local treatment site and have consisted of swelling, induration, and redness with or without urticaria. Antihistamine and systemic steroid therapy has usually resulted in temporary improvement. The general health of the patients has not been affected, and all adverse reactions ultimately subside but usually persist for approximately 4 months and can last for as long as 10 months (clinical data on file, Collagen Corp.).

I have had the opportunity to follow two patients who developed late sensitization reactions. Both seemed to benefit from antihistamines and topical steroid applied to the treatment sites to minimize redness. Induration appeared to proceed to ultimate resolution unaffected by any therapeutic intervention.

Inadvertent laceration of dermal arteries during injection with occlusion, infarction, and scarring has been reported but appears to be related to the injection technique and not to the nature of the material implanted.

The occurrence of these apparent sensitization reactions is interesting, and certainly further monitoring of these reactions is warranted as further clinical experience with the material is acquired. It is significant that patients who developed sensitization reactions had antibodies that did not cross-react with human collagen Types I and III. It is hoped that there will therefore be no development of autoimmune disease based on reactivity to Zyderm. Many patients who could benefit from repair of contour scarring, such as those with burned-out lupus erythematosus, morphea, or scleroderma variants, are specifically excluded at this time from participation in Zyderm treatment because of the theoretic concerns about autoimmunity to collagen.

In summary, the Zyderm collagen implant has a history of safe use in a large patient population, but there are significant limitations to what can be accomplished with the material. Problems in patient selection remain to be further defined by future clinical experience.

ZYDERM

Samuel J. Stegman, M.D.

The controversy concerning Zyderm collagen implantation centers on whether or not the information available thus far regarding safety and efficacy warrants endorsement of this product. My comments will be divided into three parts: efficacy, safety for the patient, and safety for the physician.

Efficacy

The available data concerning efficacy are difficult to interpret. Some of the data are based on studies from the early period, when Zyderm collagen was sometimes placed below the dermis; some of the original investigators were injecting it into scars, creases, and wrinkles, which we now know are not often corrected effectively, and some of the data are based on earlier techniques, which have since been modified. It is only within the past year that I have felt somewhat more confident in my ability to choose the lesions that have the best chance for correction. I have modified my injection technique to enhance the lasting effect.

Although these modifications in technique and lesion selection are an essential part of the growth and development of any new product, the data obtained during this developmental period are less accurate for long-term projections.

Another factor that has delayed the ability to make an accurate projection of long-term efficacy has been the realization that scarring and aging changes (wrinkles, creases, and folds) are the result of various processes. The correction of creases created by the insertion of the muscles of facial expression onto the underside of the skin is of a shorter duration than is the correction of the secondary creases that are created by the draping effect of the skin movement near those muscle insertions.

Clinical and animal studies indicate that Zyderm provides its longest-lasting correction when placed within the dermis. When it is injected into the subcutaneous fat, either by design or unbeknownst to the physician, the longevity of the implant is greatly reduced. The skin thickness, which varies with the patient and the anatomic location, greatly affects the longevity of the correction. Older women who have wrinkles and creases that seem as if they should improve but who have very thin skin will not retain the correction as long as will people who have a thicker dermis. Consequently, wrinkles in the very thin eyelid skin, folds on the cheeks of patients with thin skin, and the atrophic skin at the base of some postacne scars require a different treatment plan. Our past experience and data do not reflect this new information.

I have seen a significant correction retained for 6 to 18 months in properly selected wrinkles and creases and longer in depressed scars. At present, I am satisfied with the latest injection techniques but could not predict whether these same procedures will continue to be used. Studies of the long-term efficacy that use the newer indications for the material and the newer injection techniques are under way. It will be several years before the data from an adequate number of patients treated by a sufficiently large population of physicians can be compiled and examined.

Safety for the Patient

Because Zyderm collagen is almost always used for cosmesis, the incidence of very serious side effects must be rare and the risk/benefit ratio must be favorable.

As expected, side effects have been caused by using a needle to place the material under high pressure into the high dermis. These include ecchymosis; small vessel laceration; a low incidence of secondary infection; a low incidence of reactivation of herpes simplex virus; and a few instances of pain, ischemia, and sloughing, which is believed to be secondary to arterial spasm. These side effects are only bothersome and should become minimal as all of us become more skilled in the administration of Zyderm.

There has been one case of unilateral blindness from an injection in the glabella. For this reason, the very superficial multiple puncture technique is recommended on the central face.

Another type of associated treatment response has been the development of intermittent swelling and induration, sometimes accompanied by pruritus and erythema, at the implantation site.

To date the only other serious problem has been the late development of sensitization to the implant in those patients who have had a negative skin test. The incidence of the onset of late allergy is currently less than 1 per cent of the patients treated. The clinical manifestation has its onset between 2 weeks and 2 to 3 months after treatment. (This is after a negative skin test has been observed for 30 days and has not shown any signs of induration, erythema, or pruritus.) The allergic response takes the form of induration, erythema, pruritus, and localized swelling around the injection site. The skin test may also show similar findings. These reactions tend to last 3 to 6 months and are helped symptomatically by intralesional and systemic corticosteroids. The development of a late allergy is a nuisance for the patients and the physician. Almost always, the injections are on the face and are clearly visible, and the erythema, swelling, induration, and pruritus are no simple matter for the physician to deal with for 3 to 6 months. All of these reactions have resolved. To date, only a few of them have developed a systemic component, such as generalized urticaria, serum sickness, malaise, or arthritis. Because some of the skin test reactions did involve arthralgia, rash, generalized myalgia, fever, malaise, and swelling of the hands and the feet, one could expect that there may be patients in whom a generalized response would be manifested with the onset of a late-developing allergy.

Therefore, concerning safety, the present data indicate that the reactions (except for one) so far have been self-limiting, not serious, not life-threatening, and without any permanent sequelae. Constant vigilance and careful monitoring of all the data concerning untoward reactions is essential. As physicians we must realize that many years of treatment are needed before reliable data regarding safety can be compiled.

Safety for the Physician

The physician is safe because this is an approved medical device. The entire development of Zyderm collagen has followed the guidelines and recommendations of the federal Food and Drug Administration. During the early trials, all the requirements for new medical devices of the state of California, and, in the past year, of the Federal Drug Administration were met.

The quality of Zyderm collagen is carefully monitored, and the records are available for public inspection. The company has further insisted that all physicians using the product be board-eligible or board-certified and be trained in the use of the product. All indications support the belief that the company is committed to the careful monitoring of the quality of the product and its efficacy and safety.

Therefore, as a practicing physician, I feel that I have up-to-date and reliable information about the product, its safety, and its quality. Should there be an untoward result, either minimal or major, I can honestly represent myself as a physician who has acted in the best interests of his patients by offering a treatment that is fully approved by the state and federal drug administrations. Also, I can honestly state that the sterility, consistency, and transportation of this medical device meet the highest standards possible.

I constantly remind myself that Zyderm collagen is used almost exclusively for improvement of cosmesis. Any permanent or serious side effect would be most grievous. If I were to inflict damage on any patient, I would be upset, but I think that I would be more upset if I could not assure myself that I had been using only approved materials that have been subjected to scrutiny for quality control, infection, and consistency.

There are many patients with unsightly scars or with early isolated manifestations of aging who can be helped by intradermal implants. Previously, these patients could not be helped, because other modalities, such as dermabrasion, chemical peels, or extensive surgical procedures were either insufficient or too drastic. On the other hand, collagen implantation will often enhance the effectiveness of some of these more extensive procedures. Consequently, I feel there are good indications and needs for this product and that, to date, the efficacy and safety are such that those patients needing this material should be able to obtain it from trained and qualified physicians.

Editorial Comment

Potentially the most exciting development in treating acne is the systemic administration of 13-*cis*-retinoic acid. However, this modality is not free from drawbacks. The cost of therapy is high even in today's inflated world. The Food and Drug Administration has approved the general use of this product, but only for severe cystic acne. However, once everyone can buy this medication, we can expect to see it used for all forms and degrees of acne. This will lead to a more realistic evaluation of the benefits and hazards of this form of therapy.

Acne has never responded well to local therapy. In making this statement, I am not referring only to the traditional remedies that have been replaced by more modern products, such as retinoic acid, benzoyl peroxide, and so forth. Drying the skin leads to desquamation and, in some cases, extrusion of comedones, as exemplified by retinoic acid, but still the results leave much to be desired with regard to clearing of the eruption and prevention of recurrences. There are no careful, prolonged studies of results from the use of topical medication only.

As pointed out by Maddin, acne surgery is unnecessary and not very effective in controlling and eliminating this condition. He also stressed that opening pustules may cause scarring, which will persist much longer than the dermatosis. After all, is the scalpel less fibrogenic than the fingernail? Recurrences follow comedo removal. Furthermore, it has not been established that eradication of these sebaceous plugs minimizes the severity of the eruption or hastens its eradication.

X-ray therapy is feared by many. Although the hazards may be overemphasized, the therapeutic results leave much to be desired. Furthermore, the equipment used in such treatments is expensive, discouraging practitioners from purchasing these machines. Today's patient acceptance of this modality is yet to be adequately tested. Furthermore, the fear of x-radiation can embroil the practitioner who uses it in medicolegal entanglements that he would rather avoid.

The score on oral antibiotic therapy has not been announced as yet. Many feel that the effect of these drugs is nothing short of miraculous; others doubt their value. Certainly, these agents have become a standard method of managing acne. Although tetracycline and erythromycin can be classified as relatively safe agents, some of the other available antibiotics, such as chloramphenicol, clindamycin, and so forth, carry a substantial and serious element of danger. The value of local antibiotic preparations has not been established, despite the vociferous arguments expressed by the adherents and foes of such treatment.

These and other objections could be raised regarding the other known treatments for acne, including cryotherapy, ultraviolet light, and so forth. As of now, acne remains an enigma that we hope will clear spontaneously, when we are employing one of the methods mentioned previously. However, it is a traumatic experience (especially for girls, since many boys seem to be capable of ignoring its cosmetic disadvantages) and can lead to unsightly scarring that the sufferer may carry to his grave. We need new and (especially) better treatments for acne. The last word on this subject has not yet been uttered.

Editorial Comment on Zyderm

The injection of bovine collagen to correct deformities in the skin is too new to allow for many dogmatic statements. However, so far most users have been satisfied with the results produced in patients. Zyderm seems to be much safer than the deposition of silicones for the same purposes. The main drawback is the need for prolonged and repeated therapy. Treatment failures and cost are other influential factors limiting the acceptance of this modality by the medical profession. Sensitization and other reported reactions are few in number or easily reversible.

However, this preparation is not a panacea, even for the conditions for which it is accepted or recommended. It is too new to have established its true worth and dangers. Therefore, conservatism is recommended in the use of this agent.

Think It Over.

SECTION 5

VIRAL INFECTIONS

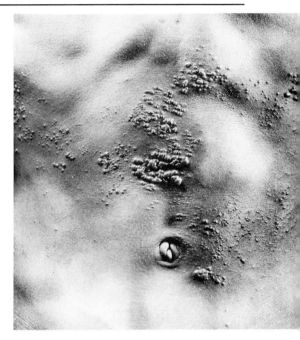

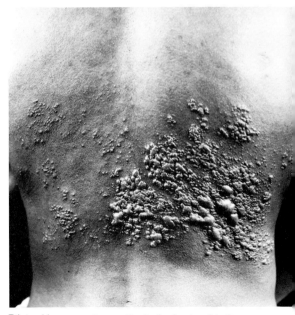

Bilateral herpes zoster meeting in the front and in the
back.

CHAPTER 19

CORTICOSTEROIDS IN THE TREATMENT OF HERPES ZOSTER

CORTICOSTEROIDS AND THE TREATMENT OF ZOSTER: SYSTEMIC ADMINISTRATION

William H. Eaglstein, M.D.

Herpes zoster represents the recrudescence of the herpes-varicella virus, and its typical painful red vesicular eruption is easily recognized. The dermatomal eruption and pain (neuralgia) may occur simultaneously, or one may precede the other; the sequence of these events carries no prognostic significance.

The eruption usually resolves spontaneously in 2 to 7 weeks. Severe scars are occasionally produced, but otherwise there are no serious side effects (from eruption), unless generalization occurs. Generalization (dissemination or spread) of the eruption is rare but may occur in the very ill patient and is associated with a mortality rate of nearly 25 per cent. Generalization is most likely to occur in people with hematopoietic neoplasms.

Although other nervous system symptoms, such as pruritus, hyperesthesia, and paralysis, may occur, neuralgia is the most common complication. The neuralgia may be mild or severe, but in people over 50 years old there is a tendency for the pain to be severe and long-lasting.[1,2] When zoster neuralgia persists beyond 6 to 8 weeks, it is termed postzoster neuralgia or chronic zoster neuralgia. These new names are based on the observation that people with neuralgia over 6 to 8 weeks in duration tend to have pain that is resistant to treatment and that may last for many years. The fundamental pathophysiologic alteration that distinguishes acute from chronic neuralgia is not known. In fact, there are no known histopathologic differences between the nerves in painful and nonpainful zoster.

It is generally accepted that chronic zoster neuralgia develops from acute zoster neuralgia. However, it is not known whether some patients with acute zoster neuralgia are affected in a way that inevitably produces resistant, long-lasting (chronic) zoster neuralgia or whether all patients have similar initial pathophysiologic alterations that only as a consequence of secondary factors (such as excessive fibrosis in response to injury) develop resistant, long-lasting chronic zoster neuralgia, which is in some way related to age. Young patients seldom develop chronic zoster neuralgia, whereas the incidence increases to nearly 50 per cent in patients 50 years old and becomes greater with each decade thereafter.[2] The location may be important, since there is a somewhat higher risk that trigeminal zoster will produce chronic zoster neuralgia compared with zoster in other distributions.

Since zoster neuralgia is so common and is often severe and able to become chronic, most therapies are aimed at stopping the pain and preventing chronic zoster neuralgia. When considering therapy, the physician must keep several points clearly in mind:

1. All treatments of acute zoster neuralgia will appear to be effective.

2. All methods of therapy for acute zoster neuralgia appear to work better when given early.

3. Therapies for chronic zoster neuralgia will tend not to be effective.

The first two points are explained by the fact that acute zoster neuralgia in its natural course resolves spontaneously. Since most people with acute zoster become pain-free early, almost any treatment will seem to be effective. Conversely, when a treatment is given later, there is a higher likelihood that the recipient is a person who is going to develop chronic zoster neuralgia and that the treatment will fail. Clearly, uncontrolled therapeutic experience in this condition is likely to be misleading. Even in control trials with zoster therapies, the question of preventing chronic zoster neuralgia usually remains unanswered. This is because the number of patients in the trial who would have developed chronic zoster neuralgia is usually too small for proper evaluation. Almost invariably, studies of zoster therapy conclude that despite the lack of statistical significance, the studied treatment seems to prevent chronic zoster neuralgia. Usually, a larger study involving several centers is recommended.

The greatest success in preventing chronic zoster neuralgia has been achieved by treating acute zoster neuralgia with systemic corticosteroids. Systemic steroid therapy does not seem to be an effective treatment for chronic zoster neuralgia, although control studies have not been reported. Treatment of acute zoster neuralgia with systemic corticosteroids has been reported in three controlled trials.[3-5] These studies specifically included older patients, who are most apt to develop chronic zoster neuralgia. In the two placebo controlled trials, almost all of the patients studied were over 50 years old, had acute painful zoster, and received either placebo or steroids (triamcinolone or prednisolone) orally for 3 to 4 weeks in doses tapering from 48 mg and 40 mg, respectively.

These two studies of 75 patients had similar results: 65 or 70 per cent of the placebo-treated patients developed chronic zoster neuralgia, compared with 15 or 30 per cent of those receiving systemic steroids. Neither study found the rapid (less than 48 hours) pain relief reported in the early small uncontrolled studies.[6-8] In one of these two studies, an increase in the rate at which the skin healed was found. In the third controlled study, early systemic steroid treatment in 30 patients was more effective in preventing chronic zoster neuralgia than was a combination of vitamins and analgesics used in ten control patients. In these prospective controlled studies, treatment was started within 10 days. The effect of systemic steroids when given later or to people with chronic zoster neuralgia was not studied.

The ideal zoster treatment might shorten the course of the skin eruptions, prevent scarring, prevent generalization or systemic spread, reduce or stop pain and pruritus, reverse motor symptoms, and prevent chronic zoster neuralgia. Systemic corticosteroids do not meet the criteria for the ideal treatment. However, considering the controlled studies and other reported investigations, it seems clear that in otherwise healthy older patients with painful acute zoster, systemic corticosteroid treatment reduces the chance that chronic zoster neuralgia will develop and does not produce a worsening, generalization, or systemic spread. Since in one study skin healing was fast and in the other studies and reports skin healing was normal, systemic steroids do not seem to retard healing and may, in fact, help. Their effect on scarring has not been determined, and their immediate effect on pain, pruritus, and motor symptoms is not impressive.

The effect of systemic corticosteroid treatment for zoster in patients with neoplasms or depressed immune systems has not been determined. Even without systemic corticosteroid treatment, these patients have an increased risk of developing zoster and having it disseminate. My own uncontrolled, but successful, experience with the development of zoster or disseminated zoster in patients with leukemia who are taking systemic steroids has been to continue the steroids either at the maintenance dose or at increased doses. Usually, these patients have been taking a small daily dose of steroid. It seems more physiologic to increase the dose of systemic corticosteroids (approximately 60 mg prednisone) rather than to discontinue administration of these agents during the stress of a painful zoster attack.

It is not known how or why systemic corticosteroids prevent chronic zoster neuralgia. Some have postulated that systemic steroids act by preventing neural inflammation, thereby averting postinflammatory fibrosis in the root ganglia or the sensory roots. Steroids are known to suppress collagen synthesis, and this might be an alternate or added mechanism of preventing fibrosis. However, since evidence linking fibrosis and chronic neuralgia is lacking, this attractive explanation is unsupported. Nevertheless, knowledge of the site, if not the mechanism, of action might be important when one considers the best route of steroid administration. For example, unless the site of action is superficial, topically applied steroids are not likely to be effective. Intralesional steroid therapy might be advantageous if high steroid levels are administered at the proper site. Similarly, epidural steroid administration might be most effective.

Although control studies have not been reported, success has been claimed for intralesional (intracutaneous) steroid therapy of both acute and chronic zoster neuralgia. Local skin atrophy and local skin bleeding are the primary reported side effects of this treatment. Steroid blood levels and pituitary adrenal axis function have not been studied following this steroid therapy for zoster.

The advantages of intralesional therapy compared with oral therapy would presumably be the absence of systemic steroid exposure and any special effect related to higher local steroid concentration. However, until controlled studies of the effect of intralesional steroid therapy in zoster are reported and it is determined that this is not another form of systemic administration of corticosteroids, only oral systemic corticosteroid therapy can be recommended. Therapy should be given to older patients with acute painful zoster who are otherwise healthy. Treatment should begin early and should last for 3 to 4 weeks, with doses starting in the range of 40 to 60 mg of prednisone or the equivalent.

References

1. de Morgas, J. M., and Kierland, R. R.: The outcome of patients with herpes zoster. Arch. Dermatol. 76:193, 1957.
2. Burgoon, C. F., Burgoon, J. S., and Baldridge, G. D.: The natural history of herpes zoster. JAMA 188:680, 1957.
3. Eaglstein, W. H., Katz, K., and Brown, J. A.: The effects of early corticosteroid therapy on the skin eruption and pain of herpes zoster. JAMA 211:1681, 1970.
4. Liquornik, M.: The results of systemic corticosteroid therapy in the prevention of algia following herpes zoster. Dermatology Proceedings of the XIV International Congress, Padua-Venice, May 22–27, 1972.
5. Keczkes, K., and Basheer, A. M.: Do corticosteroids prevent post-herpetic neuralgia? Br. J. Dermatol. 102:551, 1980.
6. Sulzberger, M. B., Sauer, G. C., Hermann, F., Baer, R. L., and Milberg, I. L.: Effects of ACTH and cortisone on certain diseases and physiological functions of the skin. I. Effects of ACTH. J. Invest. Dermatol. 16:323, 1951.
7. Gelfand, M. L.: Treatment of herpes zoster with cortisone. JAMA 154:911, 1954.
8. Appleman, D. H.: Treatment of herpes zoster with ACTH. N. Engl. J. Med. 253:693, 1955.

TREATMENT OF ACUTE HERPES ZOSTER WITH INTRALESIONAL GLUCOCORTICOIDS

Ervin Epstein, Jr., M.D.

Patients consult dermatologists most commonly because of dissatisfaction with the appearance of their skin, frequently with itching of their skin, and commonly because of fear that a lesion might be malignant. In contrast, dermatologists seldom treat that most unpleasant of sensations—pain. Therefore, given this lack of experience, it may not be surprising that they bumble frequently when they do see herpes zoster, the one dermatologic condition in which ongoing pain may consume the rest of the life of the patient.

The relative inefficacy of treatment as recently as 1957 prompted the authors of the then-standard American dermatologic textbook to conclude their discussion of the treatment of such pain with the following statement: "In many instances of postherpetic neuralgia, a relaxed vacation regimen in a warm climate seems to be as helpful as anything else."[1] Since neither Blue Cross nor Medicare provides reimbursement for trips to the seaside, it is fortunate that we now have at hand a treatment that prevents such pain with nearly uniform success—intralesional injections of suspensions of triamcinolone in saline.[2]

The physician should administer such injections daily subcutaneously to the inflamed or painful sites, using as much as 30 ml of a 2 mg per ml suspension each day. Generally, only two or three treatments in a single area are needed to eliminate the pain from that area, although occasionally more may be required. It is our practice currently to continue injections until the pain is gone or, if pain is minimal, until lesions have become dried and crusted. Like many useful techniques, this was found serendipitously, and the reason for its effectiveness is unclear. Certainly it is attractive to postulate that the glucocorticoids act by reducing inflammation and preventing scarring around peripheral nerves that are infected by virus, but evidence for this or other hypotheses is lacking.

Assessing the effectiveness of this treatment by comparison with other published therapies is difficult because of the small number of such papers, the differing definitions of postherpetic neuralgia, and the varying patient populations studied. The most cited paper on the subject described the 916 patients seen at the Mayo Clinic from 1935 to 1949 in whom herpes zoster or postherpetic neuralgia had been diagnosed.[3] This paper emphasized particularly clearly the more frequent occurrence in older patients of pain during acute zoster and of postherpetic neuralgia, although it was not the first to point this out. Unfortunately, it is not possible actually to calculate incidence figures from the data presented, because patients with herpes zoster and those with postherpetic neuralgia were lumped together, and it would be expected that the patient distribution in this referral center would be weighted heavily toward those with chronic rather than acute problems. Thus, 68 per cent of patients aged 61 or older with acute zoster or postherpetic neuralgia had pain of more than 1 month's duration (as did 28 per cent of those aged 31 to 50), but presumably many, if not most, of those with postherpetic neuralgia were not seen at the Mayo Clinic when their eruption was acute.

A smaller, but more useful, retrospective review of 206 patients with acute herpes zoster seen in dermatology, ophthalmology, and pediatrics clinics in Philadelphia in the 1940s and 1950s also concluded that older patients are more likely to develop postherpetic neuralgia.[4] Thus, 33 per cent of the 42 patients aged 60 years or older had postherpetic neuralgia, as compared with 2 per cent of the 57 patients aged 30 to 49.

Similarly, in a group of 253 Swedish patients replying to a mailed questionnaire, the incidence of postherpetic neuralgia was much greater in those 60 years of age or older as compared with those 20 to 49 years old—50 per cent versus 26 per cent for pain of at least 1 month in duration and 31 per cent versus 4 per cent for pain lasting at least 2 months.[5]

In a yet smaller, but prospectively and carefully studied, series of 34 patients in Miami, none of nine patients aged 21 to 59 had postherpetic neuralgia, whereas 14 of 25 (56 per cent) of those aged 60 to 91 had this complication.[6]

Thus, it is important to consider in particular the results of therapy in older patients when one assesses the prevention of postherpetic neuralgia. In a large, prospectively studied group of 272 individuals with acute herpes zoster treated with intralesional triamcinolone, 141 patients were at least 60 years old.[2] Of these, 7 patients (5 per cent) developed postherpetic neuralgia, a marked reduction from the 33 per cent and 31 per cent that represent the "natural history" in Philadelphia and Stockholm, respectively.

What other treatments are available for acute herpes zoster? The most commonly recommended therapy is administration of systemic glucocorticoids. Indeed, in the Miami study, the incidence of postherpetic neuralgia was significantly reduced in older patients who were randomly selected to receive oral triamcinolone as compared with those receiving placebo—3 of 10 patients (30 per cent) versus 11 of 15 (73 per cent).[6]

There was a similarly marked reduction in postherpetic neuralgia in a series of 15 patients aged 60 or older treated in Hull, England for 10 days with oral prednisolone as compared with 15 patients treated with oral carbamazepine as a placebo (20 per cent versus 80 per cent).[7] It is disturbing, however, that the incidence of postherpetic neuralgia in older patients in Miami who were treated with oral triamcinolone was as high as was the incidence in patients treated without steroids decades earlier in Philadelphia, but few would argue seriously that the lesson of the Miami and Hull studies is that oral lactose or carbamazepine induces postherpetic neuralgia. In any case, the published results are inferior to those achieved with intralesional triamcinolone, thus confirming the common-sense view that it is possible to deliver more drug to a site directly by a needle than indirectly by the blood stream.

In summary, then, intralesional triamcinolone appears so effective in preventing postherpetic neuralgia that John Dryden's lines, "For all the happiness mankind can gain it is not in pleasure, but in rest from pain" seem a direct advertisement for its widespread use.

References

1. Pillsbury, D. M., Shelley, W. B., and Kligman, A. M.: Dermatology. Philadelphia, W. B. Saunders Co., 1956.
2. Epstein, E.: Treatment of herpes zoster and postzoster neuralgia by subcutaneous injection of triamcinolone. Int. J. Dermatol. 20:65, 1981.
3. deMoragas, J. M., and Kierland, R. R.: The outcome of patients with herpes zoster. Arch. Dermatol. 75:193, 1957.
4. Burgoon, G. F., Burgoon, J. S., and Baldridge, G. D.: The natural history of herpes zoster. JAMA 164:265, 1957.
5. Molin, L.: Aspects of the natural history of herpes zoster—a follow-up investigation of outpatient material. Acta Derm. Venereol. 49:569, 1969.
6. Eaglstein, W. H., Katz, R., and Brown, J. A.: The effects of early corticosteroid therapy on the skin eruption and pain of herpes zoster. JAMA 211:1681, 1970.
7. Keczkes, K., and Basheer, A. M.: Do corticosteroids prevent post-herpetic neuralgia? Br. J. Dermatol. 102:551, 1980.

Editorial Comment

In my hands, the sublesional injection of corticosteroids in zoster has been more beneficial than the oral administration of these agents. In these few paragraphs, I would like to compare my results with those reported by Eaglstein and associates[1] and by Keczkes and Basheer.[2] The effect of therapy on zoster is difficult to interpret, since we are dealing with a self-limited disease. However, there are certain parameters that can be measured and that are important in this comparison.

Control of Lesions and Pain. Eaglstein and colleagues admitted that administration of triamcinolone orally according to their technique did not affect the healing of the cutaneous manifestations or the alleviation of the pain. Keczkes and his coworkers, on the other hand, felt that the oral administration of prednisolone shortened the course of the condition from 5.25 weeks to 3.65 weeks. In those treated by the subcutaneous administration of triamcinolone, the pain and the lesions cleared in 3.4 days.

Prevention of Postzoster Neuralgia. Eaglstein stated that his regimen reduced the incidence of postzoster neuralgia to 30 per cent compared with the incidence of 73 per cent reported in his control series. Keczkes and associates found that the use of prednisolone according to their technique resulted in the development of this unpleasant complication in only 15 per cent of the treated subjects, whereas 65 per cent of the control group suffered this fate. With the sublesional injection, the incidence was reduced to 3 per cent.

Dosage of Corticosteroids. It would seem reasonable to suppose that toxicity increases with larger doses and better absorption. Oral administration would give a higher blood level than would the use of a depot medication, such as Kenalog-40. In their articles, Eaglstein and coworkers recommended a total dosage of 618 mg of triamcinolone administered orally over a period of 3 weeks. Keczkes and Basheer recommended 40 mg of prednisolone per day for 10 days followed by successive reduction in the daily intake until total discontinuation is reached in 3 weeks. Even if one were to count only the first 10 days, the total oral dose would be 400 mg. A dose of up to 60 mg per day was recommended for those receiving sublesional injections. However, the actual total dose in this series was only 130 mg.

Number of Cases. Eaglstein and coworkers treated 10 hospitalized cases and 15 controls. Keczkes and his associate treated 20 cases and 20 controls. Those treated subcutaneously numbered 350 (plus 150 with postzoster neuralgia).

Duration of Studies. The study that evaluated the oral administration of prednisolone had a follow-up period of 2 years. Those receiving triamcinolone orally were treated during a period of 3 years. I have been using the sublesional injection of triamcinolone for 13 years.

Age of Patients. The incidence of postzoster neuralgia increases in patients over the age of approximately 50 years. All of the individuals evaluated by Keczkes and Basheer were older than 50 years of age. As far as can be determined from the published article, 71.4 per cent (25 patients) of the patients and controls studied by Eaglstein and his associates were older than 60 years of age. Of those treated by the sublesional injection of triamcinolone in saline, 50.6 per cent (191 patients) were more than 60 years old.

Think It Over.

References

1. Eaglstein, W. H., Katz, R., and Brown, J. A.: The effects of early corticosteroid therapy on the skin eruption and pain of herpes zoster. JAMA 211:1781, 1970.
2. Keczkes, K., and Basheer, A. M.: Do corticosteroids prevent post-herpetic neuralgia? Br. J. Dermatol. 102:551, 1980.

CHAPTER **20**

NECESSITY FOR LABORATORY CONFIRMATION

HERPES ZOSTER AND HERPES SIMPLEX INFECTIONS: THE CASE FOR LABORATORY CONFIRMATION OF RECURRENT ZOSTERIFORM ERUPTIONS

Neil Heskel, M.D.
Jon M. Hanifin, M.D.

Cutaneous herpes zoster and herpes simplex virus eruptions are frequently and correctly diagnosed and treated by physicians without the aid of laboratory tests. We propose that viral cultures and other laboratory methods are sometimes necessary to distinguish a clinical diagnosis of *recurrent* herpes zoster from herpes simplex virus infection.

Herpes simplex virus infections often mimic zoster. In 1950, Slavin and Ferguson reported five cases of zoster-like disease caused by the virus of herpes simplex.[1] They reviewed 16 other similar cases in the literature and concluded that "recurrent zoster" can be caused by herpes simplex virus. In 1971, Music, Fine, and Togo diagnosed and documented, via culture, a zosteriform herpes simplex virus skin infection in a 12-day-old infant. They noted that, though "neonatal zoster" had been reported ten times since 1889, varicella-zoster virus had never been cultured from a lesion.[2] We have cared for three patients with recurrent zosteriform herpes simplex virus infections that mimicked "recurrent herpes zoster" in several ways: (1) dermatomal distribution, (2) incidence of erythema and pain, and (3) prolonged intervals between attacks. All three patients had been diagnosed to have "typical" herpes zoster before we saw them and cultured herpes simplex virus from their skin lesions. Other authors have commented on the difficulty of distinguishing infections caused by herpes simplex virus from those caused by varicella-zoster in the skin.[1-5]

In spite of numerous such reports, some authors have continued to consider all zosteriform eruptions to be due to varicella-zoster. An early example of this sort of reasoning was made by Elliot, who, in 1888, diagnosed herpes zoster in a 39-year-old man who suffered from a recurrent vesicular eruption. In his words:

> . . . the diagnosis of zoster is one which offers no difficulty. It is to be based on the unilateral eruption—composed of groups of vesicles, situated on a reddened base and following the distribution of one or more nerves. It is sometimes preceded by fever and often by severe pain in the affected nerve . . .[6]

Since then, there have been reports of 64 patients with recurrent varicella-zoster skin infections. Estimates of the recurrence rate of varicella-zoster cutaneous infection range from 0.75 to 8 per cent.[3,4,6-20] However, none of these reports documented varicella-zoster by culture or other confirmatory laboratory techniques.

There have been attempts to distinguish between herpes simplex virus and varicella-zoster infections based on lesion localization and distribution. Freund and, later, Slavin and Ferguson noted that zosteriform herpes simplex virus eruptions favored areas supplied by the trigeminal nerve and sacral roots of the spinal cord, whereas varicella-zoster typically erupted on skin supplied by dorsal roots.[1,21] This difference is not consistent. To reduce clinical error, scientists sought reproducible laboratory methods to distinguish herpes simplex virus from varicella-zoster.

In the 1940s, several groups noted that herpes simplex virus would produce keratoconjunctivitis and encephalomyelitis when inoculated onto scarified rabbit corneae, whereas varicella-zoster did not cause lesions in laboratory animals. Complement fixation tests and neutralization tests have also helped to distinguish herpes simplex virus from varicella-zoster. In many laboratories, the most reliable method of documenting herpes simplex virus infection is via tissue culture. When cultured on substrates such as human diploid fibroblasts, herpes simplex virus is distinguishable from varicella-zoster in a number of ways. Herpes simplex virus shows a cytopathic effect that is initially focal and then rapidly spreads to involve the entire cell sheet within 24 to 48 hours. There is rapid progression on subculture; the cytopathic effect is apparent within 24 hours with complete destruction of the cell culture by 72 hours. The cells become rounded with some "ballooning." Varicella-zoster virus demonstrates a strictly focal cytopathic effect with slow progression, first appearing approximately 8 days after inoculation. After subculture there is a strictly focal cytopathic effect with slow progression. The cells become "flattened," or epithelioid, and have bizarre intranuclear inclusions. A chloroform sensitivity test distinguishes herpes simplex virus and varicella-zoster (both chloroform-sensitive) from adenoviruses and most pox viruses, which are chloroform-resistant. Finally, harvested cells are stained with hematoxylin and eosin for presence of inclusion bodies and multinucleated keratinocytes.

There is interest in developing a more rapid and reliable laboratory technique to verify the presence of herpes simplex virus or varicella-zoster. Rapid diagnosis is sometimes possible by use of immunofluorescence to demonstrate virus stained by fluorescein isothiocyanate conjugated to antibody to herpes simplex virus or varicella-zoster.[22,23] Frey, Steinberg, and Gershon have adapted countercurrent immunoelectrophoresis for detection of varicella-zoster antigen in vesicular fluid. This method reportedly achieves close correlation with serology and culture and takes only 2 hours.[24]

There are historical and morphologic features that may help to distinguish herpes simplex virus from varicella-zoster infections. A preceding sunburn, lesions on mucous membranes, a history of atopic dermatitis or recurrent cold sores, and a distribution of lesions over more than one dermatome all suggest the clinical diagnosis of herpes simplex virus. These clinical clues are not always present and are not infallible. On occasion, it can be very difficult to distinguish between herpes simplex virus and varicella-zoster with certainty; that zosteriform herpes simplex virus has fooled good clinicians has been amply documented earlier.[1,2,25] We recommend that viral cultures be done to help diagnose vesicular eruptions when correct diagnosis is critical for initiating proper therapy in: (1) patients with ophthalmic lesions, (2) newborns, (3) immunosuppressed patients, (4) patients with recurrent zosteriform eruptions, and (5) patients who might have simultaneous "dual" infections with herpes simplex virus and varicella-zoster,[24] among others.

Confirmatory laboratory testing is necessary in clinical research and in certain treatment situations. Studies on the natural history and response to therapy of varicella-zoster and herpes simplex virus infections would be more believable if clinical diagnoses were supported by positive cultures.

References

1. Slavin, H. B., and Ferguson, J. J., Jr.: Zoster-like eruptions caused by the virus of herpes simplex. Am. J. Med. 8:456, 1950.
2. Music, S. I., Fine, E. M., and Togo, Y.: Zoster-like disease in the newborn due to herpes-simplex virus. N. Engl. J. Med. 284:24, 1971.
3. Burgoon, C. F., Burgoon, J. S., and Baldridge, G. O.: The natural history of herpes zoster. JAMA 164:265, 1957.
4. Molin, L.: Aspects of the natural history of herpes zoster. Acta Derm. Venereol. 49:569, 1969.
5. Brehmer-Andersson, E.: Diagnostic importance of punch biopsy and cytologic examination in herpes zoster and herpes simplex. Acta Derm. Venereol. 45:262, 1965.
6. Elliot, G. T.: Relapsing double zoster. J. Cutan. Genito-Urinary Dis. 6:324, 1888.
7. Hope-Simpson, R. E.: The nature of herpes zoster: A long term study and a new hypothesis. Proc. R. Soc. Med. 58:9, 1965.
8. Seiler, H. E.: A study of herpes zoster particularly in its relationship to chicken pox. J. Hyg. 27:253, 1949.
9. Epstein, E., and Jacobson, H. P.: Bilateral herpes zoster complicating cutaneous, osseous and pulmonary tuberculosis. Arch. Dermatol. Syph. 34:989, 1936.
10. Head, H., and Campbell, A. W.: The pathology of herpes zoster and its bearing on sensory localization. Brain 23:353, 1900.
11. Nordlund, J. J.: Letter. Cutis 27:40, 1981.
12. Epstein, E.: Recurrences in herpes zoster. Cutis 26:378, 1980.
13. Sayer, A.: Recurrent herpes zoster (femoralis). Report of a case with unusual features. Arch. Dermatol. Syph. (Chicago) 33:348, 1936.
14. Stern, E. S.: The mechanism of herpes zoster and its relation to chicken pox. Br. J. Dermatol. Syph. 49:263, 1937.
15. Norris, F. H., Jr., Oramov, B., and Johnson, S. G.: Neuromyositis in a patient with recurring herpes zoster. Trans. Am. Neurol. Assoc. 93:253, 1968.
16. Leuren, J.: A case of recurrent herpes zoster. Br. J. Dermatol. 69:282, 1957.
17. Von Burckhardt, W., and Szechy, H.: Beobachtungen über den Verlauf und Bemerkungen über die Therapie des Herpes Zoster. Dermatologica 108:295, 1954.
18. Touraine, M. M., and Gole, L.: Zona redux. Bull. Soc. Fr. Derm. Symp. 42:498, 1935.
19. Barnard, R. O., and Jellinek, E. H.: Multiple sclerosis and amyotrophy complicated by oligodendroglioma: History of herpes zoster. J. Neurol. Sci. 5:441, 1967.
20. Guss, S. B., Sober, A. J., Rosenberg, M. D., and Arndt, M. O.: Local recurrence of generalized herpes zoster following x-irradiation. Arch. Dermatol. 103:513, 1971.
21. Freund, H.: Über den Nachweis des Herpeserregers bei zosteriformen Eruptionen (Savin) und Seine differentialdiagnostische Bedeutung. Arch. F. Dermat. U. Syph. 154:278, 1928.
22. Gardener, P. S., McQuillan, J., Black, M. M., et al.: Rapid diagnosis of herpesvirus hominis infections in superficial lesions by immunofluorescent antibody techniques. Br. Med. J. 4:89, 1968.
23. Taber, L. H., Brasier, F., Couch, R. B., et al.: Diagnosis of herpes simplex virus infections by immunofluorescence. J. Clin. Microbiol. 3:309, 1976.
24. Frey, H. M., Steinberg, S. P., and Gershon, A. A.: Diagnosis of varicella-zoster virus infections. *In* Nahmias, A. J., Dowdle, W. R., and Schinazi, R. F. (eds.): The Human Herpes Viruses: An Interdisciplinary Perspective. New York, Elsevier-North Holland Inc., 1980, pp. 351–362.
25. Forrest, W. M., and Kaufman, H. E.: Zosteriform herpes simplex. Am. J. Ophthalmol. 81:86, 1976.

CAN HERPES ZOSTER BE CAUSED BY THE VIRUS OF HERPES SIMPLEX?

Ervin Epstein, M.D.

The difference in the experiences of practicing dermatologists and teaching academicians has led to many of the controversies presented in this book. An outstanding example of this dichotomy was brought to mind by a contribution to the *Schoch Letter*.[1] I included a short paragraph in the monthly publication pointing out that recurrences in herpes zoster are not as unusual as we once thought. I stated that I had seen eight such recurrences in 350 patients suffering from zoster. This inspired a letter from a professor who stated that such reports needed laboratory confirmation in the form of cultures, because the eruption of zoster may be produced by the virus of herpes simplex. The way in which such a culture would prove that the first attack was actually due to zoster was unexplained. He quoted a paper from the *American Journal of Medicine* published in 1950.[2] This communication will be discussed later.

The clinical diagnosis of herpes zoster is one of the simplest and most accurate that can be made. The error rate is probably much less than 1 per cent. However, for the inexperienced, I will compare the exanthem of zoster with that of herpes simplex. The former is usually a unilateral painful eruption. There is a prodrome that may last for a day or even for a few weeks. This is marked by pain and burning in the area of the infection and may be accompanied by hyperesthesia to pin pricking. The lesions follow the course of nerves—often more than one in a single dermatome or multiple dermatomes. Bilateral involvement does occur but is very rare. There are usually multiple plaques with tense, unruptured vesicles and bullae. Regional lymphadenopathy is common. The bullae may be clear, purulent, or hemorrhagic. The lesions may eventuate in areas of necrosis and localized gangrene. Scarring is a frequent sequela of this infection. Postzoster neuralgia is characterized by continued pain, burning, itching, and numbness. This may be noted after the exanthem has subsided and may persist for years. The untreated eruption usually lasts from 4 to 6 weeks, although it may clear sooner. Recurrences are uncommon, and some even claim that they do not occur. Exposure to this disease may result in an eruption of varicella in susceptible contacts.

Herpes simplex appears most commonly on the face, especially on the lips as "cold sores" or fever blisters. It may be noted on any portion of the body, especially on the genitalia, the buttocks, and the fingers. The lesions consist of one or more erythematous plaques with a myriad of small, easily ruptured vesicles. Recurrences are usually prompt and frequent. Attacks may be precipitated by a variety of agents, including sun, wind, nervousness, and infections. The lesions usually heal without scarring. The disease is transmitted to susceptible contacts as herpes. Itching and burning are much more common than pain. Sequelae are seldom encountered, although recurrent genital herpes may predispose to cervical cancer. Infection with this virus in the newborn or following dermabrasion is a serious complication. Herpes is classified as the most common venereal disease because of its tendency to spread to sexual partners. The eruption is frequently bilateral and does not follow the course of a nerve. Hemorrhagic, necrotic, and gangrenous changes are seldom seen, except in patients with blood dyscrasias. The lesions clear spontaneously in 7 to 10 days in most cases without therapeutic intervention.

So, one may ask, how can two such diverse eruptions be confused? Of course, there are cases in which it is difficult to make a definite differential diagnosis, because some of the features with which the sufferers present may suggest a diagnosis of zoster and others may point to herpes simplex. Yet, in nearly all cases, the clinical diagnosis is definite, simple, and accurate.

I will review the two main articles that question the preceding statement. Slavin and Ferguson quoted from the literature descriptions of 16 instances of zoster-like eruptions produced by the virus of herpes simplex and reported five instances of their own.[2] In the latter group, recurrences were noted in four patients during periods ranging from days to months. The fifth individual had herpes labialis with an attack of meningitis plus a vesicular eruption diagnosed as zoster on a finger. Heskel and Hanifin added three cases to the literature—two recurred rapidly, but the third recurred only after a hiatus of 20 years.[3] However, lesions of herpes labialis developed repeatedly in the last woman over a period of many years. Although the physicians involved may have considered the eruptions with which these patients presented as zoster-like but proved by laboratory methods to be produced by herpes simplex virus, an experienced clinician would have made the proper diagnosis on the basis of recurrences with only a short period of freedom between attacks. Also, the lesions that occurred on the finger would probably have been considered to be herpes simplex by an experienced clinician.

Table 1 demonstrates the difference between the two conditions. I have seen eight cases of recurrent herpes zoster in approximately 350 patients with this disease.[1] This is an incidence of 2.3 per cent. All of these cases fulfilled the criteria for this diagnosis listed in Table 1. In other words, approximately 2 per cent of individuals who develop zoster will suffer a second attack years later. This is the same incidence as that of the development of an initial attack of this infection in unaffected people. Hence, one can say that a person who has had zoster has the same chance of suffering a second attack as an unaffected person has of developing a first eruption. The period of immunity lasts much longer in zoster than in herpes simplex. This long period of immunity (8 to 50 years in this series) probably prevents a third attack, although the possibility that a third eruption could occur cannot be ignored.

In conclusion, the following case history should be considered. A 28-year-old man consulted me on September 18, 1981. He presented an eruption that resembled herpes zoster to a surprising extent. However, the patient stated that this was the fourth annual attack that he had suffered. The lesions healed spontaneously in approximately 1 week in each instance. There was no pain, but a burning sensation was noted. The vesicles were small and superficial. Despite the resemblance, I doubt if an experienced clinician would consider seriously the diagnosis of zoster. He would realize that he was dealing with a zosteriform eruption of herpes simplex rather than a true zoster because of the frequent recurrences. A laboratory study could confirm the diagnosis, but its use would not be

Table 1. CLINICAL DIFFERENTIATION BETWEEN ZOSTER AND HERPES SIMPLEX

	Herpes Simplex	**Zoster**
Time of recurrences	Weeks or months	Years (none known under 8 years)
Number of recurrences	Many	One only
Prodrome	Hours to days	Days to weeks
Lesions		
Vesicles	Small, superficial, easily ruptured	Small to large, deep, tense, difficult to rupture; may be hemorrhagic, gangrenous, necrotic
Fluid	Clear, purulent (rare)	Clear, purulent, hemorrhagic
Patches	Usually one	Usually multiple, may coalesce
Sequelae	Usually none	Scarring common
Distribution	Unilateral or bilateral, usually does not follow a nerve	Unilateral (nearly always), follows nerve distribution, multiple nerves involved commonly

necessary to suggest or prove that this eruption is due to herpes simplex and not to the virus of chicken pox.

References

1. Epstein, E.: Recurrent herpes zoster. Schoch Letter 31:20, 1981.
2. Slavin, H. B., and Ferguson, J. J., Jr.: Zoster-like eruptions caused by the virus of herpes simplex. Am. J. Med. 8:456, 1950.
3. Heskel, N., and Hanifin, J. M.: Recurrent herpes Zoster: An unproven entity. J. Am. Acad. Dermatol. (in press).
4. Epstein, E.: Recurrences in herpes zoster. Cutis 26:378, 1980.

LABORATORY DIFFERENTIATION OF HERPES SIMPLEX AND HERPES ZOSTER

Edwin H. Lennette, M.D.

Varicella is primarily a disease of childhood. It is highly contagious and is readily diagnosed clinically when patients present with the classic symptoms and signs. Prodromes are generally absent, but when they are of sufficient magnitude to attract notice, they consist of malaise, anorexia, pharyngitis, rhinitis, myalgia, and a low-grade fever (usually below 102°F). The highly characteristic exanthem of varicella offers the basic clue to the nature of the illness; the typical vesicular rash appears in successive crops over a matter of several days, so that the picture becomes one of a mixture of macules, papules, vesicles, and scabs. The lesions begin chiefly on the trunk and the proximate extremities and then spread centrifugally, with a gradual diminution in numbers, on the limbs. In some cases, lesions may appear first on the face and then may spread to the trunk.

Until recently, the primary consideration in a differential diagnosis of varicella was smallpox, but because of the eradication of the latter disease, it is no longer an outstanding potentiality to be ruled out. However, vaccinia acquired through autoinoculation or contact (or therapeutic inoculation!) still constitutes one of the group of diseases to be considered. Perhaps the most important distinction to be made in instances of atypical presentation is that between herpes zoster and herpes simplex. In addition, hand, foot, and mouth disease; other enteroviral infections; rickettsialpox; and impetigo should be ruled out.

Herpes zoster, generally attributed to reactivation of the varicella agent (hence, the designation varicella-zoster virus), occurs primarily in older individuals (from age 50 upward). It may, however, occur at any age. The cutaneous lesions present essentially the same pathologic picture seen in varicella, except that their distribution is along one or more dermatomes and is usually unilateral, reflecting the pathogenesis of the condition (viz., inflammation of dorsal ganglia that harbor the virus as a latent infection). The reactivated virus subsequently passes from the ganglion to the periphery of the nerve and its cutaneous ending, where the painful vesicular lesions are induced. As in varicella, lesions occur in successive crops, but in the case of herpes zoster the vesicles are clustered along one or more dermatomes. Aberrant presentations, such as zosteriform herpes simplex, may make differentiation of herpes simplex from herpes zoster impossible, although a history of recurrent herpetic attacks points to herpes simplex.

It is in dealing with the atypical, and even aberrant, clinical pictures that the assistance of a diagnostic laboratory becomes desirable—not only because it provides a definitive etiologic diagnosis, but also because specifically active antiviral agents are being developed. At present, this is well exemplified by the intense effort to develop more potent antivirals against herpes simplex virus, and specific therapy against this virus is an achievable objective.

Before I delve into the laboratory aspects, I must remind the clinician that to achieve a laboratory diagnosis, it is desirable that he work closely with a laboratorian and seek the suggestions and advice of the laboratory staff.

The traditional approach to the laboratory diagnosis of varicella-zoster virus has been isolation of the agent from vesicular fluid or lesions and its identification by immunologic tests. The alternative (or complementary) approach is based upon the appearance of antibodies or their increase in titer during the course of the illness, as detected by complement-fixation or by some of the newer immunologic methods, which include immunofluorescence, fluorescent antibody to viral-induced membrane antigen, immune adherence hemagglutination, radioimmunoassay, and enzyme-linked immunosorbence. Since varicella-zoster virus is a cell-associated and slow-growing agent, an appreciable delay is involved before definitive identification of the virus can be achieved. Serologic diagnosis also involves a considerable lapse of time, inasmuch as demonstration of increases in antibody titer requires examination of serum specimens taken early after onset of the illness and during the recovery or convalescent stages.

Evidence of a herpetic infection can be obtained by microscopic examination of scrapings from the base of freshly developing vesicles. The so-called Tzanck smear, which is made by spreading the cell scrapings on a microscope slide and staining with one of the polychrome stains (such as the Giemsa or Wright stains) and examined by light microscopy, will reveal the presence of Cowdry Type A eosinophilic intranuclear inclusion bodies. Examination of the vesicular fluid by electron microscopy will show the presence of the typical, enveloped herpesvirus virions. *In both cases the structures seen by light and by electron microscopy point only to herpetic infection but do not distinguish between herpes simplex and varicella-zoster virus.* Newer immunologic methods now provide tools for permitting distinction between these two viruses. One that affords a definitive answer involves the examination of biopsy or vesicular smear material by the fluorescent antibody technique, using either the direct or indirect methods. The union of antibody with viral antigens induced in the infected cell is detected by fluorescence under ultraviolet light of the fluorescein dye used as a tag for the antibody. The development of antisera containing monoclonal antibodies to specific viral determinants should provide a highly specific means of distinguishing between herpes simplex and varicella-zoster viruses. Such definitive etiologic diagnoses, as mentioned earlier, are highly desirable in view of the concerted effort that is being made to develop antiviral agents that are effective against both viruses.

References

1. Lennette, E. H., and Schmidt, N. J. (eds.): Diagnostic Procedures for Viral, Rickettsial and Chlamydial Infections, 5th ed. Washington, D.C., American Public Health Association, 1979.
2. Glaser, R., and Gotlieb-Stematsky, T. (eds.): Human Herpesvirus Infections: Clinical Aspects. New York, Marcel Dekker, 1981.
3. Hoeprich, P. D. (ed.): Infectious Diseases, 2nd ed. Hagerstown, MD, Harper and Row, 1977.
4. Schmidt, N. J.: Further evidence for common antigens in herpes simplex and varicella-zoster viruses. J. Med. Virol. 9:27, 1982.

CHAPTER 21

IMMUNITY IN HERPES SIMPLEX BY SMALLPOX VACCINATION

HERPES SIMPLEX: THERE IS AN IMMUNITY TO IT AND SMALLPOX VACCINATIONS CAN PRODUCE IT

Ervin Epstein, M.D.

Herpes simplex is the most common of all the venereal diseases and is possibly encountered more frequently than any other viral infection. The aim of therapy of this condition should be to prevent recurrences, since the acute attack heals quickly with or without indicated therapy. Unfortunately, most therapeutic measures merely alleviate the symptomatology and clear the eruption. So, the initial question is: Can the sufferer with recurrent herpes develop an immunity to this infection? The production of immunity by exogenous influences is not merely possible; rather, it is probable, or even certain. However, it must be recognized that the immunity produced by such measures is only temporary and not permanent, in contrast with that produced by so many vaccines targeted against other viral infections. For instance, a person receiving artificial hyperpyrexia therapy for resistant gonorrhea, central nervous system syphilis, or Reiter's disease develops a very severe herpes infection of the face following his first treatment. Succeeding treatments given at daily or weekly intervals are not accompanied by a recurrence of this disease. After a hiatus of 6 to 12 months, another course of treatment may be instituted. The first treatment again results in a very severe eruption of the herpes infection, and again the following treatments are free from this complication.

Many practitioners of dermatology believe that smallpox vaccinations given in a course of three or more treatments also confer immunity. Reported double-blind studies fail to confirm this clinical impression. However, these investigations are based on recurrence rates without consideration of the time that has elapsed. Therefore, they are not designed to demonstrate temporary immunity, and, consequently, they do not disprove the development of temporary immunity—they merely indicate that smallpox vaccination does not produce a permanent immunity. No one disagrees with this, and this is not the basis for the controversy.

My technique is to give three smallpox vaccinations with an interval of 2 weeks between treatments. The vaccinations are administered with more trauma than that employed in the usual smallpox vaccination. This results in a higher proportion of inflammatory reactions, although these may well be of a nonspecific nature. In at least 80 per cent of the cases, the patient remains free of recurrences for 1 to 5 years. Even those who suffer recurrences in a shorter period usually note that the disease recurs after longer intervals of freedom, the exanthem heals more quickly, and the eruptions are of lessened severity. When recurrences appear, the patient is given another course of three vaccinations, and this can be repeated as necessary at indicated intervals.

But what happened? We were warned about severe reactions to these vaccinations. There is no question that Kempe's photographs are frightening. But these cases are rarities and occur mainly in children receiving their first vaccination. Experience indicates that these horrendous complications do not occur in those who have had a previous vaccination. Now that children no longer receive prophylactic injections, when these individuals reach adulthood, treatment for herpes may result in serious reactions. In nearly 50 years of giving series of vaccination for herpes, I have not seen any severe reactions.

In addition, it is claimed that there is no smallpox in the world today and therefore there is no need for the manufacture of these vaccines. As the volume of sales decreased, the commercial pharmaceutical producers stopped making the vaccine. As a result, patients whose immunity to herpes simplex has expired are contacting practitioners for repeat vaccinations and are being told that the vaccine is no longer available. These patients are a disappointed group, indeed.

A few years ago, Conant delivered a paper before the American Dermatological Association advocating the withdrawal of the vaccine from the market, since there is no need for it. He claimed that its application is hazardous and ineffective in herpes simplex. Perhaps this paper inspired the most lengthy discussion of any presentation made before that august body. However, nearly every discussant disagreed with Conant's views on the matter.

Certainly, herpes simplex is more common than variola. Therefore, why should this valuable agent be withdrawn from the market merely because of the worldwide disappearance of smallpox when herpes simplex still exists?

SMALLPOX VACCINATION IS NOT A TREATMENT FOR HERPES SIMPLEX

Marcus A. Conant, M.D.

Smallpox vaccination has no place in the modern treatment of herpes simplex virus. Simply stated, it does not work and, contrary to the often fanatical support that it has received by its proponents, it has never been shown to work in the treatment of herpes simplex virus. Further, the use of smallpox vaccine presents three real dangers. It is of danger to the patient, since it may result in serious complications. It is of danger to the physician, because if some adverse reaction were to occur following his use of this dangerous placebo, he would encounter great difficulty in defending himself against a malpractice action. Finally, it is of danger to the profession. The use of dramatic placebos with no demonstrable scientific value should be left to faith healers and charlatans who become rich on the scientific ignorance of their devoted followers.

Smallpox vaccine for the treatment of herpes simplex virus became popular many years ago for a variety of understandable, but unscientific, reasons. Edward Jenner, the famed British physician who in 1796 showed that cowpox infection protected individuals from acquiring smallpox, is often cited as the first to use smallpox vaccine for the treatment of recurrent herpes infections. This is not correct. In a letter to his friend Dr. Walsham in 1821, Jenner said, "Dr. W. may be assured that the greatest of all impediments to correct vaccination is that which arises from an herpetic state of the skin." The significance of Jenner's comment was reviewed in a scholarly article in the *New England Journal of Medicine* by Kibrick and Kunz in 1958.[1] These authors pointed out that Jenner was in no way concerned with the treatment of herpes simplex and was merely indicating those cutaneous conditions that he felt would interfere with proper vaccination. Indeed, if you read Jenner's entire statement, you will find that he goes on to say that such conditions as dandruff and sore eyelids will also affect vaccination. Kibrick and Kunz also point out that Jenner did not even know what herpes simplex was. The lexicons of the nineteenth century used the term "herpes" to mean anything from impetigo to ringworm.

Since there was, and is to this day, no effective treatment for recurrent herpes simplex virus, smallpox vaccination gained wide popularity among practicing physicians during the first seven decades of this century. Patients were usually subjected to vaccination every 2 to 3 weeks for a series of eight to ten treatments. During this time, patients ceased to have recurrent herpes, as they often do anyway, and glowing testimonials appeared, stating that since people got better, the treatment obviously must have worked.[2-4]

Then, in 1954, a paper appeared by Drs. Schiff and Kern[5] that unfortunately suggested that smallpox vaccination was useful in the prevention of recurrent herpes simplex. This study suffered from the same deficiency that had characterized all of the previous reports; that is, there was no indication as to how frequently the patients had been experiencing herpes simplex before the study began, and there was no attempt to treat a similar group of patients with a placebo. In 1959, Drs. Schiff and Kern[6] performed a controlled study comparing active smallpox vaccine with heat-inactivated smallpox vaccine for the treatment of recurrent herpes. Seventy-six per cent of the patients treated with active vaccine improved, and 52 per cent of those treated with heat-inactivated vaccine improved. The investigators drew the erroneous conclusion that these data showed that vaccination was useful in the treatment of recurrent herpes simplex virus, when their own data showed no statistically significant difference in the two groups of patients. Fortunately, in 1964 they corrected the conclusion they had reached in 1959 and stated that the active vaccine was obviously not beneficial.[7] In this paper, they studied the usefulness of a herpes simplex vaccine that had been prepared by an American pharmaceutical house. Seventy per cent of the patients improved after treatment with the vaccine, and 75 per cent of the patients improved after treatment with placebo.

I performed a similar study in 1977[8] in which I compared smallpox vaccine, heat-inactivated smallpox vaccine, and a saline control placebo. Fifty-nine per cent of the patients receiving smallpox vaccination improved, 69 per cent of the patients receiving heat-killed vaccine improved, and 60 per cent of the patients receiving a saline placebo improved. The only possible conclusion from these studies is that smallpox vaccination for the treatment of herpes simplex is nothing more than a placebo.

The use of this placebo is of danger to the patient. Mild reactions, such as infection at the site of vaccination, urticaria, erythema multiforme, and multiple accidental vaccinations,[1] can all occur in the normal patient. Unusual reactions, such as malignant tumors in smallpox vaccination scars,[9] photosensitivity secondary to smallpox vaccination, and recurrent herpes simplex infections at a smallpox vaccination site,[10] have been reported. Of greater concern are cases of vaccinia necrosum,[11,12] eczema vaccinatum, generalized vaccinia,[13] and postvaccinial encephalitis.[14] These complications often lead to the death of the patient.

The indiscriminate use of smallpox vaccine is even more dangerous today than it was a few years ago. Previously, if an adult was being given repeated smallpox vaccinations as a treatment for recurrent herpes simplex, the live viral eschar produced on the patient's arm was of little danger to the patient's family and friends. Today, when prophylactic vaccination is no longer given, most children are at risk for developing primary vaccination if live virus from the eschar on the patient's arm is inoculated onto their skin. Thus, a child with eczema on his face who rubs against the smallpox vaccination on his mother's arm is in great danger of an accidental primary smallpox vaccination of the face with subsequent scarring.

The physician who uses smallpox vaccine for the treatment of recurrent herpes is engaged in a clinical folly that could easily lead to a serious malpractice judgment against him. Although the chance of adverse reaction is slight, the examples just cited clearly indicate that it can occur. The package insert for smallpox vaccine prepared by the Wyeth Company states that "smallpox vaccine is indicated for, and should only be used for, immunization against smallpox." A jury would be less than sympathetic to a physician who harms his patient with a treatment that has been shown to be nothing more than a placebo. Indeed, adverse judgments have already been made against physicians for using smallpox vaccine for the treatment of recurrent herpes simplex. In a disciplinary action against a physician from northern California, the California Board of Quality Assurance charged "gross negligence in using contraindicated smallpox vaccine to treat rash and herpes on a patient with chronic leukemia, resulting in hospitalization for potentially life-threatening complications."[15]

Finally, the continued use of an agent that has been shown to have no demonstrable benefit is a great disservice to science in general and to our specialty in particular. Recurrent herpes simplex is a self-limiting disease that frequently goes into spontaneous remission and in which any placebo can be clearly shown to give a 60 to 70 per cent reduction in the severity of the disease and the frequency of recurrences. The physician should tell the patient that we have no cure for recurrent herpes simplex infection and that treatment will consist of a trial of various topical agents to lessen the discomfort, to shorten the course of the disease, and, it is hoped, to reduce the frequency of recurrence. The physician should then attempt to choose agents that effectively and safely achieve those goals.

Old ideas do not die easily. A study performed at the University of California Medical Center in 1977[8] showed that 14 per cent of primary care physicians who were attending continuing education courses at the university were still using smallpox vaccination for the treatment of recurrent herpes simplex. If we wish medicine to be a science, we must base our therapy on well-controlled scientific studies rather than testimonials.

The unscientific mind is easily persuaded by a post hoc ergo propter hoc argument. The logic goes something like this: I have a cold on Friday, I take vitamin C on Saturday, my cold is better on Sunday—therefore, the vitamin C must have killed the cold virus. It is this type of nonscientific argument that the proponents of smallpox vaccine are using, and they should be called to task to produce scientific, repeatable results rather than testimonials.

Smallpox vaccination does not work for the treatment of recurrent herpes simplex, and it is dangerous. I agree with Lane[16] that its use should be abandoned and that it should join a growing list of treatments, such as blood letting and autohemotherapy, that did not stand up to the scrutiny of scientific evaluation.

References

1. Kibrick, S., and Kunz, L.: Vaccinia of the lip. N. Engl. J. Med. 258:421, 1958.
2. Freund, H.: Die Behandlung des rezidivierenden Herpes mit Kuhpockenlymphe. Dtsch. Med. Wochenschr. 54:356, 1928.
3. Wise, F., and Sulzberger, M.: The 1934 Year Book of Dermatology and Syphilology. Chicago, The Year Book Publishers, Inc., 1934, p. 426.
4. Foster, P., and Abschier, A. B.: Smallpox vaccine in the treatment of recurrent herpes simplex. Arch. Dermatol. Syph. 36:294, 1937.
5. Schiff, B., and Kern, A.: Multiple smallpox vaccinations in the treatment of recurrent herpes simplex. Postgrad. Med. 15:32, Jan. 1954.
6. Kern, A., and Schiff, B.: Smallpox vaccinations in the management of recurrent herpes simplex: A controlled evaluation. J. Invest. Dermatol. 33:99, 1959.
7. Kern, A., and Schiff, B.: Vaccine therapy in recurrent herpes simplex. Arch. Dermatol. 89:844, June 1964.
8. Conant, M. A.: A Federal ban on smallpox vaccine. Presentation, American Dermatological Association, Phoenix, 1977.
9. MacMelzat, W.: Malignant tumors in smallpox vaccination scars. Arch. Dermatol. 97:400, 1968.
10. Mintz, L.: Recurrent herpes simplex infection at a smallpox vaccination site. JAMA 247:2704, 1982.
11. Neff, J., and Lane, M.: Vaccinia necrosum following smallpox vaccination for chronic herpes ulcers. JAMA 213:123, 1970.
12. Funk, E., and Strausbaugh, L.: Vaccinia necrosum after smallpox vaccination for herpes labialis. South Med. J. 74:383, 1981.
13. Chudwin, D., et al.: Lung involvement in progressive vaccinia. West. J. Med. 134:446, 1981.
14. Lane, M. J., et al.: Deaths attributable to smallpox vaccination: 1959 to 1966 and 1968. JAMA 212:441, 1970.
15. Department of Consumer Affairs: Action Report #20, California Board of Medical Quality Assurance, Oct. 1981.
16. Lane, J. M.: Hazards of smallpox vaccination. JAMA 247:2709, 1982.

SECTION 6

HAIR TRANSPLANTATION

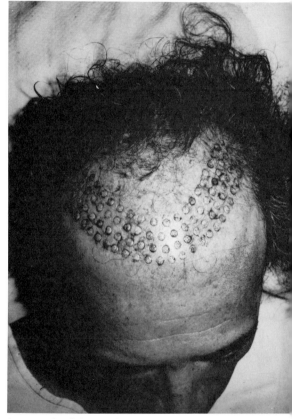

An example of the punch method of hair transplantation. (Courtesy of Dr. Samuel Ayres, III.)

CHAPTER **22**

DIFFERENCES IN TECHNIQUE

HAIR TRANSPLANTATION: PUNCH AUTOGRAFT METHOD

D. Bluford Stough, III, M.D.

The punch autograft technique for hair transplantation, employed for the past 25 years, remains the basic procedure for correction of most forms of permanent alopecia. However, because surgical adjuncts for the more severe problems of hair loss have improved significantly, it is now expedient for the hair transplant surgeon to restructure his approach when hair replacement surgery is considered.

Over 1 million patients have undergone hair transplantation during the past two decades. The majority of these have been recipients of punch autografts, primarily for correction of receding hairlines.[1] Today's hair transplant surgeon must be circumspect, since an increasingly large segment of these patients now elects to supplement the basic punch autograft procedure with certain surgical adjuncts. These may include scalp reductions and various types of hair-bearing transposition flaps. The patient should also be involved in these decisions during the initial consultation. At this time, the surgeon will analyze and recommend the procedures that will be most beneficial. Significant considerations are type of baldness, density and texture of hair, anticipated future hair loss, age, quality of donor grafts, and intended hair style.

Motivation of the patient remains an essential factor. After an evaluation of the patient's salient physical features, it is customary to determine the type of hairline configuration that will complement the patient's physiognomy. This will involve determination of the most compatible frame for the face by proper assessment of both the frontal view and the profile. Taken into this analysis should be any asymmetric features, especially the basic principles of harmonious proportions of the facial structure which, in some patients, have been disregarded or ignored.[2] The rounded or oval hairline provides a more acceptable appearance than does the widow's peak, which is no longer in vogue.

Before implantation of hair-bearing grafts, it is important that the etiology of the alopecia be recognized. For those with mild hereditary male pattern alopecia, in which no disease is involved, the baldness may progress, and additional hair replacement surgery may be required at a later date. In cases in which the hair loss is caused by a pathologic process, quiescence of the disease is mandatory, and there must be no anticipation of its reactivation. In this instance, punch autografting is usually the preferred method.

An organized pattern of graft excision and implantation is essential to a successful hair transplant. Ordinarily, the donor area is the occipital region on the side opposite the part. The alternate side is used as the donor site for the following session. Effective and prolonged anesthesia is obtained with 0.5 per cent lidocaine and 1:200,000 epinephrine injections followed by 0.25 per cent bupivacaine and 1:200,000 epinephrine, in contrast with a single and more concentrated local anesthesia. After the anesthetic has taken effect, 20 to 50 ml of saline, injected subcutaneously, in the prepared donor area produces a distention that results in increased tissue stability.[3] This bulging effect allows a better angle of excision, resulting in grafts of superior quality, especially where the donor hair is fine and limited.

With rare exceptions, the power punch is far superior to the hand punch in extracting donor grafts. However, incision of recipient sites is performed with a hand punch 0.25 to 0.5 mm smaller than grafts to be implanted. This method insures closer adherence of the graft to its cavity. A larger space may cause more visible scarring, whereas a smaller space may result in pressure necrosis. When the hair is fine, delicate, and sparse, the punch should be larger and exceptionally sharp. Minimal pressure should be used to incise the grafts. This will prevent distortion and transection of the roots. As the punch edge angles down the hair shaft, one may minimize rotation of the graft within the punch cylinder by pressing the punch firmly against the caudal and proximal wall of the incision. When a restricted amount of grafting is anticipated and there is an abundance of donor hair, extraction of grafts may be taken along a horizontal strip 1.0 to 2.0 cm in width. The adjacent hair easily covers and obscures the donor site. This may not be practical when a large number of grafts is taken.

After donor grafts are cleansed and trimmed, they are implanted in the anterior frontal hairline. Initial grafts are usually the best and therefore should be used accordingly. Since an adequate frame for the face is our aesthetic objective, the majority of treatment time should be concentrated on the first 3.0 cm of the frontal margin. This is in contrast with the method of placing the initial grafts more posteriorly and advancing anteriorly on subsequent visits, which is preferred by some. The latter method is more time-consuming and may result in a less desirable frontal margin.

In our experience, with few exceptions, we have found the following "strip punch" pattern to be preferable in this frontal region: In Row 1, the grafts are placed in spaces that are separated only by half the diameter of the implant. In remaining rows, the spaces between all grafts are at least the full diameter of the implant. This method will not compromise the blood supply, and, when tissue edema is controlled, there is no pressure necrosis. In contrast with the smaller 3.0- to 4.0-mm grafts that may be advocated, we prefer 4.25- to 4.5-mm hair-bearing implants for the majority of our patients. On rare occasions, for patients who have fine, sparse hair, grafts up to 5.0 mm in size may be preferable. The smaller implants are used for blenders in these cases. Through this method, accelerated coverage is satisfactorily acquired in three sessions rather than the previously established four-session minimum. It is our opinion that a test graft, or "trial run," session for a new patient is unnecessary for the skilled surgeon. Taking into consideration the growth yield and patient psychology, we have found that the ideal interval between graft sessions is approximately 4 weeks.

The surgeon should encourage the patient to return for the number of sessions required to achieve maximal coverage in the shortest time feasible. Blenders and fillers in conjunction with the normally sized hair-bearing grafts may be used for the most desirable results. In blender grafts, the fineness of the donor hair is often more important than the size of the blender graft in achieving a more becoming and natural hairline. Since a dense donor region does not necessarily yield finer hair, better blender grafts are often found in the lower occipital area, from which 2.0- to 4.0-mm grafts may be extracted. These should be implanted no farther than 1.0 cm into the anterior margin, because this placement concentrates a greater number of grafts for a more natural appearance in the all-important frontal region. The effect and degree of improvement with blender grafts depend upon the patient's skin and hair color, follicular density and texture of hair, degree of natural curl, and hair style. Recently, there has been a noticeable decline in the request for blender grafts. This is perhaps a result of improved grooming methods and adjunctive hair replacement procedures.

For those with fine, sparse, or limited donor hair, the punch autograft method may require numerous sessions with less than satisfactory coverage. Under these conditions, or in more severe forms of permanent alopecia and extensive baldness, it may be desirable for the surgeon and the patient to discuss and consider some of the advanced surgical procedures in conjunction with the punch autograft technique.

There are certain precautionary measures that may be advisable. One may usually avoid punch autograft complications by using an extremely sharp punch for both donor and recipient areas. Steroids are frequently administered to prevent pressure necrosis that may result from postoperative edema. When an extensive area of the scalp is treated, preoperative antibiotics are used as a precaution. When a vascular nevus (which is seldom encountered) is observed in the donor area, these grafts should not be placed near the frontal margin. The practice of implanting hair-bearing autografts only in the midvertex region is not recommended, since it does not attain a suitable frame for the face or adequate coverage in the crown area.

A disadvantage of the punch autograft technique is the time involved for the regrowth of hair. In an average hair transplant patient, the beginning of hair growth is usually observed at approximately the second or third month, with hair readily apparent around the sixth month. Within 9 months, the patient is ready to groom his newly acquired hair, in contrast with the "instant" hair that can be attained through the more advanced surgical adjuncts now being offered and used.

The punch autograft technique has certain advantages over a hair piece. First, the initial cost of a good wig is considerable, since it is advisable to have two available—one as an alternate. Adequate maintenance (conditioning and styling) may become quite expensive. In addition, a hair piece must ordinarily be replaced every 2 to 3 years. The cumulative cost over a period of approximately 8 years will usually exceed the surgical fee for obtaining one's own hair through the hair transplantation method. A hair piece is not permanent, in contrast with the growth of hair resulting from the punch autograft technique, which is a lifetime acquisition. Some physicians may anchor a hairpiece to the scalp through hair weaving or by introducing Teflon-coated stainless steel wire and Prolene monofilament sutures into the scalp tissue at various entry points. These methods of fixation often become a source of chronic irritation and subsequent infection and are not recommended by experienced consultants.[4] Growing and having one's own hair not only may result in personal satisfaction but also often makes active participation in sports more feasible. This is especially true for those who have felt restricted and apprehensive because of their insecurity when wearing a hair piece. Also, the punch autograft technique is a simple office procedure, in comparison with the more complicated surgical adjuncts, which in some cases may be performed in the office. (In other cases, however, hospitalization is required.)

Grooming is often a neglected aspect of hair transplant surgery. There is little question that hair obtained from suitably designated areas through punch autografts or ancillary procedures can be expected to last a lifetime. Although the hair replacement surgery may be a success, the patient will certainly be better satisfied with his newly acquired hair if it is properly styled and groomed to complement his features. Probably the most significant improvements in grooming are the "curly permanent" and the "body wave." Either will create a look of density and is especially recommended for those with straight or fine sparse hair. The use of hair conditioners that prevent entanglement and give the hair a natural and healthy sheen is encouraged. This may be an elective for most but is certainly a necessity for others. Also, an electric hand-styling dryer may be employed to assist in proper shaping while increasing the illusion of greater thickness. The hair may be kept neatly arranged through use of a non-oily spray. These modalities should be used after all phases of hair replacement surgery. It should be the obligation of the surgeon to encourage the patient to secure the advice of a competent stylist for proper grooming.

Fundamentally, the punch autograft method remains the procedure of choice for those patients with a dense donor region from which to obtain desirable grafts to correct a moderately receding hairline. In most patients, improvement may be expected, and complications are rarely encountered. However, when hair loss is more severe and punch autografts will not attain good coverage, the patient should be made aware of the improved surgical adjuncts now available. This comprehensive approach complements the basic punch autograft technique and often achieves the ultimate improvement.

References

1. Orentreich, N.: Autografts in alopecias and other selected dermatological conditions. Ann. N.Y. Acad. Sci. 83:463, Nov. 1959.
2. Patterson, C. N., and Powell D. G.: Facial analysis in patient evaluation for physiologic and cosmetic surgery. Laryngoscope 84:1, 1974.
3. Stough, D. B., III: Hair transplantation. *In* Epstein, E., and Epstein, E., Jr. (eds.): Techniques in Skin Surgery. Philadelphia, Lea & Febiger, 1979, pp. 149–163.
4. Stough, D.B., III, and Cates, J. A.: Contemporary techniques of hair replacement. Postgrad. Med. 69:53, April 1981.

ALOPECIA REDUCTION

Walter P. Unger, M.D.
Martin G. Unger, M.D.

Purpose and Effectiveness of Alopecia Reduction

The most obvious purpose of alopecia reduction is to excise an area of bald skin with correction of the resulting defect by advancement and rotation principles. The amount of bald skin that is removed has been reported as varying from 21 cm^2 to 135 cm^2. The benefits derived can be best demonstrated by simple mathematics. It takes approximately nine 4-mm^2 grafts placed into recipient sites, each of which is 3.5 mm^2, to fill every square centimeter of bald skin. If 40 cm^2 of skin is excised, for example, a "savings" of approximately 360 grafts will be achieved if one had intended to transplant the area solidly (four sessions of punch transplantation). Even if only two sessions had been planned for the site, there would still be a savings of at least 180 grafts. In the first 60 patients on whom we performed surgery, we reported the excision of an average of 40 cm^2. It is worth emphasizing that this average was composed of patients who had large excisions made as well as those who had alopecia reductions in relatively small spaces, such as the vertex area alone. Excisions of 60 to 90 cm^2 are common when one is dealing with large areas of alopecia, but significant savings are possible even when one is concerned with a limited area, such as the vertex (Figs. 1 through 4). The question has occasionally been raised as to whether or not there is a partial loss of the savings achieved with the procedure when the scalp characteristically "loosens" after an alopecia reduction. In answer to this question, we must first emphasize that in our particular technique only redundant skin and scalp tissues are removed, as opposed to any deliberate stretching of the skin itself. Furthermore, tension on closure is confined to the galeal plane alone. Under these conditions, the laxity returns to the scalp primarily through the "loosening" of the galea aponeurotica rather than through the stretching of overlying skin. The accepted efficacy of serial excisions for large defects[10,15] reinforced by Schultz and Roenigk's article[7] and by our own experience with well over 2000 alopecia reductions is in keeping with this view.

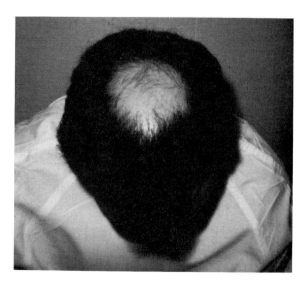

Figure 1. Patient before punch transplanting. In our practice, this vertex bald area normally would require approximately 300 grafts done in three sessions of approximately 100 grafts per session.

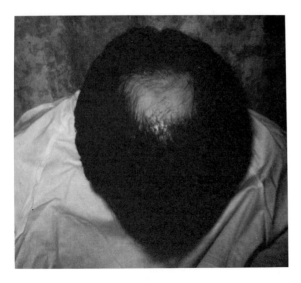

Figure 2. The patient in Figure 1 shown after one Y-shaped alopecia reduction. (The scar can be seen in the center of the bald site.) The area has been reduced by approximately 50 per cent.

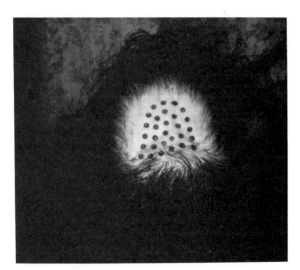

Figure 3. Twenty-eight recipient sites have been drilled out, leaving a U-shaped area of relatively sparse hair surrounding the recipient sites laterally and anteriorly. This U-shaped area will be excised in a second alopecia reduction 3 months after the sessions shown here.

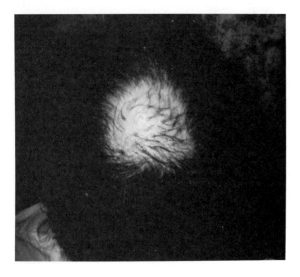

Figure 4. The U-shaped area has been excised, and growth from the initial punch transplant grafts has begun. This photograph shows the area 5 months after punch transplanting was begun. Two more sessions of approximately 28 grafts (resulting in a total of 84 grafts) were planned to complete an area that would have consumed approximately 300 grafts.

On the other hand, several factors could conceivably cause a partial loss of the savings achieved initially. If galeatomies are carried out, the spaces in the galea are replaced by fibrous scar tissue. If contracture of this tissue occurs after the surgery, it would in all probability lead to contracture of the overlying hair-bearing skin and associated stretching of the bald area. In addition, excessive tension on the skin closure or stretching of the skin would likely result in a wide scar as well as a loss of the savings. However, even under these less favorable conditions, a substantial permanent reduction of the area of alopecia would occur in virtually all patients.

Movement of the Part Medially

One of the disadvantages of punch transplanting is that the hair growth in the recipient area is not evenly distributed over the skin surface. As a result, it is only the rare patient who can part his hair through a transplanted site without "tufting" showing in a rather obvious fashion.

Hair stylists state that the part should normally begin at a point on the forehead that falls no farther laterally than a perpendicular line drawn superiorly from the lateral third of the eyebrow. Although one can move the part more medially without affecting the natural-ness of the appearance, moving it more laterally results in a "combed-over" appearance. It also broadens and tends to exaggerate the length of the forehead from side to side and is not pleasing to the eye.

Despite the aforementioned recommendations, parts in patients who have undergone transplantation often must begin at a point well lateral to the ideal location because that is the point to which the fringe of hair has receded or will recede. When an alopecia reduction is performed, this point will be moved more medially. Repeated alopecia reductions are often able to move what was initially a very unnatural lateral beginning of the part to a much more acceptable or normal position. The importance of this function of alopecia reduction cannot be overemphasized. In a patient with narrow fringes of hair, alopecia reduction becomes almost a necessity rather than an option if the individual wishes his hair to appear as natural as possible. In some individuals, a hair style that does not use a part (e.g., the Caesar style or, even better, a short, curly style) is a reasonable alternative to alopecia reductions performed for the purpose of moving the part more medially.

Correction of Unsatisfactory Punch Transplantation

Alopecia reductions are useful in improving the appearance of patients who have pre-viously undergone punch transplanting. For example, the following defects can be cor-rected:

1. Poor graft survival or hair direction in areas of previous punch transplanting.

2. Inadequate density of hair growth in transplanted sites because coverage of too large an area was attempted.

3. Extension of male pattern baldness lateral to previous punch transplanting, result-ing in a hairless gap between the narrower fringe and the transplanted area.

For the first two defects just described, a portion of the transplanted site may be excised. Prior to its excision, adequate grafts are punched out from the strip to be removed and are implanted (for a second time) into the remaining transplanted area. Not only does this result in a thickening of hair in the remaining transplanted portion, but also a cosmet-ically unsatisfactory area is eliminated. Extension of male pattern baldness lateral to pre-vious transplanting can usually be corrected by one or more alopecia reductions in which any hairless gaps are excised.

Alopecia Reduction Before or During Hair Transplanting

The advantages and disadvantages of performing alopecia reductions before punch transplanting have been covered elsewhere.[9,13] The only disadvantages that need elaboration are as follows:

1. Alopecia reductions result in thinning out of the donor hair, especially in the temporal region and if galeatomies have been performed under the hair-bearing "rim." Grafts taken from these sites will have fewer hairs per surface area.

2. If large amounts of bald scalp are removed in a serial fashion, especially if an elliptic shape is used for the reductions, the angle of growth of the fringe hair can be significantly altered to a more lateral direction, producing a permanently unnatural effect and a grooming problem.

We prefer to start with two sessions of punch transplanting and perform the first alopecia reduction during the 4-month interval between the second and third punch transplanting session.[13] We often carry out another alopecia reduction between the third and fourth hair transplanting procedures. As the experience of the practitioner increases, it becomes easier for him to decide in advance how an alopecia reduction will affect the initially drawn hairline as well as the optimal alopecia reduction pattern for particular patients. This approach allows hair to grow as quickly as possible after the initial procedure and still allows the alopecia reductions to be incorporated at an early stage in the program.

"Early" Alopecia Reductions

Some controversy surrounds the question of whether one should perform an alopecia reduction through an area of hair-bearing skin that is in the process of going bald. No single answer is satisfactory for all individuals. In general, however, the presence of hair in an area that can be removed by an alopecia reduction is not an absolute contraindication to an alopecia reduction at that time. Other factors must also be taken into account. These include:

1. The desire on the part of a patient to complete the entire hair replacement and alopecia reduction program as quickly as possible.

2. The desire of the patient to carry out all operations on hair-bearing skin so as to avoid the disfigurement that would be produced by similar operations at a later date, when the scalp would have no hair left to camouflage the scarring.

3. The desirability of moving the part more medially.

4. The willingness of the patient to accept a temporary telogen effluvium, which may occur after an alopecia reduction through an area of hair-bearing skin.

It should be remembered when the last factor is being considered that if a telogen effluvium occurs at one point, it is also likely to occur at a later point, and the sooner one does the alopecia reduction the more hair will be present to camouflage the area, even after the telogen effluvium. Telogen effluvium therefore is not a contraindication to perform an alopecia reduction in hair-bearing areas. Rather, it is an inconvenience that, if it occurs, is better tolerated earlier than later, unless the decision is made to operate only when an area is totally bald.

Some physicians believe that early alopecia reductions might hasten the rate of hair loss in any given site. This has not occurred in any of the several hundred patients on whom we have operated. It is, however, possible that other practitioners who use significantly more tension in closing their wounds might cause a permanent hair loss on either side of the incision line, just as occurs in some patients after face or brow lifts when considerable tension has been present at the suture line. As has been noted earlier, we generally try to avoid such tension and therefore have not caused any exacerbation of the rate of hair loss.

Patterns of Alopecia Reduction

We have described six basic patterns of alopecia reductions.[1,13] Many variations of these suggestions have been employed to suit the requirements of specific individuals. We stressed in our original article that by describing different patterns we intended to emphasize that no single design is optimal for all patients.

Others have described an S-shaped pattern and a lateral crescent-shaped pattern.[2] We continue to use the Y pattern most often, because it allows for large excisions yet leaves the hair direction in the vertex area relatively unaffected and the vertex area unscarred. It therefore does not force one to transplant this area to cover the scar. We also frequently employ U-, C-, J-, and lateral crescent-shaped patterns of reduction whenever they seem more advantageous in given cases.

Despite theoretic concerns about moving the hairline posteriorly or severing the majority of neurovascular bundles of the scalp when a U-shaped pattern is used (and, to a lesser extent, when C- and J-shaped patterns are employed),[2] these patterns do not cause significant problems. Closing of the defect in the U pattern involves advancement of the skin not only in an anteroposterior direction but also (more importantly) in the lateral area toward the midline. In addition, the punch-transplanted U is often to a large extent fixed by the grafts to the periosteum, making it more resistant to movement. As a result, the anterior hairline does not move significantly superiorly. On the other hand, the future part line, as explained previously, moves more medially, producing a much more pleasing aesthetic effect.

More recently, we have modified the original U-shaped pattern, as shown in Figure 5, to take maximal advantage of medial movement. In addition, this modified pattern uses even less anteroposterior movement and results in a reduced likelihood of formation of a temporary "bump" just anterior to the anterior portion of the suture line.

In patients who undergo U-, C-, or J-shaped excisions, the majority of the scalp nearly always will be transplanted, and virtually all available donor grafts will be harvested. In this situation, all of the major neurovascular bundles and arteries will be transected, whether by the alopecia reduction pattern chosen or by the punch during harvesting. Hypesthesia is temporary and should not be a contraindication to what might be the optimal alopecia reduction pattern for an individual patient. Tension, as noted earlier, is best limited to the galeal plane and not to the "skin edges." To date, we have had no problems in healing of our suture lines in over 600 cases of U-shaped alopecia reductions.

Technique

Details of technique in alopecia reduction have been dealt with in previous articles.[1,2,13] Our discussion here will be limited to areas of some controversy.

Anesthesia.   Unless the technique that is being used involves the use of considerable tension maneuvers or is associated with a great deal of bleeding, general anesthesia is of little benefit in carrying out alopecia reductions. When we have used general anesthesia, we have usually had more problems from its postoperative effects than from the surgery itself. We therefore continue to reserve it for patients who psychologically cannot accept consciousness during the procedure.

Surgery.   As indicated earlier, we do not in general use relaxing incisions in the deep surface of the galea aponeurotica. It is worth emphasizing that if one is merely

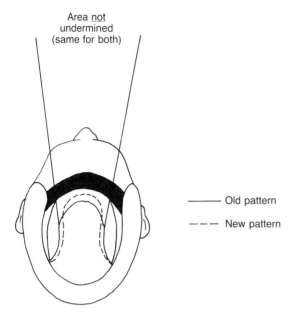

Area <u>not</u>
undermined
(same for both)

——— Old pattern

– – – New pattern

■ Area punch transplanted

Figure 5. Modification of the original U pattern alopecia reduction. The pattern has been made somewhat narrower anteriorly, and the "arms" of the U have been made wider. This pattern takes maximal advantage of medial movement and minimizes any movement of the hairline posteriorly.

stretching the bald skin, there is no advantage to be gained, and therefore galeatomies should be limited to the undersurface of the permanently hair-bearing regions. Those who need wide alopecia reductions the most (those who have the widest bald areas) have the narrowest fringes and therefore can have fewer relaxing incisions and will benefit from them less.

As has been noted previously, when the skin is stretched over hair-bearing areas that either have been donor sites or will be donor sites in the future, hair growth is made sparser in these regions. This will affect the quality of grafts (specifically, the number of hairs per surface area) or the number of grafts that one may remove from a given donor area without overdepleting it. Fewer grafts can be removed from a sparse hair-growing area than from a more densely covered site. This latter drawback occurs whether alopecia reductions are performed before or after the grafts have been taken. Some of the benefit gained by galeatomy is therefore lost, since lower-quality grafts or fewer grafts can be harvested, especially in the temple areas.

We prefer to avoid galeatomies because of the aforementioned reasons and because they pose additional risks for hemorrhage during the procedure as well as for postoperative bleeding. Insofar as our objective is to remove redundant skin rather than to stretch it, galeal incisions are reserved for those patients in whom we may overestimate what can be reasonably excised. In such individuals, galeatomies provide a valuable margin of safety.

Systemic Corticosteroids. Our patients are given oral prednisone (5-mg tablets) with or without parenteral corticosteroids, such as 125 mg of methylprednisolone sodium succinate (Solu-Medrol—Upjohn) and 120 mg of methylprednisolone acetate (Depo-Medrol—Upjohn). The following regimen is used: Day 1, six tablets; Day 2, five tablets; Day 3, four tablets; Day 4, three tablets; Day 5, two tablets; Day 6, two tablets; Day 7, one tablet. Habal and Powell showed that experimental facial edema was markedly reduced in experimental pigs following the intravenous injection of methylprednisolone sodium succinate.[12] Inflammation, discomfort, tension, and, therefore, vascular embarrassment are reduced postoperatively when corticosteroids are used.

Intervals Between Alopecia Reduction and Hair Punch Transplanting.   Alopecia reductions are generally carried out 6 weeks or more before or after a punch transplanting operation.[13] It is not unusual to use the same pattern repeatedly, each time excising the scar from the previous alopecia reduction. When alopecia reductions are carried out prior to any punch transplanting, Bosley has stated that 6-week intervals between repeat alopecia reductions give almost as good results as do longer intervals.[8] Despite this reassurance, we do not feel confident that intervals of less than 3 months will produce comparable results. Figure 6 outlines the typical sequence of events that we might use in a patient undergoing both punch transplanting and alopecia reductions.

Concomitant alopecia reductions and punch transplants can frequently be carried out,

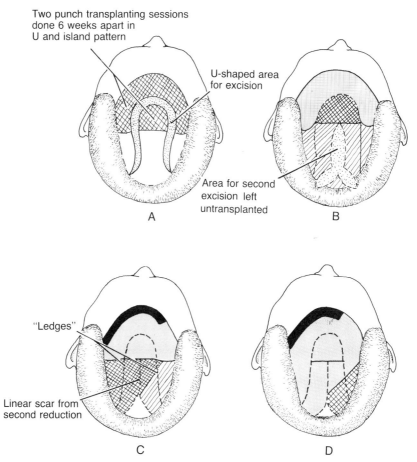

Figure 6.   A. U-shaped area to be excised 6 weeks after the second punch transplant.
   B. The third session takes place 14 weeks after the second session (i.e., approximately 8 weeks after excision) and involves the anterior U. *Above:* Six weeks later, "ledges" are created on the mid-scalp area. A space is left for reduction in a Y shape.
   C. Eight weeks later, a session involving the "island" and the part-side "ledge" as well as the anterior hairline in the area of the part is conducted. An additional alopecia reduction is performed 6 weeks later.
   D. After 6 weeks, another session, which involves the "ledges" on each side (*shown above*) or the "ledge" only on the part side, is usually performed. At this time, the procedure for the remaining vertex is begun. If the remaining vertex is still too large, a portion can be left untreated. An additional reduction may be performed there at a later date.

especially if an elliptic alopecia reduction is used in the midline and the pattern of punch transplanting is such that the blood supply to the grafts is not impaired.[13]

Complications

Hematomas (especially if galeatomies are used), infection (including osteomyelitis of the skull[14]), and skin edge necrosis are all potential complications of alopecia reductions; however, these have not occurred in our experience (over 2000 operations).

"Catgut reaction" occurred in 12 of our patients before we discontinued the use of buried catgut sutures for the galeal closure. Temporary postoperative facial edema has occurred in approximately 20 per cent of our patients. The incidence of postoperative edema is far higher in those individuals who refuse to take or cannot receive systemic corticosteroids.

CONCLUSION

In our opinion, alopecia reduction is probably the most important advance in punch hair transplanting since the inception of this modality.

References

1. Unger, M. G., and Unger, W. P.: Management of alopecia of the scalp by a combination of excisions and transplantations. J. Dermatol. Surg. Oncol. 4:670, 1978.
2. Alt, T.: Scalp reduction. Cosmetic Surg. 1:1, 1981.
3. Blanchard, G., and Blanchard, B.: Obliteration of alopecia by hair-lifting: A new concept and technique. J. Natl. Med. Assoc. 69:639, 1977.
4. Stough, D. B., and Webster, R. C.: Esthetics and refinement in hair transplantation. The International Hair Transplant Symposium, Lucerne, Switzerland, Feb. 4, 1978.
5. Sparkuhl, K.: Scalp reduction: Serial excision of the scalp with flap advancement. The International Hair Transplant Symposium, Lucerne, Switzerland, Feb. 4, 1978.
6. Bosley, L. L., Hope, C. R., and Montroy, R. E.: Male pattern reduction (MPR) for surgical reduction of male pattern baldness. Curr. Ther. Res. 25:281, 1979.
7. Schultz, B. C., and Roenigk, H. H., Jr.: Scalp reduction for alopecia. J. Dermatol. Surg. Oncol. 5:808, 1979.
8. Bosley, L. L., Hope, C. R., Montroy, R. E., and Straub, P. M.: Reduction of male pattern baldness in multiple stages: A retrospective study. J. Dermatol. Surg. Oncol. 6:498, 1980.
9. Unger, M. G., and Unger, W. P.: Alopecia reduction. In Unger: Hair Transplantation. New York, Marcel Dekker Inc., 1979, pp. 102–108.
10. Palletta, F. X.: Surgical management of the burned scalp. Clin. Plast. Surg. 9:167, April 1982.
11. de Jong, R. H., and Heavner, J.: Diazepam prevents and aborts lidocaine convulsions in monkeys. Anesthesiology 3:226, 1971.
12. Habal, M. B., and Powell, R. D.: Experimental facial edema: Treatment with methylprednisolone. J. Surg. Res. 24:353, 1978.
13. Unger, W. P., and Unger, M. G.: Alopecia reduction, In Epstein, E., and Epstein, E., Jr. (eds.): Skin Surgery, 5th ed. Springfield, IL, Charles C Thomas, 1982.
14. Jones, J. W., Ignelzi, R. J., Frank, D. H., and Blacklock, J. B.: Osteomyelitis of the skull following scalp reduction and hair plug transplantation. Ann. Plast. Surg. 5:480, 1980.
15. Vallis, C. P.: Surgical treatment of cicatricial alopecia of the scalp. Clin. Plast. Surg. 9:179, April 1982.

FLAP OPERATIONS FOR BALDNESS

Sheldon S. Kabaker, M.D.

The revival of flap operations for baldness can be attributed to Juri, who in 1975 published his experience and technique with twice-delayed temporoparieto-occipital flaps used in the treatment of baldness.[1] He interested others in this technique and its modifications. Soon thereafter, Elliott[2] reawakened interest in smaller, nondelayed temporoparietal flaps, similar to those described by Passot in 1931.[3]

Currently, scalp flap surgery involves delayed temporoparieto-occipital flaps based on the posterior branch of the superficial temporal artery or nondelayed temporoparietal flaps that are similarly based. Narrow and superiorly based preauricular and postauricular flaps have been described[4] but do not seem to be reliable and have few proponents.

The delayed temporoparieto-occipital flaps are 3.4 to 4.2 cm in width and are designed to be long enough (22 to 29 cm) to result in a complete, continuous hairline. Juri described this operation as involving two delays, 1 week apart. Others[4-6] (this author included) perform only one delay procedure. Without any delay, it is extremely unlikely that a flap with this length-to-width ratio would be so predictably viable. The transposition of this flap is performed approximately 14 days after the first (or only) delay. The donor site defect is closed by advancement and rotation of the adjacent scalp edges after the adjacent scalp and neck tissues have been sufficiently undermined to provide for a relatively tension-free closure.

Usually, the temporoparietal flaps are not delayed. Two of these flaps are required to complete a hairline. The flaps are 2.5 to 3.0 cm in width and are usually 14 to 20 cm in length. There should be a 6- to 12-week interval between the performance of these flap operations. The operative technique is quite similar to that of the transposition of the delayed temporoparieto-occipital flap.

Advantages

The major advantage of flaps is the transfer of large areas of hair-bearing scalp to regions aesthetically appropriate for hair styling. The flap operations provide a larger amount of hair in the shortest period. The hair transposed on the flap continues to grow, and the lag phase of hair growth that is experienced with the plug grafting technique is eliminated. For instance, a flap with hair of 5 inches in length would yield an immediate result—hair that is 5 inches in length. Plug grafting, on the other hand, would entail at least four operative sessions, 4 to 6 weeks apart, and an average time of 13 months (3-month telogen phase, hair growth at ½ inch per month) would be involved in order for 5 inches of hair length to be achieved.[7]

The density of flap hair is equal to that of the donor site and is much greater than the density that can be achieved by plug grafts. This advantage allows the hair to be styled with greater variety. The result of the flap operation is especially advantageous to those patients desiring a backward-combed type of hair style. Also, the hair quite often can be curled to provide still another popular style.

Disadvantages

In comparison with the plug graft method, flaps are more difficult to perform, require advanced training, and have a greater variety and incidence of complications.[8] The means of treatment for the inherent problems and potential complications of these operations must be known by the surgeon. At present, these skills are not formally taught and must be acquired by the surgeon through trial and error or through association with the few practitioners who are skilled in scalp flap surgery. One must always consider having to perform at least one minor revisional procedure, e.g., to correct widened scars, dog-ears, uneven hairlines, or a scalp reduction. Therefore, the patient is subjected to multiple procedures, and there is no advantage over plug grafting with regard to the number of operative procedures. Also, the overall cost at the time of completion is usually no less than that of equivalent coverage achieved through plug grafting, with or without scalp reductions.

Most surgeons and patients feel that the backward growth of hair causes no significant problem; however, flap procedures have come under some criticism because of this factor.

The extreme density and regularity of the frontal hairline can at times look unnatural, especially with straight black hair on a fair-skinned individual. This minor disadvantage is overcome by hair styling that covers the front hairline (permanent waves or forward-combing) or by dyeing the hair a lighter or a salt-and-pepper color.

Another disadvantage is that the flap patient will likely have a convalescent period of 7 to 10 days after his flap has been rotated. During this time, he is away from his occupation and social activities. On the other hand, the patient who has undergone plug grafting can return to his normal environment 1 to 2 days after each of the multiple procedures. Also, forehead edema and ecchymoses are more frequent and severe after the flap operation. Hospitalization, which is recommended by many proponents of flap operations, will increase the costs. With a highly skilled and efficient surgical team, however, flap operations can be performed as an outpatient procedure, thereby negating this disadvantage of hospitalization.

Indications

Six and one half years of experience have revealed few, if any, *absolute* indications for the flap operations. The pattern and extent of the baldness and the age of the patient are the most important factors involved in the selection of a particular procedure for a particular patient. As a rule, patients who are less bald are better candidates for hair transplantation, either by plugs or by flaps. For instance, patients with crown or crown and mid-scalp coverage will be better candidates for surgical hair restoration. It is important to be able to estimate the ultimate mature balding pattern when one evaluates or classifies the patient on consultation. As an example, it should be presumed that a 20-year-old patient with frontal balding will progress to a severe balding pattern, so that the surgical plan and result will not yield a disastrous appearance 20 years later. Conversely, a 40-year-old patient with limited frontal baldness will not likely progress further and is an excellent candidate for hair transplantation, especially by the flap method. Thus, the surgeon can safely plan a complete, full hairline.

Among the more favorable candidates for flap operations are the wearers of hair pieces who want hair transplantation. They are usually agreeable to having a flap operation, as opposed to plug grafting, because they want a result that can look nearly as dense and as full as their hair piece and will therefore cause them a less embarrassing transition when they discard their hair piece. The hair piece wearer will also have the advantage of being able to wear his wig during the healing phases of his surgery and will therefore have an acceptable cosmetic appearance during this period.

The black person is much better served by the flaps than by plug grafting. Some of the coiled hair follicles in a plug graft from a black patient are transected in the cutting process and give a poor yield of hair growth, whereas there is no such problem with flaps. Curly hair spreads out and covers a greater area than straight hair, giving an added benefit to the black patient. This inherent advantage of the black patient can be simulated in the white patient, whose hair can be styled with a permanent to gain more favorable coverage.

Flaps are indicated over the plug graft method in the repair of scalps damaged by fiber implant procedures. Also, the rare male-to-female transsexual desiring hair transplantation can readily acquire a full, dense, feminine hairline with flap operations. Flaps are indicated for reconstruction of the scalp where there has been loss of tissue from burns,[9] neoplasms, or trauma. These flaps are designed with greater individuality than are those for patients with male pattern baldness. It was in this area of reconstructive scalp surgery that the principles of scalp flaps were developed.

Nondelayed temporoparietal flaps may be the choice for patients with limited stable balding patterns. In other situations, these flaps need to be combined with a program of scalp reduction and plug grafting. Two of these flaps should not be performed during the same operative session; the only exception is if the flaps are short, as in filling in of frontotemporal recessions in a stable balding pattern with a strong forelock. In this situation, the scalp must be very flexible to allow for bilateral donor closure without complication.

Temporoparietal flaps can be the treatment of choice in patients who previously have undergone punch grafting, since the temporal and parietal scalp is usually less scarred from donor graft harvesting and may provide for a viable flap. One must consider a delay procedure, even with short temporoparietal flaps if there has been some scarring as a result of plug grafting.

The long-delayed temporoparieto-occipital flaps are my strong preference when flaps are chosen over plug grafts. The exceptional cases in which temporoparietal flaps are favored have been presented previously. The temporoparieto-occipital flaps yield more hair, create a continuous unbroken hairline, and involve only slightly more technical difficulty and operating time. They allow for use of a flap from the contralateral side to repair a lost initial flap or to be placed behind the first flap to provide for greater coverage. The delay offers an advantage of splitting up the operative planning time into two sessions. Since the delay procedure involves most of the thought processes and a commitment to a flap and hairline design, the transposition procedure becomes more of a technical exercise.

Contraindications

The contraindications to performing flap operations are generally the same as those to punch grafting.[7] The main contraindications are insufficient or poor-quality donor hair, an exceptionally tight scalp, and unrealistic expectations on the part of the patient.

The patient with severe baldness might be served better with a cluster of plug grafts to create a thinning, posteriorly placed forelock. This could look more natural than a dense flap, which would have an inadequate aesthetic relationship to a posteriorly displaced temporal hairline and a low fringe. This situation may create an even greater contraindication if the scalp is especially tight. The scalp would therefore allow for little in the way of reduction and may present a problem during donor site closure. If a flap operation is to be performed on a patient with a tight scalp, the flap should be designed to be 3 to 5 mm narrower than the flap for someone with normal scalp laxity.

The performance of simultaneous bilateral flap operations is contraindicated, except in the rare situation in which limited bilateral, frontotemporal coverage is desired and the scalp is very flexible.

The patient who has had a face-lift operation may have had the superficial temporal arteries ligated. If no superficial temporal artery pulse can be palpated or detected with a Doppler ultrasound transducer, flap operations should not be considered.

Patients who have undergone extensive punch grafting should be approached with caution for flap surgery. As mentioned before, the temporoparietal flap may be preferable. A temporoparieto-occipital flap can be performed if the occipital area is not scarred extensively or if suture repair in this area has not resulted in a linear closure. A flap taken from a punch grafted donor area has a better chance for survival if the plug grafting technique has involved superficial cuts, spaces left between the grafts, and no suturing. In all patients who have previously undergone punch grafting, a flap (whether temporoparietal or temporoparieto-occipital) should be delayed at least one time before being transferred. A patient in poor physical or emotional health should not be considered as a candidate for hair flap surgery.

Complications

The list of potential complications of flap surgery for alopecia must include bleeding, infection, cysts or ingrown hairs at the hairline, scarring, partial flap necrosis, permanent or temporary hair loss in the flap or donor area, and all dangers associated with anesthetics or other medications that are used.[8]

The management of complications should involve the lessening of their potential incidence. Bleeding has not been a problem, since sufficient skills have been acquired to reduce the operative time to an average of 1½ hours. During this time, the vasoconstrictor injected into the scalp maintains its function, and bleeding is further controlled with ligature or cautery of major vessels and by the tension of the wound closure. Drains should be placed underneath the transposed flap and beneath the donor closure site. The few hematomas that have occurred have been treated by drainage and irrigation and have left no unfavorable sequelae.

It is my practice to place the patient on prophylactic antibiotics before and for 5 days after the surgery. Infection problems have been insignificant.

The management of significant complications can be described only in general for this article. In almost all situations, conservative measures are to be instituted. One can best treat necrosis of a flap portion or a donor closure area by allowing healing to occur by secondary intention. Sufficient time should then be allowed for the return of scalp laxity, so that revisional surgery can be performed easily.

Occasionally, telogen effluvium may occur in different areas of the flap or around the donor closure site. Again, conservative management (mostly reassurance) is necessary for 3 to 4 months, during which time the hair should grow back.

Unfavorable scarring, cysts or ingrown hairs, or asymmetry of the frontal hairline can usually be treated by minor revisional surgery after 3 months.

Diminished scalp sensation as well as the need for correction of a dog-ear or an asymmetric hairline must be anticipated after a flap operation. These factors are *not* complications but are inherent aspects of scalp flap surgery. Dog-ears are usually adjusted 4 to 5 weeks after the flap transfer, at which time the pedicle of the flap can be transected safely if necessary.

Results

I have been performing scalp flaps for baldness since late 1975. My preference is for the delayed temporoparieto-occipital flap. In the more extensive cases of baldness, greater (if not full) coverage can be attained with a second (contralateral) flap operation performed 3 months after the first procedure. Thereafter, a series of scalp reductions can be performed to reduce the baldness further. The results have been gratifying to both the surgeon and the patient. Dense, full hairlines have been created with a significant shortening of the time before an acceptable cosmetic result is achieved, in comparison with the plug grafting method. Flaps have been used successfully to revise plug grafted hairlines and to reconstruct alopecia of traumatic origins in addition to surgery on the patient with primary, untreated male pattern baldness.

Greater experience has resulted in more consistently good results, and skills have been acquired in handling various adjustment and refinement procedures. No surgeon should attempt these operations without having proper training in related reconstructive surgery and, especially, without having observed and studied the specific flap operations that he wishes to perform.

References

1. Juri, J.: Use of parieto-occipital flaps in the surgical treatment of baldness. Plast. Reconstr. Surg. 55:456, 1975.
2. Elliott, R. A.: Lateral scalp flaps for instant results in male pattern baldness. Plast. Reconstr. Surg. 60:699, 1977.
3. Passot, R.: Chirurgie Esthetique Pure: Technique et Resultats. Paris, G. Doin et Cie., 1931.
4. Stough, D. B., III, Cutes, J. A., and Dean, A. J.: Updating reduction and flap procedures for baldness. Ann. Plast. Surg. 8:287, 1982.
5. Kabaker, S.: Flap procedures in hair replacement surgery. *In* Epstein, E., and Epstein, E., Jr. (eds.): Skin Surgery, 5th ed. Springfield, IL, Charles C Thomas, 1982.
6. Lauzon, G.: Transfer of a large, single, temporo-occipital flap for the treatment of baldness. Plast. Reconstr. Surg. 61:23, 1978.
7. Vallis, C. D.: Hair Transplantation for the Treatment of Male Pattern Baldness. Springfield, IL, Charles C Thomas, 1982.
8. Kabaker, S.: Juri flap procedure for the treatment of baldness: Two year experience. Arch. Otolaryngol. 105:509, 1979.
9. Kabaker, S.: Experiences with parieto-occipital flaps in hair transplantation. Laryngoscope 538:73, 1978.

Editorial Comment

The punch method of hair transplantation is a very popular procedure among dermatologists. Several of them confine their practice to this single modality and have been very successful indeed in doing this. The punch technique is the most widely accepted method of transplanting hair. Its proponents claim that it is the best method, producing superior cosmetic results, the highest percentage of successful "takes," and the least trauma to the patient. In addition, it affords another important plus. Compared with scalp reduction and flap operations, the punch method requires less surgical skill. Therefore, the last two modalities will probably not replace the punch method as means of transplanting scalp hair. However, this should not be construed as berating the reduction and flap procedures. In the hands of experts, the results of these two techniques are very satisfactory. Most dermatologists, however, do not have the requisite skill for flap and reduction operations.

Today, the punch method is often used in conjunction with one of the other two techniques, especially scalp reduction, which was originated and popularized by dermatologists.

There is a real demand for hair transplantation among patients. Furthermore, unlike certain other cosmetic surgical procedures, hair transplantation is successful. Performed with skill, any of the three techniques can give the person who is distressed by the paucity of hair on his scalp an excellent replacement for his natural "crowning glory." Another advantage is that hair transplantation is reasonably permanent. Although regrowth is slow after punch transplantation, it is sure in most instances.

The tyro in dermatology would be well advised to acquire training and experience in hair transplantation during his 3 years of preparation for the American Board examination and his entry into practice. He will have many demands for this procedure.

Think It Over.

SECTION 7

LUPUS ERYTHEMATOSUS

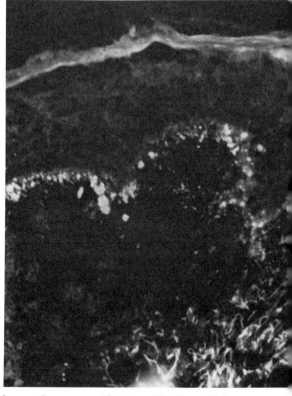

Immunofluorescence. (Courtesy of Dr. Denny Tuffanelli.)

CHAPTER 23

DISCOID AND SYSTEMIC LUPUS ERYTHEMATOSUS AS ONE DISEASE

ARE DISCOID AND SYSTEMIC LUPUS ERYTHEMATOSUS THE SAME DISEASE?

Neville R. Rowell, M.D.

In any discussion of the relationship between discoid lupus erythematosus and systemic lupus erythematosus, one has to consider the question, "Is there a single disease, lupus erythematosus, of which discoid and systemic lupus erythematosus are variants, or are they separate diseases?"

First, however, one has to ask, "What is a disease?" Philosophers distinguish between the nominalistic (or patient-oriented) concept and the essentialistic (or "demonic") concept.[1] The former is based on the idea that there are no diseases but only ill patients and that diseases are merely collections of patients with similar features. Classification of diseases has altered over the centuries as the sciences of pathology and (more recently) immunology have been added to the methods of assessment known to older physicians. Nevertheless, according to the nominalistic view diseases consist only of groups of patients.

The essentialistic, or demonic, concept suggests that diseases are entities in their own right and are like demons, which attack people. Wulff[1] examined the definitions of systemic lupus erythematosus in major textbooks and found that they were really short descriptions of the disease. (I have been guilty of a similar crime.[2]) Nevertheless, he thinks that most authors consider that there is a disease called systemic lupus erythematosus and that "it is one of those mischievous demons who like disguising themselves by producing a variety of manifestations." If one believes the forbidden clone theory, which states that autoaggression is a factor in the etiology of systemic lupus erythematosus[3] or discoid lupus erythematosus,[4] then perhaps the demonic concept is valid. On the other hand, to improve our ability to advise on the prognosis and treatment of patients, we have to define a disease by giving a name to a group of patients who fulfill specified criteria. These may include clinical, pathologic, immunologic, or genetic features.

Twenty-five years ago it was thought to be easy to distinguish discoid lupus erythematosus, a cutaneous disorder in which well-defined erythematous scaling plaques are present on the skin either localized to the head and the neck or widely scattered over the skin surface, from systemic lupus erythematosus, a multi-syndrome disorder affecting the joints, the heart, the lungs, the kidneys, the central nervous system, and the skin. Later, however, dermatologists and physicians became aware that there were similarities between the two diseases, and people started to talk about a spectrum of diseases. Although many people still believe that the concept of a spectrum is valid, others believe not only that discoid lupus erythematosus differs from systemic lupus erythematosus but also that neither discoid nor systemic lupus erythematosus is in itself homogeneous. It is currently fashionable to talk about subsets in disease to describe these differences. A subset is a group of patients with a disease who have similar clinical features, similar laboratory abnormalities, similar pathologic changes, a similar genetic pattern, or a combination of these. Consequently, is there one disease (lupus erythematosus), two disorders (discoid lupus erythematosus and systemic lupus erythematosus), or numerous disorders that are really subsets of one entity (which we call lupus erythematosus) or of two entities (which we call discoid lupus erythematosus and systemic lupus erythematosus)?

Evidence for Discoid and Systemic Lupus Erythematosus as the Same Disease

There is considerable evidence that discoid lupus erythematosus and systemic lupus erythematosus are the same disease. If patients with discoid lupus erythematosus are examined and investigated to the same extent as patients suspected of having systemic lupus erythematosus, then both groups show the same types of abnormalities, although the irregularities are less frequent in discoid lupus erythematosus. In a series of 120 patients with discoid lupus erythematosus whom I evaluated, 55 per cent had abnormalities similar to those found in systemic lupus erythematosus.[5] Clinically, lesions in both types of patients can look alike and can be histologically indistinguishable by conventional techniques. Moreover, the same hematologic, biochemical, and immunologic features can be found in both diseases. In some patients, discoid lupus erythematosus may become overt systemic lupus erythematosus, and 15 per cent of patients with systemic lupus erythematosus may have lesions of discoid lupus erythematosus at some time. Conditions such as lupus erythematosus panniculitis, which is a recognizable clinical and pathologic entity, occur in both discoid and systemic lupus erythematosus, which might tend to suggest that lupus erythematosus is a disease spectrum.

Evidence for Discoid and Systemic Lupus Erythematosus as Different Diseases

The aforementioned evidence seems to support a unitary theory, but the situation is not as straightforward as it seems. The risk that a patient with discoid lupus erythematosus will develop overt systemic lupus erythematosus is only approximately 5 to 6 per cent. The remaining discoid lupus erythematosus cases do not convert to overt systemic lupus erythematosus, despite exposure to stress, infections, sunlight, or drugs. Moreover, although immunoglobulin and complement are present in lesional skin in both conditions, they are absent from the uninvolved skin in discoid lupus erythematosus but not in systemic lupus erythematosus. Anti-DNA antibodies are not found in discoid lupus erythematosus, although antinuclear factor is present in a proportion of patients. The pattern of age at onset and sex distribution is different in the two disorders.[3,4] A study of age-specific incidence rates has suggested that certain diseases are confined to genetically predisposed individuals and that each disease is characterized by one or more specific genotypes. Dominant X-linked inheritance factors determine the greater incidence of the disease in females and account for the markedly different sex distribution in discoid and systemic lupus erythematosus. Approximately two females are affected for every male in discoid lupus erythematosus, compared with eight females to one male in systemic lupus erythematosus.

Professor Burch and I predicted that discoid and systemic lupus erythematosus were genetically different disorders, that discoid lupus erythematosus was not homogeneous, and that there were at least three genotypes, related to early, middle, and late onset. In an attempt to produce further evidence in favor of this hypothesis, HLA typing of patients was carried out.[6] In a group of patients with discoid lupus erythematosus there was no change in any HLA type but, when typing was related to age at onset, it was possible to show that HLA-B7 was associated with onset between 15 and 39 years of age in both sexes. There was a significant difference in the incidence of HLA-B7 in patients with onset between 15 and 39 years of age and those with onset after age 40. There was thus some evidence in favor of differences related to age at onset. We found that HLA-B8 was significantly raised in systemic lupus erythematosus and, when the same age at onset group (15 to 39 years) was analyzed, there were significant differences in the incidence of HLA-B8 among discoid and systemic lupus erythematosus patients. This is also evidence that discoid and systemic lupus erythematosus are genetically different.

Clinical Subsets of Discoid Lupus Erythematosus

A follow-up study performed after 16 years, in which 110 patients with discoid lupus erythematosus were evaluated,[7] showed that 5.5 per cent of cases had converted to overt systemic lupus erythematosus during the period, but there were differences between patients with discoid lupus erythematosus, who had lesions localized to the head and the neck, and patients with so-called disseminated lupus erythematosus, who in addition had lesions below the neck. Remissions occurred in 52 per cent of patients with discoid lupus erythematosus originally confined to the head and the neck, 13 per cent of cases became disseminated, and 1.2 per cent of the patients developed systemic lupus erythematosus. Remissions occurred in only 13 per cent of patients with disseminated discoid lupus erythematosus, and 22 per cent of cases went on to become systemic lupus erythematosus. This underlines the differences in the prognoses of these two subgroups of discoid lupus erythematosus. Patients with discoid lupus erythematosus who develop systemic lupus erythematosus are predominantly female, and the cases are mainly of the disseminated discoid type. Central nervous system complications and renal disease are frequent. Patients in whom this conversion occurs usually have had persistently abnormal laboratory investigations for a long period. There is an increased likelihood that they will have HLA-B8, and the presence of HLA-B8 in a female who develops discoid lupus erythematosus under the age of 40 years is a risk factor for systemic lupus erythematosus.

Prognostic subsets can also be recognized by consideration of the type and site of lesions. In our experience, patients with the rosaceous type of discoid lupus erythematosus do well compared with the poor outcome in patients with chilblain lupus erythematosus and in those with plaques in front of the ears. Lesions on the palms of the hands and the soles of the feet and those on the trunk do not heal as quickly as do those on the face. Subsets may be related to sex; for example, chilblain lupus erythematosus predominates in females and preauricular plaque lesions occur commonly in males.

If we look at the relationship from the other perspective, do patients who have systemic lupus erythematosus with discoid cutaneous lesions have particular characteristics? Most of these patients have lesions that are widely disseminated over the body. Arthritis, Raynaud's phenomenon, and periungual telangiectasia are common, and all such patients have immunologic abnormalities consistent with systemic lupus erythematosus. Renal disease is mild, but there is a considerable risk of central nervous system involvement. Such studies confirm that the risk that overt systemic lupus erythematosus will develop in patients with disseminated discoid lupus erythematosus is much higher than the probability that it will occur in individuals who have discoid lupus erythematosus confined to the head and the neck.

Classification of Cutaneous Lupus Erythematosus

In the past, lupus erythematosus has been divided into two categories: (1) discoid lupus erythematosus, which is either localized to the head and the neck or disseminated above and below the neck, and (2) systemic lupus erythematosus. Gilliam and Sontheimer[8] suggested that lupus erythematosus could be divided into three groups according to the cutaneous lesions without consideration of the systemic aspects of the disease. These three groups are: (1) chronic cutaneous lupus erythematosus, which is equivalent to discoid lupus erythematosus of the localized, disseminated, or hypertrophic variety; (2) subacute cutaneous lupus erythematosus, which can be subdivided into papulosquamous and annular-polycyclic groups; and (3) acute cutaneous lupus erythematosus, in which erythematous rashes are localized to the face or are more widespread elsewhere. This is a valuable contribution, because it provides a basis for future research.

The group of patients described by Sontheimer and coworkers[9] as having "subacute cutaneous lupus erythematosus" had either papulosquamous or annular-polycyclic lesions in association with mild systemic illness. Approximately half the cases met the criteria of the American Rheumatism Association for systemic lupus erythematosus, but renal or central nervous system disease was not a feature. Patients with this type of lupus erythematosus had an increased frequency of HLA-B8 and HLA-DR3.[10] Patients with HLA-DR3 are particularly prone to the annular subgroup of subacute cutaneous lupus erythematosus. There is also a link between subacute cutaneous lupus erythematosus and the type of circulating antibody. Patients frequently have anti-Ro or anti-La antibodies.

The lupus erythematosus/erythema multiforme syndrome described in 1963[11] is probably a variant of subacute cutaneous lupus erythematosus. This syndrome occurs in both discoid lupus erythematosus and systemic lupus erythematosus but was first described in patients with discoid lupus erythematosus. In this group, episodes of annular lesions occur over many years in association with discoid lupus erythematosus or systemic lupus erythematosus. Patients have speckled antinuclear factor, rheumatoid factor, and a precipitating antibody to saline extract of human tissue called SjT, now thought to be identical with anti–SS-B. The cases of discoid lupus erythematosus and erythema multiforme–like lesions may convert to systemic lupus erythematosus after some years.

Serologic Subsets of Discoid Lupus Erythematosus

This field has been much less actively researched than has systemic lupus erythematosus. Antinuclear antibodies in low titer may be present in up to 35 per cent of patients, but antibodies to native DNA are absent. However, 25 per cent of patients with discoid lupus erythematosus without evidence of systemic disease have antibodies to single-stranded DNA,[12] but it is not known whether the prognosis of these patients differs from that of patients without the antibody. Patients with the lupus erythematosus/erythema multiforme syndrome have speckled antinuclear factor and antibodies now thought to be anti-Ro.

Clinical Subsets of Systemic Lupus Erythematosus

Despite the fact that this is a multi-system disease, patients often appear to have a disorder affecting predominantly the kidneys, the central nervous system, or the lungs. Whether these represent subsets with different genetic factors is not yet known.

Serologic Subsets of Systemic Lupus Erythematosus

Several serologic subsets have been defined in systemic lupus erythematosus in recent years.[13] For example, high levels of circulating anti-DNA antibodies and low serum complement levels are associated with patients with active renal disease. On the other hand, patients with anti-Sm antibodies have mild renal or central nervous system disease. The antibody to nuclear ribonucleoprotein identifies a subset with overlapping features of systemic lupus erythematosus in association with dermatomyositis and systemic sclerosis. This has been called "mixed connective tissue disease," although some believe that it is really a subset of systemic lupus erythematosus. Patients with widespread cutaneous involvement and severe renal disease without anti-DNA antibodies may have an antibody to a soluble nuclear antigen called Ma. Not all patients with systemic lupus erythematosus have antinuclear factor, but such ANA-negative patients often have antibodies to cytoplasmic antigens called Ro and La. Clinically, such patients have prominent photosensitivity and rheumatoid factor, and their disease has a benign course. Anti-Ro and anti-La antibodies are frequent in subacute cutaneous lupus erythematosus. This is in contrast with discoid lupus erythematosus, in which these antibodies are rare.

SUMMARY

Where does all this leave us? The problem is much more complex than had been thought originally, and I think that, although there is evidence that discoid and systemic lupus erythematosus in the main behave differently, they must be variants of the same disease process. The profound difference, in my view, is that each represents a different genetic subgroup, and if there is a conversion from discoid to systemic lupus erythematosus, the patient must have the genetic predisposition to both disorders. On the other hand, the two main divisions each consist of many subsets, and the same type of concept can be applied to these subsets. It is likely that each subset may be represented by different genetic factors, and it seems that the subsets are related to type, site, sex, prognosis, and immunologic abnormalities. When one considers that the local and central defense mechanisms of the body are also probably under genetic control, the permutations and combinations with respect to an individual patient are many. This is compatible with our theory that both discoid and systemic lupus erythematosus arise as the result of somatic mutation in lymphocytic stem cells of predisposed individuals with the development of forbidden clones of lymphocytes. These lymphocytes attack complementary target tissues, and the distribution of the attack is also determined by central and local defense mechanisms, which can be impaired by environmental factors.

Nevertheless, it is important to distinguish clinical and immunologic subsets, because they are related to prognosis and, probably, to response to treatment. Unfortunately, subsets cannot always be defined accurately, but Gilliam and Sontheimer's approach[8] has shown what can be done with classification of the cutaneous aspects of lupus erythematosus. The clinical importance is that patients with chronic scarring discoid lupus erythematosus are not frightened by being given incorrect advice. They should be informed that they have a long-lasting cutaneous condition, but all the possible complications should not be mentioned, because it is unlikely that these problems will develop. Patients with persistent laboratory abnormalities should be kept under regular observation.

Lasagna, in his preface to *Controversies in Therapeutics,* said, "A perverse characteristic of the human race is its preference for spurious simplicity as opposed to truthful complexity."[14] This remark is especially true with regard to the controversy concerning lupus erythematosus.

References

1. Wulff, H. R.: What is understood by a disease entity? J. R. Coll. Physicians 13:219, 1979.
2. Rowell, N. R.: Lupus erythematosus, scleroderma and dermatomyositis. *In* Rook, A., Wilkinson, D. S., and Ebling, F. J. G. (eds.): Textbook of Dermatology, 3rd ed. Oxford, Blackwell Scientific Publications, 1979.
3. Burch, P. R. J., and Rowell, N. R.: Systemic lupus erythematosus: Etiological aspects. Am. J. Med. 38:793, 1965.
4. Burch, P. R. J., and Rowell, N. R.: Lupus erythematosus: Analysis of the sex and age distribution of the discoid and systemic forms of the disease in different countries. Acta Derm. Venereol. 50:293, 1970.
5. Beck, J. S., and Rowell, N. R.: Discoid lupus erythematosus. A study of the clinical features and biochemical and serological abnormalities in 120 patients with observations on the relationship of this disease to systemic lupus erythematosus. Q. J. Med. 35:119, 1966.
6. Millard, L. G., Rowell, N. R., and Rajah, S. M.: Histocompatibility antigens in discoid and systemic lupus erythematosus. Br. J. Dermatol. 96:139, 1977.
7. Rowell, N. R., and Millard, L. G.: Proceedings of the 16th International Congress of Dermatology. Tokyo, University of Tokyo Press (in press).
8. Gilliam, J. N., and Sontheimer, R. D.: Distinctive cutaneous subsets in the spectrum of lupus erythematosus. J. Am. Acad. Dermatol. 4:471, 1981.
9. Sontheimer, R. D., Thomas, J. R., and Gilliam, J. N.: Subacute cutaneous lupus erythematosus. Arch. Dermatol. 115:1409, 1979.
10. Sontheimer, R. D., Stastny, P., and Gilliam, J. N.: Human histocompatibility antigen associations in subacute cutaneous lupus erythematosus. J. Clin. Invest. 67:312, 1981.
11. Rowell, N. R., Beck, J. S., and Anderson, J.: Lupus erythematosus and erythema multiforme–like lesions. Arch. Dermatol. 88:176, 1963.
12. Reichlin, M.: Proceedings of the 16th International Congress of Dermatology. Tokyo, University of Tokyo Press (in press).
13. Provost, T. T.: Subsets in systemic lupus erythematosus. J. Invest. Dermatol. 72:110, 1979.
14. Lasagna, L.: Controversies in Therapeutics. Philadelphia, W. B. Saunders Co. 1980.

THE RELATIONSHIP BETWEEN CHRONIC CUTANEOUS (DISCOID) AND SYSTEMIC LUPUS ERYTHEMATOSUS

Denny L. Tuffanelli, M.D.

The relationship between discoid and systemic lupus erythematosus has long been debated. In general, clinicians who see patients in the entire spectrum of lupus erythematosus are less apt to regard the issue as controversial than are those who see primarily outpatient cutaneous disease or inpatient systemic disease. There is little doubt that the conditions are related, but the nature of the relationship is not completely understood.

Lupus erythematosus is a chronic inflammatory disease of unknown etiology. Usually, there are multiple target organs, but occasionally only one (e.g., skin or kidney) is involved. Discoid lupus erythematosus represents the chronic cutaneous form of the disease. The term "discoid" is confusing because it has two usages. On the one hand, it is a morphologic description of a "disc-shaped" lesion. On the other hand, it describes a form of lupus erythematosus that is limited to the skin. We prefer the term "chronic cutaneous lupus," realizing that most of these lesions are "discoid" in appearance. Acute and subacute cutaneous lupus erythematosus are other well-defined variants of cutaneous lupus erythematosus.

Discoid lupus erythematosus is the same disease as systemic lupus erythematosus. It is merely at the benign end of the lupus erythematosus spectrum. All variations occur between the cutaneous and systemic forms of the disease. The American Rheumatism Association has set definite, although arbitrary, criteria for the diagnosis of systemic lupus erythematosus. There is a "gray zone" between pure discoid lupus erythematosus and systemic lupus erythematosus. In this area are patients with discoid lupus and serologic or clinical symptoms of systemic disease.

However, before I discuss the relationship of discoid to systemic lupus erythematosus, a definition of discoid lupus is indicated. Classically, discoid lupus demonstrates well-defined plaque-like lesions with persistent erythema, telangiectasia, follicular plugging, scarring, and atrophy. The pathology of cutaneous lupus erythematosus usually relates to the age of the lesion. Hyperpigmentation and depigmentation frequently occur. Lesions are usually limited to the face, the scalp, and sun-exposed areas but may involve the mucous membranes and non–sun-exposed areas, such as the inner ear. Discoid lesions may be limited to one or two areas or may be generalized.

The relationship of pure discoid lupus to systemic lupus has long been questioned. Kaposi in 1872 contended that chronic discoid lupus erythematosus and systemic lupus erythematosus were the same disease.[1] Discoid lupus erythematosus can be divided into localized, with lesions only above the neck, and generalized forms, in which the lesions are present on the trunk and the extremities. Dubois and Martel demonstrated that clinical and serologic abnormalities are greater in generalized discoid lupus.[2]

The relationship of discoid to systemic lupus erythematosus varies, as previously noted, with the patient population studied. We have had the opportunity to study lupus erythematosus in the context of private practice dermatology, a university referral clinic, and a county hospital inpatient population. The extent of the relationship between discoid and systemic lupus varied widely in each instance. Chronic discoid lesions were the initial manifestation of systemic lupus erythematosus in 56 (10.8 per cent) of 520 systemic lupus erythematosus patients we studied with Dubois.[3] In addition, chronic discoid lesions occurred during the course of the disease in 149 (28.6 per cent) of the patients. The incidence of patients who present with discoid lesions and later develop systemic lupus erythematosus varies from 2 to 20 per cent. Again, the percentage varies directly with the patient population studied. In addition, it is not unusual for patients with typical systemic lupus erythematosus to go into remission and for the cases to be transformed into purely chronic cutaneous discoid lupus erythematosus.[4] Most observers agree that that subset of systemic lupus erythematosus patients who have discoid lesions represents individuals with a more benign form, and survival is increased when their condition is compared with that of systemic lupus erythematosus patients without discoid lupus erythematosus lesions.

In all cases of discoid lupus, potential systemic progression is present. Occasionally, patients without any abnormal findings are observed. Most commonly serologic or clinical abnormalities suggestive of systemic lupus are present, although the American Rheumatism Association criteria for the diagnosis of systemic lupus erythematosus are not fulfilled. Clinical signs in such patients may include malaise, fatigability, and mild arthralgias, and serologic abnormalities may include anemia, leukopenia, raised erythrocyte sedimentation rate, biological false positive reaction for syphilis, and so forth. In our experience, the discoid form of the disease may be transformed into the active systemic variety slowly or acutely following some stress or insult. Sera from systemic lupus erythematosus patients almost invariably have ANA, as do sera from significant numbers of discoid lupus erythematosus patients. The incidence varies with the substrate used.[5] Anti–double-stranded DNA antibodies are found in over half of systemic lupus erythematosus patients and are very specific. They and antibodies to SS-DNA occur in an occasional patient with discoid lupus, but these individuals frequently develop systemic lupus erythematosus.[6] In addition, there is a group of patients with negative ANA with rat liver substrate, cutaneous lupus erythematosus, and photosensitivity who subsequently develop systemic lupus erythematosus. These patients are often characterized by the presence of the cytoplasmic antigens Ro and La.

The occurrence of IgG and complement at the dermal/epidermal junction in cutaneous lesions, both in chronic cutaneous (discoid) lupus erythematosus and in systemic lupus erythematosus, is a further argument for a similar pathogenesis. This aspect of lupus erythematosus will be discussed in another article.

Another argument supporting the concept that discoid and systemic lupus erythematosus are the same disease is the fact that numerous well-defined variants can occur with both forms. For example, lupus-like syndromes have been reported in patients with complement deficiencies, including C1q, C1r, C1s, C2, C4, C5, C6, C7, C8, C9.[7–9] The syndrome is most common in homozygous C2-deficient females. Most of the patients have photosensitivity, discoid lesions, and features of systemic lupus erythematosus. Although children of mothers with lupus erythematosus are usually normal, newborn infants can demonstrate features of both discoid and systemic lupus. In the children with discoid lupus, leukopenia and thrombocytopenia are frequently noted.[10–12] Lupus panniculitis is another variant that occurs in both discoid and systemic lupus.[13] Subacute cutaneous lupus erythematosus is another variant with features of both systemic and discoid lupus erythematosus. Although these patients usually have annular or psoriasiform lesions, scarring discoid lesions can also be present. These patients often have mild systemic disease and the B cell alloantigen HLA-DR3.

Common etiology also suggests a relationship between discoid and systemic lupus erythematosus. Ultraviolet light, for example, can induce cutaneous lupus erythematosus and exacerbate systemic lupus erythematosus. Springtime flares of cutaneous lupus erythematosus are common. Cutaneous lupus erythematosus can be reproduced by ultraviolet light with rays between 2900 Å and 3200 Å. Photosensitivity is more common in systemic lupus erythematosus but can occur in patients with discoid lupus.

Similarly, the response to therapy, including treatment with steroids (topical and systemic), antimalarials,[14] and immunosuppressives would again suggest a common pathogenesis.

Thus, it appears that lupus erythematosus is one disease, with a spectrum of clinical, serologic, and pathologic findings. Chronic cutaneous (discoid) lupus is at the most benign end of the spectrum. Patients with discoid lupus have a protective mechanism, probably immunologic, which prevents progression and multi-system involvement.

References

1. Kaposi, M.: Neue beiträge zur kenntnis des lupus erythematodes. Arch. Dermatol. Syph. 4:36, 1872.
2. Dubois, E. L., and Martel, S.: Discoid lupus erythematosus: An analysis of its systemic manifestations. Ann. Intern. Med. 44:482, 1956.
3. Tuffanelli, D. L., and Dubois, E. L.: Cutaneous manifestations of systemic lupus erythematosus. Arch. Dermatol. 90:377, 1964.
4. Ganor, S., and Sagher, F.: Systemic lupus erythematosus changing to the chronic discoid type. Dermatologica 125:81, 1962.
5. Tuffanelli, D. L.: Connective tissue diseases. *In* Malkinson, F. D., and Pearson, R. W. (eds.): Year Book of Dermatology. Chicago, Year Book Medical Publishers, 1978, pp. 9–36.
6. Kulick, K. B., Provost, T. T., and Reichlin, M.: Antibodies to SS-DNA in patients with discoid lupus erythematosus. Invest. Dermatol. 76:309, 1981.
7. Lupus erythematosus–like syndrome with selective complete deficiency of C1q. Ann. Intern. Med. 95:322, 1981.
8. Douglass, M., Lamberg, S. I., Lorincz, A. L., Good, R. A., and Noorbibi, K. D.: Lupus erythematosus-like syndrome with a familial deficiency of C2. Arch. Dermatol. 112:671, 1976.
9. Belin, D. C., Bordwell, B. J., Einarson, M. E., McLean, R. H., Weinstein, A., Yunis, E. J., and Rothfield, N. F.: Familial discoid lupus erythematosus associated with heterozygote C2 deficiency. Arthritis Rheum. 23:898, 1980.
10. Esscher, E., and Scott, J. S.: Congenital heart block and maternal systemic lupus erythematosus. Br. Med. J. 1:1235, 1979.
11. McCuistion, C. H., and Schoch, E. P., Jr.: Possible discoid lupus erythematosus in a newborn infant. Arch. Dermatol. Syph. 70:782, 1954.
12. Kephart, D. C., Hood, A. F., and Provost, T. T.: Neonatal lupus erythematosus: New serologic findings. J. Invest. Dermatol. 77:331, 1981.
13. Tuffanelli, D. L.: Lupus erythematosus panniculitis (profundus). Clinical and immunologic studies. Arch. Dermatol. 103:231, 1971.
14. Koranda, F. C.: Antimalarials. J. Am. Acad. Dermatol. 4:650, 1981.

Editorial Comment

Most clinicians consider discoid lupus erythematosus to be distinct from systemic lupus erythematosus and believe that the former is merely a cosmetic defect and the latter is a serious systemic disease with cutaneous manifestations. After all, the discoid type rarely progresses to the systemic form. Even when it does, one can usually find clues suggesting that the condition was the systemic disease from the start. The patient may have had general malaise and, especially, easily induced tiredness and weakness. Renal derangements may have been noted. A persistent leukopenia, a rapid sedimentation rate, an albuminuria, or other laboratory evidence suggestive of dissemination may have been manifested. The lesions, although characterized by the cardinal signs of discoid lupus erythematosus, such as atrophy, telangiectasia, follicular plugging, sharp margination, and peripheral hyperpigmentation, may have been much more widespread than those that are usually encountered in a pure discoid eruption. Photosensitivity may have been more marked than in the usual discoid case.

Dr. Tuffanelli presents strong arguments to support his thesis that the two conditions are really one. Because he is a serious student of this disease and one of the outstanding experts in this field, one cannot dismiss his beliefs lightly. It is not my intention to question him, but from the practical side it seems that these two diseases (or these two manifestations of the same disorder) are different and definitely divisible. Actually, it must be admitted that nearly all experts in this field agree with Dr. Tuffanelli. Yet there seems room for the two schools to coexist, since there is a great deal of truth on both sides of this controversy.

Think It Over.

CHAPTER 24

IMMUNOFLUORESCENCE

IMMUNOFLUORESCENCE MICROSCOPY IN THE DIAGNOSIS OF LUPUS ERYTHEMATOSUS

Denny L. Tuffanelli, M.D.

Cutaneous immunopathology should be routinely used in the diagnosis of lupus erythematosus. The cutaneous immunopathology laboratory at the University of California has processed over 10,000 biopsies thus far, and the most common clinical usage is in the diagnosis of lupus erythematosus. For example, the diagnosis of facial erythema involves differentiating cutaneous lupus erythematosus, rosacea, seborrheic dermatitis, poststeroid erythema, and polymorphic light eruption. Often the immunopathology is critical for diagnosis. Similarly, one must make a differential diagnosis of lupus erythematosus and scarring alopecia or photodermatitis. The differentiation of lupus erythematosus from lichen planus, psoriasis, and actinic keratosis can also be difficult and is an indication for immunopathology. These are some examples of the wide range of clinical problems involving lupus erythematosus that may require cutaneous immunopathology for diagnosis.

In all of these clinical situations, a definite deposition of IgG, IgM, and complement can be diagnostic. I recently reviewed the data on 200 consecutively submitted specimens in which the problem of ruling out lupus erythematosus was posed. Obviously, the slides submitted were largely from problem cases. The immunopathology in 53 was highly suggestive of lupus erythematosus. In 28 it was suggestive, but not diagnostic, of lupus erythematosus, and in 119 it was negative. Thus, in 40 per cent of these problem cases, immunopathology was probably the diagnostic procedure of most value.

Skin immunopathology is also of use in the diagnosis and management of systemic lupus erythematosus. In our experience, the major usefulness in systemic lupus erythematosus is in diagnosis. In patients with multi-system disease, in whom the diagnosis of lupus erythematosus is possible, deposition of IgG-complement immune complexes at the dermal/epidermal junction in non–sun-exposed skin is a major criterion for the diagnosis of lupus erythematosus.

The literature on the value of the test for prognostic information is variable, and there are many conflicting data. Certainly, deposits may be present in the skin during periods of clinical remission and when serologic abnormalities have disappeared. They may also be absent in active disease. Some authors[1-3] claim that the test is useful prognostically, whereas others[4,5] do not. I feel that there are numerous tests that are better for determining the prognosis. It is true that patients with IgG, IgM, and complement in non–sun-exposed normal skin usually have more active disease, low serum complement, and high anti-DNA. The prognostic value, however, is less than that of tests such as determination of complement (C_3, CH_{50}) levels and anti-DNA antibody titers. However, in a thorough work-up performed on a lupus erythematosus patient, biopsy of uninvolved, non–sun-exposed skin does give information of value. Deposition of immune complexes certainly has adverse prognostic implications. The question as to whether a positive test correlates with the incidence and severity of renal disease also has proponents on both sides.[4-7]

In our published material, we report that immunopathology results in 90 per cent of discoid lupus erythematosus lesions are positive, as they are in 90 per cent of systemic lupus erythematosus lesions, 50 per cent of uninvolved, non–sun-exposed systemic lupus erythematosus lesions, and 70 per cent of uninvolved, sun-exposed systemic lupus erythematosus skin lesions.[8,9] When one studies a patient with possible systemic lupus erythematosus without cutaneous lesions, I advocate a biopsy of sun-exposed skin (arm) for diagnosis and of non–sun-exposed skin (lower back) for prognostic information.

IgG, IgM, IgA, and the complement components are present at the dermal/epidermal zone. Fibrin and properdin can also often be found. In general, early lesions usually demonstrate granular, speckled, or thready deposition. Old discoid lupus erythematosus lesions have a broad, homogeneous, PAS-positive IgG deposition. Their presence in normal-appearing skin in systemic lupus erythematosus suggests that in some situations the depositions represent antigen-antibody complexes.

Sun-damaged skin can show immunoglobulins at the dermal/epidermal junction. False positives can be identified because of the weak intensity and irregular patterns of the band. Other diseases in which IgG and complement can be demonstrated at the dermal/epidermal junction include cutaneous porphyria, pemphigoid, rosacea, leprosy, facial telangiectasia, and hypocomplementemic vasculitis. In other connective tissue diseases, IgG and complement are rarely found at the dermal/epidermal junction. However, in inflammatory scleroderma and linear scleroderma, IgM is frequently found at the dermal/epidermal junction.

Other immunofluorescent findings have been reported in cutaneous lupus. Ovoid "hyalin" bodies are often found in the epidermis and the subepidermal papillary layer. They are not specific for lupus erythematosus and are frequently seen in other diseases, particularly lichen planus and dermatomyositis. When high-titer antinuclear antibodies, particularly of the speckled or nucleolar type, are present, they may be noted in the epidermis.[10] This occurs most commonly in mixed connective tissue disease when ENA antibodies of the Rnp type are present. These ENA antibodies also are found in scleroderma when high-titer nucleolar antibodies are present. However, they are occasionally noted in lupus erythematosus skin biopsies. Their significance is unknown.

The technology of immunopathology is improving continuously. Our understanding of the antigens and antibodies involved in the depositions at the dermal/epidermal junction is still rudimentary. Recent advances in antinuclear antibody immunofluorescence have shown that the morphologic patterns of the past (speckled, granular, homogeneous, outlined, particulate, and so forth) represent specific antigens. Thus, we now recognize antibodies to centromere, centriole, nucleolus, mitochondria, histone, DNA, mRNA, and so forth. The list of specific antigens to which patients form antibodies will enlarge continuously. Similarly, the usefulness of skin biopsy immunopathology in studying lupus erythematosus will increase rapidly when the specific antigens and antibodies involved are known. For the present, immunopathologic study of cutaneous lupus erythematosus as a clinical tool has withstood the test of time. In our laboratory, the number of specimens from lupus erythematosus patients submitted has increased yearly for the past 15 years. Cutaneous immunopathology is still in its infancy, and greater discoveries lie ahead.

References

1. Burnham, T. K., and Fine, G.: The immunofluorescent "band" test for lupus erythematosus. III. Employing clinically normal skin. Arch. Dermatol. 103:24, 1971.
2. Provost, T. T., Andres, G., Maddison, P. J., and Reichlin, M.: Lupus band test in untreated SLE patients: Correlation of immunoglobulin deposition in the skin of the extensor forearm with clinical renal disease and serologic abnormalities. J. Invest. Dermatol. 74:407, 1980.

 3. Rothfield, N., and Marino, C.: Studies of repeat skin biopsies of nonlesional skin in patients with systemic lupus erythematosus. Arthritis Rheum. 25:624, 1982.
 4. Wertheimer, D., and Barland, P.: Clinical significance of immune deposits in the skin in SLE. Arthritis Rheum. 19:1249, 1976.
 5. Caperton, E. M., Jr., Bean, S. F., and Dick, F. R.: Immunofluorescent skin test in systemic lupus erythematosus: Lack of relationship with renal disease. JAMA 222:935, 1972.
 6. Gilliam, J.N., Cheatum, D.E., Hurd, E.R., Stastny, P., and Ziff, M.: Immunoglobulin in clinically uninvolved skin in systemic lupus erythematosus. J. Clin. Invest. 53:1434, 1974.
 7. Brown, M. M., and Yount, W. J.: Skin immunopathology in systemic lupus erythematosus. JAMA 243:38, 1980.
 8. Pohle, E. L., and Tuffanelli, D. L.: Study of cutaneous lupus erythematosus. Arch. Dermatol. 97:520, 1968.
 9. Kay, D. M., and Tuffanelli, D. L.: Immunofluorescent techniques in clinical diagnosis of cutaneous disease. Ann. Intern. Med. 71:753, 1969.
10. Prystowsky, S. D., and Tuffanelli, D. L.: Speckled (particulate) epidermal nuclear IgG deposition in normal skin. Arch. Dermatol. 114:705, 1978.

LIMITATIONS OF
IMMUNOFLUORESCENCE TESTING

Stefania Jabłońska, M.D.

Immunofluorescence is the most reliable method for establishing a diagnosis and prognosis of bullous diseases, collagenoses, and vascular disorders.[1] Some of the cases of bullous diseases cannot be recognized without immunofluorescence testing, and some varieties of bullous disorders have been distinguished on the basis of immunofluorescence findings. However, in the 18 years since immunofluorescence tests were introduced by Beutner and associates,[2] as experience has been accumulated, limitations of the method (i.e., the difficulties in the interpretation and evaluation of the tests) have become more evident.

Bullous Diseases

Immunofluorescence tests are of basic diagnostic significance in these disorders.

Pemphigus.   The immunofluorescence pattern of pemphigus is characteristic and diagnostic. However, in a small proportion of cases, the results of indirect immunofluorescence testing are negative, and the diagnosis is based on the positive direct immunofluorescence test (i.e., in vivo fixed intercellular antibodies).

Circulating intercellular (pemphigus) antibodies parallel the disease activity according to some authors,[3,4] but others disagree.[5,6] This disagreement might be partially caused by technical problems (different substrates and reagents used for immunofluorescence tests) and partially caused by the formation of immune complexes with no antibodies in circulation or the presence of pemphigus lesions in the larynx, the vagina, and so forth that are overlooked by the physicians. Thus, although periodic serum examinations in pemphigus seem to be useful in monitoring the treatment, their value is still a subject of controversy.

Another controversial problem is the appearance of complement-fixing pemphigus-like antibodies,[7,8] which cannot be differentiated from true pemphigus antibodies by routine tests.[9] However, in contrast with pemphigus antibodies, they fix complement, have a low titer, and are transient.[8] They appear in response to burns, drug reactions, and various insults to the epidermis. These antibodies may be responsible for false positive immunofluorescence tests in pemphigus.

Another subject of controversy is complement fixation in pemphigus lesions in the direct (tissue) immunofluorescence test.

Although it has been shown in tissue culture that acantholysis is induced by pemphigus antibodies without participation of the complement,[10] there are still differences of opinion concerning whether in vivo complement fixation initiates pemphigus lesions[11] or whether it is not needed for the reaction.[12] The presence of complement in untreated, very early, or ultraviolet-induced pemphigus lesions[13] would favor the theory of some pathogenic role of complement binding in the tissue after acantholysis has been induced by pemphigus antibodies.

Direct immunofluorescence studies in bullous diseases have disclosed a pemphigus pattern in some cases that has not shown any clinical characteristics of the disease. For example, pemphigus herpetiformis, a new form of pemphigus, has been identified. This disease is clinically similar to dermatitis herpetiformis and is responsive to sulfones. However, its immunopathology and histology are characteristic of pemphigus.

In addition, without immunofluorescence it would not be possible to diagnose a form of pemphigus resembling erythema annulare and some other atypical varieties whose relationship with the true pemphigus would otherwise be rather dubious.

Some other limitations of the immunofluorescence method are caused by technical problems and, especially, species specificity. In these cases, intercellular antibodies can be detected only on some substrates (for instance, on the monkey esophagus) but not in human skin.[14]

Bullous Pemphigoid. The immunopathology is highly characteristic (i.e., deposits of immunoglobulins and complement are invariably present at the basal membrane zone), and basal membrane zone antibodies are detectable in approximately 70 per cent of the cases. With the use of immunofluorescence it has been shown that bullous pemphigoid has variable clinical features, and the histopathology, although characteristic, not infrequently is not diagnostic.

The controversy concerns mainly the diagnostic significance of immunofluorescence findings. Should vesicular and erythematous eruptions (in which the only immunopathologic markers are complement deposits at the basal membrane zone with no circulating and in vivo fixed antibodies) be classified as bullous pemphigoid? What relationship does the localized form at pretibial areas have with bullous pemphigoid? There are usually negative immunofluorescence findings, although single cases have been reported to have immune deposits at the basal membrane zone.[15] On the other hand, cicatricial pemphigoid, in which the clinical features are rather distinct, has essentially the same immunopathologic pattern as do other varieties of bullous pemphigoid, although immune deposits are often detectable only in repeated biopsies. This form of bullous pemphigoid differs also in the presence of IgA deposits in as high as 23 per cent of the cases (unpublished data).

Immunopathologic studies have disclosed cases of bullous pemphigoid induced by drugs, mainly those used in treating scabies and psoriasis. How closely these bullous eruptions, which are often transitory and not infrequently have exclusive complement basal membrane zone deposits, are related to true bullous pemphigoid is a matter of controversy. The same is true of the bullous eruption that accompanies various skin diseases, especially lupus erythematosus and lichen planus. Is it a coexistence of two diseases or a transient immune response to the destruction of the basal membrane, which is characteristic both of lupus erythematosus and lichen planus? Bullous lesions accompanying systemic lupus erythematosus either have all the characteristics of bullous pemphigoid or are similar to IgA linear dermatosis (prevalent IgA deposits at the basal membrane zone, polymorphonuclear papillary microabscesses, response to sulfones), and their classification is not infrequently quite arbitrary.[16] It is also not entirely clear whether herpes gestationis should be included in the bullous pemphigoid group or regarded as a separate entity.[17] The immunopathology is quite characteristic, with complement usually as the exclusive component at the basal membrane zone and with no circulating antibodies in the routine indirect immunofluorescence technique. However, in approximately 20 per cent of bullous pemphigoid cases, complement is also the only detectable component in the direct immunofluorescence test, and indirect immunofluorescence tests are negative. On the other hand, in a proportion of herpes gestationis cases IgG is bound in vivo, and circulating IgG antibodies occur at one time or another, not infrequently after the delivery.

The so-called herpes gestationis factor (i.e., in vitro complement fixation by the serum of patients with no detectable IgG antibodies) has been proved to be a basal membrane zone antibody at a level below the sensitivity of the routine immunofluorescence procedure, with a high complement-binding capacity, very much as in bullous pemphigoid. Evidence for the relationship of herpes gestationis and bullous pemphigoid is that the immune electron microscopic patterns are similar, i.e., immune deposits are present in the lamina lucida.

More controversial is the relationship of bullous pemphigoid and epidermolysis bullosa acquisita. The immunopathologic patterns of these diseases are quite similar at the light microscopy level.[18] The important difference, however, is that immune deposits can be localized below the basal lamina[19] in immune electron microscopy. This can also be confirmed in the tissue culture.[20] Thus, in spite of the identical immunopathology of bullous pemphigoid and epidermolysis bullosa acquisita both in direct immunofluorescence and in indirect immunofluorescence, the diseases should be regarded as separate entities. Immunofluorescence at the microscopy level is not contributory, whereas the diagnosis may be made by immune electron microscopy.

Dermatitis Herpetiformis. Direct immunofluorescence is disease-specific (granular, papillar IgA deposits).[21] However, if IgA deposits are in linear arrangement, the problem becomes controversial. Some authors believe these cases to be dermatitis herpetiformis with some atypical clinical and histologic features.[22,23] Others regard them as a variety of bullous pemphigoid because of a similar immunofluorescence pattern.[24] Still others believe that these cases are a separate entity: IgA linear bullous dermatosis, in which the immunofluorescence hallmark is linear IgA basal membrane zone deposits.[25,26] The controversy is still greater in the childhood form, chronic bullous disease of childhood, which was separated from both dermatitis herpetiformis and bullous pemphigoid of childhood primarily because of negative immunofluorescence findings.[27] However, the immunofluorescence marker of this bullous dermatosis is linear IgA deposits at the basal membrane zone and, in some cases, circulating basal membrane zone antibodies of the IgA class. A controversial problem remains as to whether this disease is related to bullous pemphigoid or to dermatitis herpetiformis or whether it is a separate entity—a counterpart of IgA linear bullous dermatosis of adults.

Although the controversy is far from settled, the identification of this disease seems to be of practical importance, because such cases usually respond to sulfones combined with small doses of corticosteroids. On the other hand, there are cases with both IgG and IgA basal membrane zone deposits and no circulating basal membrane zone antibodies that defy any classification. Such borderline cases are arbitrarily classified as either bullous pemphigoid or IgA linear bullous dermatosis. There are also highly controversial cases that more closely resemble dermatitis herpetiformis, with granular immune deposits, but that are located in a continuous pattern along the basal membrane zone. In our experience, such cases have to be classified as granular dermatitis herpetiformis.

Immunopathology in this group of bullous diseases is of decisive diagnostic importance. Cases with granular IgA deposits should be studied for the presence of gluten-sensitive enteropathy, and patients should be placed on a gluten-free diet.[28] In cases with a continuous homogeneous pattern of IgA deposits, on the other hand, there are no jejunal abnormalities, and the diet is not helpful.

Lupus Erythematosus

Immunofluorescence is a basic diagnostic procedure for lupus erythematosus—both the cutaneous and the systemic varieties. Immune deposits at the dermal/epidermal junction of the lesional skin are a characteristic finding in both discoid lupus erythematosus and systemic lupus erythematosus, whereas their presence in seemingly uninvolved skin is highly characteristic of systemic lupus erythematosus. Whatever the scope, the limitations of immunofluorescence are even greater here than in bullous diseases.

Discoid Lupus Erythematosus. In the cutaneous form, the results may be negative, especially in recent (less than 6 to 8 weeks' duration) and edematous lesions; in those localized to covered areas on the trunk, the arms, or elsewhere; and after a prolonged application of corticosteroids. Thus, the immunofluorescence tests may be negative in many typical cases of discoid lupus erythematosus. On the other hand, there may be false positive immunofluorescence results in cases of rosacea, lichen planus, and some other diseases. Recently, IgM dermal/epidermal junction deposits were found even in linear scleroderma, especially in children. Therefore, immunofluorescence findings, although very helpful, are not decisive in clinically and histologically atypical cases.

Systemic Lupus Erythematosus. The limitations of immunofluorescence in the detection of dermal/epidermal junction immune deposits in the lesional skin are the same as for discoid lupus erythematosus. Positive immunofluorescence findings in the seemingly uninvolved skin are in general of diagnostic significance. However, negative findings may be obtained in covered areas or may result from systemic corticosteroid or immunosuppressive treatment. On the other hand, we have seen dermal/epidermal junction deposits in the uninvolved skin of single cases of Hodgkin's disease and severe juvenile diabetes with kidney involvement.

Positive results have been reported in mixed connective tissue disease[29] and other overlap syndromes. In these cases the pattern of ANA is mostly speckled or, rarely, nucleolar on tissue substrate and small and speckled on Hep 2 cell culture, whereas in systemic lupus erythematosus the pattern is often homogeneous or peripheral. In the differentiation of systemic lupus erythematosus from systemic sclerosis, the positive immunofluorescence *Crithidia luciliae* test for d–s DNA is of importance. Immunofluorescence tests for ANA are not sufficient for differentiating various collagen diseases, especially systemic lupus erythematosus, mixed connective tissue disease, and systemic sclerosis, and additional serologic (mainly immunodiffusion) tests for antibodies against extractable nuclear and cytoplasmatic antigens are an important supplement.

The prospective tests are essentially serologic, with strictly defined antigens against separated components of nuclear DNA, RNA, cytoplasmatic organelles, and so forth. The antibody Sm, highly characteristic of systemic lupus erythematosus, has been found to be directed on the molecular level against small nuclear RNAs.[30,31] Some newly described antibodies may be detected by immunofluorescence (e.g., anticentromeres, centrioles); however, others are detectable mainly by immunodiffusion. Thus, limitations of immunofluorescence tests in collagenoses and other autoimmune diseases are rather significant.

Vascular Diseases

Another field in which immunofluorescence tests are very useful is vascular disorders.[32] However, here the limitations of the immunofluorescence method are especially prominent. The false negative results may be caused by the removal by polymorphonuclears of immune complexes fixed in the vessel walls, and the false positive results are usually related to the nonimmunologic trapping of immunoglobulins and complement components by destroyed vessel walls. To overcome this, one should perform the biopsy preferably in the seemingly uninvolved skin, possibly after injection of histamine solution.[33] Despite the limitations of immunofluoresence tests, characteristic findings are vascular IgA immune deposits in Schönlein's purpura, IgG and complement deposits in leukocytoclastic vasculitis, and IgM deposits in lymphocytic vasculitis.

Positive immunofluorescence results in the vessel walls are also characteristic in pyoderma gangrenosum and have been reported in erythema multiforme and in some cutaneous disorders.

Porphyria Cutanea Tarda. Positive homogeneous immunofluorescence deposits in and around the vessel walls in porphyria cutanea tarda are characteristic of the disease and are seen even in inactive cases. To a lesser extent, immune deposits are also present at the dermal/epidermal junction.[34] It appears that the immunoglobulins are nonimmunologically trapped within the vessel walls because of the reduplication of the vascular basal lamina. Thus, although deposits of immunoglobulins and complement seem to be unrelated to immune responses, the immunofluorescence tests are useful for diagnostic purposes.

Lichen Planus. Fluorescent cytoid bodies are a characteristic, but not a disease-specific, phenomenon and seem to be a secondary event. Whatever the limitations, immunofluorescence findings might be useful in differentiating lichen planus and lichen planus–like eruptions.

Psoriasis

Direct immunofluorescence tests in psoriasis consist of detecting immunoglobulins (mainly IgG and IgA) and complement fixed in vivo in the stratum corneum in a pattern characteristic of stratum corneum antibodies fixed on the specific substrate.[35,36] The significance of these findings is highly controversial, since similar patterns are sometimes observed in other cutaneous disorders. It is not clear whether this is a basic immunologic event or an epiphenomenon.

CONCLUSIONS

Immunofluorescence tests, although indispensable in modern dermatology (specifically in the diagnosis of bullous and collagen diseases), have important limitations. These concern mainly the pathogenic significance of immune deposits, the evaluation of the results, and the role of the findings in monitoring treatment.

References

1. Beutner, E. H., Chorzelski, T. P., and Bean, S. F.: Immunopathology of the Skin. New York, John Wiley & Sons, 1979.
2. Beutner, E. H., and Jordon, R. E.: Demonstration of skin antibodies in sera of pemphigus vulgaris patients in indirect immunofluorescence staining. Proc. Soc. Exp. Biol. Med. 117:505, 1964.
3. Chorzelski, T. P., von Weiss, H. F., and Lever, W. F.: Clinical significance of autoantibodies in pemphigus. Arch. Dermatol. 93:570, 1966.
4. Sams, W. M., and Jordon, R. E.: Correlation of pemphigoid and pemphigus antibody titers with activity of the disease. Br. J. Dermatol. 84:7, 1971.
5. Judd, K. P., and Lever, W. F.: Correlation of antibodies in skin and serum with disease severity in pemphigus. Arch. Dermatol. 115:428, 1979.
6. Fitzpatrick, R. E., and Newcomer, V. D.: The correlation of disease activity and antibody titers in pemphigus. Arch. Dermatol. 116:285, 1980.
7. Heine, K. G., Kumar, A., and Jordon, R. E.: Pemphigus-like antibodies in bullous pemphigoid. Arch. Dermatol. 113:1693, 1977.
8. Kumar, V., Beutner, E. H., Chorzelski, T. P., and Jablońska, S.: Letter to the editor. Arch. Dermatol. Res. 263:239, 1978.
9. Nishikawa, T., Kurishara, S., and Hatano, H.: Comparison of in vivo and in vitro capability of complement fixation by pemphigus antibodies. Dermatologica 159:290, 1979.
10. Schiltz, J. R.: Pemphigus acantholysis: A unique immunological injury. J. Invest. Dermatol. 74:359, 1980.
11. Jordon, R. E.: Complement activation in pemphigus. J. Invest. Dermatol. 74:357, 1980.
12. Jordon, R. E., Sams, W. M., Jr., Diaz, G., and Beutner, E. H.: Negative complement immunofluorescence in pemphigus. J. Invest. Dermatol. 56:407, 1971.
13. Cram, D. L., and Fukuyama, K.: Immunochemistry of ultraviolet-induced pemphigus and pemphigoid lesions. Arch. Dermatol. 106:819, 1972.
14. Chorzelski, T. P., and Beutner, E. H.: Factors contributing to the occasional failures of detection of pemphigus antibodies by indirect immunofluorescence test. J. Invest. Dermatol., 53:188–191, 1969.
15. Person, J. R., Rogers, R. S., and Perry, H. O.: Localized pemphigoid. Br. J. Dermatol. 95:531, 1976.
16. Hall, R. P., Lawley, T. J., Smith, H. R., and Katz, S. I.: Bullous eruption of systemic lupus erythematosus. Ann. Intern. Med. 97:165, 1982.

17. Provost, T. T., Yaoita, H., and Katz, S. I.: Herpes gestationis. *In* Beutner, E. H. Chorzelski, T. P., and Bean, S. F. (eds.): Immunopathology of the Skin. John Wiley & Sons, 1979, pp. 273–282.
18. Wilson, B. D., Birnkrant, A. F., Beutner, E. M., and Maize, J. C.: Epidermolysis bullosa acquisita: A clinical disorder of varied etiologies. J. Am. Acad. Dermatol. 3:280, 1980.
19. Yaoita, H., Briggaman, R. A., Lawley, T. J., Provost, T. T., and Katz, S. I.: Epidermolysis bullosa acquisita: Ultrastructural and immunological studies. J. Invest. Dermatol. 76:288, 1981.
20. Chorzelski, T., Petkow, L., Dąbrowski, J., Kraińska, T., Sulej, J., Jablońska, S., and Beutner, E. H.: Epidermolysis bullosa acquisita. Hautarzt 32:487, 1981.
21. Katz, S. I., and Strober, W.: The pathogenesis of dermatitis herpetiformis. J. Invest. Dermatol. 70:63, 1978.
22. Yaoita, H., Hertz, K. C., and Katz, S. I.: Dermatitis herpetiformis: Immunoelectronmicroscopic and ultrastructural studies of a patient with linear depositon of IgA. J. Invest. Dermatol. 67:691, 1976.
23. Pehamberger, H., Konrad, K., and Holubar, K.: Circulating IgA anti–basement membrane antibodies in linear dermatitis herpetiformis (Duhring): Immunofluorescence and immunoelectronmicroscopic studies. J. Invest. Dermatol. 69:490, 1977.
24. Provost, T. T., Maize, J. C., Ahmed, A. R., Strauss, J. S., and Dobson, R. L.: Unusual subepidermal bullous diseases with immunologic features of bullous pemphigoid. Arch. Dermatol. 115:156, 1979.
25. Jablońska, S., Chorzelski, T. P., Beutner, E. H., Maciejowska, E., and Rzesa, G.: Dermatitis herpetiformis and bullous pemphigoid. Intermediate and mixed forms. Arch. Dermatol. 112:45, 1976.
26. Chorzelski, T. P., and Jablońska, S.: IgA linear dermatosis of childhood (chronic bullous disease of childhood). Br. J. Dermatol. 101:535, 1979.
27. Jordon, R. E., Bean, S. F., and Triftshauser, C. T.: Childhood bullous dermatitis herpetiformis. Arch. Dermatol. 101:629, 1970.
28. Fry, L., and Seah, P. P.: Dermatitis herpetiformis. *In* Fry, L., and Seah, P. P. (eds.): Immunological Aspects of Skin Diseases. New York, John Wiley & Sons, 1974, pp. 22–65.
29. Sharp, G. C.: Mixed connective tissue disease. *In* McCarty, D. J. (ed.): Arthritis and Allied Conditions, 9th ed. Philadelphia, Lea & Febiger, 1979, pp. 737–741.
30. Lerner, M. R., and Steitz, J. A.: Antibodies to small nuclear RNAs complexed with proteins are produced by patients with systemic lupus erythematosus. Proc. Natl. Acad. Sci. U.S.A. 76:5495, 1979.
31. Takano, M., Golden, S. S., Sharp, G. C., and Agris, P. F.: Molecular relationships between two nuclear antigens, ribonucleoprotein and Sm: Purification of active antigens and their biochemical characterization. Biochemistry 20:5929, 1981.
32. Sams, W. M.: Leukocytoclastic vasculitis. *In* Beutner, E. H., Chorzelski, T. P., and Bean, S. F. (eds.): Immunopathology of the Skin. New York, John Wiley & Sons, 1979, pp. 463–470.
33. Braverman, I. M., and Yen, A.: Demonstration of immune complexes in spontaneous and histamine-induced lesions and in normal skin of patients with leukocytoclastic angitis. J. Invest. Dermatol. 64:105, 1975.
34. Epstein, J. M., Tuffanelli, D. L., and Epstein, W. L.: Cutaneous porphyrias and porphyria-like cutaneous changes induced by drug photosensitization. *In* Beutner, E. H., Chorzelski, S. F., and Bean, S. F. (eds.): Immunopathology of the Skin. New York, John Wiley & Sons, 1979, pp. 445–463.
35. Beutner, E. H., Jablońska, S., Jarzabek-Chorzelska, M., Maciejowska, E., Rzesa, G., and Chorzelski, T. P.: Studies in immunodermatology. VI. IF studies of autoantibodies in the stratum corneum and of in vivo fixed IgG in stratum corneum of psoriatic scales. Int. Arch. Allergy Appl. Immun. 48:301, 1975.
36. Jablońska, S., Beutner, E. H., Jarzabek-Chorzelska, M., Maciejowska, E., Rzesa, G., Chowaniec, O., and Chorzelski, T. P.: Clinical significance of autoimmunity in psoriasis. *In* Milgrom, F., and Albini, B. (eds.): Immunopathology. Basel, S. Karger, 1979, pp. 148–153.

SECTION 8

PATCH TESTS

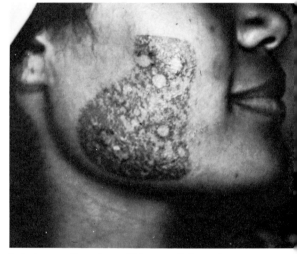

A do-it-yourself patch test. This young lady was ironing clothing when the telephone rang. Instead of putting the receiver to her ear, she picked up the hot iron and absent-mindedly touched it to her face.

CHAPTER 25

SAFETY

THE SAFETY OF PATCH TESTING

Alexander A. Fisher, M.D.

In patch testing, as in making love, if proper precautions are taken, the results can be quite beneficial and free of adverse reactions.

Indeed, the greatest hazard in the management of patients with certain dermatoses is the omission of patch testing procedures. Such omission dooms these patients to repeated attacks of avoidable contact dermatitis.

The great importance of patch testing has been most recently re-emphasized by Sulzberger.[1] In answer to the question in the *Schoch Letter*—"What are the five most important advances in clinical dermatology during the twentieth century?"—Sulzberger replied:

(1) *The increased use and usefulness of the patch tests and the international standardization of test concentrations and methods.** (2) The effectiveness of topical steroids in inflammatory and itching dermatoses. (3) The life-saving effect of systemic steroids in pemphigus vulgaris and their effectiveness in treatment of amny other dermatoses. (4) Immunofluorescent techniques in diagnosis of different bullous and other dermatoses. (5) The demonstration of the role of Langerhans' cells in allergic contact dermatitis and the potential roles of these cells in the prevention of allergic contact dermatitis, homograft rejection resistance to cancer.

It should be noted that Sulzberger lists patch tests as the *first* most important advance in clinical dermatology. Obviously, such a clinically important diagnostic procedure should not be withheld because certain rare, and mostly minor, adverse reactions may occur.[2] Table 1 lists such reactions.

Active Sensitization from Patch Tests

A response that occurs after 7 days or later with no preceding effect is a late reaction caused by the interaction of residues of the allergen with the newly sensitized tissues. This type of reaction is sometimes called a "spontaneous flare." The sign of such active sensitization is either that the patch test becomes positive 10 to 14 days after application (flare-

Table 1. ALLEGED ADVERSE
PATCH TEST REACTIONS

Active sensitization
Irritant patch test reactions
"Ectopic" flare of dermatitis
Koebner phenomenon
Persistence of a positive reaction
Hyper- and hypopigmentation at the sites of
  positive patch test reactions
Anaphylactoid reaction
The "angry back" syndrome

*Emphasis added.

367

Table 2. ROUTINE "STANDARD SCREENING PATCH TEST SERIES"*

Nickel sulfate 2.5%
Ethylenediamine dihydrochloride 1%
Paraphenylenediamine 1%
Benzocaine 5%
Paraben mixture 15%
Thimerosal (Merthiolate) 0.1%
Ammoniated mercury 1%
Wool alcohols 30%
Formaldehyde 2% aqueous
Mercaptobenzothiazole 1%
Tetramethylthiuram disulfide 2%
Potassium dichromate 0.025%
Neomycin sulfate 20%
Balsam of Peru 25%
Epoxy resin 1%

---

*All are tested in petrolatum vehicle, except formaldehyde.

up) and is positive when repeated in 2 to 4 days or that reactions occur in patients who are systematically retested after an interval.

I have used the "Standard Screening Patch Test Series" (Table 2) on hundreds of patients in the past 10 years, and I am not aware of having sensitized a single patient by the patch test procedure. It should be emphasized that for all the "standard" allergens, the correct patch test concentrations are known, and lists have been published.[3-7] The most frequent cause of active sensitization is the use of an excessively high concentration of the test substance; of lesser importance are the amount applied and the length of time that the patch is worn. However, since the proper concentration of each "standard" chemical has now been determined after thousands of patients have been tested, sensitizing reactions are currently being avoided.[8-10]

Cronin[3] correctly states,* "Active sensitization is a *complication* of patch testing *but is not a hazard* and it should not be used as an excuse by the *indolent* for eschewing this investigation. To reject patch testing is the greater disservice to the patient."

Agrup[11] reported the results of a retest of 379 hand eczema patients with 11 substances that had first been applied 6 to 21 months previously. In 281 (74 per cent) the results were unchanged, in 73 (19 per cent) tests had become positive, in 19 (5 per cent) tests had become negative, and in 6 (2 per cent) some tests had become positive and others had become negative. The allergens for which there was a statistically significant change were potassium dichromate (0.29 per cent in water), cobalt chloride (2.4 per cent in water), paraphenylenediamine (2.2 per cent in ethanol), para-aminoazobenzene (0.9 per cent in methyl ethyl ketone), and diaminophenylmethane (2 per cent in methyl ethyl ketone).

Among the 79 patients thought to have been sensitized by the patch tests, 20 per cent had healed, 52 per cent had improved, 20 per cent were the same, and 8 per cent were worse. Agrup concluded that the course of the hand dermatitis was the same whether or not the patients had become sensitized by the tests. In these patients, therefore, the clinical course was unaffected by patch testing, and they were not harmed by the investigation.

It should be noted that even though this investigative patch test procedure exposed the patients to "nonstandard" vehicles, no marked adverse reactions occurred. For example, Agrup tested paraphenylenediamine 2.2 per cent in alcohol, but the present "standard" is 1 per cent in petrolatum, a much "safer" concentration and vehicle. Also, Agrup employed a powerful solvent, methyl ethyl ketone, as a vehicle for para-aminobenzene and diaminophenylmethane, which are now tested with the much "safer" petrolatum vehicle. The margin of "safety" was thus shown to be quite great, since such unorthodox vehicles did not sensitize the patient.

---

*Emphasis added.

As far as paraphenylenediamine is concerned, in the "old" days, when patients were tested with various concentrations of this dye (even as high as 8 per cent), active sensitization did occur. At present, testing this dye in a 1 per cent concentration is eminently "safe" and free of the hazard of sensitizing the tested patient.

To study the risk of sensitization from patch testing, Meneghini, Rantuccio, and Lomuto[12] retested 181 patients with eczema and 100 patients with noneczematous dermatoses. New positive patch tests were found in 31 patients with eczema and in four of the other group. These authors concluded that sensitization had been caused by further environmental exposure rather than active sensitization from the patch test. In a follow-up study, Meneghini and Angelini[13] emphasized that patch testing does not cause new sensitizations to any significant extent, provided that proper techniques are used.

Adams,[2] stating that active sensitization is, fortunately, rare with "standard" allergens, warns that testing with substances of unknown composition that are brought in by patients presents the greatest hazard of the patch test procedure.

Malten[7] states that the following "nonstandard" substances (if applied in sufficient concentration) undoubtedly have a sensitizing capacity: DNCB (2,4-dinitro-1-chlorobenzene), NDMA (p-nitrosodimethylaniline), and certain natural products of plants, e.g., leaves of poison ivy and of *Primula obconica*. Malten emphasizes that precisely because they are such potent sensitizers, these substances will not be used industrially, which makes their patch testing in search of the cause of contact eczema unnecessary.

Irritant Patch Test Reactions

The correct concentration of an allergen will give a moderate reaction in a sensitized person but none in controls. With bland chemicals, this concentration is easy to determine, but for the many allergens that also are irritants, the concentration necessary to elicit an allergic reaction may differ very little from that producing an irritant response. Failure to appreciate this causes misinterpretation of results and is a major stumbling block in patch testing.

In the standard screening patch test series, even the 1 per cent aqueous solution of formaldehyde will give a mild, noneczematous erythema, which is not an allergic reaction. Also, nickel occasionally will produce a nonspecific pustular reaction that is of no significance.

When tests are performed with a "nonstandard" allergen, the correct concentration has to be determined for most chemicals. An initial test concentration of 0.1 to 1.0 per cent is suitable for clinical use, but for known irritants it should be weaker. If the results are negative, the concentration can be increased. One should check a positive reaction that looks allergic by using this same concentration to test approximately ten controls. Many substances used in daily life, such as cosmetics and medicaments, can be used without dilution, but under the occluded conditions of patch testing some are mild irritants. Testing should not be performed with undiluted solvents, gasoline, soaps, or detergents.

One can avoid serious irritations by using standard procedures. These include pretesting of substances of unknown composition in a number of volunteers (including the investigator). Substances should be toxicologically and allergologically investigated before they are used in industrial work. This also involves an assay of possible dermatologic toxicity.

Irritant and allergic reactions to the patch test materials and to adhesive tape were formerly quite common. With the advent of the modern aluminum patch, the Finn chamber, and nonrubber acrylate adhesives (Dermicel, Scanpore), such reactions have been greatly minimized.

"Ectopic" Flare of Dermatitis

On rare occasions, a positive patch test reaction may be accompanied by a flare-up of an existing or pre-existing dermatitis caused by the test allergen. Thus, a positive patch reaction to nickel sulfate may produce a flare-up of a pre-existing nickel ear lobe or wrist dermatitis.

I have found that when such a flare-up occurs it has proved to be a beneficial, educational experience for both the patient and the physician, because it emphasizes the importance of the avoidance of the contact allergen by the sensitized patient.

The Koebner Phenomenon

A positive patch test reaction in a patient with active psoriasis or lichen planus may reproduce the dermatoses at the patch test site. The application of a corticosteroid preparation usually clears this localized ''hazard'' quickly.

Persistence of a Positive Patch Test Reaction

In my experience, the only patch test reaction that has persisted for more than a month is one that was caused by a 0.5 per cent aqueous solution of gold chloride in a gold-sensitive individual. Allergic contact gold dermatitis is known to persist even when there has been no re-exposure to gold. The persistence of the positive gold patch test reaction merely confirms the clinical phenomenon. Intralesional injections of a corticosteroid into the patch test site quickly control the persistent reaction.

Alteration in Pigmentation

I have encountered hyperpigmentation from patch tests only in black skin. Such hyperpigmentation may last for several weeks and usually responds well to 1 per cent hydrocortisone. Hydroquinone should not be used, since it may produce depigmentation (contact leukoderma).

Also, sunlight exposure immediately following removal of patches where coal tar or fragrance materials have been tested may also result in hyperpigmentation. Sometimes a severe reaction may cause hyperpigmentation or total depigmentation. Hyperpigmentation may result from irritant reactions in certain patients from the inflammation alone, independent of the responsible allergen.

Since patch testing is usually performed on the back, which is covered by clothing, these temporary pigmentary changes do not present serious hazards. Preparations such as Covermark may be used until the pigmentation clears.

Anaphylactoid Reaction from Patch Testing

Very rarely, anaphylactoid reactions are seen within 30 minutes after topical testing with certain antibiotics, such as penicillin, neomycin, gentamycin, or bacitracin. Nitrogen mustard may also produce such a reaction.[14]

In addition to these specific allergic reactions, ammonium persulfate used as a ''booster'' of hydrogen peroxide for bleaching ''platinum blondes'' may extremely rarely produce a nonspecific, idiosyncratic release of histamine with a resulting anaphylactoid reaction. Patch testing with ammonium persulphate is not advised. If the test is performed under unusual circumstances, e.g., a medicolegal procedure, readily available injectable epinepherine should be on hand.[15]

The "Angry Back" Syndrome

Many years ago, Max Jessner would state that certain patients had a "crazy back." Such patients are now labeled as having an "angry back," or "excited" skin syndrome.

Mitchell[16] described the "angry back" as a regional phenomenon caused by the presence of a strongly positive reaction. The reaction produces a state of skin hyper-reactivity in which other patch test sites become reactive (especially marginal irritants, such as formalin or potassium dichromate). Mitchell believes that these concomitant "positive" reactions are unreliable. He tested 35 patients who showed 90 positive 1+ reactions to 28 substances at 48 hours. He then retested them on Day 7. On Day 9, 42 per cent of the reactions were negative, suggesting that false positive reactions were common when one strong positive reaction occurred. Mitchell suggests that the true index of sensitivity is falsely exaggerated by concomitant testing. To confirm or deny the significance of individual reactions found on the "angry back," Mitchell recommends sequential testing performed later with each substance alone.

I have found that nickel sulfate and potassium dichromate are the two "standard" patch test allergens that are most likely to engender nonspecific reactions in adjacent patch test materials. These strongly positive patch test reactions may be confused with allergic responses. Whenever the clinical history strongly suggests that either one of these common allergens may produce a positive reaction, I have placed the nickel or dichromate on the arm, away from the other patches, and have thus avoided the "angry back."

References

1. Sulzberger, M.: Important advances in clinical dermatology. Schoch Letter 31, no. 10, item 14, 1981.
2. Adams, R. M.: Patch testing—a recapitulation. J. Am. Acad. Dermatol. 5:637, 1981.
3. Cronin, E.: Contact Dermatitis. London, Churchill Livingstone, 1980.
4. Fisher, A. A.: Contact Dermatitis, 2nd ed. Philadelphia, Lea & Febiger, 1973.
5. Fregert, S.: Manual of Contact Dermatitis. Copenhange, Munksgaard, 1974.
6. Rook, A., Wilkinson, D. S., and Ebling, F. J. G.: Textbook for Dermatology, vol. 1. Oxford, Blackwell Scientific Publications, 1979.
7. Malten, K. E., Nater, J. P., and van Ketel, W. G.: Patch Testing Guidelines. Nijmeager, Dekker en Van de Vegt, 1976.
8. Brun, R.: Epidemiology of contact dermatitis in Geneva (1000 cases). Contact Dermatitis 1:277, 1975.
9. Rudner, E. J.: North American group results. Contact Dermatitis 3:208, 1977.
10. Romaguera, C., and Grimalt, F.: Statistical and comparative study of 46,000 patients tested in Barcelona (1973–1977). Contact Dermatitis 4:301, 1978.
11. Agrup, G.: Sensitization induced by patch testing. Br. J. Dermatol. 80:631, 1968.
12. Meneghini, C. L., Rantuccio, F., and Lomuto, M.: A propos de réactions de sensibilisation active après l'execution des tests diagnostiques épicutanes: Observations sur 281 cas. Ann. Dermatol. Syph. 99:161, 1972.
13. Meneghini, C.L., and Angelini, G.: Behavior of contact allergy and new sensitivities on subsequent patch tests. Contact Dermatitis 3:138, 1977.
14. von Krogh, G., and Maibach, H.: The contact uritcaria syndrome. An updated review. J. Am. Acad. Dermatol. 5:328, 1981.
15. Fisher, A. A., and Dooms-Goossens, A.: Persulfate hair bleach reactions. Arch. Dermatol. 112:1407, 1976.
16. Mitchell, J. G.: The angry back syndrome: Eczema creates eczema. Contact Dermatitis 1:1934, 1974.

PATCH TESTING: HAZARDS

Robert A. Snyder, M.D.
Howard I. Maibach, M.D.

Since the introduction of patch testing eight decades ago, its use has become widespread as a means of investigating causes of exogenous dermatoses in human beings. When comparing patch testing with other, more invasive, diagnostic methods in modern medicine, few would argue that it is a low-risk procedure. When patch testing is performed properly, its potential benefit outweighs the potential risk to the patient. Nonetheless, adverse reactions as a result of patch testing are not uncommon. We will summarize the possible complications that may arise in the course of patch testing.

Severe Reactions to Test Substances

The most common adverse reaction to patch testing is a severe eczematous response at test sites that results in patient discomfort. An excessive irritant reaction not infrequently occurs when unknown chemical substances are taken out of the work place for use in patch tests. Occasionally, an exuberant allergic response to a test substance (i.e., a strongly positive test) can result in significant discomfort at the test site. False positive severe and, sometimes, ulcerative irritant reactions occur with a frequency directly related to the physician's (and the nurse's) experience (or lack thereof) with patch testing. These reactions occur early in the dermatologist's career; the resultant horror leads either to abandonment of the method or to a more serious approach to the complexity of technique. With the advent of training fellowships and dermatology departments with rotations through contact dermatitis clinics, the incidence of such errors should be minimized. The novitiate choosing the route of self-education may greatly decrease the risk to the patient by thorough and repeated study of Malten's classical guidelines to patch testing with "environmentals"—a euphemism for the contents of the various bottles, bags, and boxes that patients bring in. (The task is further complicated by smudged and handwritten or inadequate labels.) Malten's text is not widely available but is worth seeking, because it is the only such guideline.[1] An alternative approach consists of patch testing with the well standardized routine series only—and referring patients who need to be tested with "environmentals" to an appropriate center. Another method consists of discussing the case with an experienced colleague. This is best not performed as a curbstone consultation, since the exact details (concentration, vehicle, and so forth) are critical in minimizing ulceration as well as false positive and false negative reactions.

In addition to the local discomfort that can result from excessive patch test reactions, we have recently seen a patient with tender lymphadenopathy draining a strongly positive patch test. One can sometimes minimize unusually severe reactions by instructing patients to remove patch tests when high degrees of discomfort develop. Additionally, use of the Finn chamber has been helpful in localizing severe reactions when they do occur.

"Flare-up"

"Flare-up," or "focal flare," refers to the phenomenon of reactivation of an eczematous process at its original site by a positive patch test. Such reactions are occasionally severe enough to require administration of systemic corticosteroids. In addition, a strongly positive test can at times result in a state of skin hyperactivity in which other patch test sites become positive, adding to the patient's discomfort. This phenomenon, referred to as the "angry back," or "excited skin," syndrome, has recently been reviewed.[2]

Adhesive Tape Reactions

Mild adhesive tape reactions are not uncommon. One can generally avoid severe eczematous tape reactions by use of nonocclusive acrylic tapes. Nonocclusive tapes should be used especially for patients with a previous history of adhesive tape sensitivity. The patches that currently are used (the Al test and the Finn chamber) are themselves occlusive, and therefore occlusive tapes are not required.

Pigmentary Changes

Strongly positive patch tests may result in postinflammatory hyperpigmentation[3] or, occasionally, depigmentation. These reactions are more common in heavily pigmented individuals. Patch testing with known depigmenting agents (e.g., monobenzyl ether of hydroquinone) may result in depigmentation.

Keloid Formation

The formation of a scar or keloid at the site of a patch test is a rare complication of patch testing.[4] This reaction is likely to be related to the extent of the inflammatory response as well as to individual susceptibility. We have observed two such lesions that gradually disappeared without treatment, suggesting that they were not keloids but hypertrophic scars.

Systemic Absorption of Toxic Materials

At dosages usually used in routine patch testing, sufficient systemic absorption of test substances resulting in toxicity is an unlikely, but theoretically possible, occurrence. This is most apt to occur when unknown substances are used for testing. Several examples of probable systemic effects as a result of systemic absorption of test substances from patch tests will be described in this section. Gastrointestinal symptoms of nausea and diarrhea have been reported to occur in association with contact dermatitis to hydroxyethylmethacrylate. These symptoms were reproduced with patch testing of the substance.[5] Periorbital edema, flushing of the face and the neck, and gastrointestinal upset were reported to occur during the course of patch testing in a patient with contact urticaria to teak.[6] Nausea, vomiting, weakness, vertigo, and diaphoresis developed in a patient who underwent patch testing of a spray containing nicotine.[7] Finally, respiratory symptoms were reported to develop in a patient with contact dermatitis to piperazine following patch testing of this substance.[8]

Although partially anecdotal, the aforementioned reports suggest that systemic reactions to test substances can occur as a result of patch testing. We therefore attempt to obtain acute toxicity information concerning materials with significant pharmacologic activity. This is especially important in dealing with pesticides, some of which are highly potent toxins for human beings as well as insects. It thus may be necessary to limit the applied dose to decrease the risk of systemic toxicity. Since most pure allergens will elicit a positive allergic reaction in relatively small amounts, this should only infrequently lead to a false negative patch test response.

Infectious Complications

Inoculation herpes simplex infection at a patch test site has been reported in a patient who had an incompletely healed herpetic infection of the lip at the time of patch testing.[9] Candidal infections and furunculosis are also known to develop at the site of occluded patch tests. When observing an unusual adhesive tape or patch test reaction, we consider not only *Candida* but also other fungal infections as well as staphylococcal and streptococcal lesions. Many such pustules contain only gram-positive rods (*Propionibacterium acnes*). We emphasize that most candidal and bacterial infections induced by tape or occlusion clear without antimicrobial therapy; *P. acnes* folliculitis does so routinely.

Active Sensitization

Patch testing entails a risk of sensitization to the test material. Sensitization often manifests itself by a delayed reaction ("flare-up") at the patch test site 10 to 14 days after testing. When this occurs, retesting at a later date can document the development of sensitization. Active sensitization has been reported with potent allergens, such as poison ivy, *Primula obconica*, streptomycin, reactive diluents for epoxy resins, beryllium, and azo compounds. When testing with such materials, one should use low concentrations to minimize the risk of sensitization. The importance of the concentration of patch test material has been emphasized in one study that documented an increased incidence of sensitization to *p*-phenylenediamine 8 per cent in petrolatum when compared with 2 per cent in petrolatum.[10]

The exact risk of active sensitization is not known. One study of 379 patients with hand eczema showed 21 per cent to have positive reactions to patch test substances to which they had not reacted 6 to 21 months previously.[11] Although some have interpreted this relatively high rate of sensitization to active sensitization during patch testing, others have provided some evidence that the development of new positive tests on retesting is more likely the result of further occupational exposure during the period between patch tests.[12] To date, no study has documented an adverse effect on the course of a patient's eczema as a result of active sensitization to a substance during patch testing. Although this phenomenon presumably can occur, it must be uncommon.

Anaphylaxis, Angioedema, and Asthma

Most patients with delayed hypersensitivity reactions do not also have *clinical* manifestations of immediate sensitivity, i.e., contact urticaria, angioedema, asthma, and anaphylaxis (i.e., the contact urticaria syndrome). Most cases worked up for this syndrome are first identified on the basis of clinical history and are followed up with appropriate open, scratch, or prick testing. When the history suggests anaphylaxis, full precautions should be taken to protect the patient. Rarely, the patient may develop the contact urticaria syndrome when patch tested, even though there may have been no previous indication that this would occur. For this reason, a patch test clinic should have appropriate therapeutic facilities available. In any instance, the risk that the patient will develop contact urticaria syndrome in a controlled environment is much lower than the risk that is involved if the physician does not test and does not make the diagnosis; the latter choice places the patient in greater danger of inadvertent challenge at a time when therapy is not available. In 1981, von Krogh published a series of recommendations on contact urticaria testing; a careful review of this article should minimize the hazard of such testing.[13]

CONCLUSION

Patch testing, like many diagnostic methods, is not without hazard. The risk is greatly decreased by expertise with the method. In any instance, the risk of not identifying the allergen is greater than that of performing such testing.

References

1. Malten, K. E., Nater, J. P., and van Ketel, W. G.: Patch Testing Guidelines. Nijmegen, Dekker en Van de Vegt, 1976.
2. Mitchell, J. C., and Maibach, H. I.: The angry back syndrome—the excited skin syndrome. Semin. Dermatol. 1:9, 1982.
3. Rudzki, E., and Gryzwa, Z.: Hyperpigmentation from irritant patch tests. Contact Dermatitis 3:138, 1977.
4. Calnan, C. D.: Keloid formation after patch tests. Contact Dermatitis 7:279, 1981.
5. Mathias, C. G. T., Caldwell, T. M., and Maibach, H. I.: Contact dermatitis and gastrointestinal symptoms from hydroxyethylmethacrylate. Br. J. Dermatol. 100:447, 1979.
6. Schmidt, H.: Contact urticaria to teak with systemic effects. Contact Dermatitis 4:176, 1978.
7. Epstein, E.: Untoward reactions to patch tests. J. Invest. Dermatol. 5:55, 1942.
8. Fregert, S.: Respiratory symptoms with piperazine patch testing. Contact Dermatitis 2:61, 1977.
9. Calnan, C. D: Inoculation herpes simplex as a complication of patch tests. Contact Dermatitis Newsletter, 10:232, 1971.
10. Skog, E.: Sensitization to p-phenylenediamine. Arch Dermatol., 92:276, 1965.
11. Agrup, G.: Sensitization induced by patch testing. Br. J. Dermatol. 80:631, 1968.
12. Meneghini, C. L., and Agelini, G.: Behavior of contact allergy and new sensitivities on subsequent patch tests. Contact Dermatitis 3:138, 1977.
13. von Krogh, G., and Maibach, H. I.: The contact urticaria syndrome—an updated review. J. Am. Acad. Dermatol. 5:328, 1981.

Editorial Comment

In all probability, nothing in medicine is completely free of hazards. However, patch tests are reasonably safe. Furthermore, since the dangers are basically caused by human error, the procedure itself is benign. One should not forget that ignorance and carelessness can create problems and make the test harmful to the subject.

False interpretation of tests can lead to difficulties that may haunt a patient for the rest of his life. A reaction resulting from a primary irritant may cause the patient to believe that he is sensitive to a certain substance. In some cases, this supposed sensitivity can interfere with his employability or his life style. Also, it may prevent the performance of further tests that might establish the correct diagnosis. Over-reading of the test results may have the same effect. In other words, crediting a 1+ reaction with the same significance as a 4+ reaction might lead to serious errors in interpretation. Primary irritant reactions may result from applying a substance that is basically irritating (such as an acid or an alkali) under occlusion, using too strong a concentration, or keeping the test on the skin for too long. It is wise to remove a test in less than the prescribed amount of time if the patient complains of a severe itching or burning sensation.

Primary irritants may cause not only erythema but also blisters containing purulent or clear fluid, necrosis, ulceration, hyperpigmentation or hypopigmentation, slow healing, and scarring, all of which are complications to be avoided.

Patch tests may lead to the development of hypersensitivity. One of the methods of sensitizing an individual is applying a foreign substance repeatedly. Sometimes, a single patch test will result in sensitization in a local area, or the changes may be widespread and may cause a dermatitis plus other signs of sensitivity at the next application.

Absorption of a test substance may lead to irritation of the present dermatitis or relapse of one that has cleared. For example, this may occur in individuals who have or who have had an exfoliative dermatitis from neoarsphenamine or related antisyphilitic agents. Although these medications are not administered for this purpose today, other allergens, including drugs that are currently used, may cause the same type of reaction.

A more serious reaction to agents applied to the skin under occlusion is the absorption of toxic substances. In my experience, a number of toxins have caused this poisoning. The outstanding example of this phenomenon occurred in a Japanese gardener who had never indulged in the smoking of tobacco. However, he did handle a number of nicotine-containing pesticides. Within 30 minutes of a patch test with these sprays, he experienced collapse, weakness, cold sweat, hypotension, vomiting, and other complications—the same symptoms that one would encounter in an individual who is smoking and inhaling his first cigar.

Most books on allergic reactions of the skin, including those that discuss industrial dermatoses, give tables of safe concentrations of various substances for patch testing. Anyone who performs these studies should have consulted such lists before subjecting a patient to the tests. Acceptance of these lists would eliminate most of the reactions mentioned in this discussion. On the other hand, patients may bring in chemicals that are new or experimental. In most cases, the safe dilution of these substances for patch testing has not been established. In such instances, one should be very conservative and should dilute the industrial compounds to a low level before applying them to the skin. Accurate interpretation of the results might require comparison with control studies performed on a normal volunteer. It might be wise to apply various concentrations to the subject in order to establish safe dilutions in case other workers or purchasers present contact dermatitides while using the suspected substance or compound.

Think It Over.

SECTION 9

VITAMIN E

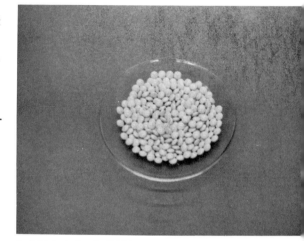

A dishful of vitamin E tablets.

CHAPTER 26

EFFECTIVENESS

VITAMIN E: AN EFFECTIVE THERAPEUTIC AGENT IN DERMATOLOGY

Samuel Ayres, Jr., M.D.

Ever since vitamin E (tocopherol) was discovered by Evans and Bishop in 1922,[1] its importance in maintaining normal physiologic processes and its value in treating various disease states have been the subject of much controversy.

Probably the most important function of vitamin E is its role as an antioxidant.[2,3] Cell membranes of all tissues are composed of lipoproteins. The lipid portion of the lipoproteins tends to combine with oxygen, and this lipid peroxidation liberates free radicals of unpaired electrons, which have a very destructive effect upon cell membranes and the membranes of intracellular organelles, including lysosomes. Damaged lysosomes release enzymes, which, according to Criep,[4] may attach themselves to normal tissues, altering them and causing the body to produce autoimmune antibodies. Since vitamin E protects cell membranes, it should be of value in treating autoimmune diseases.[5]

A variety of autoimmune diseases affecting various tissues of the body may develop as the result of lipid peroxidation of cell membranes. Under normal conditions, cell membranes are provided with adequate quantities of vitamin E to retard peroxidation to the degree involved in the normal aging process. Abnormal lipid peroxidation may be caused by various factors: inadequate supply of vitamin E, congenital requirement for much larger quantities than the average, defective absorption, or defective utilization caused by abnormal physiologic function or various diseases.

Since free radical damage to cellular structures may produce a variety of immunologic abnormalities, it would appear more effective for treatment of some uncommon diseases of unknown etiology to be centered on protection of cell membranes rather than on immunosuppression, which inhibits the body's normal defenses against diseases. In other words, one should treat the cause (lipid peroxidation of cell membranes) rather than the result (immunologic abnormalities).

According to Schwartz,[6] in addition to its function as an antioxidant, vitamin E facilitates oxygen utilization in normal metabolic processes through its relationships with certain enzymes and other vitamins and minerals. It performs a truly catalytic function in enzyme systems that are essential to normal life. One of the most important recent findings concerning this function was the discovery by Ames[7] of a strong synergism between vitamin E and vitamin A. This has proved to be of great value in several dermatoses involving defective keratinization.

The amount of lipid peroxidation and its protection by vitamin E has recently been determined by measurements of exhaled pentane.[8]

Structure and Function of Vitamin E

Vitamin E is oil-soluble, but water-miscible forms are available. It is composed of four fractions—alpha, beta, gamma, and delta—of which the alpha fraction is believed to be most effective therapeutically. The alpha fraction is available in the *d* (or natural) form, the *dl* (or synthetic) form, and the mixed form, of which the *d* form is considered the most potent. Most of our personal observations have been with *d*-alpha-tocopheryl acetate or succinate.

Successful therapy depends upon an adequate dose of an effective form of vitamin E over an extended period—in some conditions indefinitely on a maintenance basis. An average therapeutic dose might range from 800 to 1600 IU daily before meals and at bedtime. Inasmuch as vitamin E improves the tone of the heart muscle, patients with hypertension or damaged hearts should be started on 100 IU once daily. The physician can gradually increase the dose while monitoring the blood pressure.[9] Diabetics who receive insulin should also be started on 100 IU daily, since vitamin E improves glycogen storage in the tissues. One can gradually increase the dose by checking the blood sugar and adjusting the insulin dosage accordingly. Failure to do this has resulted in an insulin shock reaction.[10,11]

Inorganic iron, including white bread and cereals reinforced with iron, combines with and inactivates vitamin E and should be avoided.[12] Female hormones, including birth control pills, have an antagonistic effect on vitamin E and should not be used.[9] Diets containing excessive polyunsaturated fats increase vitamin E requirements.[13] Laxatives and mineral oil should also be avoided, since they interfere with the absorption of vitamin E.

Dermatoses Successfully Treated with Vitamin E

Pseudoxanthoma Elasticum

Vitamin E was first called to our attention in 1950 when O. M. Stout presented the case of a patient with pseudoxanthoma elasticum before the Los Angeles Dermatological Society. Two years previously, the patient, a middle-aged woman, had been presented with classical skin lesions and angioid streaks of the retina that resulted in visual disturbances sufficient to cause her to give up her work. At the time of the second presentation before the society, she had been taking vitamin E for 1 year. The skin lesions were markedly improved, her vision had recovered to the extent that she could read a newspaper in ordinary daylight, and she had resumed her work.[14] Approximately 1 year later, we had occasion to treat a 10-year-old girl with histologically confirmed skin lesions of pseudoxanthoma elasticum of 2 years' duration but without eye changes. Her lesions cleared almost completely after 4 months of treatment with vitamin E, and they remained clear on maintenance therapy. There have been a number of published confirmatory reports.[15]

Epidermolysis Bullosa

We have had excellent response to vitamin E in two cases of the simplex (Weber-Cockayne) type of epidermolysis bullosa: a 7-year-old girl and an 8-year-old boy. Both patients were incapacitated and could not perform normal childhood activities, but both recovered. The boy was able to play football while under maintenance therapy.[16]

There have been a number of confirmatory reports on the control of epidermolysis bullosa, including the dystrophic type, with adequate doses of vitamin E. Sehgal and associates reported the successful treatment of epidermolysis bullosa dystrophica in three family members.[17] Smith and Michener proved that vitamin E had therapeutic value in epidermolysis bullosa dystrophica in a double-blind cross-over study of twin sisters.[18] Michaelson and coworkers demonstrated that the disappearance of collagenase from the skin accompanied the clinical response to vitamin E in patients with epidermolysis bullosa.[19] There have been other favorable reports.

Raynaud's Phenomenon, Scleroderma, Morphea, and Calcinosis Cutis

We reported a series of eight patients with manifestations of one or more of these diseases whose condition markedly improved with vitamin E in daily doses of up to 1200 IU.[20] The most spectacular case was a 45-year-old man with rapidly deteriorating Raynaud's phenomenon of 6 months' duration who had ulcerations of the tips of the middle three fingers of both hands, three of which were gangrenous. Two months after the initiation of oral treatment with tocopherol, 800 IU daily, and topical application of a water-dispersible vitamin E cream, the fingers were entirely healed. One year after the initiation of vitamin E therapy, the fingers had remained clear, in spite of the trauma incurred in the patient's occupation of loading cardboard cartons onto trucks.

There have been a number of additional reports of successful treatment of this group of dermatoses with vitamin E. The degree of response of scleroderma and calcinosis cutis is related to the duration and presence of irreversible damage.

Benign Chronic Familial Pemphigus (Hailey-Hailey Disease)

Three patients healed completely while taking vitamin E in daily doses of 800 to 1200 IU. Two of them had recurrences when the dose of the vitamin was reduced or omitted. A relapse occurred in one patient when he also took medication containing inorganic iron, which inactivates vitamin E, but he recovered when proper treatment was resumed.[21]

Yellow Nail Syndrome

A 65-year-old woman had developed this rare syndrome during a period of 11 months prior to her first visit. Her symptoms included characteristic nail changes with cessation of growth, yellow discoloration, exaggerated lateral curvature, and disappearance of the lunula. She also had recurrent bronchitis, sinusitis (for which surgery had been scheduled), and transient lymphedema about the eyelids. She had experienced numbness and tingling of the fingertips, nocturnal leg cramps, and intermittent claudication over a period of years. Six months after the initiation of therapy with d-alpha-tocopheryl acetate, her nails had become normal, and all of her other symptoms had disappeared, except for an occasional bronchial cough. The sinus surgery was cancelled.[21]

Subcorneal Pustular Dermatosis

A 63-year-old woman had had a typical widespread eruption that had been histologically confirmed as subcorneal pustular dermatosis. Oral corticosteroids, which she had taken for 5 years prior to her first visit, had failed to control the eruption, and during that period she had developed diabetes, emphysema, and edema. Because of her medical complications, she was started on a small dose (100 IU) of d-alpha-tocopheryl acetate, which was gradually increased to 400 IU daily. Within a period of 4 weeks, the eruption was under complete control, in spite of the low dosage, and during a 2-year period of observation she experienced no recurrence while on a maintenance dosage.[21]

Lichen Sclerosus et Atrophicus

We have reported a series of ten female patients with lichen sclerosus et atrophicus, involving especially the genital area, who received 300 to 1200 IU of *d*-alpha-tocopheryl acetate daily, together with a vitamin E cream topically. Five improved 70 to 90 per cent, two showed moderate improvement, and three improved slightly.[21]

Granuloma Annulare

We reported the response of 12 patients with granuloma annulare to vitamin E in doses of 300 to 1600 IU daily. Six healed completely, three were much improved, two were moderately improved, and one did not respond.[21]

Vasculitis-Type Eruptions

We have reported that four patients with each of the following dermatoses responded excellently to vitamin E: pityriasis lichenoides chronica, pityriasis lichenoides et varioliformis acuta, recurrent erythema nodosum, and purpura annularis telangiectodes. All responded to vitamin E therapy; three of them remained clear over a 2-year period of observation, except on several occasions when medication was discontinued.[21]

Post–Herpes Zoster Neuralgia

We reported a series of 13 patients with chronic post–herpes zoster neuralgia, all of whom required sedation. One case had lasted for 19 years, and one had lasted for 13 years. Nine of these patients, including the two whose cases were of the longest duration, experienced complete or nearly complete relief of pain. Two had moderate relief, and two were slightly improved.[21]

Porphyria Cutanea Tarda

Two patients healed completely with simultaneous disappearance of uroporphyrin; one had a recurrence when given female hormones, which have an antagonistic effect on vitamin E. Two other patients experienced partial clearing.[22]

Lupus Erythematosus (Discoid)

We have reported a small series of seven patients with discoid lupus erythematosus who were treated with vitamin E over a period of months. Two of the patients who took only 300 IU daily showed only slight improvement, and the other five, who took 800 to 2000 IU daily, experienced complete or nearly complete clearing. We had an excellent response in one patient with subacute disseminated lupus erythematosus with a positive

ANA test, which became negative following vitamin E therapy. We have not had the opportunity to treat any patients with systemic lupus erythematosus.[23]

Synergism of Vitamins A and E

Keratosis Follicularis (Darier's Disease), Pityriasis Rubra Pilaris, Acne Vulgaris, and Ichthyosis

A strong synergism between vitamin A and vitamin E was demonstrated by Ames in a symposium on vitamin A sponsored by the Massachusetts Institute of Technology. In a group of laboratory rats on a vitamin E–deficient diet, the vitamin A blood level dropped very low and remained low regardless of the amount of vitamin A given by mouth or even by injection. The vitamin A level became normal, however, when vitamin E was added to the diet.[7]

We have confirmed this synergism in the successful control of the aforementioned four dermatoses involving defective keratinization.[24]

We have successfully treated three patients with keratosis follicularis with combined vitamin E and vitamin A therapy. One patient had a generalized eruption that had failed to respond to vitamin A alone in doses of 200,000 IU daily for 5 years but healed almost completely while the patient was taking a combination of vitamin A (100,000 IU) and vitamin E (1600 IU) daily. In a 5-year follow-up the eruption remained clear, except on several occasions when the dose was markedly reduced or discontinued.

We have had excellent results with the A and E therapy in four cases of pityriasis rubra pilaris and in one case of ichthyosis.

We have achieved excellent control of acne vulgaris over a period of 6 years by correcting the defective keratinization of sebaceous follicles by the combined administration of vitamins A and E. The ability of vitamin E to prevent lipid peroxidation of sebum damaged by bacteria has had an anti-inflammatory effect. We reported that 90 of a series of 98 patients had a good to excellent response and that, of these, 42 showed 90 to 100 per cent clearing in 2 months or less. Our acne regimen included several other modes of treatment, but no antibiotics were used either orally or topically.[25]

Our results in the treatment of the aforementioned dermatoses involving defective keratinization compare favorably with recent reports of response to oral retinoids without undesirable side effects.

Muscular Conditions Successfully Treated with Vitamin E

As the result of a serendipitous trial, we have successfully treated the following muscular conditions with vitamin E: nocturnal leg cramps, rectal cramps, exercise cramps, blepharospasm, intermittent claudication, and restless legs syndrome.[26] We also observed one patient with severe polymyositis who had deteriorated to the extent of having to be fed with a gastrostomy tube in spite of three immunosuppressive drugs. Following the discontinuation of the immunosuppressive agents, and the administration of 1600 IU of vitamin E daily, the elevated blood level of the muscle enzyme aldolase returned to normal, and most of the patient's muscle function improved markedly.[27] Incidentally, degeneration of both skeletal and cardiac muscles is one of the earliest manifestations of vitamin E deprivation in rhesus monkeys.[28,29]

SUMMARY

We have attempted to relate our own personal experiences with the value of vitamin E as a therapeutic agent in a number of dermatologic conditions. We realize that the number of cases treated is too small for any final conclusions to be drawn, but the trend is highly optimistic. There are many other conditions in which vitamin E has been found useful as well as others in which its value has not been explored. The fundamental importance of vitamin E is its protection of cell membranes from oxidation and its ability to facilitate the utilization of oxygen in normal metabolic processes.

Harman, in animal experiments, has demonstrated the ability of tocopherol to retard aging.[30] It also might help progeria, if started early, since Tuchweber and colleagues concluded that "experiments on the rat indicate that the progeria-like syndrome induced by chronic intoxication with dihydrotachysterol can be prevented by concurrent *d*-alpha-tocopheryl acetate treatment. . . ."[31]

The New York Academy of Sciences has published a collection of papers on the subject. The research was presented at an international symposium in New York in 1981.[32]

References

1. Evans, H. M.: The pioneer history of vitamin E. Symposium on vitamin E and metabolism (Zurich, Switzerland). Vitam. Horm. 20:379–397, 1962.
2. Tappel, A. L.: Vitamin E as the biological antioxidant. Symposium on vitamin E and metabolism (Zurich, Switzerland). Vitam. Horm. 20:493–510, 1962.
3. Tappel, A. L.: Where old age begins. Nutrition Today 2:2, 1967.
4. Criep, L. H.: Clinical Immunology and Allergy, 2nd ed. New York, Grune & Stratton, 1969, p. 3.
5. Ayres, S., Jr., and Mihan, R.: Is vitamin E involved in the autoimmune mechanism? Cutis 21:323, 1978.
6. Schwartz, K.: A possible site of action for vitamin E in intermediary metabolism. Am. J. Clin. Nutr. 9:71 (Part 2, Suppl.), 1961.
7. Ames, S.R.: Factors affecting absorption, transport and storage of vitamin A. Am. J. Clin. Nutr. 22:934, 1969.
8. Tappel, A. L., and Dillard, C. J.: In vivo lipid peroxidation: Measurement via exhaled pentane and protection by vitamin E. Fed. Proc. 40:174, Feb. 1981.
9. Shute, W. E.: Complete Updated Vitamin E Book. New Canaan, CT, Keats Publishing, Inc., 1975, pp. 162, 182.
10. Vogelsang, A.: Vitamin E in the treatment of diabetes mellitus. Symposium on vitamin E. Ann. N.Y. Acad. Sci. 52:406, 1949.
11. Butturini, U.: Clinical and experimental studies on vitamin E. Ann. N.Y. Acad. Sci. 52:397, 1949.
12. Goldberg, L., and Smith, J. P., Changes associated with the accumulation of iron in certain organs of the rat. Br. J. Exp. Pathol. 39:59, 1958.
13. Horwitt, M. K., et al.: Polyunsaturated lipids and tocopherol requirements. J. Am. Diet Assoc. 38:231, 1961.
14. Stout, O. M.: Pseudoxanthoma elasticum with retinal angioid streaking decidedly improved on tocopherol therapy. Arch. Dermatol. 63:510, 1951.
15. Ayres, S. Jr., and Mihan, R.: Pseudoxanthoma elasticum and epidermolysis bullosa: Response to vitamin E (tocpherol). Cutis 5:287, 1969.
16. Ayres, S., Jr., and Mihan, R.: Vitamin E (tocopherol)—a reappraisal of its value in dermatoses of mesodermal origin. Cutis 7:35, 1971.
17. Sehgal, V. N., Vadiraj, S. N., Rege, V. L., and Beohar, P. C.: Dystrophic epidermolysis bullosa in a family: Response to vitamin E (tocopherol). Dermatologica 144:27, 1972.
18. Smith, E. B., and Michener, W. M.: Vitamin E treatment of dermolytic bullous dermatoses. Arch. Dermatol. 108:254, 1973.
19. Michaelson, J. D., Schmidt, J. D., Dresen, M. H., and Duncan, W. C.: Vitamin E treatment of epidermolysis bullosa: Changes in tissue collagenase levels. Arch. Dermatol. 109:67, 1974.
20. Ayres, S., Jr., Mihan, R., Levan, N. E., Rapaport, J., and Couperus, M.: Raynaud's phenomenon, scleroderma, morphea and calcinosis cutis: Response to vitamin E. Cutis 11:54, 1973.
21. Ayres, S., Jr., and Mihan, R.: Vitamin E and dermatology. Cutis 16:1017, 1975.
22. Ayres, S., Jr., and Mihan, R.: Porphyria cutanea tarda: Response to vitamin E, a review and two case reports. Cutis 22:50, 1978.
23. Ayres, S., Jr., and Mihan, R.: Lupus erythematosus and vitamin E: An effective and nontoxic therapy. Cutis 23:49, 1979.

24. Ayres, S., Jr., Mihan, R., and Scribner, M. D.: Synergism of vitamins A and E with dermatologic applications. Cutis 23:600, 1979.
25. Ayres, S., Jr., and Mihan, R.: Acne vulgaris: Therapy directed at pathophysiologic defects. Cutis 28:41, 1981.
26. Ayres, S., Jr., and Mihan, R.: Nocturnal leg cramps (systremma): A progress report on response to vitamin E. South. Med. J. 67:1308, 1974.
27. Killeen, R. N. F., Ayres, S., Jr., and Mihan, R.: Polymyositis: Response to vitamin E. South. Med. J. 69:1372, 1976.
28. Mason, K. E.: Effects of deficiency (the tocopherols). *In* Sebrell, W. H., Jr., and Harris, R. S. (eds.): Vitamins: Chemistry, Physiology, Pathology, vol. 3. New York, Academic Press, 1957, pp. 522–530.
29. Fitch, C. D.: Experimental anemia in primates due to vitamin E deficiency. Vitam. Horm. 25:501, 1968.
30. Harman, D.: Free radical theory of aging: Effect of free radical inhibitors in the life-span of male LAF mice: Second experiment. Gerontologist 8 (Part 2):13, 1968.
31. Tuchweber, B., Gabbiani, B., and Selye, H.: Effect of vitamin E and methyltestosterone upon the progeria-like syndrome produced by dihydrotachysterol. Am. J. Clin. Nutr. 13:238, 1963.
32. Lubin, B., and Machlin, L. J.: Vitamin E: Biochemical, hematological, and clinical aspects. Ann. N.Y. Acad. Sci. 393:323, 1982.

THE VITAMIN E ENIGMA: PERSPECTIVES FOR PHYSICIANS

H. J. Roberts, M.D.

Many persons in the United States are taking large amounts of vitamin E (used here to designate the various tocopherols). Most do so for its alleged therapeutic or prophylactic value—often because of impressive features and anecdotal testimonials in health-oriented magazines. Some are advised to take megadoses of vitamin E by physicians and other professionals.

Vitamin E as Therapy

The disorders for which vitamin E is most frequently recommended include ischemic heart disease, occlusive peripheral vascular disease, thrombophlebitis, leg cramps, the vascular complications of diabetes, scleroderma, other dermatoses, polymyositis, sterility, and "aging."[1-4] The basic premise of such therapy is the presumed function of vitamin E as a biological antioxidant that limits free-radical chain reactions and protects body cells from lipid peroxidation (especially polyunsaturated fatty acids in biological membranes). Perhaps vitamin E also serves as a repressor of certain lysosomal catabolic enzymes.[5]

Although there may be some validity to vitamin E therapy in the foregoing conditions, its purported efficacy has been repeatedly denied, as it was in *The Medical Letter*.[6] Indeed, the status of clinical indications for this vitamin described over a decade ago in a *Journal of the American Medical Association* editorial[7] has hardly changed: "The story of vitamin E since its discovery in 1922 is one of repeated frustrating searching for effects of its deficiency and for its therapeutic utility." Even in their report of the apparent efficacy of vitamin E in treating dermolytic bullous dermatosis, Smith and Michener[2] commented: "Although some advocates of vitamin E therapy insist that it is good for most of man's ailments, the use of this vitamin as therapy for mechanobullous diseases must be considered empirical."

The Vitamin E Crusade

Many "nutritionists" champion vitamin E as the "granddaddy" of all vitamins because "it puts oxygen quality in each blood cell." Some have suggested that it be added to bread and other foods as a mechanism for increasing the life span on the basis of mice studies. Wellness-oriented periodicals repeatedly emphasize the repletion of antioxidants that are lost through the refining of natural grains, oils, and other foods.

Virtually any "breakthrough" involving vitamin E administration is newsworthy for the public. A few examples will suffice.

1. Many persons undoubtedly will be self-administering vitamin E (with selenium) in an attempt to prevent or minimize macular degeneration.

2. Others take tocopherol as a possible antiatheromatous measure to counteract vitamin E depletion from the use of increased polyunsaturated fats in the diet.

3. Preliminary data concerning the alleged enhancement of cytotoxic drugs for chemotherapy by vitamin E, coupled with the purported stimulation of host immunity by tocoph-

erol, will be widely misinterpreted by the public as an inherent anticancer effect of vitamin E.

Unfortunately, the vitamin E crusade has attained so much momentum that any serious challenge to its rationale or safety is likely to evoke strong criticism and rebuke—both from lay sources and from a cadre of physician-champions. I can vouch for this reflex response on the basis of considerable correspondence following publications expressing concern over the serious side effects of vitamin E.[8-10] There was violent commentary on my seemingly prudent recommendation: "Megadoses of vitamin E should be used with restraint. . . . Patients taking large amounts of vitamin E should be followed up for the foregoing listed side effects."[8] The problem is being further polarized by several foundations that spearhead vitamin E megatherapy.

Side Effects and Complications

The attitude that vitamin E intake is essentially innocuous prevails. I have emphasized that this may not be the case, especially when pharmacologic doses (arbitrarily defined as 400 units or more daily) are taken.[8-10]

The most serious problem I have noted in persons taking vitamin E over prolonged periods is *thrombophlebitis, pulmonary embolism,* or both. My series currently exceeds 90 such cases. Pulmonary embolism occurred even in patients receiving anticoagulant therapy. Several experienced exacerbation of thrombophlebitis when they resumed taking vitamin E after having been advised to discontinue it.

The virtual epidemic of deep vein thrombosis in the United States underscores the seriousness of this problem. There are an estimated 200,000 deaths from pulmonary embolism annually. It is therefore obvious that the use of *any* drug that is capable of precipitating or aggravating thrombosis and phlebitis warrants close scrutiny, especially in persons already having metabolic, cardiovascular, or endocrine disorders that predispose them to platelet aggregation, thrombosis, and small vessel disease.

There is considerable confusion concerning vitamin E and thromboembolism. Reports of the apparently beneficial effect of tocopherol in preventing postoperative thromboembolism generally involved *temporary* dosages of 200 to 600 IU (orally or intramuscularly) for a few days.[11] These results differ from the thrombophlebitis and thromboembolism following *prolonged* use of vitamin E in megadoses. Critical studies have failed to confirm an antithrombic action.[12] Furthermore, vitamin E does not alter the platelet aggregation response to varying concentrations of adenosine diphosphate and epinephrine.[13]

A list of other complications of hypervitaminosis E appears in my review article.[8] The most serious side effects include (1) aggravation of hypertension, (2) a severe fatigue syndrome, (3) gynecomastia (both in men and in women), (4) breast tumors (presumably related to an estrogen-like action of vitamin E), (5) altered changes in the metabolism and concentrations of multiple hormones (thyroid, pituitary, adrenal),[14,15] (6) increased cholesterol and triglyceride concentrations,[16,17] and (7) altered immunity. Only a few will receive further comment here.

Although the severe fatigue syndrome associated with large amounts of vitamin E has been denied, other physicians encounter it. Dr. Harold M. Cohen[18] emphasized this side effect a decade ago. He subsequently wrote:

> In my very large practice, it never ceases to amaze me how often patients taking megadoses of vitamin E experience symptoms such as you describe. After thorough history, physical and laboratory studies, I find hypervitaminosis E ranks only second to depression as a cause of fatigue in my young patients (if pharmacologic agents, such as tranquilizers, etc., are excluded) (personal correspondence, July 17, 1981).

The depressed bactericidal activity of leukocytes and mitogen-induced lymphocyte transformation in men who had ingested 300 mg *dl*-alpha-tocopherol acetate daily for 3 weeks[19] also deserves particular attention. There is little information concerning the possible role of excessive tocopherol intake in predisposing to or aggravating toxic shock associated with the menses, Legionnaire's disease, and other infections. For example, the effects of vitamin E might extend the leukocyte defect during menstruation, which is characterized by difficulty in lysing *Staphylococcus aureus*.[20] The Centers for Disease Control have no available data concerning a possible enhanced diathesis to toxic shock or Legionnaire's disease by the intake of excessive vitamin E (personal communication, May 1982).

Necrotizing gastroenteritis has been encountered in infants receiving vitamin E.[21,22] This assumes greater relevance in light of the current experimental use of vitamin E for its alleged improvement of retrolental fibroplasia.[23] The Food and Drug Administration reported a possible association between high-dose vitamin E administration and an increased incidence of necrotizing enterocolitis in premature infants who received tocopherol orally or intramuscularly.[22] This disorder developed in 30 per cent of all treated infants with vitamin E blood concentrations above 3.5 mg per dl, compared with only 4 per cent of treated infants with concentrations lower than this level. Replying to the need for such caution, Hittner[24] stated that "... maintenance of levels of 2 to 3 mg per 100 ml is sufficient to protect the retina. Higher levels are unwarranted and may tip the scale of vitamin E administration from a favorable to an unfavorable risk/benefit ratio."

Pertinent Correspondence

Many individuals have written to me about their adverse experiences from vitamin E megadoses. A few are illustrative.

1. The marketing manager for a medical equipment firm in England developed deep vein thrombosis of the right leg in August 1976 and a subsequent near-fatal pulmonary embolus in January 1978. He wrote: "No underlying reason for the embolism could be found. . . . Until two weeks ago, I had been taking 250 IU of vitamin E daily and had been so doing during most of 1976 and 1977."

2. A prominent California attorney wrote: "I have always registered within the normal readings of blood pressure, with the readings averaging 128 systolic and 80 to 84 diastolic. About two years ago, I began taking large doses of vitamin C and vitamin E. The vitamin E was taken three times a day, 800 IU per time or 2500 IU per day. I joined a gym about six months ago for exercise. . . . In the last six months I began to get higher readings—as high as 160/100."

3. A 25-year-old woman indicated that she had been hospitalized with thrombophlebitis 1 year previously, even though she had been in apparently excellent health. There was no clue to the cause until her father (a pathologist) sent her a copy of my review article. She wrote: "At the time of my hospitalization, I was consuming several vitamin E capsules per day."

4. An active 45-year-old woman stated that she had been taking 400 IU vitamin E daily "for no particular reason but with the encouragement of my husband, a chemist, who took the same dose." She was hospitalized for 12 days because of a pulmonary embolus. Concomitantly, her husband ". . . had a growing hypertension problem in spite of diet modification, discipline running, and a weight control program."

5. A prominent internist described two patients who had had three episodes of significant and extensive ecchymoses while on warfarin *each time* they took 400 or 800 IU of vitamin E. There was prompt clearing when the vitamin was discontinued.

6. A 37-year-old woman had had tender and lumpy breasts for a long time. Her

grandmother had died of carcinoma of the breast. The patient was advised to take 800 units of vitamin E "prophylactically." Although one breast "flattened out nicely," the other developed a distinct lesion 1 year later that proved to be carcinoma. In spite of her surgeon's objection to taking further vitamin E ("because it closely resembles the effects of estrogen"), several other physicians *insisted* that she continue taking it.

Related Aspects of Vitamin E Metabolism

Valid perspectives concerning vitamin E require clarification of various aspects of its requirements, absorption, and action. I shall summarize some issues that are not generally known. At the risk of being superfluous, I must insert the usual disclaimer that data from experimental animals, particularly studies involving animals on E-deficient diets, cannot be extrapolated to human beings.

1. Most healthy adults do not require more than 10 IU of vitamin E daily.

2. A deficiency of vitamin E occurs infrequently in our society, even in persons whose diets are not healthful.[25] Vitamin E exists in association with polyunsaturated fatty acids. It is therefore adequate in most conventional diets. Furthermore, the need for dietary tocopherol may decrease with increasing age.[26]

3. Many tocopherol products have limited activity. (This is probably fortunate.) Horwitt[27] has observed that *"all-rac-a-*tocopheryl acetate (the article of commerce) may have no more than half the biological potency of D-*a*-tocopheryl acetate when the commercial substance is used as a supplement for vitamin E–depleted adult subjects. The so-called DL-*a*-tocopherol is a fraction of the commercial mixture of *all-rac-a-*tocopheryl acetate, which includes eight possible stereoisomers in the form of four racemates." In a more recent correspondence, Horwitt[28] asserted: "In view of the evidence and until there is contrary information, it is reasonable to state that *all-rac-a*-TA acetate has about 50% of the biological activity of RRR-*a*-TA." (The commercial name of *all-rac-a*-tocopheryl acetate is *dl-a*-tocopheryl acetate. RRR-*a*-tocopheryl acetate was formerly called *d-a*-tocopheryl acetate.)

4. Another factor that also is probably fortunate concerns the limited ability of the gastrointestinal tract to absorb vitamin E. Its absorption under different experimental conditions ranges from 10 to 52 per cent.[46] (Approximately 1 per cent is stored in the liver.) Even when daily dosages as high as 80 IU per kg body weight are ingested, adults do not increase their serum levels more than fourfold. Although vitamin E has proved helpful in reducing transfusion requirements in homozygous β-thalassemia,[29] this benefit could be obtained only by parenteral administration.

5. The serum alpha-tocopherol concentration reaches a plateau after approximately 3 weeks of oral supplementation.[30] This suggests a feedback mechanism involving the absorption of vitamin E.

6. Vitamin E is an excellent antioxidant in vitro. On the other hand, the real magnitude of its in vivo ability to prevent peroxidation of polyunsaturated fatty acids in membranes remains debatable. *Nutrition Reviews*[31] concluded its discussion of vitamin E action on prostanoid biosynthesis by stating: "There is clearly a difference between in vivo and in vitro antioxidants, and there is doubt that vitamin E modulates prostaglandin synthesis via its antioxidant property."

7. Witting[32] attempted to determine vitamin E requirements for individuals consuming diets high in polyunsaturated fatty acids. He wrote: "The kinetics of antioxidant action by vitamin E in vitro are rather complex, since the efficiency of the antioxidant decreases as the concentration of vitamin E increases beyond the optimum. . . . Excessive intake of vitamin E would therefore appear to be undesirable."

8. There is marked confusion regarding the antioxidant effect of vitamin E and the

superoxide dismutases within the context of human physiology. The relative importance of the superoxide dismutases in the antioxidant hierarchy and the true significance of "free radicals" remain nebulous. T. L. Dormandy[33] emphasized: "Free radicals never exist for more than fractions of a second." He also stressed that the meaning of the terms auto-oxidation and antioxidants to the biologist is different from the meaning of the terms to the industrial chemist. (I am skeptical of the current promotion of superoxide dismutase supplements as "free radical superoxide scavengers." Inasmuch as the dismutase enzymes are proteins, they probably do not remain biologically intact when taken orally.)

9. The purported synergism of vitamin A and E administration[34] requires further analysis and confirmation. As a case in point, vitamins E and A have opposite effects on testicular cells in culture.[35] Vitamin E increases cell growth and does not affect the gonadotropin receptor levels. On the other hand, vitamin A (retinoic acid) eliminates the growth response to follicle-stimulating hormone and decreases the human chorionic gonadotropin receptors in Leydig cell cultures.

Other observations must be considered relative to the suggested benefit of megadoses of vitamins A and E in skin disorders resulting from defective keratinization.[34] The findings of normalized serum vitamin A concentrations following vitamin E administration occurred in E-deficient rats.[47] Data in humans also exist—e.g., patients on total parenteral nutrition cannot sustain normal plasma vitamin A concentrations in the absence of vitamin E. Vitamin A appears to be stored more efficiently when adequate vitamin E is taken orally or given by injection.[46] The mechanisms for this sparing effect may involve increased intestinal absorption or decreased oxidative loss of vitamin A. If so, the administration of large amounts of vitamins A and E could cause hypervitaminosis A (see later). (Normal persons absorb at least 80 per cent of vitamin A from the gastrointestinal tract. Thirty to 50 per cent of the dose is then stored in the liver.)

10. The interactions of E and other vitamins also require scrutiny, especially when advocated as polypharmacy. In the chick, vitamin E increases the requirements for vitamins D and K.[36] Keith[37,38] was unable to demonstrate a rise in plasma tocopherol levels during vitamin C supplementation in male volunteers who had ingested 300 mg of ascorbic acid for 3 weeks. Another report asserted: ". . . the adverse effect of the high supplementation of vitamin C on tissue antioxidant potential may be overcome by increasing the supplementation level of vitamin E and suggests that vitamin E requirement may be increased with increased vitamin C supplementation."[39]

11. The pharmacologic effects of vitamin E in diabetics must be considered in attempts to treat this disorder and its complications with tocopherol. Bensley and associates[40] failed to demonstrate improvement of diabetes with vitamin E, even though plasma tocopherol levels doubled. The slight reduction of serum glucose concentrations in maturity-onset diabetics must be weighed against the concomitant significant rise of serum cholesterol and triglyceride concentrations.[41] McMasters and coworkers[42] found a relative increase of adipose tissue tocopherol levels coupled with a more rapid rate of depletion in diabetics after the subjects had ingested vitamin E. The investigators also noted higher adipose tissue tocopherol levels in response to oral hypoglycemic medication during and following administration of vitamin E.

Some Sources of Confusion and Misinformation

The promotion of nutritional misinformation has fostered a multi–billion-dollar business that capitalizes on the public's fears, hopes, and misplaced back-to-nature attitudes. The *Dairy Council Digest*[43] emphasized: "Less well known is what happens when normal healthy individuals consume large amounts of a variety of vitamins and nutritional supplements. . . . Megadoses of vitamins provide no benefit, are costly, and potentially are harmful, yet there are no regulations to limit vitamin dosage in over-the-counter multivitamin capsules.'' The extent to which people are confused is evidenced by the ongoing intense promotion of ''vitamin B_{17}'' (Laetrile) and ''vitamin B_{15}'' (pangamic acid), neither of which has been demonstrated to be a true vitamin.

Professional confusion and misinformation concerning vitamin E exists. For example:

1. I received correspondence from a vigorous proponent of vitamin E megadosage in which he offered the following ''reference'': ''Dr. Donald J. Dalessio of the Scripps Clinic/Research Foundation in LaJolla, California states, 'There is a substantial increase in platelet aggregation during the preheadache stage of migraine.' He then points out that any substance which might interfere with platelet aggregation could act as a protective measure against recurrent migraines as well as stroke.'' Replying to my query on the matter, Dr. Dalessio (personal correspondence, September 29, 1978) asserted: ''I am not aware of any significant studies which suggest that vitamin E is effective as a platelet antagonist. There is some suggestion that vitamin E may inhibit the oxidative production of prostaglandins, but whether this is an important effect is not clear to me. I have never seen any studies relating vitamin E to interference with platelet aggregation specifically. . . . I know of no control studies relating vitamin E to migraine prophylaxis.''

2. Vitamin E has purported value in minimizing the severity of retrolental fibroplasia among preterm infants. In advocating such therapy, Hittner and associates[23] asserted: ''Oral administration of vitamin E has never been associated with toxicity even when megadoses have been given. . . . It may be ill-advised to withhold vitamin E until after oxygen has been administered and after neovascularization into the vitreous has been identified—that is, to use vitamin E as a therapeutic agent.'' Along with others, I am concerned about the misinterpretation of this report. Hillis[21] commented: ''Unless clinicians are provided some balanced guidance, this report may be overinterpreted, to the detriment of the medical community and that of infants who may be subjected to an unproved and possibly harmful treatment. . . . If all deaths are eliminated from the analysis, the protective effect of vitamin E is no longer statistically significant.'' The possible role of such therapy in necrotizing enterocolitis among infants was mentioned earlier.

3. In a case of polymyositis responding to vitamin E,[3] steroid therapy *was* continued. Therefore, the improvement observed might not have been solely ascribable to vitamin E. (My analysis of the case report indicates that cyclophosphamide and azathioprine were stopped on approximately June 2 following the appearance of mucocutaneous erosive lesions and an acute thrombophlebitis. Thereafter, ''. . . the dosage of prednisone was tapered off over a period of several weeks.'' Vitamin E had been started on May 26; ''improvement was noted within a period of a few weeks. . . .'')

4. There has been a stream of unconfirmed reports concerning other clinical and biochemical benefits of vitamin E. For example, an impressive redistribution of cholesterol in the lipoproteins—especially the increased percentage of high-density lipoprotein cholesterol—was reported among subjects who ingested 600 IU alpha-tocopheryl acetate daily for 30 to 45 days.[44] Subsequent investigations[30] failed to confirm such an effect in both normal subjects and patients with hypercholesterolemia or hypertriglyceridemia—even with 800 IU tocopherol or tocopheryl acetate for 6 weeks.

CONCLUDING COMMENTARY

There may be a place for vitamin E therapy, even if the vitamin is administered only on an empiric basis. Perhaps judicious amounts might benefit some persons with intrinsic difficulties in metabolizing vitamin E, altered vitamin E receptors, or diets extremely high in polyunsaturated fats. I do not know how to define a ''dependency'' state in clinical terms, however. Furthermore, there are reasonable grounds for doubt concerning the safety of prolonged vitamin E ingestion, especially in large doses. Accordingly, physicians who recommend such a regimen have the responsibility of (1) carefully following their patients and (2) seeking out the cited side effects and any others. Certainly, megadoses of vitamin E ought to be restrained until more data are in in the case of sophisticated pregnant women who seek to prevent retrolental fibroplasia or bronchopulmonary dysplasia. (Other fat-soluble vitamins are also potentially teratogenic.)

Dermatologists understandably are interested in the reported dramatic improvement of challenging skin diseases involving defective keratinization after administration of megadoses of vitamins A and E.[34] However, it is imperative that patients receiving 100,000 to 150,000 IU of vitamin A and 1200 to 1600 IU of vitamin E daily be carefully monitored for hypervitaminosis A if vitamin A absorption and transport are potentiated by vitamin E.

Perhaps vitamin A and E synergism could prove beneficial as *topical therapy* to patients with selected skin disorders. Impressive results were reported by Tereno and Harrison[48] in 30 cases of trophic ulcers and gangrene of the feet after local administration of vitamin E oil (28,000 units per ounce) and vitamin A and D ointment.

Hypervitaminosis E is *not* a benign state. This issue becomes one of mounting concern in light of the widespread use of the vitamin generated by glowing reports in health-oriented periodicals. Physicians need not apologize to avant-garde "nutritionists" for their conservative stand on this and related issues. They are entitled to proof that any purported "breakthrough" within the emotionally charged realms of vitamin, mineral, and "organic" food therapeutics is *both* effective and safe. For example, the advocacy of tocopheryl nicotinate for scleroderma by a private foundation—including its distribution "on a first-come, first-served basis"[45]—is disturbing, since this product is neither made nor marketed in the United States. I reiterate the warning by *Nutrition Reviews*[49]: "The fat-soluble vitamins as a group are two-edged swords, life-saving at physiological levels and dangerous at megavitamin levels."

Addendum

The widespread use of vitamin E was demonstrated in an analysis of 2451 survey questionnaires (a 70 per cent response) received from persons in seven states.[50] Twenty per cent were using vitamin E, commonly up to 1000 IU per day "for a variety of unfounded reasons."

English and Carl[51] also reported on the extraordinary use of nutritional supplements by family practice patients. Although these supplements were taken by 67 per cent of the patients, 62 per cent had never discussed such self-medication with their physicians.

In a prospective study, Enstrom and Pauling[52] analyzed the responses of 479 elderly Californians to a 1974 questionnaire carried in *Prevention* magazine. A significantly higher mortality was associated with high vitamin E intake in the 1977 follow-up. Indeed, the rate was almost *double* for those taking 1000 IU or more when compared with the three categories of users taking between 100 and 999 IU (P = 0.02).

Baehner and associates[53] studied polymorphonuclear cell metabolism and function following the administration of 1600 IU vitamin E to humans. They found a decrease in the bactericidal potency of polymorphonuclear cells, marked impairment of hydrogen peroxide release from polymorphonuclear cells, and decreased hexose monophosphate shunt activity (which is dependent on intracellular hydrogen peroxide) during phagocytosis.

References

1. Ayres, S., Jr., and Mihan, R.: Vitamin E and dermatology. Cutis 16:1017, 1975.
2. Smith, E. B., and Michener, W. M.: Vitamin E treatment of dermolytic bullous dermatosis: A controlled study. Arch. Dermatol. 108:254, 1973.

3. Killen, R. N. F., Ayres, S., Jr., and Mihan, R.: Polymyositis: Response to vitamin E. South. Med. J. 69:1372, 1976.
4. Shute, E.: The Heart and Vitamin E. Shute Foundation for Medical Research, London, Ontario, 1969.
5. Olson, E. E.: Are we looking at the right enzyme systems? Am. J. Clin. Nutr. 20:604, 1967.
6. Vitamin E. The Medical Letter, August 15, 1975, p. 69.
7. Editorial: Target for tocopherol. JAMA 217:1545, 1971.
8. Roberts, H. J.: Perspective on vitamin E as therapy. JAMA 246:129, 1981.
9. Roberts, H. J.: Vitamin E and thrombophlebitis. Lancet 1:49, 1978.
10. Roberts, H. J.: Thrombophlebitis associated with vitamin E therapy: With a commentary on other medical side effects. Angiology 30:169, 1979.
11. Konafsky, J. D., and Konafsky, P. B.: Prevention of thromboembolic disease by vitamin E. N. Engl. J. Med. 305:173, 1981.
12. Olson, R. E.: Vitamin E and its relation to heart disease. Circulation 48:179, 1973.
13. Gomes, J. A. C. P., Venkatachalapathy, D., and Haft, J. I.: The effect of vitamin E on platelet aggregation. Am. Heart J. 91:425, 1976.
14. Carpenter, M. P., and Howard, C. N., Jr.: Vitamin E, steroids, and liver microsomal hydroxylations. Am. J. Clin. Nutr. 27:966, 1974.
15. Tsai, A. C., Kelley, J. J., Peng, B., et al.: Study on the effect of megavitamin E supplementation in man. Am. J. Clin. Nutr. 31:831, 1978.
16. Nikkilä, E. A., and Pelkonen, R.: Serum tocopherol, cholesterol, and triglyceride in coronary heart disease. Circulation 27:919, 1963.
17. Bieri, J. G.: Vitamin E. Nutr. Rev. 33:161, 1975.
18. Cohen, H. M.: Effects of vitamin E: Good and bad. N. Engl. J. Med. 289:980, 1973.
19. Prasad, J. S.: Effect of vitamin E supplementation on leukocyte function. Am. J. Clin. Nutr. 33:606, 1980.
20. Repine, J. E.: Cited by Medical World News, March 15, 1982, p. 39.
21. Hillis, A.: Vitamin E in retrolental fibroplasia. N. Engl. J. Med. 306:867, 1982.
22. Sobel, S., et al.: Vitamin E in retrolental fibroplasia. N. Engl. J. Med. 306:867, 1982.
23. Hittner, H. M., et al.: Retrolental fibroplasia: Efficacy of vitamin E in a double-blind clinical study of preterm infants. N. Engl. J. Med. 305:1365, 1981.
24. Hittner, H. M.: Vitamin E in retrolental fibroplasia. N. Engl. J. Med. 306:867, 1982.
25. Baker, H., Frank, O., Thind, I. S., et al.: Vitamin profiles in elderly persons living at home or in nursing homes, versus profile in healthy young subjects. J. Am. Geriatr. Soc. 27:444, 1979.
26. Grinna, L. S.: Effects of dietary a-tocopherol on liver microsomes and mitochondria of aging rats. J. Nutr. 106:918, 1976.
27. Horwitt, M. K.: Relative biological values of D-a-tocopheryl acetate and all-rac-a-tocopheryl in man. Am. J. Clin. Nutr. 33:856, 1980.
28. Horwitt, M. K.: Bioequivalence of RRR-a-tocopheryl and all-rac-a-tocopheryl acetate. Am. J. Clin. Nutr. 34:1634, 1981.
29. Giardini, O., Cantini, A., and Donfrancesco, A.: Vitamin E therapy in homozygous β-thalassemia. New Eng. J. Med. 306:644, 1981.
30. Hatam, L. J., and Kayden, H. J.: The failure of a-tocopherol supplementation to alter the distribution of lipoprotein cholesterol in normal and hyperlipoproteinemic persons. Am. J. Clin. Pathol. 76:122, 1981.
31. Review article: Effect of vitamin E on prostanoid biosynthesis. Nutr. Rev. 39:317, 1981.
32. Witting, L. A.: The role of polyunsaturated fatty acids in determining vitamin E requirement. Ann. N. Y. Acad. Sci. 203:192, 1972.
33. Dormandy, T. L.: Free-radical oxidation and antioxidants. Lancet 1:647, 1978.
34. Ayres, S., Jr., Mihan, R., and Scribner, M.D.: Synergism of vitamins A and E with dermatologic applications. Cutis 23:600, 1979.
35. Mather, J. P., and Haour, S. G.: The effects of vitamins A and E on testicular cells in culture: Growth and cell specific function. Abstract 241, 62nd Annual Meeting of the Endocrine Society, Washington, D.C., June 18, 1980.
36. Bieri, J. G.: Vitamin E. Nutr. Rev. 33:161, 1975.
37. Keith, R. E.: Dietary vitamin C supplementation and plasma vitamin E levels in humans. Am. J. Clin. Nutr. 33:2394, 1980.
38. Keith, R. E., Chrisley, B. M., and Driskell, J. A.: Dietary vitamin C supplementation and plasma vitamin E levels in humans. Am. J. Clin. Nutr. 33:2394, 1980.
39. Chen, L. H.: An increase in vitamin E requirement induced by high supplementation of vitamin C in rats. Am. J. Clin. Nutr. 34:1036, 1981.
40. Bensley, E. H. A., Fowler, A. F., Creaghan, M. V., et al.: Trial of vitamin E therapy in diabetes mellitus. Can. Med. Assoc. J. 61:260, 1949.
41. Bierembaum, N. L.: Cited by Internal Medicine News, 14:3, May 1981.
42. McMasters, V., Howard, T., Kinsell, L. W., et al.: Tocopherol storage and depletion in adipose tissue and plasma of normal and diabetic human subjects. Am. J. Clin. Nutr. 20:622, 1967.
43. Nutrition misinformation. Dairy Council Digest, July-August 1981, pp. 19–24, 1981.
44. Hermann, W. J., Ward, J., and Faucett, J.: The effect of tocopherol on high-density lipoprotein cholesterol. A clinical observation. Am. J. Clin. Pathol. 72:848, 1979.
45. Newsletter Number 1: Double E Medical Foundation, Incorporated, April 1982.
46. McKenna, M. C., and Bieri, J. G.: Tissue storage of vitamins A and E in rats drinking or infused with total parenteral nutrition solutions. Am. J. Clin. Nutr. 35:1010, 1982.

47. Ames, S. R.: Factors affecting absorption, transport and storage of vitamin A. Am. J. Clin. Nutr. 22:934, 1969.
48. Tereno, I., and Harrison, H. B.: A preliminary report on polytherapy of gangrene and trophic ulcers in geriatric patients. Curr. Podiatry 28:15, June 1979.
49. Feature: Vitamin D intoxication treated with glucocorticoids, clinical nutrition cases. Nutr. Rev. 37:323, 1979.
50. Read, M. H., et al.: Vitamin use: A survey. Nutr. Rep. Int. 24:1133, 1981.
51. English, E. C., and Carl, J. W.: Use of nutritional supplements by family practice patients. JAMA 246:2719, 1981.
52. Enstrom, J. E., and Pauling, L.: Mortality among health-conscious elderly Californians. Proc. Natl. Acad. Sci. 79:6023, 1982.
53. Baehner, R. L., Boxer, L. A., Ingraham, L. M., et al.: The influence of vitamin E on human polymorphonuclear cell metabolism and function. Ann. N.Y. Acad. Sci. 393:237, 1982.

Editorial Comment

This controversy can be considered from several viewpoints. It is possible that this agent is a therapeutic marvel. A friend of mine, a physician, complained of hardening of the nails of the fingers and the toes to a degree that it was nearly impossible for him to cut them. Someone recommended a large daily dose of vitamin E, and he consumed it religiously for a period of months. The nails softened remarkably, but in addition the hair on his scalp thickened, a therapeutically resistant synovial cyst on his finger disappeared, and Dupuytren's contracture of his palm showed considerable improvement. This, of course, is characteristic of the reports we receive. The series are small and uncontrolled. Basically, they are of an anecdotal nature and offer little scientific proof of the efficacy of the medication. This is true even of such conditions as acne, for which there is no shortage of clinical material. Furthermore, the treatment must be prolonged. It is difficult to convince people to spend the money and to endure the nuisance of daily dosing to obtain the hoped-for results. Therefore, the clinical efficacy of this approach must remain sub judice for the time being.

Many people believe that vitamins are a "natural product" and as such are perfectly safe to apply to the skin or to ingest per os. Nothing could be farther from the truth. I have encountered *severe* systemic reactions from hypervitaminosis A and D. Local reactions following the topical application of vitamin E creams and lotions are not unusual, although these eruptions may be caused by the bases in which the vitamin is incorporated. There is no reason to assume that the use of large doses of vitamin E for prolonged periods cannot result in undesirable effects that may be more important than the derangements for which the vitamin is taken.

Both Dr. Roberts and Dr. Ayres must be congratulated for their impressive presentations on both sides of this disagreement.

Think It Over.

SECTION 10

SÉZARY SYNDROME (MYCOSIS FUNGOIDES)

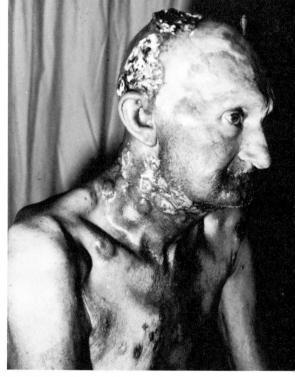

Mycosis fungoides, or Sézary syndrome, may be a severe, disfiguring dermatosis. (Courtesy of Dr. Ervin Epstein, Jr.)

CHAPTER **27**

THE NATURE OF SÉZARY SYNDROME (MYCOSIS FUNGOIDES)

CONTROVERSIES IN T CELL SKIN DISEASE: MYCOSIS FUNGOIDES AND SÉZARY SYNDROME

R. K. Winkelmann, M.D.

It is both fashionable and easy to combine mycosis fungoides and Sézary syndrome into lymphoproliferative T cell skin disease and to consider them as variable sides of the same problem, similar to the relationship between lymphoma and leukemia. The same cerebriform lymphocyte with helper T cell function is observed commonly in the skin in both diseases and in the blood, the lymph nodes, and the viscera in progressive disease. The diseases may have a chronic course and a later accelerated course as tumors of lymphoma, frequently T cell in type, develop.

This unity of the T cell lymphoproliferations of the skin may be considered with some legitimate skepticism, as emphasized by Winkelmann and Caro[1] and by Zackheim.[2] The lymphocytic cell types and functions observed in these diseases are heterogeneous. There are distinctive patterns of disease development as well as multiple forms of lymphoma-leukemia development from cutaneous T cell diseases. The recent finding of a relationship between C retrovirus and the Japanese adult T cell leukemia implies a unique etiology of some T cell lymphoma-leukemia.[3,4] The varied skin and visceral presentations of adult T cell lymphoma-leukemia imply that one must exercise caution in disease interpretation. I have observed T cell leukemia with massive skin involvement and a separate syndrome of cutaneous T cell lymphoma without bone marrow changes or epidermotropism. Clendenning and associates[5] have recently reported an adult with T cell lymphoma and marked epidermotropism in the skin and later in the viscera. They termed this condition a true mycosis fungoides d'emblée.

The past decade has seen the publication of large series involving patients with mycosis fungoides (Epstein and associates,[6] 1972, 144 patients; Fuks and coworkers,[7] 1973 and Hoppe and colleagues,[8] 1979, 140 patients; Van Scott and Kalmanson,[9] 1973, 243 patients; and the United States Mycosis Fungoides Study Group, Lamberg and associates,[10] 1979, 376 patients) and Sézary syndrome and pre-Sézary syndrome (Winkelmann,[11] 1974, 28 cases; Broder and associates,[12] 1979, 12 cases; Hamminga and coworkers,[13] 1979, 8 cases; Buechner and Winkelmann,[14] 1982, 39 cases Sézary syndrome, 18 cases pre-Sézary syndrome). These series plus the immunologic, cytologic, and etiologic study of the problem will be reviewed here to give emphasis to the consistencies and inconsistencies of the developing data relating to cutaneous T cell lymphoproliferative disease.

Patterns of Disease

The typical early mycosis fungoides picture is that of a chronic superficial inflammatory, sharply localized parapsoriasis. This often involves the hips or the trunk. Atrophic, poikilodermatous, or pigmented lesions may be present in chronic disease. Thickened, infiltrative plaques or tumors may occur episodically or as a general evolution of the process.[15] Ulceration accompanies massive nodule development. Spontaneous healing occurs.[16] Rare cases of accelerated mycosis fungoides in which all three stages occur acutely have been reported.[17] Mycosis fungoides d'emblée was the name given to mycosis fungoides in the eruptive tumor stage. Most cases of mycosis fungoides d'emblée have been recognized as B or T cell systemic lymphoma involving the skin,[18] but one recent case of T cell disease was epidermotropic at the onset and justified the use of this term.[5] Erythrodermic mycosis fungoides may occur in many ways: by coalescence of localized mycosis fungoides lesions to universal erythroderma, by allergic reaction as contact dermatitis or drug-induced exfoliative dermatitis superimposed on mycosis fungoides, by irritation with therapy or ultraviolet light, and by evolution of dermatologic disease as psoriasis. Such erythrodermic mycosis fungoides cases have a poorer prognosis than localized or generalized plaque mycosis fungoides[19] and are usually mistaken for Sézary syndrome clinically.

The evolution of a typical Sézary syndrome is from a dermatitis. The dermatitis is commonly chronic contact dermatitis, but atopic dermatitis and photosensitivity dermatitis have been described as precursor states.[20] Drug-reaction erythroderma can evolve into Sézary syndrome. Cases of lymphomatoid contact dermatitis with circulating Sézary cells have been reported.[21] Similarly, actinic reticuloid and erythroderma[22] and Sézary syndrome with photoreactivity have been noted.[20] Buechner and Winkelmann[23] have observed seven cases of pre-Sézary syndrome that developed over many years into a chronic Sézary syndrome.

Four Sézary-type phenomena have been described:

1. *Pre-Sézary syndrome*—an erythroderma developing chronically from dermatitis without significant adenopathy and with circulating cyclic Sézary cells below 1000 per mm³.

2. *Sézary syndrome*—an erythroderma with adenopathy and with circulating Sézary cells above 1000 per mm³. General tissue pathology is negative.

3. *Sézary phenomenon*—transient sézaremia with dermatitis or with lymphoproliferative disease, as Hodgkin's disease.

4. *T cell leukemic erythroderma*—erythroderma with Sézary cells, leukocytosis, adenopathy, and bone marrow involvement. The general tissue pathology is usually positive.

These terms should not be, but often have been, used interchangeably. Thus Sézary syndrome is often considered by many authors to be the equivalent of either erythrodermic mycosis fungoides or T cell leukemic erythroderma. I believe it is usually possible to make separate diagnoses.

A second pattern of erythematous infiltrative skin lesions leading to Sézary syndrome occurs.[20] The prognosis and later evolution of such cases are not clearly different from those of cases of Sézary syndrome beginning as dermatitis. There remains a continuing belief, however, that such cases should be primary cutaneous or visceral lymphoproliferative disease, or both, even if studies of the cytology, histology, and course of disease do not discriminate. These cases should be similar to the rare erythrodermic cases of adult onset T cell leukemia that involve the skin.

Circulating Cells

Cycles of circulating cerebriform cells occur within the normal white count of patients with pre-Sézary and Sézary syndromes. Elevation of total white count and lymphocytosis indicate systemic T cell malignant disease. Epstein and associates[6] also found lymphocytosis a poor prognostic sign in mycosis fungoides. The white cell count and circulating cells are usually not abnormal in mycosis fungoides.[26] Studies with concentrated buffy coat and electron microscopy have shown that cerebriform cells may be found by such methods in many patients with mycosis fungoides,[24] but they also may be found in those with normal buffy coat.[25] Bone marrow studies in both mycosis fungoides and Sézary syndrome are normal until a diagnosis of advanced lymphoproliferative disease can be made. Occasional mycosis fungoides and lymphoma patients do have elevated Sézary counts (Sézary phenomenon) or combined Sézary syndrome. Rare cases of parapsoriasis with transient sézaremia have also been reported.[26]

The cycles of Sézary cells are considered to be longer than diurnal. Sézary counts should be performed in patients in whom circulating Sézary cells may be anticipated for a minimum of 3 days and sometimes for a longer period in order for significant numbers of Sézary cells to be detected.[27] I have found that 2 weeks of daily Sézary counts performed in the morning are necessary in order to demonstrate the quantitative cyclic nature of the tides of circulating Sézary cells. The cycles of Sézary cells usually occur once or twice a week. This rate of frequency explains why leukapheresis is necessary twice weekly in order to bring the Sézary cell counts under control, and it partially explains the requirement for cyclic chemoterapy in some cases. Treatment may cause a rise in circulating Sézary cells, as occurred in the patient of Weinerman and Lu, who was treated with local nitrogen mustard,[28] and as occurred after electron beam therapy in a patient of Miller and coworkers.[29] I have observed increased Sézary cell counts with PUVA therapy (Fig. 1).

Lymphoid cells in the skin originate from lymph nodes or visceral lymphoid tissue and circulate to the skin. The question to be answered is whether the transformation to Sézary cells occurs in the skin or primarily in the viscera. Tritiated thymidine uptake studies indicate that some cell proliferation occurs in the dermis.[30,31] Sauglier-Guedon, Prunieras, and colleagues[32] suggest that evidence shows more thymidine uptake in epidermal Sézary cells. This implies that normal lymphocytes may invade the epidermis, become stimulated by interaction with Langerhans' cells and antigen, and then recycle into the dermis. Turnover studies with radiolabeled Sézary cells showed circulation from blood to skin and no significant entrance of skin cells into the blood over periods of up to 2 days.[29]

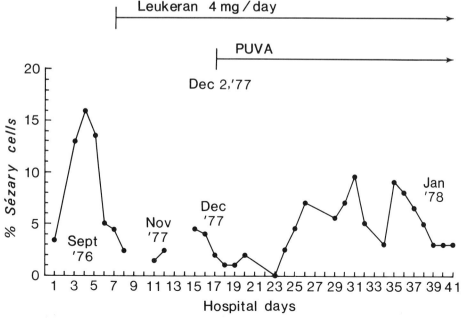

Figure 1.   Cycles of Sézary cells showing the effect of Leukeran and later increase with PUVA therapy.

Circulating Sézary cells do not show a significant uptake of tritiated thymidine and are therefore not proliferative.[33] If the antigen or transforming agent is absorbed into the lymphoid organs, then visceral formation of altered cells could be a primary event in the disease. The rare drug-reaction erythroderma that develops into Sézary syndrome could support this. The homing of the Sézary cells to the skin could be related to the basic T cell nature of the cells.

Because of the onset of Sézary syndrome with dermatitis and the multiple allergens related to that dermatitis, it is attractive to believe that the skin may be a major source of antigen stimulation and cell transformation. Perhaps systemic disease would not develop until adequate antigen or stimulated cells reached the central lymphoid tissue. The skin pathology of the lymphoid infiltrate could develop in a manner similar to that of the tissue culture of Sézary cells cited later, in which cell proliferation under the influence first of antigen and T cell growth factor and then of T cell growth factor alone occurs.

Histology

All stages of mycosis fungoides are characterized by epidermotropism of lymphoid cells. The lymphocytes may be perivascular or band-like in the papillary and subpapillary dermis, but they invade the epidermis as individual cells, as a form of lymphocytic basal layer liquefaction, in focal collections (Pautrier's abscesses), or by diffuse swarming of lymphocytes into the epidermis. The first two patterns are characteristics of Stage I parapsoriasis disease, and the latter two forms relate to more active, aggressive stages of mycosis fungoides. The epidermis thickens in response to this invasion, and the chronic and neurodermatitis, lichenoid, and psoriasiform histologies may develop in mycosis fungoides. The invasion of the cells produces parakeratosis and loss of the barrier.

Sanchez and Ackerman[34] suggest that the diagnosis of mycosis fungoides may be made in its earliest clinical stage by microscopic examination; most authors do not agree.[35] Whereas small, round, or cerebriform lymphocytes characterize the parapsoriasis phase, the greater variability of cell sizes in later stages suggests that small cell and large cell populations are routinely present. Meyer and coworkers[25] found small benign and large cell populations of cerebriform cells in mycosis fungoides and Sézary syndrome. Varying numbers of noninflammatory cells, including eosinophils and histiocytes, are observed. Absence of involvement of the epidermis may occur over mycosis fungoides lymphoma tumors, and it has been suggested that this is a progression from epidermal to dermal disease.[36] Usually, however, lesions with epidermotropism coexist in patients with such tumors, implying that dermotropism is a natural feature of malignant growth patterns. Similarly, it might be argued that epidermotropism is a sign of benign lesions, but of course visceral T cell disease in mycosis fungoides is frequently epidermotropic.[37]

The microscopic picture of Sézary syndrome consists of dermatitis, lymphocytic band, and lymphomatoid band histology.[38,39] The dermatitis involves thickening of the epidermis without significant lymphoid cell changes and with varying keratin layer changes. Rarely, acute dermatitis may be seen. The lymphocytic band is a subpapillary band of mature lymphocytes with occasional cerebriform cells. The lymphomatoid band is a subpapillary band of which the major component is cerebriform cells; cell size varies, and hyperchromatism is present. Epidermotropism is absent to rare in the first two histologic patterns and is only occasionally found in lymphomatoid band. Buechner and Winkelmann[39] found that 15 per cent of lymphomatoid band patients showed a significant epidermotropism. Because the majority of these features were observed consistently in only two patients in that series, the possibility arises that these two patients had true erythrodermic mycosis fungoides with massive circulating Sézary cells. Of the other 39 patients with Sézary syndrome, single-specimen epidermotropism was observed only rarely. Progressive histology from dermatitis to lymphocytic band to lymphomatoid band was observed in some cases. Well-differen-

Table 1. FEATURES OF THE
SÉZARY CELL

Reactive Cell
  Associated with benign disease
  Produced by lectin stimulation
  Polyclonal chromosome changes

Neoplastic Cell
  Increased DNA
  Chromosome markers
  Aneuploidy
  Monoclonal chromosome abnormalities

tiated infiltrates of the skin in patients with erythrodermic T cell disease did not predict the course. No histology except clear lymphoma did predict the course of the disease, and patients with all of the different histologies developed visceral T cell disease. Response to treatment was indicated by diminished cell infiltrate, vascular and fibrous changes, and the presence of giant cells.

Cytology

The cerebriform cell is observed in both mycosis fungoides and Sézary syndrome. It was first described in the blood of Sézary patients by Lutzner and Jordan[40] and has been detected repeatedly by many methods, including phase contrast and freeze fracture techniques. The cerebriform cell is a lymphocyte with a large (10 to 18 micra), expanded, folded nucleus with homogeneous chromatin and no apparent nucleolus. The blue cytoplasm is abundant and often vacuolated, and occasional pseudopods are seen. Zucker-Franklin[41] states that 8-nm cytoplasmic fibrils are typical. The cell is cytologically benign and may be seen in inflammatory dermatoses.[42] Similar cells may appear with immunologic stimulation of lymphocytes (Table 1).[43]

Cerebriform cells characterize mycosis fungoides in the skin, and such cells are observed in the dermis and in the epidermis. Because the larger "mycosis fungoides cell" is so hyperchromatic, this distinctive larger cell cannot be absolutely equated with the smaller cerebriform cell, but a relation seems obligatory from current knowledge.[2,44] The mycosis fungoides lymphoma in the skin is usually composed of larger cerebriform cells in which the nucleus contains heterochromatin and in which the nucleolus is often large and prominent. The nuclear-to-cytoplasmic ratio is increased. Mycosis fungoides lymphoma is the diagnosis when these signs of cellular malignancy and the uniform character of the cell mass are observed. Mycosis fungoides lymphoma cells do not always show surface antigens of T cell type in monoclonal antibody studies. These large cerebriform malignant cells compose the mycosis fungoides lymphoma observed in the viscera, where epidermotropism may also be seen in the urinary, respiratory, and gastrointestinal tracts. Cerebriform cells are observed in both the pre-Sézary and the Sézary syndromes, although they are noted in significant numbers only in the Sézary syndrome. The large cerebriform cell of mycosis fungoides lymphoma occurs occasionally in skin biopsies of Sézary syndrome. Touch preparations of skin biopsies of Sézary syndrome show atypical lymphocytes in half the cases, but not lymphomatoid or lymphoblastoid cells.[38]

Immunology

Crossen and associates were the first to demonstrate that lymphoid cells of the skin in mycosis fungoides and Sézary syndrome are T cells.[45] Sheep cell rosettes, absence of globulin and complement receptors, and specific responses to T cell antibodies have con-

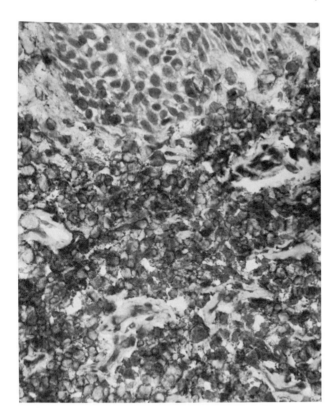

Figure 2. T helper cells constitute most of the subpapillary cell mass in this patient with mycosis fungoides. Immunoperoxidase method. T helper cell monoclonal antibody LEU-3 × 400.

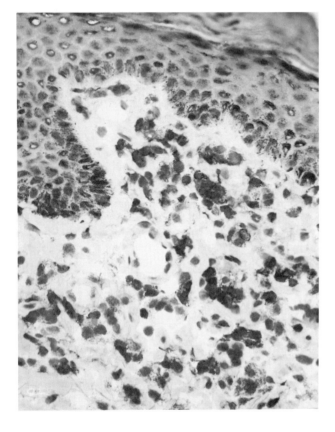

Figure 3. T cells in the subpapillary dermis in Sézary syndrome. Immunoperoxidase method. PAN T cell monoclonal antibody LEU-1 × 400.

Table 2.   REPORTED TYPES OF SÉZARY CELL
MEMBRANE PROPERTIES

Cell Properties	Test Result Combinations Reported	
T cell properties	Rosettes +	Anti-T serum +
	Rosettes −	Anti-T serum +
T and B cell properties	Ig +	Complement +
	Ig −	Complement +
T and B cell properties absent	Null cells	—

firmed the T cell nature of the cerebriform lymphocyte (Figs. 2 and 3).[46] Although this T cell population in both diseases is a unifying feature, further studies have revealed variability in the T cell antigen expression (Table 2). Prunieras[47] summarized the variability of cell surface receptors, indicating that (rarely) B cell markers and, particularly, complement receptors may be expressed on the populations of some Sézary cells.

Broder and coworkers[48] demonstrated that the T cell was a helper T cell, but the latest report has shown that only 7 of 12 patients demonstrated this mature T cell function.[49] T suppressor cell Sézary cases have now been reported.[50] Studies with monoclonal antibodies have shown that the majority of Sézary cells in the skin are T helper cells.[52] However, T suppressor cell populations are seen in large numbers in some cases,[50] and suppressor T cell leukemia involving skin has been reported.[51] T cell monoclonal antibody studies of mycosis fungoides have demonstrated the presence of T helper cells in most cases of this disease, but there are also rare cases of T suppressor cell mycosis fungoides.[52] A more important case may occur when the T cell does not differentiate into the mature helper, for it may be that the T helper cell activity is another sign of differentiated function in a cell.

The response of Sézary cell populations to lectin stimuli reveals two populations of cells. Braylan and colleagues[53] and Kirkpatrick and associates[54] found an absence of Sézary cell response to lectin. Taswell and Winkelmann[55] and other authors[47] showed normal Sézary cell response to lectins (Table 3). The patients in whom there was no response are those with progressive systemic T cell disease. It has been proposed that this difference represents a distinction between the Sézary syndrome and progressive T cell leukemia;[1] in any event, it indicates progressive disease.

The helper T cell population of Sézary patients and mycosis fungoides patients may be associated with elevated IgE values found in some individuals.[56,57] Atopic disease that can lead to Sézary syndrome may be only one reason for the elevated IgE values. Polyclonal gammopathy may also be the result of helper cell activity. The relation of monoclonal protein production to helper T cell function in Sézary syndrome has been suggested, but the two reported cases[58,59] and my two cases do not support this. A B cell clone of

Table 3.   RESPONSE OF THE SÉZARY CELL TO MITOGENS

Authors	No. of Cases	Response	
		Normal	*Minimal to None*
Crossen et al.[45]	1	1	0
Zucker-Franklin[41]	6	4	2
Lutzner et al.[40]	4	4	0
Brouet et al.[46]	6	5	1
Edelson et al.[54]	3	1	2
Braylan et al.[53]	3	0	3
Taswell and Winkelmann[55]	8	7	1
Kirkpatrick et al.[54]	8	2	6

plasma cell proliferation must underlie this entity. I found plasma cells in the skin in my patients, and one of these individuals developed multiple myeloma. It appears that the absence of control (suppression?) of B cell proliferation is basic to monoclonal protein appearance.[60]

Circulating macrophage-inhibiting factor, a lymphokine derived from activated lymphocytes, was observed in the blood of Sézary patients by Yoshida and coworkers[61] and by Umbert, Belcher, and Winkelmann.[62] Circulating macrophage-inhibiting factor was not found in Stage I or Stage III mycosis fungoides in the study by Umbert and colleagues but was present in Stage II mycosis fungoides. Thulin[63] did not find macrophage-inhibiting factor in the serum of mycosis fungoides patients. This macrophage-inhibiting factor material represents the result of T cell stimulation (by antigen?), and it appears logical that dermatitis-evolving Sézary syndrome should demonstrate this and that mycosis fungoides should show macrophage-inhibiting factor only when epidermal interaction is extensive and maximal. When mycosis fungoides tumor formation has occurred and overt malignant cell transformation is present, the fall in macrophage-inhibiting factor could be related to these changes or to additional immune suppression.

T cell–stimulating factor, another lymphokine, has been found in the blood of patients with mycosis fungoides and Sézary syndrome by Poiesz and associates.[64] Normal lymphocytes do not respond to the T cell–growth, or stimulating, factor unless previously stimulated by lectin or antigen. The fact that Sézary cells do respond directly to the T cell factor implies that these cells are chronically stimulated by antigen or are transformed. Gazdar and colleagues[65] also showed propagation in culture of Sézary cells by lectins. It may be supposed that T cell–stimulating factor is being produced by the T cell of the disease process, thus permitting this response.

Safai and coworkers[66] found increased levels of serum thymus factor in 15 of 23 patients with mycosis fungoides but not in Sézary patients. This factor also was elevated in rheumatoid arthritis and psoriasis and is probably a nonspecific response.

Cytogenetics

Crossen and associates[45] described tetraploid cerebriform cells in Sézary syndrome. The presence of increased numbers of chromosomes and of marker chromosomes appears to support the concept of transformed and malignant cells. Whang-Peng and coworkers[67] studied 36 patients, 22 with mycosis fungoides and 14 with Sézary syndrome, and found two stages of disease. The first stage is characterized by lack of clone formation and a wide range of heteroploidy and marker chromosome formation; the later stage consists of abnormal clonal cell development. Dewald and colleagues[68] reported a long-term Sézary patient who died without systemic lymphoid disease but with an hypodiploid chromosome number and three consistent chromosome markers. One appeared to be a translocation between chromosomes 6 and 2. Goh and associates[69] found chromosome 2 abnormalities in a case of Sézary syndrome. The most recent study by Shah-Reddy and coworkers[100] showed a 14:14 (q12–q31) translocation in an unusual Sézary syndrome or advanced T cell disease. This translocation is found frequently in ataxia-telangiectasia. Whang-Peng and colleagues found seven patients with chromosome 1 changes. A recent review of 16 Mayo Clinic patients showed that most had normal chromosomes but that marker chromosomes, translocation, and polyploidy were observed in some patients.

Goh and associates[69] found chromosomal changes in mycosis fungoides to be different from those in Sézary syndrome. The mycosis fungoides patients were characterized by a consistently abnormal karyotype. Erkman-Balis and Rappaport[70] had earlier reported consistently abnormal karyotypes in the skin, nodes, and viscera of mycosis fungoides patients, indicating clonal proliferation in all organs. Goh and coworkers found chromosome abnormalities in B cells as well as T cells in mycosis fungoides, indicating that transformation could affect all lymphocytes in this disease. Edleson and colleagues[71] found consistent karyotypes from extracutaneous sites of three patients, supporting the concept of monoclonal cell proliferation.

The cell DNA content, which reflects chromosome number changes, has been studied extensively by Van Vloten and associates[72,73] and confirmed by Hagedorn and Kiefer.[74] DNA abnormalities in skin and nodes correlate with cytology and with prognosis. For most patients with abnormal DNA histograms, a positive diagnosis of lymphoproliferative disease could be made on follow-up. The presence of increased DNA correlates with progressive disease from plaque to tumor stage. DNA cytometry showed two cell populations in mycosis fungoides and Sézary syndrome: a small-sized, normal cell population and a generally larger altered cell population with increased proliferative and late T cell malignancy.

Associated Diseases

Alopecia mucinosa or follicular mucinosis has a definite relationship to mycosis fungoides. It is so indicative of mycosis fungoides in the adult that it is considered often as a skin manifestation of mycosis fungoides. However, it occurs frequently in children, and in adults it may be a benign, limited skin disease. A study of the cells in alopecia mucinosa might be revealing and might enable investigators to predict which cases may be part of the T cell spectrum. A relationship between mycosis fungoides and Kaposi's sarcoma has been reported, and rare cases of xanthoma lesions have been noted. No relation to other systemic disease is recognized.

There is a high incidence of contact dermatitis, drug reactions, and even atopic dermatitis with Sézary syndrome. Two cases of lymphocytoma have been reported accompanying or preceding Sézary erythroderma. Alopecia mucinosa has not been reported with Sézary syndrome. One of my patients had localized xanthomatous lesions. Skin and visceral carcinoma may be observed, as was also noted by Epstein and associates[6] and by DuVivier and coworkers[75] after nitrogen mustard therapy in mycosis fungoides. Tinea infections are not uncommon. Late mycosis fungoides and evolving Sézary syndrome may be accompanied by herpes simplex or other cutaneous infections.

Evolution

It is important to note that parapsoriasis–mycosis fungoides can progress to malignant lymphoma tumor formation, which occurs in 25 per cent of the cases.[15] Self-healing lesions and rapid response of localized lesions to many forms of therapy indicate that lymphoma-leukemia development does not always occur. The progressive disease is most frequently a T cell malignancy that may develop first in regional nodes or may rapidly develop in visceral organs. For the past 5 years, cases of Hodgkin's disease in lymph nodes together with parapsoriasis and mycosis fungoides of the skin have been reported.[76] Recently, Scheen and coworkers[77] reported seven cases of large cell lymphoma (B and T cell) and six cases of Hodgkin's disease in the lymph nodes and viscera of patients with mycosis fungoides. Cases of myelomonocytic leukemia evolving in mycosis fungoides in which therapy is not related indicate a general potential for hematopoietic malignancies in the patient.[78] The finding of chromosomal abnormalities in B cells of mycosis fungoides patients by Goh and colleagues[69] is additional evidence for the possibility of diverse malignant changes. The finding of Hodgkin's disease as a frequent malignancy in relatives of patients with mycosis fungoides is additional confirmation of this supposition.[79]

Evolution of Sézary syndrome to T cell lymphoma-leukemia is a common course.

However, most patients die of septicemia and cardiorespiratory disease without such systemic lymphoma-leukemia evolution. Only 4 of one series of 27 patients developed lymphoma, and one of these patients had Hodgkin's disease.[11] Our more recent series of 39 patients shows 8 of these patients alive or in remission. Of the 31 patients who died, it was possible to determine the cause of death in 28. The primary cause of death in 12 patients was sepsis, pneumonia, or cardiovascular disease. Three patients died of widespread Sézary cell infiltration of visceral organs and lymph nodes. High-grade lymphoma was present in six patients: lymphosarcoma in three, Hodgkin's disease in one, lymphocytic leukemia in one, and multiple myeloma in one. Three patients developed an unknown visceral granulomatosis.

Comment

The development of the unifying concept of T cell cutaneous disease has had a great impact on ideas and practice of dermatologic oncology. The monoclonal methods for demonstration of T cell subsets in blood and tissues have provided a tool to confirm the ideas and (it is hoped) to aid the practice. To date, however, it has not been possible to state definitely by clinical, histologic, or immunocytologic methods the benign or low-risk T cell lymphoproliferative disease that will develop aggressive T cell or other lymphoma. Even staging laparotomy is not adequate as a predictor: Variakojis and coworkers[80] and Doyle and Winkelmann[81] found that even after negative laparotomies and aggressive local therapy (electron beam and nitrogen mustard), malignant lymphoma could develop years later.

Cerebriform and variable atypical cells characterize all the syndromes listed in Table 4. Unusual forms of T cell lymphoma in which position is less certain include the erythrophagocytic T lymphoma described by Kadin and colleagues[82] and the visceral T cell lymphoma with polylobed nuclei described by Pinkus and associates.[83] Circulating Sézary cells may characterize some of them. The cytology is another unifying feature of these clinical states, but differences abound. There are many major differences between Sézary syndrome and mycosis fungoides; these are listed in Table 5. The purpose of this list is to emphasize the separation—the reasons to consider these conditions as one disease process are clear and have been repeatedly emphasized. The differences listed may be a result of antigen presentation, host response, or carcinogenic transforming agents—viral or chemical.

A C-type virus in culture of cells from mycosis fungoides and Sézary patients was originally considered to be a possible contaminant. Cells from most patients did not demonstrate the virus. The presence of a T cell growth factor in the blood of Sézary and

Table 4. SYNDROMES OF T CELL PROLIFERATION

Benign Disease
    Lymphomatoid contact dermatitis
    Actinic reticuloid
    Pre-Sézary syndrome
    Parapsoriasis

Low-Risk Malignancy
    Mycosis fungoides
    Sézary syndrome

High-Risk Malignancy
    Acute T cell leukemia—child
    T cell leukemia—adult
    T cell lymphoma—adult
    T cell mycosis fungoides d'emblée

Table 5. COMPARISON OF MYCOSIS FUNGOIDES AND SÉZARY SYNDROME

	Mycosis Fungoides	Sézary Syndrome
Preceding lesion	Parapsoriasis	Dermatitis
Clinical presentation	Plaque, tumor, rare erythroderma	Erythroderma, rare tumor
Course	Chronic	Chronic
Histology	Epidermotropic, lymphomatoid band	Dermatitis, lymphocytic or dermal lymphomatoid band
Circulating cells	Rare Sézary cells	Significant cycles of Sézary cells
Immune reactions	Delayed tests positive	Delayed tests negative
Allergic reaction	Occasional	Frequent
Chromosome studies	Clonal changes	Nonclonal changes

mycosis fungoides patients implied some cell transformation.[84] The discovery of a C retrovirus in cells of adult Japanese T cell lymphoma-leukemia and its similarity to the American T cell virus provided a strong rationale for additional viral studies.[85] The DNA of the isolated viruses is unique and unlike other viral DNAs.[86,87] It has been noted that the Japanese T cell disease occurs in two localized areas of Japan. Antibodies to the virus are present in the blood of the patients and in some of their family members. Both American and Japanese patients may have the same antibody.

A satisfactory model for progressive inflammatory and malignant lymphoid disease is the graft versus host reaction. Injection of lymphoid cells to promote the graft versus host reaction results in a lichenoid, T cell, lymphocytic band inflammation of the skin. This inflammation can involve the epidermis. Following graft versus host inflammation, malignant lymphoma may develop in surviving animals.[88] The presence of a virus in the lymphoma has been confirmed in some instances.[89]

It is probable that unique skin-oriented low-grade T cell malignancy is related to the later development of high-grade malignancy in Sézary and mycosis fungoides patients.[90] A virus present in the tissue of patients with mycosis fungoides or Sézary syndrome could be activated by chronic dermatitis or inflammation of the skin. Because Sézary patients have many recurrent sensitivity reactions in the skin, it is also possible that this renders the patient susceptible to later virus infections and cell transformation. Mycosis fungoides has been proposed to be the result of antigen stimulation by Tan and coworkers,[56] Schuppli,[91] and Bazex.[92] Patch tests were positive in 15 per cent of mycosis fungoides patients tested and studied by me in the last 5 years. Multiple allergic sensitivities were noted by Green and associates.[79] More studies of this kind are necessary in mycosis fungoides.

The autopsy study of mycosis fungoides by Rappaport and Thomas[37] demonstrated the great unity in the pathology of cases of mycosis fungoides in which the patients died of lymphoma, and this study supported the central T cell concept of primary lymphoid skin disease. The problem of mycosis fungoides is broader than this unity achieved in autopsied patients, as I have tried to emphasize. Only a percentage of patients with mycosis fungoides develop tumors or die of this malignant progression. Two opposing philosophies that affect how we consider and treat patients with mycosis fungoides and Sézary syndrome are apparent. One considers all mycosis fungoides cases malignant—at all times. That is, malignant transformation occurs at the time of the first clinical manifestations and when the first histologic signs of the problem can be recognized. The second view considers that these diseases represent benign, transitional, and malignant phases of T cell disease. I believe that this latter approach has been successfully documented by classical descriptions of cases, by progressive changes in the pathology and cytology, and by the development of overt systemic lymphoma in patients with extensive skin disease, regional lymph node involvement, and immune suppression.

Sophisticated studies of staging can demonstrate as many as 80 per cent of patients to have systemic disease.[93] This may be attributed to patient selection in specialized centers.

Table 6. SEZARY SYNDROME: TREATMENT AND DURATION OF REMISSION
IN 42 PATIENTS

	No. of Patients	No. of Negative Responses	Remission	
			4–8 Mos.	>1 Yr.
Prednisone and chlorambucil	29	6	16	7
X-irradiation	7	3	3	1
Electron beam therapy	3	1	2	0
Leukapheresis	3	0	3	0
Total no.	42	10	24	8
%	100	24	57	19

Another possibility is that it may be the result of application of sophisticated technology that can detect minor circulating abnormal cell levels, which light microscopy and ordinary technology cannot recognize (and which may not always be clinically relevant). Does it mean, as the authors suggest, that all cases of mycosis fungoides are systemic and should be treated by systemic means—that is, polychemotherapy—before the pathology can determine the presence of lymphoma? Current practice calls for suppression and definitive therapy only to the skin in mycosis fungoides, and aggressive chemotherapy only when high-risk malignancy is identified. More selective and safe chemotherapy will be necessary before anyone can feel comfortable about using massive systemic chemotherapy in a patient with an intact hematopoietic and immune system by all clinical and laboratory measurement. Sézary patients have died from therapy rather than from the disease.[94]

A therapy that is safe for Sézary syndrome and particularly effective for pre-Sézary syndrome is the combination of leukapheresis, low-dose prednisone, and chlorambucil (Leukeran) advocated by Winkelmann and coworkers (Table 6).[13,94] The leukapheresis may be used as the only treatment in patients with normal white counts, and 6 of 16 patients in the literature have shown a good response to the therapy.[95] Rather than perform aggressive chemotherapy for mycosis fungoides, it might be most useful to attempt to use these safer regimens that have been developed to help Sézary syndrome in mycosis fungoides. Specific anti–T cell therapy may also be tried when it is possible to use it without danger. Antithymocyte globulin will reduce Sézary cells in some,[96] but not all, patients.[97] Tilorone has produced good improvement in pre-Sézary erythroderma with a decrease in circulating cells and improvement in skin biopsies and clinical findings.[98] Monoclonal T cell antibodies have had a preliminary trial with definite but minimal improvement in mycosis fungoides.[99] Treating these patients safely and effectively in the benign and low-risk stage will provide the best opportunity for clinical response.

References

1. Winkelmann, R. K., and Caro, W. A.: Current problems in mycosis fungoides and Sézary syndrome. Annu. Rev. Med. 28:251, 1977.
2. Zackheim, H.: Cutaneous T cell lymphoma. Arch. Dermatol. 117:295, 1981.
3. Poiesz, B. J., Ruscetti, F. W., Reitz, M. S., Kalyanaraman, V. S., and Gallo, R. C.: Isolation of a new type C retrovirus (MTLV) in primary uncultured cells of a patient with Sézary T-cell leukemia. Nature 294:268, Nov. 1981.
4. Kalyanaraman, V. S., Sarngadharan, M. G., Bunn, P. A., Minna, J. D., and Gallo, R. C.: Antibodies in human sera reactive against an internal structure protein of human T-cell lymphoma virus. Nature 294:271, Nov. 1981.
5. Clendenning, W. E.: Mycosis fungoides d'emblée. A rare presentation of cutaneous cell lymphoma. Cancer 49:742, 1982.

6. Epstein, E. H., Jr., Levin, D. L., Croft, J. D., Jr., and Lutzner, M. A.: Mycosis fungoides: Survival, prognostic features, response to therapy, and autopsy findings. Medicine 51:61, 1972.

7. Fuks, Z. Y., Bagshaw, M. A., and Farber, E. M.: Prognostic signs and the management of mycosis fungoides. Cancer 32:1385, 1973.

8. Hoppe, R. T., Fuks, Z. Y., and Bagshaw, M. A.: Radiation in the management of cutaneous T cell lymphoma. Cancer Treat. Rep. 63:625, 1979.

9. Van Scott, E. J., and Kalmanson, J. D.: Complete remission of mycosis fungoides lymphoma induced by topical nitrogen mustard. Cancer 32:18, 1973.

10. Lamberg, S. I., Green, S. B., Byar, D. P., Block, J. B., Clendenning, W. E., Epstein, E. H., Golitz, L. E., Lorincz, A. L., Michel, B., Roenigk, H. H., Van Scott, E. J., Vonderheid, E. C., and Thomas, R. J.: Status report of 376 mycosis fungoides patients at 4 years. Cancer 63:701, 1979.

11. Winkelmann, R. K.: Clinical studies of T cell erythroderma in Sézary syndrome. Mayo Clin. Proc. 49:519, 1974.

12. Broder, S., Uchiyama, T., and Waldmann, T. A.: Current concepts in immunoregulatory T-cell neoplasms. Cancer Treat. Rep. 63:607, 1979.

13. Hamminga, L., Hartgrink-Groeneveld, C. A., and van Vloten, W. A.: Sézary's syndrome: A clinical evaluation of eight patients. Br. J. Dermatol. 100:291, 1979.

14. Buechner, S. A., and Winkelmann, R. K.: Sézary syndrome and pre-Sézary syndrome. Unpublished results.

15. Samman, P. D.: Cutaneous reticuloses. Trans. St. Johns Hosp. 61:11, 1975.

16. Samman, P. D.: The natural history of parapsoriasis en plaques. Br. J. Dermatol. 87:405, 1972.

17. Schmoeckel, C., Burg, G., Braun-Falco, O., and Klingmuller, G.: Mycosis fungoïde à forte malignité avec transformation cytologique. Ann. Dermatol. Venereol. 108:231, 1981.

18. Schmoeckel, C., Burg, G., and Braun-Falco, O.: Quantitative analysis of lymphoid cells in cutaneous low-grade malignant B cell lymphoma. Arch. Dermatol. Res. 266:239, 1979.

19. Ficks, Z., Bagshaw, M. A., and Farber, E. M.: Prognostic signs and the management of the mycosis fungoides. Cancer 32:1385, 1973.

20. Winkelmann, R. K., and Linman, J. W.: Erythroderma with atypical lymphocytes (Sézary syndrome). Am. J. Med. 55:192, 1973.

21. Ecker, R. I., and Winkelmann, R. K.: Lymphomatoid contact dermatitis 7:84, 1981.

22. Ive, F. A., Magnus, I. A., Warin, R. P., and Wilson-Jones, E.: Actinic reticuloid. Br. J. Dermatol. 81:469, 1969.

23. Buechner, S. A., and Winkelmann, R. K. Pre-Sézary erythroderma evolving to Sézary syndrome, a report of seven cases. Arch. Dermatol. 119:285. April 1983.

24. Guccion, J. G., Fischmann, A. B., Bunn, P. A., Jr., Schechter, G. P., Patterson, R. H., and Mathews, M. J.: Ultrastructural appearance of cutaneous T cell lymphomas in skin, lymph nodes and peripheral blood. Cancer Treat. Rep. 63:565, 1979.

25. Meyer, C. J. L. M., Van Leeuwen, A. W. F. M., Van der Loo, E. M., Van de Putte, L. B. A., and Van Vloten, W. A.: Cerebriform (Sézary-like) mononuclear cells in healthy individuals. Virdi. Arch. B Cell Path. 25:95, 1977.

26. Winkelmann, R. K., and Hoagland, C. A.: Circulating Sézary cells in mycosis fungoides. Dermatologica 160:73, 1980.

27. Duncan, S. C., and Winkelmann, R. K.: Circulating Sézary cells in hospitalized dermatology patients. Br. J. Dermatol. 99:171, 1978.

28. Weinerman, B. H., and Lu, L. C.: Sézary syndrome: An unusual case. Cancer 47:2946, 1981.

29. Miller, R. A., Coleman, C. W., Fawcett, H. D., Hoppe, R. T., and McDougall, I. R.: Sézary syndrome: A model for migration of T lymphocytes to skin. N. Engl. J. Med. 303:89, 1980.

30. Bosman, F. T., and Van Vloten, W. A.: Sézary syndrome: A cytogenetic, cytophotometric, and autoradiographic study. J. Pathol. 118:49, 1976.

31. Chandra, P., Chana, A. D., Chickappa, G., and Cronkite, E. P.: Cytokinetic characteristics of Sézary cells. Blood 48:996, 1976.

32. Sauglier-Guedon, I., Prunieras, M., Durepaire, R., and Grupper, C.: Preferential replication of Sézary cells in the epidermis. Bull. Cancer 64:259, 1977.

33. Shackney, S. E., Edelson, R., and Bunn, P. A., Jr.: The kinetics of Sézary cell production. Cancer Treat. Rep. 63:659, 1979.

34. Sanchez, J. L., and Ackerman, A. B.: The patch stage of mycosis fungoides. Am. J. Dermatopathol. 1:5, 1979.

35. Clendenning, W. E., and Rappaport, H. W.: Pathology of cutaneous T cell lymphomas. Cancer Treat. Rep. 63:719, 1979.

36. Edelson, R. L.: Cutaneous T cell lymphomas. J. Am. Acad. Dermatol. 2:89, 1980.

37. Rappaport, H., and Thomas, B.: Mycosis fungoides: The pathology of extracutaneous involvement. Cancer 34:1198, 1974.

38. Holdaway, D. R., and Winkelmann, R. K.: The histopathology of Sézary syndrome. Mayo Clin. Proc. 49:541, 1974.

39. Buechner, S. A., and Winkelmann, R. K.: Clinopathiological correlation of 39 patients with Sézary syndrome. Unpublished results.

40. Lutzner, M. D., and Jordan, H. W.: The ultrastructure of an abnormal cell in Sézary's syndrome. Blood 31:719, 1968.

41. Zucker-Franklin, D.: Thymus dependent lymphocytes in lymphoproliferative disorders. J. Invest. Dermatol. 67:412, 1976.

42. Flaxman, B. A., Zelazny, G., and Van Scott, E. J.: Nonspecificity of characteristic cells in mycosis fungoides. Arch. Dermatol. 104:141, 1971.

43. Yeckley, J. A., Weston, W. L., Thorne, E. G., and Norris, D.: Production of Sézary-like cells from normal human lymphocytes. Arch. Dermatol. 111:29, 1975.

44. Brehmer-Anderson, E.: Mycosis fungoides and its relation to Sézary's syndrome. Acta Dermatol. Venereol. 56:1, 1976.

45. Crossen, P. E., Mellor, J. E. L., and Finley, A. G.: The Sézary syndrome. Am. J. Med. 50:24, 1971.

46. Brouet, J. C., Flandrin, G., and Seligmann, M.: Indication of the thymus derived nature of the proliferating cells in six patients with Sézary syndrome. N. Engl. J. Med. 289:314, 1973.

47. Prunieras, M.: The Sézary syndrome. Trans. St. Volum. 61:1, 1975.

48. Broder, S., Edelson, R., and Lutzner, M. A.: The Sézary syndrome: A malignant proliferation of helper T cells. J. Clin. Invest. 58:1297, 1976.

49. Broder, S., Uchiyama, T., and Waldman, T. A.: Current concepts in immunoregulatory T-cell neoplasms. Cancer Treat. Rep. 63:607, 1979.

50. Kansu, E., and Hauptman, S.: Suppressor cell activity in Sézary syndrome. Blood 50 (Suppl.):221, 1977.

51. Uchiyama, T., Sagawa, K., and Takatsuki, K.: Effect of adult T cell leukemia cells on pokeweed mitogen induced normal B-cell differentiation. Clin. Immunol. Immunopathol. 10:24, 1978.

52. Buechner, S. A., Winkelmann, R. K., and Banks, P. M.: Characterization of T cells in cutaneous lesions of Sézary syndrome and T cell leukemia by monoclonal antibodies. Arch. Dermatol. (in press).

53. Braylan, R., Variakojis, D., and Yachnin, S.: The Sézary syndrome lymphoid cell: Abnormal mitogenic responsiveness and surface properties. Blood 42:1024, 1973.

54. Edelson, R. L., Kirkpatrick, C. H., Shevach, E. M., Schein, P. S., Smith, R. W., Green, I, and Lutzner, M.: Preferential cutaneous infiltration by neoplastic thymus-derived lymphocytes: Morphologic and functional studies. Am. Intern. Med. 80:685, 1974.

55. Taswell, H., and Winkelmann, R. K.: Mitogen response of Sézary cells. Unpublished results.

56. Tan, R. S. H., Butterworth, C. M., and McLaughlin, H.: Mycosis fungoides, a disease of antigen persistence. Br. J. Dermatol. 91:607, 1974.

57. Mackie, R., Sless, F. R., and Cochran, R.: Lymphocyte abnormalities in mycosis fungoides. Br. J. Dermatol. 94:173, 1976.

58. Kovary, P. M., Niedorf, H., and Sommer, G.: Paraproteinemia in Sézary syndrome. Dermatologica 154:138, 1977.

59. Joyner, M. V., Cassuto, J. P., and Dujardin, P.: Cutaneous T-cell lymphoma in association with a monoclonal gammopathy. Arch. Dermatol. 115:326, 1979.

60. Kermani-Arab, W., Roberts, J. L., and Hanifin, J. M.: Lack of functional immunoregulatory cells in a patient with mycosis fungoides and circulating Sézary cells. J. Natl. Cancer Inst. 60:1295, 1978.

61. Yoshida, T., Edelson, R., Cohen, S., and Breen, I.: Migration inhibitory activity in serum and cell supernatant in serum of patients with Sézary syndrome. J. Immunol. 114:915, 1975.

62. Umbert, P., Belcher, R. W., and Winkelmann, R. K.: Macrophage inhibitor factor (MIF) in cutaneous lymphoproliferative diseases. Br. J. Dermatol. 95:475, 1976.

63. Thulin, H.: Absence of leukocyte migration inhibitory factor in serum from patients with mycosis fungoides. Arch. Dermatol. Res. 257:157, 1976.

64. Poiesz, B. J., Ruscetti, F. W., Mier, J. W., Woods, A. M., and Gallo, R. C.: T cell lines established from human T lymphocytid neoplasias by direct response to T cell growth factor. Proc. Natl. Acad. Sci. U.S.A. 77:6815, 1980.

65. Gazdar, A., Carney, D. N., Bunn, P. A., Russell, E. K., Jaffe, E. S., Schechter, G. P., and Guerion, J. G.: Mitogen requirements for in vitro propagation of cutaneous T cell lymphomas. Blood 55:409, 1980.

66. Safai, B., Dardenne, M., Incefy, G. S., and Good, R. A.: Circulating thymic factor in mycosis fungoides and Sézary syndrome. Clin. Immunol. Immunopathol. 13:402, 1979.

67. Whang-Peng, J., Bunn, P. A., Jr., Knutsen, T., Schechter, G. P., Gazdar, A. F., Mathews, M. J., and Minna, J. D.: Cytogenetic abnormalities in patients with cutaneous T cell lymphoma. Cancer Treat. Rep. 63:575, 1979.

68. Dewald, G., Spurbeck, J. L., and Vitek, H. A.: Chromosomes in a patient with the Sézary syndrome. Mayo Clin. Proc. 49:553, 1974.

69. Goh, K., Reddy, M. M., and Joishy, S. K.: Chromosomes and B and T cells in mycosis fungoides. Am. J. Med. Sci. 276:197, 1978.

70. Erkman-Balis, B., and Rappaport, H.: Cytogenetic studies in mycosis fungoides. Cancer 34:626, 1974.

71. Edelson, R. L., Berger, C. L., and Raafat, J.: Karyotype studies of cutaneous T cell lymphoma: Evidence for a clonal origin. J. Invest. Dermatol. 73:548, 1979.

72. Van Vloten, W. A., Schalberg, A., and Van der Ploeg, M.: Cytophotometric studies in mycosis fungoides and other cutaneous reticuloses. Bull. Cancer 64:249, 1977.

73. Van Vloten, W. A., Scheffer, E., and Meijer, C. J. L. M.: DNA-cytophotometry of lymph node imprints from patients with mycosis fungoides. J. Invest. Dermatol. 73:275, 1979.

74. Hagedorn, M., and Kiefer, G.: DNA content of mycosis fungoides cells. Arch. Dermatol. Res. 258:127, 1979.

75. DuVivier, A., Von der Heid, E. C., Van Scott, E. J., and Urbach, T.: Mycosis fungoides, nitrogen mustard, and cancer. Br. J. Dermatol. 99(Suppl. 16):61, 1978.

76. Chan, W. C., Griem, M. L., Grozea, P. N., Freel, R. J., and Variakojis, D.: Mycosis fungoides and Hodgkin's disease occurring in the same patient. Cancer 44:1408, 1979.

77. Scheen, S. R., Banks, P. M., and Winkelmann, R. K.: Heterogeneity of malignant lymphomas arising in mycosis fungoides. Presented at Int. Acad. Pathol., Chicago, 1981.
78. Lofgren, R. K., Wiltse, J. C., and Winkelmann, R. K.: Mycosis fungoides evolving to myelomonocytic leukemia. Arch. Dermatol. 114:916, 1978.
79. Green, M. H., Dalager, A. A., Lamberg, S. I., Argyropoulos, C. E., and Fraumeni, J. F., Jr.: Mycosis fungoides: Epidemiologic observations. Cancer Treat. Rep. 63:597, 1979.
80. Variakojis, D., Rosas-Uribe, A., and Rappaport, H.: Mycosis fungoides: Pathologic findings in staging laparotomies. Cancer 33:1589, 1974.
81. Doyle, J. D., and Winkelmann, R. K.: Staging procedures in cutaneous T-cell disease. Arch. Dermatol. 117:543, 1981.
82. Kadin, M. E., Kamoun, M., and Lamberg, J.: Erythrophagocytic T gamma lymphoma. N. Engl. J. Med. 304:648, 1981.
83. Pinkus, G. S., Said, J. W., and Hargreaves, H.: Malignant lymphoma, T-cell type: A distinct morphologic variant with large multilobulated nuclei. Am. J. Clin. Pathol. 72:540, 1979.
84. Poiesz, B. J., Ruscetti, F. W., Drier, J. W., Woods, A. M., and Gallo, R. C.: T-cell lines established from human T-lymphocytic neoplasias by direct response to T cell growth factor. Proc. Natl. Acad. Sci. U.S.A. 77:6815, 1980.
85. Miyoshi, I., Kulsonishi, I., Yoshimoto, S., Akagi, T., Ohtsuki, Y., Shiraishi, Y., Nagata, K., and Hinuma, Y.: Type C virus particles in a cord T-cell line derived by cocultivating normal human cord leukocytes and human leukemia cells. Nature 294:770, 1981.
86. Poiesz, B. J., Ruscetti, F. W., Gazdar, A. F., Bunn, P. A., Minna, J. D., and Gallo, R. C.: Detection and isolation of type C retrovirus particles from fresh and cultured lymphocytes of a patient with cutaneous T cell lymphoma. Proc. Natl. Acad. Sci. U.S.A. 78:7415, 1980.
87. Poiesz, B. J., Ruscetti, M. S., Kalyanaraman, V. S., and Gallo, R. C.: Isolation of a new type C retrovirus in primary uncultured cells of a patient with Sézary T cell leukemia. Nature 294:268, 1981.
88. Schwartz, R. S.: Immunoregulation, oncogenic viruses, and malignant lymphomas. Lancet 1:1266, 1972.
89. Melief, C. J. M., Datta, S., Louis, S., and Schwartz, R. S.: Immunologic activation of murine leukemia viruses. Lancet 34:1481, 1974.
90. Büchner, S., and Rufli, T.: Manifestation eines malignen Lymphoms von hohem Malignitätsgrad im Spätstadium der Mycosis fungoides. Enzymzytochemische und immunzytologische Untersuchungen. Dermatologica 159:125, 1979.
91. Schuppli, R.: Is mycosis fungoides an immunoma? Dermatologica 153:1, 1976.
92. Bazex, J.: Mycosis fungoides: Can continuous antigen stimulation be its cause? Nouv. Presse Med. 22:1410, 1978.
93. Huberman, M., Bunn, P., Mathews, P., Fischmann, B., Guccion, J., Drinnick, R., Ihde, D., Cohen, M., and Minna, J.: Extracutaneous Involvement in patients with cutaneous T cell lymphomas: Mycosis fungoides and Sézary syndrome. Proc. Am. Assoc. Cancer Res. 20:410, 1979.
94. Winkelmann, R. K., Perry, H. O., Muller, S. A., Schroeter, A. L., Jordon, R. E., and Rogers, R. S., III: Treatment of Sézary syndrome. Mayo Clin. Proc. 49:590, 1974.
95. Revuz, J., Touraine, R., and Thivolet, J.: Leukapheresis for Sézary syndrome. Presented at the International Congress of Dermatology, XVI, Tokyo, May 22–27, 1982.
96. Edelson, R. L., Raafat, J., and Berger, C. L.: Antithymocyte globulin in the management of cutaneous T cell lymphoma. Cancer Treat. Rep. 63:675, 1979.
97. Gould, D. J., Rowell, N. F., and Anthony, H.: Failure of antithymocyte globulin treatment in T cell lymphoma. Lancet 2:1365, 1977.
98. Crotty, C., and Winkelmann, R. K.: Tilorone treatment of mycosis fungoides and Sézary syndrome. J. Am. Acad. Dermatol. 7:468, 1982.
99. Muller, R. A., and Levy, R.: Response of cutaneous T cell lymphoma to therapy with hybridoma monoclonal antibody. Lancet 2:226, 1981.
100. Shah-Reddy, I., et al.: Sézary syndrome with a 14:14 (q12:q31) translocation. Cancer 1:75, 1982.

MYCOSIS FUNGOIDES IS A CANCER*

Ervin Epstein, Jr., M.D.

In general, mycosis fungoides today is *defined* as a malignant lymphoma, most commonly (and perhaps always) being an excess proliferation of helper T lymphocytes.[1] In recent years, only Winkelmann and Caro[2] have been bold enough to question the prevailing wisdom that mycosis fungoides is a distinct malignancy which, albeit of uncertain prognosis, is a cancer at the very start. Even they admit that in its late stages mycosis fungoides is a lymphoma, but they suggest that the usual patient with cutaneous mycosis fungoides or the Sézary syndrome has some sort of "transitional" disease between the benign parapsoriasis and the truly malignant late-stage "lymphoma."

The Sézary syndrome initially was defined in patients with erythroderma and peculiar large, circulating leukocytes. Subsequently, at least three types of data have shown to all but the most die-hard "hair splitters" that the Sézary syndrome is merely a leukemic variant of mycosis fungoides. Thus, circulating abnormal cells like those of the Sézary syndrome can be found in most patients with mycosis fungoides if the detection system is sufficiently sensitive, irrespective of whether or not erythroderma is present. Furthermore, the same patient may have typical mycosis fungoides with plaques and tumors at one time and erythroderma at another time. Finally, the circulating cells in patients with "classical" Sézary syndrome, like those in the skin in "classical" mycosis fungoides, are helper T lymphocytes and appear, at least in some patients, to migrate between skin and blood compartments.

I shall argue that mycosis fungoides is a cancer because it resembles other diseases that we call cancer. I also believe that there is overwhelming evidence that mycosis fungoides is a malignancy at its very onset. Arguing by resemblance may be unsatisfying to some, for there will be persons who expect evidence to be open to many interpretations (for example, galloping hooves may belong to herds of zebras rather than to horses). However, in the absence of a fundamental understanding of cancer, it is most reasonable to consider that diseases that resemble cancers indeed are cancers. Such resemblance falls into three categories: clinical behavior of the disease, in vitro growth characteristics of the cells, and changes in the chromatin of the cells.

Cancer. It is to be expected that definitions of cancer may change, just as will diagnostic criteria for mycosis fungoides itself. Currently it seems best to define cancer as a disease in which there is a cellular overgrowth that is limited eventually only by the death of the patient. At present, we know of no way to reverse such disorderly growth other than to kill the affected cells. However, it appears that our understanding of the causes of such growth is now expanding enormously.

The current theory is that it is excessive expression of growth-regulatory genes ("oncogenes," or "transforming genes") within the cell that causes cancer and that these genes either are or resemble closely normal cellular constituents.[3] The excess expression might be caused by transposition of the gene to a site that normally promotes high-level transcription of a less harmful gene (e.g., one coding for an antibody), by the unlucky insertion of a viral promoter near the oncogene, by duplication of the chromosome or the appropriate part of the chromosome carrying the transforming gene, or by some other mechanism.

---

*I prefer to use the term "mycosis fungoides" rather than the now more fashionable "cutaneous T cell lymphoma"[1] for the sake of tradition, in order not to frighten the patient unduly by the use of "lymphoma," and so as not to exclude unnecessarily the patient whose cell type has not been defined.

Thus, viral infection, contact with carcinogenic chemicals, or exposure to damaging irradiation all may produce cancer by a final common pathway—by increasing the production of specific proteins that cause disordered growth of cells. Obviously, such new understanding holds the promise that some way of reversing specifically the effects of the proteins or of remodulating the gene expression might be found someday.

Mycosis fungoides currently is somewhat unique in that, at least in some forms, it is the human malignancy most clearly associated with an RNA tumor virus (retrovirus). Such RNA tumor viruses are associated strongly with lymphomas and leukemias in subhuman mammals. This virus can be isolated from cell lines in some patients with T cell malignancies[4] and appears to be able to transform normal human T lymphocytes to malignant-appearing cells.[5] Relatives and close contacts of these patients have an antibody to core proteins purified from the human T cell leukemia virus.[6,7]

Thus, it may be necessary to consider some forms of mycosis fungoides to be infections caused by a virus that produces cellular proliferation rather than cellular death. However, irrespective of the cause, it is the proliferation that is typical of the disease and that is detrimental to the patient.

Clinical Behavior.   We now believe that mycosis fungoides is an overproliferation of thymus-derived lymphocytes that normally circulate through the epidermis, the lymphatics, and the blood. When relatively well differentiated, they maintain their epidermotropism and invade the epidermis, where they may be recognized histologically as scattered cells or as the clusters described by Pautrier. When they are less well differentiated, so many cells may accumulate in the lymph nodes that normal cells are replaced. The number of these cells in the blood is so great that the disease is said to be in a leukemic phase—the Sézary syndrome. Clinically, the excess accumulation is manifested in the skin by progressively thicker patches, plaques, and tumors. Early in the course, most of the cells appear histologically to be normal inflammatory cells, whereas later the infiltrate assumes a more monomorphous pattern, with sheets of malignant cells. It is uncertain whether the inflammatory cells somehow regulate the growth of the malignant cells. However, one should not make the logical error that because inflammatory cells respond to nonmalignant stimuli, their response in mycosis fungoides is to something other than malignant cells. In late-stage mycosis fungoides, when tumors are filled with abundant abnormal-appearing cells, lymph nodes are replaced by abnormal cells, and internal viscera are infiltrated by abnormal cells, it is hard to mistake the disease for something other than an uncontrolled growth of cells.

Cell Growth in Vitro.   Cells from patients with mycosis fungoides can form long-lived cell lines in vitro when cultured with partially purified human T cell growth factor (pp-TCGF or Interleukin 2).[8] T cells from normal persons cannot be grown in this manner unless they are first activated by mitogens, such as phytohemagglutinin, or by antigen. Some cell lines from mycosis fungoides patients have lost their requirement for pp-TCGF and are able then to continue to grow rapidly without it. This seemingly indefinite life span in vitro is typical of malignant, but not of benign, cells.

Chromosomal Abnormalities.   There is abundant evidence that cells in patients with mycosis fungoides usually have abnormal DNA content (aneuploidy). Again, this finding is typical of malignant cells. Two techniques are used to measure DNA content. The first, karyotyping, involves stimulating the cells to divide in vitro, inhibiting the mitoses in metaphase, and staining and examining the individual chromosomes directly. At least nine groups of investigators have examined tissues from patients with mycosis fungoides and have found at least some chromosomal abnormalities.[9-18] Although aneuploidy generally is found more commonly in cases in which cells are abnormal histologically, some patients with apparently localized disease have aneuploid cells at sites where no histologically abnormal cells are seen.[13-14] No chromosomal abnormality specific for mycosis fungoides has been found. Although one group found that the karyotype of abnormal blood cells in each individual patient is heterogeneous,[16] other groups have found that many of the abnormal cells in an individual patient have the same karyotype, even when cells are taken from different sites.[12,15,17,18] This finding suggests that, at least in the stage at which those patients were studied, the abnormal cells represented a clone derived from a single malignant progenitor cell. Such clonal expansion would not be expected in a benign proliferative process but, rather, is typical of a malignancy.

The second method of measuring DNA content, DNA cytophotometry, involves the use of the Feulgen stain, which binds to DNA, and the measurement of the amount of stained DNA per cell. Cells from patients with mycosis fungoides studied by DNA cytophotometry both in suspension[19] and after imprinting onto slides[20,21] have a high incidence of abnormalities. As with karyotyping, these abnormalities often are found even when no abnormal cells are detectable histologically. These studies are of absolutely central importance to the concept that mycosis fungoides is a cancer—not only are abnormalities found in patients with mycosis fungoides at sites not apparently involved, but also (most importantly) abnormalities are found in patients in whom the diagnosis of mycosis fungoides has not yet been made with certainty.[20] Specifically, 12 of 24 patients with parapsoriasis had normal findings on DNA cytophotometry, and none developed mycosis fungoides during the period in which they were followed. In contrast, of those with parapsoriasis who had abnormal findings, 10 of 12 subsequently developed histologically identifiable mycosis fungoides. Thus, one could argue that not only is histologically identifiable mycosis fungoides a cancer but also that even pre–mycosis fungoides has malignant cells. Such objective findings support the contention that it is possible to make a diagnosis of mycosis fungoides even in its early stages with careful examination by light microscopy[22] or by electron microscopy.[23]

In summary, then, I believe that mycosis fungoides is best considered a cancer from its early stages because of (1) the unchecked growth of abnormal-appearing cells that leads to death in late stages, (2) our ability to establish long-lived cell lines in culture from tissues of patients under conditions in which such lines cannot be established from tissues of normal persons and the association of RNA "tumor" viruses with some such cell lines, and (3) the findings of abnormal chromosomes in tissues of patients with pre–mycosis fungoides who develop histologically proved mycosis fungoides only later.

When early-stage disease evolves to late-stage disease, the chromosomal abnormalities are detectable even before the characteristic histologic abnormalities are present. How, then, can we explain that some patients with minimal skin disease appear not to develop progressive lesions when they are treated with current modalities and observed for several years?[24–26] First, it is possible that current therapy actually prevents the spread of mycosis fungoides, since earlier studies depicted the course of mycosis fungoides as more inexorably progressive, even when patients were seen initially with mild skin involvement.[27] Second, it may be that mycosis fungoides in these patients indeed will progress eventually and that longer observation is necessary. Third (and most interesting) is the possibility, or even the probability, that the very long course of this cancer and the great variability in its aggressiveness in fact may be quite typical of many other cancers. The difference is that in mycosis fungoides the early acts of the drama are played in front of the audience, whereas the early stages of visceral cancer are hidden from observation by an opaque skin.

Study of the skin affords the student an unparalleled opportunity to learn biological principles that cannot be discovered elsewhere. Certainly we do not puzzle over the fact that most infections with *Mycobacterium tuberculosis* heal spontaneously, and we do not claim that it is not an infection because it has not become disseminated. Why, then, should we doubt our observations of patients with mycosis fungoides? Columbus was correct in challenging the prevailing wisdom of his time. Those who claim today that the world is flat will miss out on some marvelous voyages. The opinion of a large group of experts most usually is correct.

References

1. Schein, P. S., MacDonald, J. S., and Edelson, R.: Cutaneous T-cell lymphoma. Cancer 38:1859, 1976.
2. Winkelmann, R. K., and Caro, W. A.: Current problems in mycosis fungoides and Sézary syndrome. Annu. Rev. Med. 28:251, 1977.
3. Klein, G.: The role of gene dosage and genetic transpositions in carcinogenesis. Nature 294:313, 1981.
4. Poiesz, B. J., Ruscetti, F. W., Reitz, M. S., Kalyanaraman, V. S., and Gallo, R. C.: Isolation of a new type C retrovirus (HTLV) in primary uncultured cells of a patient with Sézary T-cell leukaemia. Nature 294:268, 1981.
5. Miyoshi, I., Kubonishi, I., Yoshimoto, S., Akagi, T., Ohtsuki, Y., Shiraishi, Y., Nagata, K., and Hinuma, Y.: Type C virus particles in a cord T-cell line derived by co-cultivating normal human-cord leukocytes and human leukaemic T cells. Nature 294:770, 1981.
6. Kalyanaraman, V. S., Sarngadharan, M. G., Bunn, P. A., Minna, J. D., and Gallo, R. C.: Antibodies in human sera reactive against an internal structural protein of human T-cell lymphoma virus. Nature 294:271, 1981.
7. Kalyanaraman, V. S., Sarngadharan, M. G., Nakao, Y., Ito, Y., Aoki, T., and Gallo, R. C.: Natural antibodies to the structural core protein (p24) of the human T-cell leukemia (lymphoma) retrovirus found in sera of leukemia patients in Japan. Proc. Natl. Acad. Sci. U.S.A. 79:1653, 1982.
8. Poiesz, B. J., Ruscetti, F. W., Mier, J. W., Woods, A. M., and Gallo, R. C.: T-cell lines established from human T-lymphocytic neoplasias by direct response to T-cell growth factor. Proc. Natl. Acad. Sci. U.S.A. 77:6815, 1980.
9. Crossen, P. E., Mellor, J. E. L., Finley, A. G., Ravich, R. R. M., Vincent, P. C., and Gunz, F. W.: The Sézary syndrome: Cytogenetic studies and identification of the Sézary cell as an abnormal lymphocyte. Am. J. Med. 50:24, 1971.
10. Fukuhara, S., Rowley, J. D., and Variakojis, D.: Banding studies of chromosomes in a patient with mycosis fungoides. Cancer 42:2262, 1978.
11. Goh, K. O., Reddy, M. M., and Joishy, S. K.: Chromosomes and B- and T-cells in mycosis fungoides. Am. J. Med. Sci. 276:197, 1978.
12. Edelson, R. L., Berger, C. L., Raafat, J., and Warburton, D.: Karyotype studies of cutaneous T cell lymphoma: Evidence for clonal origin. J. Invest. Dermatol. 73:548, 1979.
13. Whang-Peng, J., Bunn, P., Knutsen, T., Schechter, G. P., Gazdar, A. F., Matthews, M. J., and Minna, J. D.: Cytogenetic abnormalities in patients with cutaneous T-cell lymphomas. Cancer Treat. Rep. 63:575, 1979.
14. Bunn, P. A., Jr., Huberman, M. S., Whang-Peng, J., Schechter, G. P., Guccion, J. G., Matthews, M. J., Gazdar, A. F., Dunnick, N. R., Fischmann, A. B., Ihde, D. C., Cohen, M. H., Fossieck, B., and Minna, J. D.: Prospective staging evaluation of patients with cutaneous T-cell lymphomas—demonstration of a high frequency of extracutaneous dissemination. Ann. Intern. Med. 93:223, 1980.
15. Liang, J. C., Gaulden, M. E., and Herndon, J. H., Jr: Chromosome markers and evidence for clone formation in lymphocytes of a patient with Sézary syndrome. Cancer Res. 40:3426, 1980.
16. Van Vloten, W. A., Pet, E. A., and Geraedts, J. P. M.: Chromosome studies in mycosis fungoides. Br. J. Dermatol. 102:507, 1980.
17. Nowell, P. C., Finan, J. B., and Vonderheid, E. C.: Clonal characteristics of cutaneous T cell lymphomas: Cytogenetic evidence from blood, lymph nodes, skin. J. Invest. Dermatol. 78:69, 1982.
18. Shah-Reddy, I., Mayeda, K., Mirchandani, I., and Koppitch, F. C.: Sézary syndrome with a 14:14 (q12:q31) translocation. Cancer 49:75, 1982.
19. Bunn, P. A., Jr., Whang-Peng, J., Carney, D. N., Schlam, M. L., Knutsen, T., and Gazdar, A. F.: DNA content analysis by flow cytometry and cytogenetic analysis in mycosis fungoides and Sézary syndrome—diagnostic and prognostic implications. J. Clin. Invest. 65:1440, 1980.
20. Van Vloten, W. A., Schaberg, A., and van der Ploeg, M.: Cytophotometric studies on mycosis fungoides and other cutaneous reticuloses. Bull. Cancer 64:249, 1977.
21. Van Vloten, W. A., Scheffer, E., and Meijer, C. J. L. M.: DNA-cytophotometry of lymph node imprints from patients with mycosis fungoides. J. Invest. Dermatol. 73:275, 1979.
22. Sanchez, J. L., and Ackerman, A. B.: The patch stage of mycosis fungoides: Criteria for histologic diagnosis. Am. J. Dermatopathol. 1:5, 1979.
23. Meijer, C. J. L. M., van der Loo, E. M., Van Vloten, W. A., van der Velde, E. A., Scheffer, E., and Cornelisse, C. J.: Early diagnosis of mycosis fungoides and Sézary's syndrome by morphometric analysis of lymphoid cells in the skin. Cancer 45:2864, 1980.
24. Vonderheid, E. C., Van Scott, E. J., Wallner, P. E., and Johnson, W. C.: A 10 year experience with topical mechlorethamine for mycosis fungoides: Comparison with patients treated by total-skin electron-beam radiation therapy. Cancer Treat. Rep. 63:681, 1979.
25. Hoppe, R. T., Cox, R. S., Fuks, Z., Price, N. M., Bagshaw, M. A., and Farber, E. M.: Electron-beam therapy for mycosis fungoides: The Stanford University experience. Cancer Treat. Rep. 63:691, 1979.
26. Lamberg, S. I., Green, S. B., Byar, D. P., Block, J. B., Clendenning, W. E., Epstein, E. H., Jr., Fuks, Z. Y., Golitz, L. E., Lorincz, A. L., Michel, B., Roenigk, H. H., Jr., Van Scott, E. J., Vonderheid, E. C., and Thomas, R. J.: Status report of 376 mycosis fungoides patients at 4 years: Mycosis fungoides cooperative group. Cancer Treat. Rep. 63:701, 1979.
27. Epstein, E. H., Jr., Levin, D. L., Croft, J. D., Jr., and Lutzner, M. A.: Mycosis fungoides: Survival, prognostic features, response to therapy, and autopsy findings. Medicine 15:61, 1972.

SECTION 11

RHUS DERMATITIS

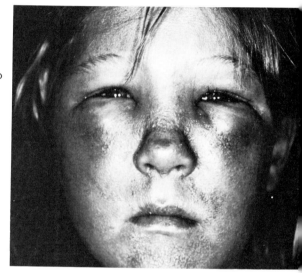

A characteristic but severe example of an acute *Rhus* reaction.

CHAPTER 28

IMMUNITY TO POISON OAK

ADULTS CANNOT BE IMMUNIZED AGAINST *RHUS* SENSITIVITY . . . AND CERTAINLY NOT WITH CURRENTLY AVAILABLE EXTRACTS

Earl R. Claiborne, M.D.

A number of years ago, a physician specializing in industrial diseases stated that contractors were hiring blacks to work in poison oak–infested areas, since these individuals were immune to the ravages of the noxious weed. This was deemed unlikely, because many of the black patients in Dr. Ervin Epstein's private practice had this contact dermatitis. However, it did inspire an investigation that lead us into new vistas and to potentially important discoveries.

We first studied the prevalence of poison oak dermatitis in approximately 12,000 patients who were seen in Dr. Epstein's private practice and then calculated the percentage of members of various ethnic groups seen in this practice. We were unable to show any difference in the incidence of *Rhus* dermatitis among whites compared with blacks. However, there were no cases of this cutaneous disorder in Orientals, although 456 (3.8 per cent) of Dr. Epstein's patients were of Oriental extraction. There should have been 13 cases in this group, but actually there were none.

The study was expanded to include other institutions in the East San Francisco Bay area. Allington* noted that of 430 patients hospitalized because of poison oak dermatitis at Cowell Memorial Hospital (the infirmary at the University of California at Berkeley), only six were Orientals, and four of these individuals had been born and raised in the United States. Urrere* reviewed the records at Mills College in Oakland and found that none of her 417 cases occurred in Orientals or Hawaiians. Both Mills College and the University of California at Berkeley have many students from the Orient and Hawaii. Combining these two groups, we find that of a total of 1184 cases of poison oak, only 0.5 per cent occurred in Orientals and Hawaiians, and only 0.17 per cent of these individuals were born outside the continental United States.

Letters were sent to several dermatologists who practiced in Hawaii or the Orient, and some of the replies were of interest. Johnson* noted that in 15 years of practice in Hawaii, he had never seen a case of *Rhus* or mango dermatitis in an Oriental, a Filipino, or a Hawaiian or in a white person born in the Hawaiian Islands. He credited the latter findings to the fact that white people born in Hawaii handle mangos extensively as children, since this fruit grows in every back yard in the islands. Arnold* confirmed that mango dermatitis

---

*Personal communications to authors.

is rare in natives of Hawaii. Fujinami,* of Japan, and Reiss,* who practiced in China, agreed that lacquer workers eventually become immune to urushi (lacquer) dermatitis.

Although medical histories are not always accurate, they can be significant and interesting. It was found that 40 per cent of the blacks, 39.8 per cent of the Chinese, 72.6 per cent of the Japanese, 60 per cent of the Filipinos, and 73 per cent of the Hawaiians knew or believed that they had been exposed to the poison oak plant. However, when the same individuals were questioned about previous attacks of *Rhus* dermatitis, it was learned that 23 per cent of the whites, 17.6 per cent of the blacks, 5.5 per cent of the Hawaiians, and 12.7 per cent of the Japanese and the Filipinos claimed that they had experienced such an eruption. Of those Orientals born in the continental United States, the incidence was about 19 per cent (approximately the same as that for blacks and whites), but among those born elsewhere, there was a single case of poison oak dermatitis in a Hawaiian (0.17 per cent)— a very substantial difference.

When one compares the incidence of actual cases of poison oak dermatitis with the number of individuals exposed to the plant, one finds that 43 per cent of the patients born in the continental United States were affected, but only 3 per cent of those born elsewhere suffered from this dermatitis. The findings are summarized in Table 1, which shows the marked difference in dermatitis and positive patch tests for each ethnic group and compares those born in the continental United States with those who first saw the light of day in other countries.

A group of 899 patients were patch tested with a commercial extract obtained from Graham Laboratories. Among those born in the continental United States, the incidence of strongly positive reactions varied from 20 to 35 per cent in the different racial groups. However, among those born in Hawaii or the Orient, the incidence decreased to 1.3 per cent.

What is the significance of this study with regard to the question of immunizing adults against *Rhus* dermatitis? In the first place, the only persons to develop an immunity to *Rhus* dermatitis were those born in the Orient (including the Philippine Islands) or Hawaii. These areas are not infested with poison oak, poison ivy, or poison sumac plants, as are the continental United States. Instead, they have other *Rhus* plants—Oriental lacquers and mangos. Therefore, it is likely that mangos and lacquers are better immunizers against *Rhus* dermatitis than are the *Rhus* plants that are indigenous to the continental United States.

Secondly, only those born in the Orient or Hawaii and who lived there for several

---

*Personal communications to authors.

Table 1.   SUMMARY OF STUDIES OF EXPOSURE AND DERMATITIS AND PATCH TESTS*

		Cases	Exposed to *Rhus*	Cases of *Rhus* Dermatitis	Relationship Cases: Exposure	Positive Patch Tests
Whites		250	100(40%)	58(23.2%)	58%	78(31.2%)
Blacks		159	64(40%)	28(17.6%)	43.5%	36(22.1%)
Chinese	Born in U.S.A.	84	22(26.2%)	10(11.9%)	45.5%	18(21.4%)
	Born in China	97	50(59.5%)	0	0	1(1.0%)
Japanese	Born in U.S.A.	60	50(83.4%)	13(21.7%)	26.0%	21(35%)
	Born in Japan	50	30(60%)	1(2%)	3.3%	0
Filipinos	Born in U.S.A.	76	50(65.8%)	13(17.2%)	26%	14(18.4%)
	Born in Philippine Islands	34	16(47.1%)	1(2.9%)	6.6%	0
Hawaiians	Born in continental U.S.A.	43	30(70%)	14(32.5%)	46.8%	12(27.9%)
	Born in Hawaii	46	35(74.0%)	2(4.7%)	5.77%	2(4.3%)

*From Epstein, E., and Claiborne, E. R.: Racial and environmental factors in susceptibility to *Rhus*. Arch. Dermatol. 75:197, 1957. Copyright 1957, American Medical Association. Used by permission.

years before migrating developed and maintained this immunity. This was true even for those coming to the continental United States and becoming exposed to *Rhus* plants on a continuing and intimate manner, such as Japanese gardeners. Gardening is a very common occupation for Japanese in the San Francisco Bay area.

American adults migrating to the Oriental countries or to Hawaii do not become immune to these noxious plants when they return to the continental United States. Therefore, it seems likely that one can be immunized to these plants only in utero or early in childhood. However, it would seem reasonable to attempt immunization with lacquer or mango extracts, especially in children. Of course, it would take many years indeed to establish the efficacy or worthlessness of such an approach. On the other hand, present-day medicine does not offer another viable approach to the problem of producing artificial immunity to these ubiquitous toxic plants.

WHAT FACTORS DETERMINE UNRESPONSIVENESS TO POISON OAK/IVY?

William L. Epstein, M.D.

In 1957, Epstein and Claiborne published a provocative paper, "Racial and Environmental Factors in Susceptibility to *Rhus*." [1] Initially, they extracted information from the records of a busy private practice, noting simply the race of patients who presented themselves for treatment of poison oak dermatitis. The population was composed primarily of whites, 3.2 per cent of whom were diagnosed as having a *Rhus* rash. Of approximately 1300 blacks, only 0.9 per cent were so diagnosed, and of the 348 Orientals, none complained of contact dermatitis to poison oak. This must have been moderately surprising, because the investigators quote an unpublished communication from Fujinami in Japan to the effect that "urushi dermatitis" is common, especially in Japanese lacquer makers.

This prompted a further study of the records of two hospitals in Berkeley and Oakland that deal primarily with young college students. Again, an absurdly small number of Orientals had been hospitalized for treatment of poison oak dermatitis. Encouraged, Epstein and Claiborne then carried out a prospective study, patch testing 899 volunteers with a commercially available *Rhus* extract. The results showed 31 per cent positive reactions in whites and 22 per cent in blacks. Most fascinating, however, were the findings in Orientals, which included Chinese, Japanese, Filipinos, and Hawaiians. Of the 263 Orientals born in the continental United States, 50, or 19 per cent, were found to be sensitive by patch testing, whereas only 4, or 0.02 per cent, of the 227 foreign-born Orientals had positive patch test reactions.

Neither dismayed nor deterred by the inherent weaknesses in their lines of evidence, the authors sought further data by contacting their colleagues in Hawaii. The reply proved supportive, in that mango dermatitis was restricted to poison ivy/oak–sensitive visitors from the mainland and was virtually unknown among natives. This "fourth wall" completed the "house of cards" and emboldened the authors to speculate about the reason for their curious findings: "It seems possible, therefore, that the mango of Hawaii and the lacquer plants of the Far Orient are more potent immunizers than are the domestic plants." They concluded, "It may be necessary to administer these extracts in childhood to get the desired results."

As a young investigator interested in the experimental aspects of allergic contact dermatitis, I was appalled at the audacity of my favorite uncle to draw such broad, wide-sweeping conclusions from the trivial information he had gathered. Each wall of evidence was rife with intellectual termites and could easily be attacked. For instance, the office-based data are retrospective and do not consider why the few Orientals might choose to go to a dermatologist's office in the first place. The hospital histories have the same limitation and in addition might mean that Orientals have less severe dermatitis or other habits and mores. The patch test study is more interesting but was done by amateurs. Thus, the test sites were examined in 24 and 48 hours and not at 4 and 6 days, as required for accurate assessment of sensitivity. Furthermore, there was no follow-up at 2 weeks to detect possible flare-ups, indicating recall of weak or marginal sensitivity. For this reason or because of the inherent weakness of the commercial extract, the investigators found less than one third positives in the white population. In most large studies, 50 per cent of the subjects

Table 1.   POSITIVE PATCH TEST REACTIONS TO A POISON OAK
EXTRACT AND 1:100 PDC*

Subjects	Extract (%)	PDC (%)
Orientals (Japanese, Taiwanese, Filipinos)	8/16 (50)	10/14 (71)
South Americans (not Mexican)	8/22 (36)	18/18 (100)
Age-matched concurrent controls	14/23 (61)	18/19 (95)

General concurrent
  controls
    (all ages)
	77/153 (50)	117/135 (87)

PDC = Pentadecylcatechol.

in the United States have positive skin test reactions.[2] Under the circumstances, Epstein and Claiborne's method would not detect less reactive individuals and would give misleadingly low results. How could such frail data lead to such a magnificent and important proposal for immunization against poison ivy/oak dermatitis? This is the stuff of which controversy is made.

For the next 5 years I assiduously patch tested every immigrant from the Orient and South America that I could within 1 to 2 months of the arrival of these individuals in the United States. The method involved a commercial extract applied as an open patch with a glass applicator and 1:100 pentadecylcatechol (PDC) in acetone, also applied as an open patch, 0.25 ml in the area of a ring 1.5 cm in diameter. Test sites were observed at 2, 4, and 6 days and were graded 1+ (erythema and edema) to 4+ (bullae).[3] The results (Table 1) were compared with data obtained from similar testing in adults born and raised in the United States. None of the foreign volunteers had ever had any plant-induced dermatitis, and most had never heard of poison ivy/oak dermatitis, although some knew of a nettle-like rash in their homeland.

The findings indicated that despite the negative histories, the majority had in fact been exposed to urushiol-related antigens in the past and had developed delayed hypersensitivity or cell-mediated immunity. At this point, satisfied that the published data[1] were not truly representative, I abandoned further study in this area without bothering to publish my admittedly limited observations. Alas, my judgment was hasty and mistaken. The basic immunologic evidence accumulated in the past 25 years[4] clearly supports the major principle that Epstein and Claiborne attempted to adduce from their clinical investigation.

At issue is how to prevent someone from becoming contact-sensitive to poison ivy/oak or other chemicals. The available and emerging strategies are briefly reviewed in the proceedings of the Contact Dermatitis Symposium held at the XVI International Congress in Tokyo.[5] Although natural tolerance on a genetic basis can be detected in experimental animals,[4] it requires strict inbreeding and is limited to specific chemical ions, so that such occurrence in human beings, even in the relatively inbred Oriental populations, seems unlikely. On the other hand, it is now generally accepted that almost every antigenic stimulus has two opposing effects. One is immunogenic and results in specific T effector cells that set in motion a local inflammatory response upon re-exposure to the offending chemical. The other, and more complicated, response is tolerogenic and produces a series of T suppressor cells and blocking factors that interdict the immunogenic (proinflammatory) process. As indicated, the blockade system is complex. It may be specific or nonspecific. It can affect the afferent or the efferent limbs of contact sensitization, or both. It is seldom complete or long-lasting. Under the usual methods of exposure, i.e., by topical contact with chemicals, the balance of the two forces usually falls on the side of immunity (contact allergy) and away from tolerance. However, there are several ways to shift the balance toward tolerance. Any antigenic stimulus that bypasses the skin is effective. Thus, intravenous administration of antigen elicits T suppressor (T_s) cells, which block both afferent and efferent limbs of contact sensitization.[5] In addition, it is likely that the hyposensitization produced in humans by administration of urushiol[6] is caused by stimulation of additional T_s cells. This effect is temporary and requires continual feeding of a maintenance dose in order for it to persist. In the 1960s and 1970s, Lowney produced partial tolerance by administering dinitrocholorobenzene (DNCB) to human volunteers before attempted sensitization.[5,7]

Another approach supported by experimental studies is to alter the immunizing molecule chemically. It is well recognized that some related molecules are more tolerogenic than immunogenic. Thus, dinitrobenzene sulfonate ($DNBSO_3$) is more likely to produce tolerance, whereas DNCB is most likely to sensitize.[5] With regard to poison ivy/oak, recent studies have shown that there are two sites on the catechol ring of urushiol that are preferentially available for nucleophilic attack by proteins or ligands to form covalent bonds. As outlined in Figure 1, urushiol must first change to a quinone in the body before it can form covalent links with protein, an accepted requirement for it to become a complete antigen. The chemical hapten and "carrier" protein then are presented to lymphocytes and stimulate clonal T cell proliferation and differentiation of effector T cells. As indicated in the figure, the carbon 5 site on the ring is regiospecifically attacked by amide groups, and the carbon 6 site is attacked by sulfhydryl (thiol) groups on protein ligands. Furthermore, in a mouse model of allergic contact dermatitis it has been shown that urushiol is both immunogenic and tolerogenic. Blocking urushiol at the carbon 5 ring position with a methyl group produces a molecule that is primarily tolerogenic, and blocking the ring at carbon 6 in the same way results in an analog that is an immunogen.[8] This observation suggests that covalent bonding through thiol groups at carbon 6 forms a tolerogenic stimulus, and an amide linkage at carbon 5 or elsewhere produces an immunogen. Following up the original observations,[1] one might ask whether the catechols in mango rind or in Japanese lacquer contain more thiol-sensitive adducts or are more efficient in this type of covalent peptide

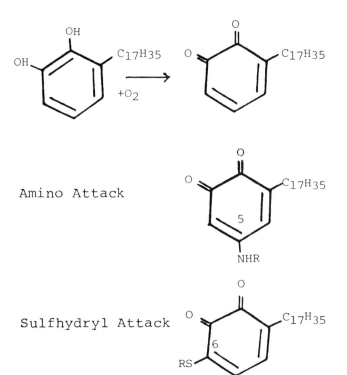

Amino Attack

Sulfhydryl Attack

Figure 1. Chemical modifications of the urushiol molecule required for it to bind covalently with proteins in vivo. Urushiol in the body becomes an intermediary quinone that is susceptible to regiospecific nucleophilic attack of the ring structure by ligands at C5 (amide) and C6 (thiol).

bonding. Certainly it should be possible to manufacture such a molecule to administer to children at risk of becoming poison ivy/oak sufferers, in keeping with the proposal of our protagonists.[1]

Perhaps more practical is a preliminary experiment we reported in which a group of children not known to be sensitive to poison oak were injected intramuscularly with very small amounts of urushiol in divided doses.[9] A matched control group of children received no injection. Then both groups were topically exposed to a sensitizing amount of urushiol. The results demonstrated sensitization in the controls and tolerance in the injected group. Furthermore, the tolerance persisted in a partial form for approximately 6 years. Thus, it appears that specific immunologic tolerance to poison oak/ivy urushiol can be induced in humans in a simple and meaningful way. The next obvious step is to extend these studies to a larger group of children at risk of developing poison oak sensitivity and to determine if booster injections can result in an adult population resistant to the scourges of those nasty poison ivy and oak weeds. More importantly, the study verifies the principle of immunologic tolerance for humans and offers hope for its use in the field of tissue transplantation and replaceable parts.

From what has been said it is clear that medical science is about to catch up with the clinician's vision. The question is whether that pertinent controversy stirred long ago will receive its due when tolerance to poison oak/ivy is finally developed. The answer is probably not, because the original proposal twists and twirls in the backwater of a clinical eddy and does not flow in the scientific mainstream. Although the field of medicine is founded upon sharp clinical observation and many advances were made in this way during the first half of this century, this is less true today. Advances now require experimental facts derived from well-planned and timely studies. The report of Epstein and Claiborne[1] comes from the older genre. Perhaps some of the later studies will achieve a lasting impact.

References

1. Epstein, E., and Claiborne, E. R.: Racial and environmental factors in susceptibility to *Rhus*. Arch. Dermatol. 75:197, 1957.
2. Epstein, W. L., Baer, H., Dawson, C. R., and Khurana, R. G.: Poison oak hyposensitization: Evaluation of purified urushiol. Arch. Dermatol. 109:356, 1974.
3. Epstein, W. L.: Contact-type delayed hypersensitivity in infants and children: Induction of *Rhus* sensitivity. Pediatrics 27:51, 1961.
4. Polak, L.: Immunological aspects of contact sensitivity. Monogr. Allergy 15:63, 1980.
5. Report on the Symposium on Contact Dermatitis. *In* Proceedings of the XVI International Congress of Dermatology (1982). Tokyo, Tokyo Press (in press).
6. Epstein, W. L., Byers, V. S., and Frankart, W.: Induction of antigen specific hyposensitization to poison oak in sensitized adults. Arch. Dermatol. 118:630, 1982.
7. Lowney, E. D.: Dermatologic implications of immunologic unresponsiveness. J. Invest. Dermatol. 54:355, 1970.
8. Dunn, I. S., Liberato, D. J., Castagnoli, N., et al.: Induction of suppressor T cells for lymph node proliferation after contact sensitization of mice with urushiol. Cell. Immunol. (in press).
9. Epstein, W. L., Byers, V. S., and Baer, H.: Induction of persistent tolerance to urushiol in humans. J. Allergy Clin. Immunol. 68:20, 1981.

Editorial Comment

In the preceding pages, academician William Epstein has paid a great compliment to clinicians E. Epstein and Claiborne for their investigation of the rarity of poison oak dermatitis in Orientals. He has pointed out that this type of research allowed discoveries to be made in the past without the time-consuming procedures demanded today. Indirectly, it is a much-needed boost for clinical and deductive research. Reading his acceptance of the thesis of Epstein and Claiborne's article, I remembered a similar experience. As a medical student in the early 1930s, I noticed that the prognosis of Hodgkin's disease was much more favorable in women during their periods of menstrual activity, (13 to 50 years of age). I contrasted this with the prognosis of the disease in women of other ages and in men of all ages. The study was based on mortality and longevity statistics and was presented in the *American Journal of Cancer* in February of 1939. In 1980, Kaplan published the second edition of a massive tome on Hodgkin's disease (published by the Harvard University Press), and on page 571 we found the following:

> The possible influence of sex on the prognosis of patients with Hodgkin's disease was first reported by Epstein (1939), who compared the longevity of 204 cases in females with that of 180 cases among males, all collated from the medical literature. His conclusion was that females have a better prognosis than males. Though founded on evidence that is clearly unacceptable by current standards, this view has nonetheless been supported by a plethora of subsequent studies (Peters, 1950; Jelliffe and Thomson, 1955; Heilmeyer et al., 1957; Croizat et al., 1958; Meighan and Ramsay, 1963; and others). The magnitude of the difference in prognosis appears to be statistically significant in the data collected by Hohl et al. (1951); Shimkin et al. (1955); Peters and Middlemiss (1958); Musshoff ct al. (1964 and 1966); Westling (1965); Peters et al. (1966); and Gross et al. (1966).

One statement made by Kaplan must be corrected, however; the cases were gathered from hospital charts. W. Epstein is right—today scientific discoveries must be established by complicated formalized research to gain any attention. The reason for this is the belief that without such confirmatory proof, fallacies may creep into our thinking. Of course, such controls and experiments do not guarantee that errors cannot become accepted as facts anyway. However, it does slow down progress, especially in the field of therapeutics, because of unreasonable demands. Despite these so-called safeguards, it is probably true that 50 per cent of what we believe today in medicine is incorrect and we do not even know which half we should discard.

Controls and experimentation often become a substitute for thinking. To me, the frightening aspect of this is that neither the article on *Rhus* dermatitis nor the one on Hodgkin's disease would be acceptable for publication today. Even worse, if these articles could not have been published in a reputable journal, it is likely that no investigator would have thought of these possibilities and performed the necessary studies to bring them to the attention of the medical profession. As a present-day example of this, I am confronted with the impossibility of convincing the editor of any prestigious journal to publish the results of the treatment of approximately 600 patients with zoster or postzoster neuralgia by the subcutaneous injection of triamcinolone, although some admit that this is an important clinical observation. So, many individuals suffering the tortures of the damned from these conditions are denied treatment with triamcinolone because of the "fallacy" in the study—the same reason that the two aforementioned articles would not be accepted if submitted for publication today.

I believe that our thinking must be attuned to reality in acceptance or rejection of new medical concepts. I still believe that the discovery of the cause and cure of cancer will result from an idea in the head of a thinker . . . not in a funded, stylized university laboratory. It is still true that you cannot solve problems by throwing money at them.

Think It Over.

SECTION 12

SCABIES

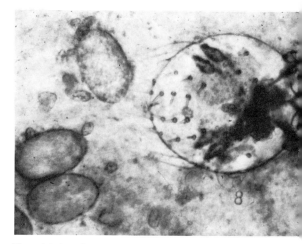

The adult female acarus in a run, including the eggs she laid and the feces she passed. (Courtesy of Dr. Milton Orkin.)

CHAPTER **29**

TREATMENT OF UNINVOLVED CONTACTS

TREATMENT OF HOUSEHOLD AND SEXUAL CONTACTS OF PATIENTS WITH SCABIES

Milton Orkin, M.D.
Dennis D. Juranek, D.V.M., M.P.H.
Howard I. Maibach, M.D.

In the 1940s, Mellanby[1] noted that "whenever possible, the whole household (of a patient with scabies) should be treated at the same time, particularly if members are living under overcrowded conditions, irrespective of whether or not every member has developed clinical symptoms." The implication was that if one person in a household becomes infested, it is likely that other family members will eventually suffer, unless all are treated simultaneously. The rationale behind this recommendation lies in understanding the long incubation period for scabies and the reproductive potential of mites during that period. In a person who has never had scabies, the time between acquiring the mite and developing pruritus or lesions may be as long as 1 to 2 months. During this period, the mites reproduce and may be transmitted to other family members or sexual contacts. Although partial immunity occurs if a patient is cured after sensitization, complete immunity is infrequently achieved, and such persons remain at risk of reinfestation if they are re-exposed.[2] A recent study has shown that in two thirds of families of patients with scabies, there was no transmission to other family members; in one third of families, two or more members became infested.[3]

To avoid "ping-pong" transmission among family members, we previously recommended that all members of a person's household as well as sexual contacts of infested persons outside the household be treated at the same time.[4] It is imperative that the physician be as certain as possible that the first family member presenting with symptoms truly has scabies. The stronger the physician's criteria for making the diagnosis, the more justified is prophylactic treatment for exposed family members and sexual contacts. Criteria for diagnosis include features suggestive of scabies (Table 1) and confirmatory procedures for identifying the mite (Table 2).[4,5] If the diagnosis is doubtful, treatment of household members and sexual contacts is difficult to justify.

Recently, we considered exceptions to the treatment of all household members. Additional information useful in making a decision includes the patient's living conditions, sexual habits, and past medical history of skin and neurologic disorders.[5] For example, if the patient (adult or child) routinely shares a bed with another person, the probability is high that transmission to that person has already occurred, and therefore treatment of the asymptomatic bed partner is justified. Similarly, infested mothers caring for young children

Table 1. FINDINGS SUGGESTIVE OF
SCABIES

Distribution of lesions—hands, wrists, elbows, anterior axillary folds, areolae of female breasts, abdomen, genitals, buttocks.

Morphology of lesions—typically polymorphic. Burrows are pathognomonic but less frequent in current epidemic.

Nocturnal pruritus.

Contact with infested person (highly suggestive).

Response to "specific" therapy.

Results of skin biopsy in inflammatory or nodular lesions.

Table 2. LABORATORY TECHNIQUES
FOR CONFIRMING THE DIAGNOSIS OF
SCABIES

Skin scrapings
Needle extraction of mite
Epidermal shave biopsy
Burrow ink test (BIT)
Curettage of burrows
Swab technique with clear cellophane adhesive
Topical tetracycline, then Wood's light
Punch biopsy

or infants have a good chance of exposing their children to scabies through such daily activities as bathing them, rubbing on baby oils or powders, and holding them in the hands and arms. It is less significant to treat those individuals who have minimal skin-to-skin contact with an infested family member.[6] Family members with a history of seizures or atopic eczema should be examined before a course of action is chosen.

Some physicians prefer to treat only the infested family member. Two reasons are most commonly advanced in support of this. First, these physicians believe that informed patients can observe other family members or sexual contacts for signs and symptoms of scabies and have these individuals treated if itching lesions develop. We have offered the counterargument that by selective treatment of asymptomatic family members who are at high risk for acquiring the infestation from a person with a confirmed case, unnecessary morbidity and anxiety can be prevented. Given the relative safety of available scabicides when dispensed and applied in an appropriate manner, the benefit of *selective* prophylactic treatment (in our opinion) outweighs the potential risk of drug side effects. The second issue of concern to some physicians is the medicolegal implications of treating individuals without seeing them and taking responsibility for such treatment. Similar criticism could be directed at the physician who does not prevent unnecessary morbidity in family members by selectively treating exposed but asymptomatic persons in the household.

Prophylactic treatment of persons exposed to fomites in contact with an infested patient is usually *not justified*. Studies of scabies transmission following exposure to bed linen previously used by persons with conventional scabies indicated a risk of less than one infestation per 200 exposures.[1] Fomites are generally disinfested at the completion of treatment by machine washing and drying using the hot cycle of each machine. However, the risk of fomite transmission is higher in those with crusted (Norwegian) scabies, in which infestation is more severe. Bed linen, underwear, and pajamas of patients with crusted scabies often harbor living mites; persons exposed to such fomites should be considered for prophylactic treatment.

Asymptomatic patients and staff in nursing homes, hospitals, and other institutions present special problems. Deciding which individuals to treat requires common sense as well as time for the physician to assess the situation personally. If the infested patient has crusted (Norwegian) scabies, then not only is it more reasonable to treat asymptomatic patients who have an exposure history, but also greater attention should be given to cleaning up the patient's environment. Bed linen and clothing in contact with the infested patient should be placed in plastic bags for transport to the laundry to avoid unnecessary exposure of other patients and employees. Floors, curtains, and furniture should be vacuumed.

Once the physician has decided whom to treat from a preventative point of view, the choice of scabicides depends on the effectiveness of the preparation, the risk/benefit ratio,

Table 3. THERAPY FOR SCABIES

Lindane* Cream or Lotion 1% (*Kwell, Kwellada, Scabene*)	Crotamiton* Cream 10% (*N-ethyl-o-crotonotoluide; Eurax*)	Precipitated sulfur* 6%
1. Apply one thin layer to entire trunk and extremities and leave on for 8 to 12 hours.	1. Massage medication into skin from neck downward nightly for 2 nights.	1. Apply preparation to trunk and extremities nightly for 3 nights.
2. At end of 8 to 12 hours, shower or bathe to remove medication thoroughly; change intimate apparel and bed linen.	2. Twenty-four hours after second application, wash off medication thoroughly; change intimate apparel and bed linen.	2. Twenty-four hours after last application, bathe to remove medication thoroughly; change intimate apparel and bed linen.

Nonrefillable prescription should be made for only amount needed.

and the possibility of resistance to the scabicide. There has been limited interest in comparative, controlled efficacy trials of scabicides; the three used most commonly in the United States are lindane, crotamiton, and precipitated sulfur (Table 3).[4] We prefer *not* to use lindane in household members (or infested patients) who are infants, small children (less than 10 years of age), or pregnant or lactating women and in patients with seizure disorders or other neurologic diseases because of cutaneous absorption (10 per cent of the amount applied to the skin is excreted in the urine). In addition, there is a potential for central nervous system toxicity (clinically limited to misuse situations). We prefer to use precipitated sulfur in infants and pregnant and lactating women and sulfur or crotamiton in older children and patients with seizure disorders or other neurologic diseases. Patients find sulfur less acceptable than modern scabicides because of odor, messiness, and staining. Lindane is the treatment of choice in adults, with the aforementioned exceptions. It is not uncommon for us to use different preparations for different age groups in the same family, e.g., lindane or crotamiton in adults and sulfur in small children.

Recent clinical experience with crotamiton in the treatment of infants and young children with scabies suggests that five daily applications may be better than the two currently recommended.[7] This should be studied further in all age groups.

References

1. Mellanby, K.: Scabies. Los Angeles, E. W. Classey Ltd., 1972.
2. Mellanby, K.: Immunology of scabies. *In* Orkin, M., et al. (eds.): Scabies and Pediculosis. Philadelphia, J. B. Lippincott Co., 1977.
3. Palicka, P.: The incidence and mode of scabies transmission in a district of Czechoslovakia (1961–1979). Folia Parasitol. 29:51, 1982.
4. Orkin, M., et al.: Treatment of today's scabies and pediculosis. JAMA 236:1136, 1976.
5. Orkin, M., and Maibach, H. I.: Scabies. *In* Holmes, K., et al. (eds.): Sexually Transmitted Diseases. New York, McGraw-Hill, 1983.
6. Juranek, D. D.: Scabies: A practical protocol for managing the pandemic. Mod. Med. 46:66, 1978.
7. Cubella, V., and Yawalkar, S. J.: Clinical experience with crotamiton cream and lotion and treatment of infants with scabies. Br. J. Clin. Pract. 32:229, 1978.

DON'T TREAT ASYMPTOMATIC SCABIES CONTACTS

Ervin Epstein, M.D.

It is common teaching and practice to subject the asymptomatic contacts of a patient with scabies to the usual application of scabicides. This procedure is of questionable necessity and limited benefit and poses hazards to the patient, to his family and other contacts, and even to the physician.

It is obvious that not all close contacts of a patient with scabies eventually manifest the signs and symptoms of infestation. This is true even of bedmates or sexual partners, although such transfer of infection is not uncommon. However, if the person does develop scabies at a later date, it can be eradicated quickly and without additional treatment (that is, no more therapy than would have been used prophylactically). In fact, the disease can be eliminated in a matter of hours. Since an attack of scabies does produce immunity (which is said to explain the waning and waxing of epidemics of this disease), the possibility of reinfecting cured individuals in a "ping-pong" manner probably does not exist or, at worst, is exceedingly unlikely.

It is obvious also that just because one member of a group, family or otherwise, has scabies and other members of the unit are itching or have an eruption, they do not necessarily all have scabies. Recently I saw a girl with scabies who stated that five other members of her family also had the same condition. Examination revealed that all of the other five had poison oak. I think we will all agree that scabicides are not effective in treating a *Rhus* dermatitis and might in fact cause considerable aggravation when applied to a vesicular, weeping contact dermatitis. Therefore, it is advocated that other contacts be examined before being subjected to antiscabetic therapy that can cause dermatitis in asymptomatic individuals and other toxic reactions in infants.

Prophylactic treatment of contacts is often performed in a blind manner. The patient is given a scabicide in a volume that is large enough to treat all contacts. These individuals are being treated for a disease that may not even be present without examination by the physician. No one knows what a jury might decide in medicolegal confrontations, but I would say that they might look askance at the treatment of an absent dermatitis sans examination. And using a scabicide for 1 to 5 nights, covering the entire body from the shoulders down with such an agent, would certainly be classified as a treatment. As an example, if I had given a scabicide to the five family members of the girl discussed previously, I could have irritated five cases of poison oak and could have possibly faced five malpractice actions.

Scabicides are not safe for indiscriminant use. The reported and observed reactions vary from central nervous system hazards to irritation of normal or dermatitic skin. Patients consult a doctor for a cure, not the production of a reaction, whether the skin is normal or pathologic. A person with normal skin using a medication in this manner who develops a chronic itching eruption might well look with disfavor at the physician who produces such a complication, and a jury might well go along with this concept.

So, why take a chance of doing harm with such rapidly acting therapeutic agents in a benign disease with little chance of reinfection? Such heroics and blind therapeutics are not for me.

SECTION 13

DERMABRASION

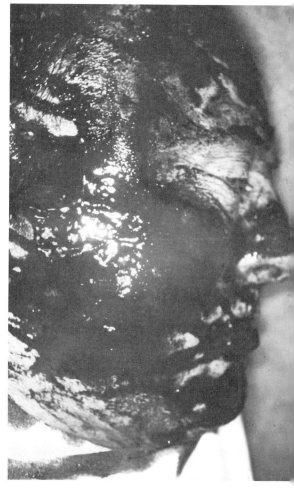

The production of such bleeding indicates that dermabrasion is not a minor procedure.

CHAPTER **30**

THE VALUE OF DERMABRASION

THE VALUE OF EFFECTIVE THERAPEUTIC AND COSMETIC DERMABRASION*

Thomas H. Alt, M.D.

Facial dermabrasion is an excellent therapeutic procedure for postacne scarring. It provides definitive and permanent improvement of abnormal contours. In some instances, it can offer cosmetic perfection. Dermabrasion produces a cosmetic result that is not attainable through the use of silicone or xenogenic collagen. These filling substances used in combination with dermabrasion constitute a therapeutic regimen that can significantly heal postacne scarring, be it mild or severe. Although somewhat less predictable, the therapeutic results for chronic or uncontrollable cystic acne have been gratifying. Facial dermabrasion offers a bright outlook for the patient who seeks improvement.

Unfortunately, the technique of facial dermabrasion has not been granted its proper place among cosmetic and therapeutic surgical procedures. In fact, some malign facial dermabrasion, stating that it gives little or no improvement. It is my observation that these critics have not encountered a surgeon who skillfully performs dermabrasion or have little personal skill in the procedure. This lack of skill may result from inexperience or a failure to understand the techniques required to perform a successful facial dermabrasion.

It is my advice that one not be a casual participant in performing facial dermabrasion. If a physician performs an average of only one dermabrasion per month, he will never gain adequate experience to attain a high degree of skill that will produce predictable and repeatable results. It is a misconception that skill can be achieved from such limited experience. It is also fallacious to judge the value of a technique based on results obtained by surgeons who have had limited experience.

How can one become a skilled surgeon in facial dermabrasion? Is there a middle ground between inexperience and demonstrated ability? Of course! If one has innate surgical ability and the desire and motivation to learn dermabrasion, one must spend time with a surgeon who has demonstrated skills in the procedure. One must learn the principles of dermabrasion and gain personal experience in the operative techniques under supervised tutelage.

Those who attain marginal results do not apply the principles of facial dermabrasion. Many physicians judge dermabrasion based upon results obtained by unskilled operators whose techniques are inadequate. Many dermabrasions are performed through the use of local or general anesthesia on unaltered skin that is insensitive to pain. Skin at normal temperature is soft and pliable. It is impossible to produce excellent results when one performs dermabrasion on soft, pliable skin; the results will be predictably inadequate.

---

*This text was presented in part as the Christian Radcliffe Memorial Lecture entitled "The Renaissance of Dermabrasion" before the Iowa Dermatological Society on April 16, 1982.

If one analyzes the physics of forces and mass that are essential to dermabrasion, certain principles become self-evident. In seminars and the literature, these rules are often poorly articulated or ignored altogether. I propose that these criteria are essential to the performance of an effective dermabrasion. The principles are: (1) The normal contour of the skin should be maintained during dermabrasion, (2) the skin should be changed to a firm, solid state to provide effective abrasion, and (3) one should be aware of danger areas that may scar readily.

The purpose of a cosmetic dermabrasion is to improve the abnormal contour of the skin. Most scars are depressed, and the adjacent normal skin is higher. Dermabrasion does not elevate skin, as does silicone or xenogenic collagen. On the contrary, dermabrasion diminishes the level of the normal skin to the greatest amount safely possible—(it is hoped) to the level of the depressed scars. The surgeon selectively abrades the higher, normal skin to the level of the lower, abnormal skin. He is a sculptor.

We are taught to stretch the skin prior to freezing. This is incorrect. To alter the abnormal skin by stretching it will flatten the contours, thus modifying and minimizing the difference in heights. When the pressure of stretching is released, the natural forces controlling the skin will spring back into effect, and pre-existing contours will reappear. Thus, the dermabrasion must be accomplished without any tension to distort the abnormal contour. There are exceptions: One must stretch areas with marked natural contours to avoid excessive abrading of their high spots while trying to abrade their low spots. These zones are the philtrum, the cleft of the chin, the angles of the mouth, the nasolabial folds, and the alar flares of the nose. Other areas with marked contouring, such as excessive wrinkling, should be treated similarly.

A second maneuver that can alter contour is the infiltration of local anesthetic. If adequate time is not allowed for the anesthetic to disperse completely, the instilled liquid will distort the pre-existing contour. I find no need to use infiltration anesthesia (even regional blocks), since the preanesthetic allays fear and the refrigerant spray, when properly used, provides total anesthesia in the area on which dermabrasion is being performed.

The second principle is the transformation of the semisolid skin into the solid state. This is the most important factor in achieving excellent results. Let us review some simple logic. Skin is soft and pliable and has a normal surface temperature of 92°F. It is a semisolid that is distorted in shape when pressure is applied to its surface by a solid object. Therefore, any solid object, such as a fingertip, a pencil or, specifically, an abrading apparatus (wire brush or diamond fraise) will distort its contour. This is contrary to our objective. One must transform the skin to a solid state in order to provide firm resistance to the abrading equipment. Imagine trying to recontour a piece of gelatin with a file. It would be impossible and would give unpredictable results. However, against a hard surface, such as a block of wood, the file can produce desired effects.

By using any of the refrigerant anesthetics (Fluoroethyl, CryOsthesia, or Frigiderm), one can transform the skin to an insensitive, solid state. It is frozen in small segments of approximately 1 square inch until it is absolutely firm. A high-pitched tone will emanate from the solid skin that is being abraded. When the tone is lost, one must refreeze the skin to perform effective dermabrasion. To prepare the skin, one should prechill any segment selected (e.g., the cheek or the forehead) with ice (frozen to 0°F inside a sterile rubber glove) for 20 to 30 minutes immediately prior to the dermabrasion. Each segment should be chilled consecutively so that dermabrasion of the segment commences immediately after removal of the ice pack. For example, one should chill the right cheek, remove the ice, and chill the left cheek while abrading the right cheek. One should then abrade the left cheek while chilling the forehead. Fresh ice packs should be used for each segment to maintain uniformity.

In order to provide a further improvement in freezing, the room temperature may be decreased from 72°F to 62°F by an independent air conditioner. This is a 50 per cent improvement in ambient air temperature when compared with the skin temperature of 92°F. Increased humidity and patient anxiety will adversely affect freezing.

Freezing the skin to a solid state is often omitted, and this is the major cause of inadequate results. I suspect that those using refrigerant anesthetics fail to do so from timidity. This is unfortunate, because it prevents adequate abrasion and reduces anesthesia, thus making the procedure uncomfortable. Many write that they can complete a full facial dermabrasion in 15 to 20 minutes. In my hands this is impossible. Freezing small segments until they are absolutely solid and applying meticulous attention to every scar and its subsequent correction are time-consuming. For me to complete a full facial dermabrasion, at least 1 hour, and usually more, is required. This additional attention to detail is rewarded by superior cosmetic and therapeutic results.

Transforming the skin to a solid state has two additional advantages. It freezes the blood in the underlying capillary loops and promotes intense vasoconstriction of the arteriolar bed, both of which provide a bloodless field during abrasion. In addition, the capillary loops in the papillary dermis are readily recognizable, providing positive identification of the depth of abrasion. Dermabrasion carried below the papillary dermis and into the deeper reticular dermis will probably result in scarring because of the paucity of epidermal appendages. It is no wonder that surgeons performing dermabrasion using general anesthesia without freezing the skin with a refrigerant or those who inadequately freeze the skin produce inadequate results. Blood obscures the depth of dermabrasion, and pliable skin is distorted and responds poorly to the abrasive surface.

The third principle in performing effective and successful facial dermabrasion is that one should be aware of danger areas that are susceptible to scarring. Skin, which has differing underlying structures, has varying but predictable freeze-thaw cycles. Skin overlying relatively avascular bone will freeze rapidly and will thaw slowly. Skin overlying abundant subcutaneous fat and muscle with a rich vascular bed will freeze slowly and will thaw rapidly. Areas that freeze rapidly and thaw slowly are the mandible (particularly at the juncture of its posterior and middle third), the bossing of the chin and the forehead, and the areas over the malar eminence and the zygomatic ridge. Caution must be taken, because correct freezing permits deep, effective abrasion.

I believe that the major mistake made by the inexperienced surgeon is to freeze an excessively large area. When a large zone is frozen, the skin overlying richly vascularized subcutaneous tissue, as compared with that overlying bone, does not freeze as firmly and thus thaws more rapidly, both of which limit the depth of the dermabrasion. When one performs dermabrasion on a large area, the abrasion is carried deeper on the firmly frozen skin over the bone, but the depth is more superficial over the subcutaneous tissue, which is not frozen as firmly. Repeated freezings and abrading of the entire area will finally carry the level of the dermabrasion to an adequate depth in the skin overlying subcutaneous tissue but may reach a level too deep in the area overlying bone, resulting in scar formation. This may also be observed when the procedure is performed using general anesthesia without refrigerant freezing, because the bone offers a greater resistance to the abrasive surface.

Although I do not consider the following adjunctive measures to be essential for attaining excellent results in facial dermabrasion, they do improve the healing phase. I have always used wet packs to remove the postoperative crust, followed by the application of sterile petrolatum to diminish re-formation of the crust. This is in accordance with the many studies that have shown that re-epithelialization under moist conditions is superior to that occurring under a desiccated crust. An additional aid is the short-term use of injectable systemic steroids, which decrease the inflammatory response and subsequent edema formation. Steroids may also have a beneficial effect on the healing phase and can assist in providing improved results.

Evaluation, both pre- and postoperative, is important in any surgical procedure. It must be remembered that the sole purpose of performing a dermabrasion is to improve the appearance of the patient. I have often seen patients who have come to me after being discouraged by their own practitioner, be it a dermatologist or someone in another discipline. Their most common comments are, ''I was told my scarring wasn't severe enough'' or ''My doctor told me my scarring was too severe.'' These patients have had mild to severe scars, *all of which have been subsequently improved by dermabrasion.*

Self-image is extremely important. Those who suffer the discomfort of scars need our understanding and corrective help. My sole judgment is made on the basis of whether I can improve the patient's anatomic defect, assuming that there are no physical or psychological contraindications. I am frank when I discuss with my patients the different responses to a change in anatomy. I do not change their personality, only their appearance. An improved self-image and a greater self-confidence may, and usually do, accompany this change.

Postoperative evaluation may be divided into three categories: short-term, midterm, and long-term. Short-term evaluation is mentioned mainly as a caution to the patient, the surgeon, and the reader of surgical literature. This is the period from complete re-epithelialization (usually the tenth to the fourteenth days) through the twelfth postoperative week. During this period, there is varying erythema and edema. The latter gives a fullness to the remaining depressed scars, and the former masks the pre-existing hypopigmented areas. In most patients, the best cosmetic appearance is achieved within this interval. As edema and erythema subside, the true results of the surgery can be appreciated. Postoperative photographs taken during this period can be grossly deceptive, and no editor should allow these pictures to represent the final results.

During this short-term phase, some patients who have undergone a dermabrasion for chronic or uncontrollable acne experience a recrudescence of their active acne with pustule and cyst formation. This is not to be confused with milia formation, which is an expected postoperative event. This flare usually subsides by the sixth postoperative month but will mask the cosmetic and therapeutic value of the surgery, at least temporarily.

Midterm results are those evaluated between the fourth and twelfth months. During the preceding short-term phase, all of the edema subsides, but some of the erythema may persist. A flare of active acne usually diminishes by 6 months, and a therapeutic benefit is almost universally achieved before the twelfth month. The compensatory seborrhea and milia formation has subsided by this time, and the patient has received maximal cosmetic and therapeutic benefit. It is at this time that I evaluate permanent improvement. I usually perform my assessment in the sixth month, but I have evaluated patients as late as 1 year following the procedure.

The long-term results are those that are evaluated more than 1 year following surgery. This may be too long an interval for objective evaluation to be possible. It is often difficult to get the patients to return, and they have difficulty in recalling their preoperative appearance. Without the aid of preoperative photographs, their evaluation is of little or no value, since it lacks objectivity. The passage of time dulls one's memory. Evaluation of results more than 1 year after the surgery, particularly with a written questionnaire and without the aid of preoperative pictures cannot provide meaningful results.

Standardized methods of evaluation are elusive. Surprisingly, however, physician and patient usually arrive at a similar percentage of improvement independently. Usually, neither the patient nor the surgeon will count the individual scars that have been completely corrected or those remaining in his estimation of the relative percentage of improvement. If the patient looks at his face and likes what he sees, it is then better, and he is improved. The old adage that ''beauty is in the eye of the beholder'' holds true. I have never seen a patient who could thoroughly recall the degree and extent of his preoperative scarring, nor could I. High-quality preoperative photographs that honestly portray the scarring are imperative. Shadowing is necessary to display scarring, but excessive shadowing distorts the natural appearance and exaggerates the defects. To recall the preoperative appearance, both the patient and I carefully review the *standardized series of 13* preoperative pictures. Then, with the aid of wall-mounted mirrors and overhead oblique light to accentuate remaining scarring, we independently arrive at a percentage of improvement. On occasion, several patients who are undergoing final evaluation of improvement and postoperative pictures participate in the evaluation. When two evaluators are involved, it is rare that the appraisal varies more than 5 per cent. When more participate, the variation is usually 10 per cent or less. It should be remembered that these evaluations are made independently, so one assessment is not influenced by another.

Although I have been performing facial dermabrasion since 1970, I have been keeping records of postoperative evaluation only for the past 5 years. It is difficult for me to evaluate adequately patients who live a great distance from Minneapolis, particularly those who reside outside the continental United States. During the past 5 years, none of my patients have evaluated their cosmetic or therapeutic improvement as less than 50 per cent. Many have rated the improvement at 100 per cent. Some of those undergoing cosmetic dermabrasion had obvious scars remaining. When they were asked why they rated their improvement as 100 per cent, their answer was, "I achieved at least 100 per cent of the improvement I had hoped for." This type of evaluation skews the statistics to the right but clearly demonstrates the patients' satisfaction with their choice of action and the results of the procedure.

To assess the cosmetic and therapeutic benefit of facial dermabrasion more closely, I reviewed 100 consecutive cases that had recently been evaluated. The ages of the patients ranged from 16 to 53, with females outnumbering males 2:1. Fifty-six per cent were between the ages of 20 and 29. Fifty-three percent of the patients were referred by their physicians. For 87 per cent of the patients, the dermabrasion being evaluated was their first procedure. For 11 per cent, the dermabrasion in question was their second procedure. One patient had undergone a third dermabrasion, and one had had a fourth procedure. Sixty-five per cent presented with some form of active acne, either under control but chronic in duration or uncontrollable with aggressive systemic and topical therapy. In addition to amelioration of the acne, most of these patients were seeking cosmetic improvement. This group is classified as therapeutic. Thirty-five per cent were receiving no acne therapy and presented with no evidence of active acne. They are classified as solely cosmetic. Therapeutic improvement was judged no sooner than 6 months following surgery. Cosmetic improvement was judged no sooner than 3 months after the procedure and usually occurred at 6 months or later. Therapeutic improvement was based on four categories, ranging from improvement with continued medication to complete control following cessation of all medication.

As stated earlier, the range for cosmetic improvement was between 50 and 100 per cent. The largest group of patients rated their cosmetic improvement as 65 per cent to 85 per cent, with the peak being 75 per cent to 80 per cent. These statistics were not compiled during the period of short-term recovery, when edema, erythema, and the flush of initial enthusiasm can result in overly optimistic evaluations.

Therapeutic improvement of chronic or uncontrollable pustular or cystic acne was also judged by the patients to range from 50 to 100 per cent. The average therapeutic benefit was less than the average cosmetic improvement, with the bulk of patients reporting from 55 to 80 per cent improvement. No significant peak was identified. These statistics for therapeutic improvement are similar to those reported by many who regularly perform dermabrasion. Unfortunately, little has been written about the therapeutic benefits of the procedure. I suspect that those who see little or no therapeutic improvement are abrading too superficially. These statistics also refute the adage that dermabrasion should not be performed until all the acne is quiescent. Although it is advisable to obtain the best possible acne control prior to dermabrasion, it is detrimental to deny the therapeutic effects of facial dermabrasion to patients with active acne, particularly uncontrollable acne. To be sure, these patients may develop more scars after dermabrasion, but the subsequent scarring will be less severe, since the active acne is ameliorated or completely controlled by the procedure. The exception is patients with active acne keloid, in whom dermabrasion should be delayed until the process is totally quiescent.

Dermabrasion for facial scarring, particularly postacne scars, provides a definitive cosmetic improvement when performed by an experienced, skilled surgeon using the principles outlined. The results are gratifying for patient and surgeon alike. There is no alternative treatment to dermabrasion. Some other procedures correct acne scarring, e.g., collagen injections, scar excision, and punch grafting. However, none of these techniques replaces dermabrasion; rather, they act as adjunctive procedures. Facial dermabrasion also provides therapeutic improvement for chronic or uncontrollable pustular or cystic acne and should not be denied during the active phase, despite the widely held belief that additional scars may form if dermabrasion is performed before the acne has subsided. In these patients the improvement of active acne is hastened by facial dermabrasion. Dermabrasion has rightfully earned a proper place in our surgical armamentarium.

DERMABRASION: AN ANACHRONISM

Ervin Epstein, M.D.

Dermabrasion has been the outstanding dermatologic bomb of the twentieth century. It streaked across the horizon like a capsule barreling toward the stratosphere, but, unfortunately, it fizzled like a defective firecracker. Probably as many as 50 per cent of the dermatologists introduced this modality into their therapeutic armamentarium, tested it in hundreds of patients in their own practice, and then discarded it. This was true despite a substantial investment in the necessary apparatus. The main reason that the dermatologists stopped using the procedure had to do with disappointment in the results obtained. It should be stressed that many of these practitioners were experienced and possessed a high degree of manual skill and even surgical dexterity.

It is claimed that the modern dermatosurgeon can perform this operation with more skill and can obtain better results. This may be true, but there are reasons to question this claim. For instance, pitted scars are not merely a loss of tissue but are produced by fibrous tissue in the dermis that pulls the epidermis or dermis down. If one were to plane deeply enough to eradicate this fibrous tissue, the surgical procedure would produce scarring of its own and might even magnify the preoperative defects. No matter how skilled the operator may be, he cannot eliminate this factor. Also, watching "modern" surgeons perform this procedure, one is struck by the fact that their planing is much more superficial than what we did in the "old days." They do little more than wipe the epidermis away, which causes a "brush burn." Can this produce the results that the fathers of dermabrasion claimed?

Some patients feel that the results obtained produce a marvelous improvement in their appearance and even change their lives. Dermabrasion could cause an improvement in their social and business lives by imparting a feeling of self-confidence. After all, beauty is in the eyes of the beholder. The edema that follows the performance of planing makes the skin look pinker and tends to erase wrinkles and scarring by the swelling of the tissues. However, this improvement is only temporary and disappears as the edema subsides. I sent a questionnaire to the first 50 patients that I had planed at least 10 years previously. Only one even bothered to reply. The others seemed to prefer to let bygones be bygones. Perhaps this soured me on dermabrasion even more than the lack of objective results. The realistic patient and the observers in his environment may wonder what has been accomplished. A physician that I know referred a patient to a dermatologic surgeon for dermabrasion to "erase" her acne scars. The patient returned to the office of the physician 2 weeks postoperatively, and the nurse greeted her with, "Oh, Miss Smith, when are you going to have your planing done?" Understandably, the patient was unhappy and discouraged when a health professional could not recognize the difference that this unpleasant procedure had produced.

Although there may be fewer scars after the operation and they may not be as deep, there are still scars present. As long as this is true, it is difficult to see the difference. When searching for cosmetic improvement, the patient usually expects cosmetic excellence—something that dermabrasion cannot produce. Patients may protest that all they expect is improvement in their appearance when they consult the physician, but they consciously or subconsciously expect to emerge with a perfect complexion. Many of the individuals seeking this modality have very minor scarring. The results are much better in those with severe scarring.

The literature is devoid of long-term follow-up studies. This makes the evaluation of this procedure even more difficult. It must be remembered also that surgical scars improve with time, so that photographs taken before dermabrasion and 10 years later may show improvement that is not really due to the procedure. The demand for dermabrasion has decreased appreciably. I am seldom consulted regarding planing any more.

One must consider the possible complications of dermabrasion. They are well known, since they occur frequently. The major problem is pigmentary alterations. Postoperative pigmentation is said to result from exposure to sunshine, and this is a potent factor. However, such alterations may occur even after minimal exposure to solar irradiation. It is interesting to note that this is less of a problem in blacks than in whites, since the pigmentary alterations tend to blend into the normal dark skin in a superior manner and are less noticeable. The hyperpigmentation disappears in most cases within 6 months. This can be hastened by the topical use of hydroquinones, although these agents have their hazards and limitations also. In some cases, hyperpigmentation appears at the periphery of the planed area, usually a year or so later, and is permanent in most instances. Depigmenation may develop in some individuals and also may be permanent.

Scarring may result from overzealous use of the planer or from slipping of the skin from the assistant's hand during the operation. This may result in hypertrophic scars, especially around the mouth. Hypertrophy responds to the usual therapeutic measures, although scarring persists. These scars are usually of the linear type and do not blend in well with the normal skin.

Infection is an unusual, but disturbing, complication. Pyogenic infection is rare. If one planes active, pustular acne, one can anticipate an exacerbation of the acne some weeks later. The more serious infection is caused by the herpes virus. This may cause a comparatively resistant and persistent infection that may increase the postoperative scarring considerably.

There are other potential, but rare, complications that should be mentioned, such as hemorrhage. A common but unimportant complication is the development of milia in the planed areas. These can be removed easily with a needle and a comedo extractor or will subside spontaneously.

Courses in planing are still popular. Many young dermatologists are still performing this procedure. The probable reason for the persistence of this anachronism is that certain training programs are still offering instruction in this procedure. As long as this continues, dermabrasion will persist and will be available to those seeking it.

SECTION 14

RESEARCH

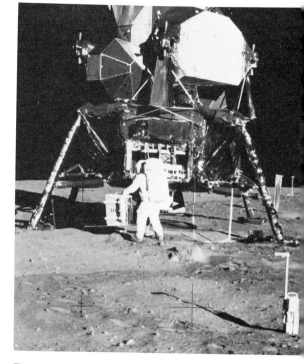

The greatest accomplishment of research during the twentieth century. (Courtesy of NASA.)

CHAPTER **31**

TYPES AND BENEFITS OF RESEARCH

THE VALUE OF ACADEMIC RESEARCH IN DERMATOLOGY*

Rudolf L. Baer, M.D.

The major aims of academic research are critical scientific investigation and experimentation leading to discovery of new facts and their interpretation and pursued in institutions of higher learning. Immediate or practical results of such investigations are not necessarily expected.[1]

The question of whether such academic research is of value to the field of dermatology must be considered in the context of today's complex world of medical and biological science and may be viewed from several vantage points. The most significant of these obviously are the general advancement of medical knowledge and the specific advancement of dermatology as a branch of medicine that intellectually and scientifically ranks high in overall performance and is influencing the training of academic and practicing dermatologists.

The principal purpose of having a separate specialty such as dermatology within the general field of medicine is to render the most advanced, effective, and economical health care with respect to the skin and to disseminate new knowledge to the medical community. This includes both the prevention and the treatment of skin diseases by dermatologists, by other physicians, and by persons in allied health fields. How can these individuals provide steadily improving care without progressive accumulation of knowledge of the skin and its diseases?

It is still possible today for nonacademic dermatologists and other physicians based in offices and clinics to make interesting and novel clinical observations and to work in certain areas of clinical research, such as applied therapeutics, without the back-up of an academic department. However, the bulk of significant discoveries and probably all of the fundamental advances in dermatology have been accomplished by researchers using the technical skills, facilities, and resources available only in academic institutions or in research divisions of large pharmaceutical companies.

My feeling unequivocally is that without active academic research in our specialty there can be no arena for the intellectual stimulation that is so essential to optimal education and health care. Particularly at this juncture in the rapid development of biological and medical sciences, academic research in dermatology must keep pace with the other disciplines to maintain its productivity and to prevent a state of stagnation. If this precept were not followed, the specialty of dermatology would remain static, and physicians receiving training in departments that are entirely clinically oriented would acquire only a

---

*Miss Diane Silberling provided editorial assistance.

package of existing know-how in diagnosis and treatment, comparable with that given in a trade school or a diploma mill. Serious efforts to prepare these individuals to delve into problems and to come up with new information to add and to integrate into the existing pool of dermatologic knowledge would no longer be possible.

Perhaps the best example of such a state of affairs is the circumstances surrounding American dermatology in the era preceding the founding of the American Academy of Dermatology and the Society of Investigative Dermatology, with its *Journal of Investigative Dermatology*—before enlightened members of the specialty, such as Donald M. Pillsbury, Stephen Rothman, and Marion B. Sulzberger, spearheaded the drive toward academic research. At that time, dermatology was barely looked upon as a true medical specialty by many physicians and members of the lay community. Throughout the country, most dermatologists were spending their time exclusively in private offices, except in large communities, where the "elite" were consultants and other dermatologists attended outpatient clinics of large hospitals.

In academic centers in this early period, although clinical departments in "important" health fields (such as medicine and surgery) were already being partially staffed by full-time faculty members, many engaged in clinical and basic research, dermatologists were still participating in relatively ancillary consultant and clinical activities. This undeveloped state of our specialty in the United States (the field was more advanced in certain other countries) produced serious consequences. Participation in vibrant and creative spheres of medical life was virtually impossible. Because of the undeveloped state of the specialty, many dermatologists in the United States who aspired to quality specialty training had to overcome additional problems. For example, as late as 1940, it appears that only four of the nine examiners on the American Board of Dermatology were trained in relatively structured programs of the type which, in the United States, were available to prospective specialists in internal medicine and surgery. The remainder had received their training either in Europe or in unstructured programs in the United States.

Striking improvements followed the founding of the two aforementioned organizations. The performance of the specialty of dermatology in the areas of clinical care and education and its efforts toward productive research and improved organizational structure now began to contribute to the upgrading of existing departments, the creation of new departments and, in some instances, the establishment of divisions of dermatology in academic departments of medicine. Full-time academic staffs were assembled, often including specialists in various aspects of basic science, and their research became an integral part of the total program. This had a pronounced effect on the quality and quantity of clinical and basic research in dermatology.

These raised standards of excellence in dermatologic performance, engendered by the establishment of "complete" departments that were concerned simultaneously with the delivery of patient care, graduate and postgraduate teaching, and clinical and basic research, opened the door to scientists in previously unrelated clinical and basic science fields. These researchers began to show a new and pronounced interest in the functions of the skin and in skin diseases. This development has been of value to the field of dermatology, because these investigators have contributed still further knowledge pertaining to the skin and its problems. Furthermore, it has encouraged a steady flow of interaction and a free exchange of information among clinical and basic science investigators in dermatology and those in numerous other specialties and fields, particularly medicine, pathology, immunology, biochemistry, physiology, cell biology, and microbiology.

Another important consequence of these advances is that dermatologists in the academic community are now able to publish in nondermatologic journals that have the most demanding standards of performance as well as in dermatologic clinical and research-oriented journals. They are also being invited more frequently to share programs with other investigators at meetings sponsored by prestigious clinical and basic science research-oriented organizations. This exchange provides opportunities not only for critical scientific discussions with nondermatologists but also for peer review, which is an essential ingredient in the furtherance of quality clinical and basic research.

I would like to cite two recent examples of fundamental advances in dermatology made through academic research. One of them has already led to important and fascinating advances in understanding the way in which the skin functions and how impairment of immunologic skin functions may have a profound impact on immunologic functions of the body itself. The other has revealed how a very rare and puzzling disease, limited to a minute part of the total skin surface of the body, basically is caused by a biochemical defect in the liver.

The first example concerns Langerhans' cells, whose existence in the epidermis has been known to us for more than 100 years. However, it was not until 1970 that a dermatologist engaged in academic research suggested that these cells serve the immunologic function of antigen presentation in the skin.[2] Subsequent research has confirmed this.[3] In addition, it was shown that first exposure to an allergen or antigen at skin sites where the number of Langerhans' cells is inadequate or where their function is defective favors the production of suppressor cells (i.e., those interfering with allergic reactivity)[4] and not the expected normal production of effector cells (i.e., sensitizing cells mediating hypersensitivity). In this way, tolerance and absence of reactivity, rather than hypersensitivity and increased resistance to the antigen, are likely to result. The tolerance produced by the many suppressor cells that are present, however, is not necessarily limited to the skin.[5] Thus, in the case of certain malignant tumors that have their origin in the skin, it is not only the skin that becomes tolerant but also the whole body, and this may favor the occurrence of metastases of the tumor to internal organs, such as the lungs.[6]

The second example concerns the pathogenesis of the Richner-Hanhart syndrome, which manifests itself with localized areas of palmar and plantar hyperkeratosis along with severe eye changes and mental retardation. Through dermatologic academic research, this disorder has been shown to be caused by a deficiency of tyrosine aminotransferase in the liver.[7] This enzyme deficiency results in tyrosinemia, i.e., flooding of the body with high levels of the amino acid tyrosine. Skin lesions are produced by the precipitation of tyrosine crystals in epithelial tissues, which initiates inflammation. Clinical manifestations of the disease can be cleared with diets low in tyrosine and phenylalanine.[8]

I have mentioned these examples of successful academic research because of their simultaneous contribution to the advancement of knowledge in dermatology and in medicine. In one instance a deficiency in the number or function of a particular type of skin cell affects the resistance of the body as a whole, and in the other a metabolic anomaly in the liver produces severe consequences in the skin.

The benefits of research conducted in academic departments of dermatology, however, are much more far-reaching and extend to the practicing dermatologist—that member of the specialty whose major responsibility is to use new knowledge in diagnosing and treating patients. It is true that some of this new knowledge has been made available through academic research conducted outside of dermatology, but there is no doubt that a substantial number of useful advances have had their roots in a dermatologic research environment. This has provided an added benefit for the practicing dermatologist, who now has an opportunity to engage in some phase of academic research if he so wishes, even if it is only on a part-time basis. Stimulating and potentially productive activities of this nature can only complement his practice and serve to counteract whatever degree of monotony is bound to be associated with routine patient care in a private office. Deepening interest on the part of private practitioners in academic research also tends to counterbalance certain weaknesses inherent in the practice of dermatology. Unfortunately, our present world of hype, hoopla, and hucksterism exploits the visibility of the skin for commercial gain, placing undue emphasis on preserving the appearance of this remarkable organ. With the tacit (and, at times, even active) cooperation of a very small segment of dermatologists, the public is constantly being bombarded with panaceas for improving the health of the skin and keeping it forever youthful. This does not add dignity to a learned profession and a serious branch of medicine!

As one who has been actively engaged in the field of dermatology for several decades, I cannot fail upon reflection to be astounded and impressed by the tremendous advances that have occurred during my lifetime. It is safe to suggest that the majority of dermatologic diagnostic and therapeutic procedures in use today were not even dreamed of 40 years ago. The direction of the present world of dermatology has changed, and the specialty now benefits not only from advances in research outside the field but also increasingly from within.

In recent years, there have been two major attempts to outline the most urgent needs for academic research in dermatology. The first was the unique effort of the National Program for Dermatology,[9] undertaken jointly in 1969 by practicing and full-time academic members of the specialty with no government support. The second attempt was made in 1979 with support from the National Institutes of Health.[10] Even such well-conceived planning for academic research, however, can provide only the skeleton, which must be fleshed out by new, original, and creative ideas.

It is gratifying to observe that dermatology today is looked upon as a truly viable, stimulating, and productive specialty. Academic research has played an invaluable and exciting role in our accomplishments, and only through its continuation will growth, productivity, and acquisition of knowledge be assured for its future.

References

1. Webster's Third New International Dictionary. Springfield, MA, G. & C. Merriam Co., 1965.
2. Silberberg, I.: Apposition of mononuclear cells to Langerhans cells in contact allergic reactions. An ultrastructural study. Acta Derm. Venereol. (Stockh.) 53:1, 1973.
3. Stingl, G., Katz, S. I., Shevach, E. M., Rosenthal, A. S., and Green, I.: Analogous functions of macrophages and Langerhans cells in the initiation of the immune response. J. Invest. Dermatol. 71:59, 1978.
4. Toews, G. B., Bergstresser, P. R., and Streilein, J. W.: Epidermal Langerhans cell density determines whether contact hypersensitivity or unresponsiveness follows skin painting with DNFB. J. Immunol. 124:445, 1980.
5. Daynes, R. A., and Spellman, C. W.: Evidence for the generation of suppressor cells by ultraviolet radiation. Cell. Immunol. 31:182, 1977.
6. Kripke, M. L., and Fidler, I. J.: Enhanced experimental metastasis of ultraviolet induced fibrosarcomas in ultraviolet irradiated syngeneic mice. Cancer Res. 40:625, 1980.
7. Goldsmith, L. A., and Reed, J.: Tyrosine induced eye and skin lesions in humans. A treatable disease. JAMA 236:382, 1976.
8. Goldsmith, L. A., Thorpe, J., and Roe, C. R.: Hepatic enzymes of tyrosine metabolism in tyrosinemia II. J. Invest. Dermatol. 73:530, 1979.
9. National Program for Dermatology, published by the American Academy of Dermatology, 1969.
10. Research needs in 11 major areas in dermatology. J. Invest. Dermatol. 73:402, 1979.

CLINICAL RESEARCH

P. Haines Ely, M.D.

Too many training programs pressure their students into mini-fields of expertise. . . . Scholarship and progress in clinical medicine cannot be mutually exclusive.

JOHN T. McCARTHY, 1982 [1]

Whoever wants a fine garden does better to consult the experience of the dull plowman and unread gardener than the profound philosopher.

THOMAS SYDENHAM, 1668 [2]

In 1980, 20 million dollars were spent on dermatologic research with approximately 11 million dollars spent in dermatology departments.[3] In spite of this largess, several articles have lamented the decline in the number of clinical investigators.[4,5] The basic premise is that "clinical research is usually conducted by the physician-investigators working in a clinical department of a medical school or in a clinical division of an institute."[4] For all practical purposes, private practitioners are excluded from consideration as clinical investigators. The argument is put forth that "worthy dermatologists-scientists, like wine, require time to develop"[6] and that during the early stages of training in clinical research "the young physician cannot know whether this will prove to be gratifying and consuming unless the research life can be sampled for a year or more without incurring unwarranted economic or professional penalties."[4] It has been suggested that promising dermatologists be funded at $30,000 per year for 3 years, lest the frustration of inadequate salary "forces them to turn to a part time practice, which erodes their research training and productivity."[6] A physician-investigator training program that covers basic laboratory techniques as well as grant application and manuscript writing has been developed at the University of Pittsburgh. It is acknowledged that graduates of this program will need external financial support.

Most published arguments center on money and imply that the clinical practice of dermatology is somehow counterproductive to scientific achievement. It should be self-evident that this is not so. Today's arguments are representative of the dichotomy of rationalism and empiricism. Galen's text "On the Medical Sects: for Beginners" clearly delineated the two schools of thought: "Experience alone is all that our art requires, while to others it seems that also reason or reflection has no small contribution to offer. Those who make experience alone the starting point are, accordingly, called empiricists, and similarly those who start from reason are called rationalists."[2] The empiricist point of view is becoming more evident in society as a whole, and this will be reflected in medicine. The trend toward family practice and holistic health care with all its attendant branches (nutritional therapy, vitamins, massage, herbs, acupuncture, and environmental allergy) has stressed human values over technologic achievement, and this may be one of the causes for the decrease in applicants to research traineeships. In 1977, 2800 postdoctoral fellowships in clinical research were authorized by the National Academy of Sciences, but only 900 positions were filled by medical degree–holders.[4]

Today's "critical mass of dermatologists-scientists"[6] represents the rationalist point of view taken too far for the good of the specialty. New ideas and techniques in clinical research are mandatory and necessary, but academic departments, whose lifeblood is money, have become dependent upon grants and growth. Grants reward rationality, benchwork laboratory techniques, frequent publication, and established trends in research. Our institutions are producing dermatologists who believe what they read and feel comfortable with scientific facts but are uncomfortable with practical observation and generation of hypotheses based on empiricism. Journals publish mostly *safe* topics of academia, and residents are trained to memorize the last 3 years' issues "to pass the boards." Each new generation is becoming increasingly myopic with regard to clinical dermatology, yet most of our recent advances in diagnosis are attributable to clinicians.

"Indeed it is well said, in every object there is inexhaustible meaning, the eye sees in it what the eye brings means of seeing."[7] As one encounters acrodermatitis enteropathica, one "sees" a zinc deficiency state. Similarly, when confronted with the glucagonoma syndrome, one "sees" an alpha cell pancreatic tumor. Cowden's disease was rediscovered by Peyton E. Weary, who described it as the "multiple hamartoma syndrome" in 1972.[8] Lives have probably been saved as a result. Lymphomatoid papulosis, bowenoid genital papules, actinic granuloma, Sweet's syndrome, Dysplstic nevus syndrome, bowel bypass syndrome, Kyrle's disease associated with renal failure, and Kaposi's sarcoma in homosexuals are examples of entities we are able to "see." The initial description or rediscovery in most cases was provided by an *individual* who was lucky enough to observe several patients with the affliction and who followed up his observations with clinical research.

However, in a very real sense, luck is hard work. "It is based on objective facts that have been observed by you and stored and processed in your mind . . . hunches do not come—and intuition does not work accurately—in areas where you have not already done an awful lot of homework and research."[9] It is not necessary to master many areas of basic science in order to conduct good clinical research. There are always workers whose specialized skills can be enlisted. As a personal example, I found that I could obtain peptidoglycan antibody assays, cryoglobulin precipitate analysis, and immunofluorescent studies at no charge merely by asking.

All dermatologists do some clinical research in their private practices, and many studies that are published under the aegis of a dermatology department were actually performed in an attending physician's private office. As a balance to the present position that scientific research is more valuable than clinical research, *I would suggest that at least half of the research funds requested by dermatology departments be devoted to proving or disproving the clinical observations or hypotheses of the attending faculty or community physicians.* Publishable permutations of previous studies or widely discussed topics would be excluded from the outset. Each new resident would undertake an in-depth 3-year project of clinical research. The first year would be devoted to a thorough historical review and an intensive question-forming period. In the second year, any scientific skills required by the project would be learned in conjunction with active clinical investigation. The results of each resident's journey might be published as a monograph as a prerequisite for graduation. A compilation of the best monographs might be published as a journal.

As an example of the value of clinical research, the disease gout will be considered. No one speaks of the *cause* of gout. It was known in 1900 that urates were elevated in the tissues and blood, but patients do not go to physicians saying, "I have a high uric acid level in my blood and deposition of sodium biurate crystals in my joints." Instead, they complain of the symptoms and signs of the disease: toe swelling, pain, tophi, or renal stones. The great biochemical development of the last 50 years has enabled us to understand uric acid metabolism, and we can inhibit xanthine oxidase with allopurinol. But after all, if a high uric acid level in the blood is the cause of gout, why do only 20 per cent of patients with an elevated uric acid level have symptoms? John Mason Good knew in 1826 that excesses of diet (meat and alcohol), exposure to cold, and fits of anger might trigger attacks. He also noted that "bodily conformation and individual peculiarities" were somehow involved in the disease. Riverius, in 1728, wrote that the cause of gout sine qua non was "weakness of the joints and the laxity of the pores."[2]

Is "weakness of the joints and laxity of the pores" relevant today? Let us make up some questions as suggestions for our residents' research project: Do gouty patients have large pores? Are large pores associated with any other conditions, such as seborrhea, acne, or rosacea? Are gouty patients afflicted with rosacea? Are they plethoric? Is rosacea a systemic disease? Do patients with rosacea have decreased stomach acidity or gastrointestinal problems, as some older studies suggest? Does a low stomach acidity allow absorption of exogenous xanthine oxidase? Is this related to skin oiliness, atherosclerosis, or serum uric acid levels? Do intestinal bacterial populations affect absorption of purines—xanthine oxidase? Are intestinal bacteria capable of synthesizing some absorbable cofactor or adjuvant for arthritogenicity? Do dietary purines or intestinal by-products initiate the production of vasoactive peptides, which influence flushing, stomach acidity, or intestinal transit time? Are the pores in any way associated with the elimination of toxins, as suggested hundreds of years ago? Are bacterial toxins in the bowel related to gout, psoriasis, or any other conditions that show elevations of uric acid? Does hyperuricemia cause gouty attacks in patients with small, visible pores? Do patients with small pores have evident seborrhea? Are they more likely to be atopic? Do patients with psoriasis and elevated uric acid levels share any physiologic similarities with patients with gout? Since emotional factors may trigger bouts of gout or psoriasis, could there be a neurohumoral factor involved in the generation of each? Would this factor be detectable in the dialysate from patients with gout and renal failure? Would this factor have any effect on tissue culture of nerves? High uric acid levels are sometimes seen in patients receiving chemotherapy for Hodgkin's disease. How does their skin differ from that of patients with gout? Are the pores different? Is there less apparent skin oil? If the skin in a patient with Hodgkin's disease or lymphoma is exceedingly dry, is this related to the production of oil, sebaceous gland size, or pore size, or are lymphocytes per se involved in the sensation of skin dryness? Are atopic patients more likely to have lymphoproliferative disorders? Is lymphocyte function related in any way to follicular keratinization, sebum production, or acne? Is there a "weakness of the joints" associated with gout? Is such a weakness associated with any skin types? Are atopic patients more flexible in the joints? Are seborrheics less flexible?

The questions are inexhaustible. At some time during the resident's question-forming period, the clinical research project should suggest itself. This project might address the ultimate cause of the disease state. Certainly the attempt would be a solid antidote for the "intellectual priggishness" described by Arthur Conan Doyle in his address to the medical students at St. Mary's Hospital in 1910. Doyle said:

> . . . there is another danger upon which I would warn you. It is intellectual priggishness. There is a type of young medical man who has all his diseases nicely tabulated, and all his remedies nicely tabulated, the one exactly fitting the other—you produce the symptom and he will produce the tabloid—who really is a very raw product. Life may turn him into a more finished article. Each generation has thought it knew all about it, each generation has in turn discovered its limitations, and yet with invincible optimism each fresh lot still thinks that they really have got to the bottom of the matter. Not only have we never got to the end of any medical matter, but it is only the truth that we have never got to the beginning of it. What we have done is to come in the middle of it, with more or less accurate empirical knowledge.[10]

References

1. McCarthy, J. T.: Achoo! Achoo! We all fall down (editorial). Cutis 29:409, 1982.
2. King, L. S.: The Philosophy of Medicine. Cambridge, MA, Harvard University Press, 1978.
3. Anderson, P. C.: Tactics. J. Am. Acad. Dermatol. 4:231, 1981.
4. Wyngaarden, J. B.: The clinical investigator as an endangered species. N. Engl. J. Med. 301:1254, 1979.
5. Levey, G. S., Lehotay, D. C., and Dugas, M.: The development of a physician investigator training program. N. Engl. J. Med. 305:887, 1981.

6. Fitzpatrick, T. B., and Blank, I. H.: A plea to help build the future of dermatology. J. Am. Acad. Dermatol. 6:112, 1982.
7. Carlyle, T.: The French Revolution, vol. 1. New York, E. P. Dutton & Co., Inc., 1973, p. 4.
8. Weary, P. E., Gorlin, R. J., Gentry, W. C., Comer, J. E., and Greer, K. E.: Multiple hamartoma syndrome. Arch. Dermatol. 106:682, 1972.
9. Schultz, D. (ed.): The xebex report. New Canaan, CT, Xebex Publications, May 1982, p. 4.
10. Doyle, A. C.: The romance of medicine. Lancet 2:1066, 1910.

DEDUCTIVE RESEARCH

Ervin Epstein, M.D.

All four types of research discussed in this section are important in the achievement of medical progress. However, we spend millions of dollars plus uncounted hours and an unbelievable amount of energy for systematized research in university laboratories. This effort has produced many worthwhile results, but many of the discoveries made by this method have not proved to be clinically important to date. The purpose of medicine is to cure or to alleviate suffering. Some of the outstanding achievements in clinical medicine during this century have resulted from old-fashioned armchair research—deductive reasoning by untrained investigators who have thought the problem through and have come up with logical answers. I am sure that the discovery of insulin would be classified as one of the greatest achievements of medicine in the 1900s.[1] Banting was a surgeon with few patients, no laboratory animals (until his investigation was far advanced), and no training in research. He had no budget or grants, yet, through reasoning and brilliant evaluation of results, he discovered insulin and its uses. Some of us have our best ideas and receive our inspiration in the bathtub, others in bed, and others by merely attempting to produce order out of chaos with our God-given intelligence.

Of the projects with which I have been concerned, two stand out in my mind because the problems were solved by deductive reasoning applied to available facts. Unfortunately, at times what seem to be facts are actually fallacies. It is often difficult to differentiate between reason and rationalization. But, as imperfect human beings, we continue the search for truth. At times we succeed, and at times we fail. I hope that the reader will find the underlying intellectual processes that were applied in these two problems interesting. These solutions were attained by an untrained investigator without a research laboratory, assistants, grants, sophisticated computers, and other tools of modern research. The axiom that one cannot solve all problems by merely "throwing money at them" is applicable in these cases.

Problem Number 1

When I was a consultant for the local veteran's hospital shortly after World War II, I was called to see a Filipino man in his forties.[2] He presented a large granulomatous lesion covering most of the left side of his face. It had been present for approximately 6 months. The clinical diagnosis was that of an infectious granuloma, such as tuberculosis, or a deep fungus infection, such as actinomycosis. A biopsy was performed, and it revealed a sarcoid histologic architecture. Unfortunately, the clinical picture did not conform to this diagnosis. One day the patient called the ward physician over to his bedside and said, "Look what came out of my left cheek." He presented the foreign body to the physician. It looked like a piece of glass—which indeed it was.

The patient then offered a more important history. Thirteen years previously, he had been in an automobile accident and was thrown through the windshield. The left side of his face was lacerated badly. The wounds were cleansed of all possible foreign matter and then sutured. The lacerations healed uneventfully, but the residual scarring was marked. Then, approximately 6 months before his admission to the hospital, the cutaneous lesions appeared. During the interval between the accident and the appearance of the dermatitis, small pieces of glass were extruded intermittently from his left cheek. The patient did not realize the significance of the relationship between the accident and the dermatosis because of the time lapse.

The histologic slides were reviewed, and, lo and behold, there were tiny clear spaces in some of the giant cells that appeared morphologically to be microscopic pieces of glass ("glass dust"). By polariscopy, it was determined that these bodies polarized light. Boiling the tissue in strong acids did not eliminate these bodies. Therefore, it was felt that these microscopic bodies were glass.

In an attempt to determine if these particles were identical to the glass in the windshield of the car, the specimens were taken to Dr. Kirk, head of the Criminology Department at the University of California in Berkeley. Dr. Kirk was a famous forensic pathologist who had solved many crimes through his brilliant investigative studies. He subjected the bodies to examination and determined their refractile index. This allowed him to identify these bodies as silica—silicon dioxide. This established the diagnosis of silica granuloma, a rare cutaneous condition.

The next problem was to determine how the silica entered the tissues and how and why it caused this sarcoid reaction. Glass contains a great deal of silicon but is one of the most inert substances. However, it seemed resonable to suppose that somehow the silica came from the windshield glass. A little reading revealed that glass is water-soluble. One can demonstrate this by filling a glass bottle with water and letting it stand for 10 or more years. If the water is poured out of the bottle at that time, etching can be seen on the inside of the container. One can accelerate this dissolution by changing the water frequently and by using water with an alkaline pH. Of course, the blood is slightly alkaline and is being changed constantly by the circulation. It was only one step further to realize that the soluble salts from the glass were excreted through the circulation, whereas the insoluble crystals were deposited in the tissues. The silicon dioxide conformed to this requirement and thus was left in the skin, whereas the other salts were washed away. As foreign bodies, they were engulfed by the scavenger giant cells.

However, this left a number of unanswered questions. First, why was there such a long incubation period between the accident and the appearance of the granulomas? Again, reading established that this was characteristic of silica granuloma. There were two possible explanations for this. First, it might be necessary to have sufficient amounts of silica present in the skin before the organ can react to this intruder. Biopsies were performed on other patients who had a history of pieces of glass, pottery, sand, and other inert substances containing silicon imbedded in the skin after traumatic incidents but in whom cutaneous lesions did not develop. Silica could be demonstrated in these tissues by polariscopy, but there was no histologic evidence of inflammation or other features of a microscopic or macroscopic reaction. Therefore, it seemed likely either that there was not enough silica present to cause pathologic changes or that it took this length of time for hypersensitivity to develop in the host. The patient was given an intradermal injection of a dilute solution of silica, which resulted in an intense local reaction. This was not the case when the same solution was injected into nonsensitized volunteers. The need to develop either or both of these mechanisms could explain the delay. It seemed reasonable to suppose that both mechanisms were operative and important in explaining the long incubation period in this disease.

Another interesting facet of this condition is that silica granuloma tends to clear spontaneously. This patient was treated with oral cortisone, and the reaction subsided. The patient was clinically well in 6 weeks. There was no recurrence over the 10 years or so that I followed this case. In an attempt to explain this condition, successive biopsies were taken after the patient's clinical recovery. In one section, I was lucky enough to find a Schaumann body extruding a crystal of silica. This made it obvious that the Schaumann bodies engulfed the crystals and extruded them from the reacting tissues into areas where they could be swept up by the circulation. This established the way in which the silica was excreted and the "cure" was obtained. It seemed possible that the cortisone accelerated this process. It certainly did more than block the reaction, since there was no recurrence. The biopsies taken after healing occurred continued to show scar tissue and sarcoid tissue for approximately 1 year. However, the proportion of cicatricial changes continued to increase as the nodules of sarcoid disappeared.

I am not saying that tests were not necessary to establish the pathogenesis of these lesions. However, this was not sophisticated research produced by full-time, trained scientists working in a laboratory with expensive equipment. The investigation was performed by a clinician who was exerting brain power to figure out what was happening, how to prove or disprove the theories, and how to interpret the findings.

Problem Number 2

This was a much more serious problem with much more important ramifications. During World War II, thousands of soldiers were incapacitated by a severe dermatitis that was characterized clinically by lesions of hypertrophic lichen planus, exfoliative dermatitis, and an eczematoid eruption.[3] It occurred mainly in New Guinea and on the nearby islands. The soldiers were ingesting quinacrine (Atabrine) as a prophylactic against infection with malaria. When this eruption became a problem, General Douglas MacArthur issued a statement that the dermatitis was caused by the quinacrine but that this information should not be disseminated. He felt that if the theory were made public, the men would discontinue taking the prophylactic medication and the infection rate with malaria would increase dramatically. Since this pronouncement received no publicity, each physician, and especially each concerned dermatologist, was forced to investigate the cause of the dermatosis independently. Most arrived at the same conclusion as General MacArthur.

However, there were some facets of the puzzle that did not fit. The use of quinacrine was widespread, but the eruption developed only in certain geographic areas. For instance, although quinacrine was also used by the soldiers in Italy, there were few, if any, cases of the dermatitis in that country. On the other hand, in the South Pacific, as much as 50 per cent of a military outfit might require evacuation to the United States because of the dermatitis. It would have been better for MacArthur to have allowed the men to get malaria if the eruption was caused by the quinacrine. This military goof probably saved the lives of more young men than penicillin did. Of course, the lucky evacuees were replaced from an endless pool of unlucky draftees that could never be depleted completely.

In addition, these soldiers suffered from systemic alterations, such as hematologic disorders, hepatic problems, and so forth. The armchair research was therefore resumed. It struck me that the toxicity manifested in these men resembled that occurring after the intravenous injection of arsenobenzols in the treatment of syphilis or the intravenous injections of gold sodium thiosulfate then in use for the treatment of discoid lupus erythematosus. This realization sent me scurrying to my physics and chemistry books to peruse the atomic tables. I found that a number of "rare elements" were closely related to gold and arsenic. These elements included vanadium, selenium, and several others with which I was not acquainted. I then went to the chemistry department of Stanford University. The professor there gave me a small vial of each of these substances. I added water to make a solution or a suspension and then patch tested the victims with these substances. To my surprise, all of the tests were negative except for a high proportion of reactions to selenium. A few normal volunteers were also patch tested to the selenium and failed to react. Therefore, it seemed possible that selenium was the actual cause of this troublesome dermatitis.

I returned to the library and learned that selenium occurs in nature mixed with various metals in ore and that some of the selenium salts are water-soluble. The next important piece of information to turn up was that New Guinea is rich in such metal ores. Also, the rainfall in that part of the world is excessive. How simple . . . the rain washed the soluble selenium out of the ores into the rivers and streams. Then the soldiers drank the water and developed the dermatitis.

I wrote a paper describing my findings. When an author is in the Army, before submitting a paper to a medical journal, he must first submit it to the Surgeon General's office for approval. After forwarding the manuscript to headquarters, I received a phone call from the dermatologic consultant for the Surgeon General. He congratulated me on my work but advised me not to publish it. He assured me that there was enough evidence to prove that this cutaneous condition was caused by quinacrine. I accepted his judgment and did not submit my work to a journal.

However, I was not really convinced, and when Abbott Laboratories brought out Selsun shampoo, I confidently expected an epidemic of South Pacific lichen planus. Despite the enthusiastic reception given this product and its widespread use, no such epidemic developed, and so I was forced to admit that perhaps my reasoning was rationalization and the evidence on which I based my conclusions was circumstantial.

As a postscript, when dermatologists adopted the quinacrine treatment for discoid lupus erythematosus, again an epidemic of this dermatitis failed to make its appearance.

I still believe that this eruption, which damaged our war effort so much, is a mystery that will never be solved. But then, you can't win 'em all.

References

1. DeKruif, P.: Banting: Who Found Insulin. New York, Harcourt, Brace and Co., 1932, pp. 59–87.
2. Epstein, E.: Silica granuloma of the skin. A.M.A. Arch. Dermatol. 71:24, 1955.
3. Epstein, E.: The lichen planus–eczematoid dermatitis complex of the Southwest Pacific: A study of 65 cases. Bull. U.S. Army Med. Dept. 4:687, 1945.

HUNCH, CHANCE, AND SERENDIPITY IN DERMATOLOGIC RESEARCH

Lawrence Charles Parish, M.D.
John Thorne Crissey, M.D.

The essence of dermatology, its *raison d'être*, resides in the realm of morphology. As disturbing as this observation may be to the more progressive practitioners of the specialty, who insist (quite properly) that we have advanced a long way beyond the mere appearance of things, it is abundantly clear that identification of skin lesions is the sole reason dermatology thrives. The ability of our specialty to maintain itself so successfully as an activity apart from general medicine lies in the fact that professional colleagues and the general public alike find it convenient to have access to physicians who can recognize and explain the significance of lesions and manage them properly. It is the presence of the lesions themselves—and nothing else—that has determined which pathologic states have been assigned to the catalog of conditions that come routinely under the care of the skin specialist. Since they range from trivial local disturbances to surface evidence of profound systemic disease, the result is the wonderfully odd, checkered, motley, and discontinuous collection of entities that has been considered in the pages of the scientific journals of the specialty since the publication of the first of them some 140 years ago.[1]

This heterogeneity is an accepted fact of life, but it makes very difficult indeed the construction of generalizations regarding the thrust and direction of dermatologic research, both past and present. Nevertheless, despite the philosophic inconsistencies and the artificiality of the selection process, the entities have been served well by the physicians who have studied them. A survey of the history of dermatology from its inception in the final decades of the eighteenth century until modern times will show that the most talented representatives of the specialty have attempted in every era to apply the best available methods to the study of the diseases that have fallen under their care.[2]

As in other branches of the biological sciences, dermatologic research activities have consisted for the most part in the collection of observations, the formation of hypotheses linking these observations together, the testing of the truth of these hypotheses, and the use of the theorems in the examination of further observations or in the re-examination of those already considered. This approach is, in short, the standard induction-deduction interaction that constitutes the contemporary concept of the scientific method. During the first decades of the nineteenth century, these activities were largely confined to the careful elaboration of clinical dermatologic entities based on the macromorphologic features of the lesions described, defined, and named by Robert Willan and Thomas Bateman in London and by their "French Willanist" followers in Paris, most notably Theodore Biett and Alphée Cazenave. Through this absolutely essential clinical research, the outlines of skin diseases were inked in well enough to allow physicians who later came into possession of powerful tools for the investigation of pathogenesis and cause to select for study reasonably homogeneous groups of patients with diseases that were genuinely sui generis.

The logical extension of macromorphology into the realm of microscopy took place in the 1840s and 1850s following the establishment of the cellular theories of life. Simon and von Baerensprung pioneered in this work and, following their lead, Auspitz, Neumann, Kaposi, Vidal, Leloir, and Unna greatly expanded the world of dermatohistopathology in the closing years of the nineteenth century.

During the same period, Bazin, Hardy, Koebner, Pick, and Tilbury Fox succeeded in identifying fungi as the cause of that strange disease, ringworm, and the dermatophytes were placed on a thoroughly modern footing in the monumental work of Sabouraud in the early years of the present century. When the exciting bacteriologic discoveries of Pasteur, Koch, and Lister burst upon the medical scene in the 1870s and 1880s, the dermatologists Albert Neisser and Augusto Ducrey added the gonococcus and the hemophilus of chancroid to the catalog of disease-producing microbes. Although the demonstration of the significance of the micrococci in the deeper pyogenic infections was largely the work of the surgeons, it was Sabouraud, Unna, and other dermatologists who provided new and valuable insights into the role of these organisms in the pyodermata.

Also central to the concerns of the specialty from the days of Willan onward has been the group of morphologically similar cutaneous reaction patterns formerly included in the term *eczema*. The separation of this unwieldy, monolithic clinical construction into the current subheadings—namely, contact dermatitis, seborrheic dermatitis, atopic dermatitis, and so forth—also occupied a large share of the time devoted to research by workers in the nineteenth century and in the early decades of the twentieth century. Such illustrious dermatologic names as Hebra, Rayer, Unna, Duhring, Devergie, Besnier, and McCall Anderson figured prominently in these important investigations.

Fortuitous Discovery

All of these, and many other research activities of earlier days, set the stage for the enormous expansion of investigative dermatology in our own time, particularly since the end of World War II, in which virtually every immunologic, histochemical, and optical innovation has been applied systematically to the study of all deviations from the normal that are characterized by the presence of a rash. The great bulk of these advances, both the older and the more recent, have clearly been made through the painstaking accumulation, linkage, and cross-comparison of information in accordance with the standard tenets of the scientific method. And yet, it has been recognized for some time that examination of the ordinary research activities of this sort fails to account for the significant number of scientific discoveries made on the inspiration of the moment, by lucky stroke, or while the investigator was looking for something else. Such events—and there are a number of dermatologic examples among them—are more properly attributed to the three closely related handmaidens of fortuitous discovery: *hunch, chance,* and *serendipity*.[3-5]

Hunch

It was a *hunch* springing from the prepared mind of Johann Lucas Schoenlein that led in 1839 to a discovery fundamental to everything that came later in the field of medical mycology, a discovery of particular dermatologic significance that ranks among the most important in the history of medicine. Schoenlein, who later achieved international fame as a pioneer in the introduction of laboratory methods into clinical medicine, was then a young man working in Zürich and interested in dermatologic problems. An admirer of the great Swiss botanist, de Candolle, he was engaged at the time (as were a number of others) in an attempt to classify skin diseases along the lines suggested by de Candolle for the classification of plants. His results, to put it charitably, were less than satisfactory.

While thus botanically preoccupied, Schoenlein had come across several other pieces of information from the world of vegetable research that prepared the way for his productive hunch. Of primary importance were the reports of Agostino Bassi of Italy and J. V. Audoin of France published between 1835 and 1837, in which a fungus was clearly identified as the cause of muscardine, a fatal disease of silkworms that threatened to destroy the European silk industry. The totally new concept put forth in these reports, the idea that a disease in animals could actually be caused by a plant, made a deep and lasting impression on Schoenlein. Somewhat earlier (1833), an influential book on plant diseases had been published by Franz Unger of Vienna in which that noted botanist fancied that he saw a resemblance between the lesions of certain human skin diseases and some of the leaf scales affecting his plants. He called the latter "plant exanthems." The idea appealed greatly to Schoenlein in his botanical frame of mind, and when he reviewed Unger's observations in the light of the muscardine discoveries, the cerebral switch was thrown. Two cases of favus on the ward of his hospital service came suddenly to mind. He scraped scutula from the heads of the pair, examined them under the microscope, and recognized that the lesions were made up of masses of mycelia. Delighted, he sent a short preliminary report of his finding to Johannes Mueller, whose journal, *Muellers Archiv*, was the *Science* of its day. In playing his hunch, Schoenlein launched singlehandedly the field of medical mycology, with all of its dermatologic ramifications.

Chance

The fame that accrues to physicians who introduce new treatment modalities into the practice of medicine is fugitive more often than not. So certain is it that new drugs and new procedures will be superceded by newer drugs and newer procedures that both the innovators and their innovations are likely to come across to later generations as something less than inspiring.

No one but an aficionado of historical matters would concern himself now with the bloody linear scarification techniques developed by England's Balmanno Squire for the treatment of lupus vulgaris or Radcliffe Crocker's intralesional thiosinamine injections, which in his hands supposedly induced prompt resolution in a great many keloids, and yet both of these were exciting therapeutic innovations a generation or two ago.

There are countless other examples. In our own time, Lawrence Goldberg of Cincinnati[6] and, later, George Andrews, Anthony Domonkos, Marion Sulzberger,[7] and Victor Witten of New York[8] introduced and popularized the use of tetracycline in the management of acne vulgaris, an approach that is still very much current. But how many who use tetracycline regularly remember the names of those who introduced the treatment? Advances of this type cast much longer shadows, of course, when they generate an enjoyable quantum of controversy along the way, as in the great griseofulvin race of 1958, in which the Miami team of Harvey Blank[9] and the London group of David Williams[10] crossed the wire in what ought to be judged a dead heat.

Another therapeutic innovation of our time furnishes a good example of *chance observation* in action in dermatologic research. Pinched for cash in 1953, William Pace of London, Ontario[11] took a stopgap job at slave wages running a skin clinic at a local Veterans Affairs Hospital, where a young soldier with severe papulopustular acne vulgaris came under his care. Scheduling conflicts made it necessary for the soldier, who had made only modest progress on a regimen of lotio alba and acne surgery, to be transferred to an alternate skin clinic, run by Dr. Ivan Price of the hospital staff. A few weeks later, when exigencies of the service once more required reassignment to the original clinic, Dr. Pace was surprised at the marked improvement in the patient's condition and even more surprised when he learned that the response followed the use of 10 per cent sulfur precipitate in Squibb's Quinolor Compound Ointment, prescribed by Dr. Price. Dr. Pace wrote:

> I could never have conceived of applying this exceptionally occlusive, foul-smelling ointment to a patient with acne vulgaris. Had I ever done so, I would have expected the occlusiveness of the medication to have made the acne much worse. I therefore realized instantly that there must be some medication in Compound Quinolor Ointment which had an incredibly different effect on acne than anything I had ever used.

After searching through and checking out the many ingredients in the Squibb preparation, Pace decided that the 10 per cent benzoyl peroxide that was present was the therapeutically active ingredient, potentiated perhaps by the added sulfur. It is true that one may quibble over the soundness of the logic that lay beneath Pace's original investigations; one may also complain about the tenuousness of the evidence on which he based his conclusion that benzoyl peroxide was the agent responsible for the improvement, and question the value of a hypothesis based on a single observation. However, no one can fault the results, which led to the development of a whole new branch of the dermatologic pharmaceutical industry. In addition, no one can fail to appreciate the Canadian's alertness in identifying the change in the patient, who passed his way twice entirely by chance, as something new and different.

Serendipity

Horace Walpole, English politico, gouty bachelor, literary luminary, and perhaps the best letter writer in the English language, introduced the word *serendipity* in 1754. It appeared first in a letter written by him to Sir Horace Mann, and Walpole used it to indicate the faculty for making fortunate discoveries by accident. The word was derived from a fairy tale, *The Three Princes of Serendip,* in which the main characters traveled about the countryside of Serendip (ancient Ceylon) and other places, making such discoveries.[12]

The most notable example of serendipity associated with dermatologic research took place in the year 1905 under the auspices of Edmund Lesser's *Klinik für Haut- und Geschlechtskrankheiten* in Berlin. At the suggestion of the German government and with the support of the German Academy of Science, a program had been organized to test the validity of an elusive, motile protozoan, *Cytoryctes luis,* proposed by one Dr. Siegel as the cause of syphilis. This imaginary microbe was only one of the more notorious among the 135 or so causative organisms that had been identified in the preceding 35 years of syphilis research, a review of which would re-educate quickly anyone naïve enough to believe for a moment that superior scientific minds are immune to folly.

Because the *Cytoryctes* was purportedly a protozoan, a zoologist of international repute, Fritz Schaudinn, was called in for the job. Erich Hoffmann, an experienced dermatologist who had access to a great many syphilis cases at Lesser's clinic and who could be depended upon to recognize a chancre when he saw one, worked with him. It took Schaudinn no more than a few days with the material brought to him by Hoffmann to identify Dr. Siegel's protozoan as nothing more than organic debris dancing about in the random rhythms characteristic of brownian movement. In the very first case examined, however, the zoologist noted something else, and it was at this point that the manifestations of serendipity became evident.

Schaudinn not only was an expert on protozoa but also had had extensive experience in the study of spirochetes, a class of organisms with which dermatologists and syphilologists who had investigated the disease so intensely in the past were not at all familiar. This special expertise enabled him to identify at once the pale spiral form of a microbe belonging to that family. If we are to believe Charles Dennie,[13] who had it straight from Hoffmann himself, this is one of the few instances in the annals of medical research in which the discoverer actually cried *"Eureka!"* (*auf Deutsch*, of course) on first observing his find. Schaudinn's identification of *Treponema pallidum* in the lesions of syphilis and the convincing evidence that he and Dr. Hoffmann were able to marshal over the next few months to establish the organism as the true cause of syphilis constitute one of the most significant discoveries in medicine. It would not have taken place at this moment and in this way, however, if a skilled observer with extra knowledge that was not essential to the problem at hand had not been able to identify something new while looking for something else. This is exactly what Walpole had in mind when he coined his fine new word.

In Retrospect

It would be nice to be able to tap at will the resources of the mind that lie beneath those advances attributable to hunch, chance, and serendipity, with a view, of course, to catalyzing similar reactions in all types of difficult research situations. Alas, the cerebral mechanisms are completely unknown, and the circumstances of each event are so special that one suspects that no useful leap from the particular to the general is going to be possible in the foreseeable future. Nevertheless, examples of the unexpected triumph can at least be employed in the defense against attacks by the omnipresent forces of reaction—those who insist that funds be allotted only to those scientific investigations that are oriented toward specific and easily identifiable goals.

References

1. Parish, L. C.: American dermatology journals: Their growth from 1870–1920. Arch. Dermatol. 96:77, 1967.
2. Crissey, J. T., and Parish, L. C.: The Dermatology and Syphilology of the Nineteenth Century, New York, Praeger Scientific, 1981.
3. Cohen, L.: The fruits of error and false assumption. Proc. R. Soc. Med. 60:673, 1967.
4. Rossman, R. E.: The history and significance of serendipity in medical discovery. Trans. Coll. Phys. Phila., 4th ser. 33:104, 1965.
5. Lembeck, F.: Successful errors and other odd ways to new discoveries. Med. Hist. 11:157, 1967.
6. Goldberg, L. C.: Personal communication, January 9, 1982.
7. Sulzberger, M. B.: Personal communication, December 29, 1981.
8. Witten, V. H.: Personal communication, February 2, 1982.
9. Blank, H.: Personal communication, December 30, 1981.
10. Williams, D.: De mortuis nil nisi bonum. J. Am. Acad. Dermatol. 6:968, 1982.
11. Pace, W. E.: Personal communication, February 3, 1982.
12. Rajam, R. V.: Serendipity in medicine. Ind. J. Hist. Med. 18:15, 1973.
13. Dennie, C. C.: A history of syphilis. Springfield, IL, Charles C Thomas, 1962, pp. 91–96.

Editorial Comment

Despite the fact that in this section we have divided research into four categories, actually they are inseparable, and all are important. Often clinical investigation and discovery are built on academic or pharmacologic research. The purpose of medical training is to bring comfort and cure to the sufferers in our society. Therefore, one cannot deny the importance of clinical research, because the determination of therapeutic effects and iatrogenic hazards is what reaches the patient.

When one visits the training centers of the world, one cannot help being impressed with the equipment and the experts working on the problems of clinical dermatology. After seeing a number of these organizations, all busy investigating our problems, one must wonder why all of the puzzles in dermatology have not been solved. There may be several reasons for this failure. As an example, one cannot solve problems by throwing money at them. Inspiration and dedication are more important than perspiration and a salary.

Serendipity, which might be loosely translated as luck, also plays a part in the problem-solving process. However, serendipity is not merely luck. It is luck plus the ability to recognize the serendipitous event when it occurs and to interpret its significance correctly. One must realize that opportunity is knocking and then must understand its meaning. Also, deductive research applied to the findings of the other three types mentioned herein is essential and often furnishes the key to the importance of a seemingly insignificant basic discovery produced by sophisticated research.

Clinical research is performed without funds or with those furnished usually by the investigator himself. Millions are spent on formal academic research, but little or nothing is donated to the solving of problems concerned with findings in living subjects. There is no question that some of the research funds should be devoted to such clinical investigations. The Dermatology Foundation promised to allot an undisclosed percentage of their donations to such studies, but when one examines their list of grants at this time, it does not seem that they donated anything to this type of study.

In some instances, pharmaceutical companies do provide funds for research. Although there are exceptions, such as donations by Westwood Pharmaceuticals, most of the money goes for clinical testing of products that the companies hope to get approved by the Food and Drug Administration and to place on the market. The results of such studies are sterile at best and slanted at worst. The conflict of interest interferes with the impartiality and the search for truth that must be inherent in all scientific endeavors.

Cooperative clinical studies, such as those performed at the Mayo Clinic, Case Western Reserve, Johns Hopkins, the University of Pennsylvania, and the University of Michigan in the evaluation of syphilis or the study that was used to evaluate PUVA, should be employed. This allows for the assessment of larger numbers of cases than can be examined by a single investigator or training center. The statistics emanating from such investigations are therefore more apt to be significant than are those gathered by a single individual or institution.

Again, it should be remembered that the purpose of research is to increase our knowledge and to restore health to the ill. Cooperation may be the best way to reach these goals in the shortest time. Furthermore, the clinician who performs important, unselfish studies should be able to raise money to pursue his projects.

Think It Over.

INDEX

Page numbers in *italics* indicate illustrations. Page numbers followed by t indicate tables.